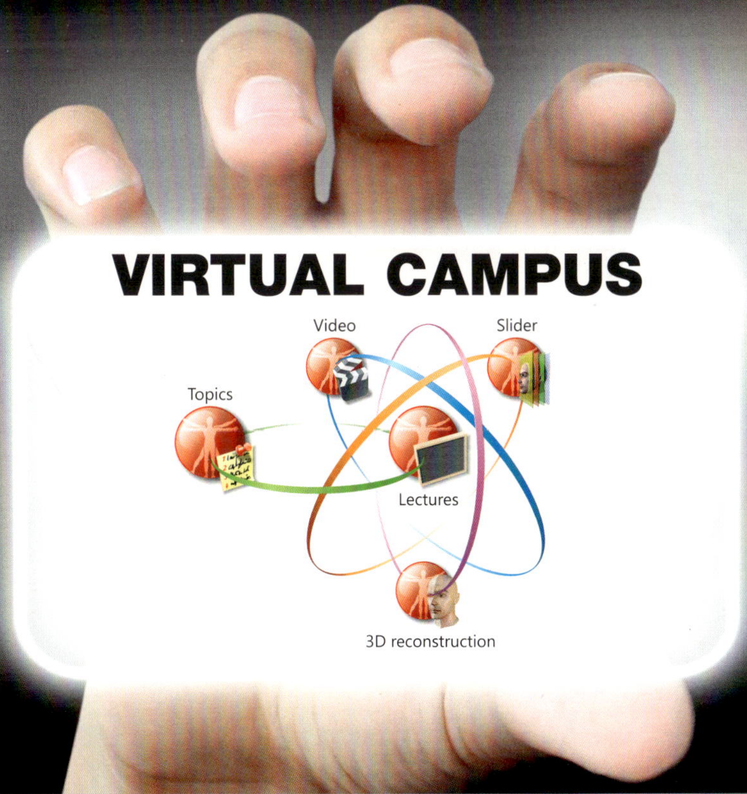

AF898450

HUMAN ANATOMY *atlas*

FOUR STEPS TO ACCESS DIGITAL CONTENTS

1 CONNECT — Go to the website indicated on the label that includes the access code

2 REGISTER — Register at the Publisher Portal (first time only) to receive a username and password

3 ACCESS — Enter your username and password to access the restricted contents

4 TYPE THE CODE — On the web page dedicated to the work, type in the personal access code hidden under the protection of the label applied to this page

After the first access, digital contents will be available on the website entering your username and password.

The **online access** grants **personal license** limited to a **single user** for each code.
The **access is limited to the individual user** and is not a library or institutional access license.

Sharing of passwords and/or code is not allowed; any misuse of the personal code will invalidate and lock it. The access cannot be shared and will expire according as indicated in the license agreement subscribed at the first access. Further details may be provided upon acceptance of the license agreement. The use of the code is subject to acceptance of the conditions. Any violation or attempted violation of code protection will not be accepted.

To remove the protection use a coin to scrape with light pressure

EE5893004599
www.evirtualcampus.com/en

Hardware and software requirements:
PC with Windows, Macintosh or Linux,
latest generation of internet browser such as Internet Explorer (version 9 onwards), Firefox, Chrome etc.; Internet connection.

Technical Help Desk: by email at support@ediermes.com

Contributors
English Edition

Editors

Giuseppe Anastasi	University of Messina, Italy
Eugenio Gaudio	University of Roma (Sapienza), Italy
Carlo Tacchetti	University Vita-Salute San Raffaele, Milan, Italy

Editor English Edition

Estomih Mtui	Weill Cornell Medicine, New York, USA

Coauthors

Paolo Castano†	University Vita-Salute San Raffaele, Milan, Italy
Sergio Castorina	University of Catania, Italy
Ottavio Cremona	University Vita-Salute San Raffaele, Milan, Italy
Raffaele De Caro	University of Padova, Italy
Guido Macchiarelli	University of l'Aquila, Italy
Mario Rende	University of Perugia, Italy
Domenico Ribatti	University of Bari, Italy
Chiarella Sforza	University of Milan, Italy

Other contributors

Demetrio Milardi, University of Messina, Italy, *3D volume rendering images*

Web contents

Estomih Mtui, Weill Cornell Medicine, New York, USA
Angelo Favaloro, University of Messina, Italy
Antonio Esposito, University Vita-Salute San Raffaele, Milan, Italy
Maurizio Vertemati, Department of Biomedical and Clinical Sciences "L. Sacco" University of Milan, Italy

Giuseppe Anastasi
Eugenio Gaudio
Carlo Tacchetti

Estomih Mtui
Editor English Edition

HUMAN ANATOMY
Atlas

Volume 2

HEAD AND NECK
THORAX

edi·ermes

HUMAN ANATOMY - Atlas - Volume 2 - Giuseppe Anastasi, Eugenio Gaudio, Carlo Tacchetti (eds)
Estomih Mtui (ed English edition)

ISBN 978-88-7051-589-3

A book is the final product of a very complex series of operations that requires numerous tests on texts and images. It is almost impossible to publish a book with no errors. We will be grateful to those who find them and notify us. For enquiries or suggestions about this volume, please use the following address:

External relations - Edi.Ermes srl - Viale Enrico Forlanini, 65 - 20134 Milan (Italy)
Phone +39.02.70.21.121 - Fax +39.02.70.21.12.83

Drawings, Edi.Ermes Archive/Andrea Rossi Raccagni, Marco Fanuli, Raffaella Stilo, Maria Acquaviva, Anna Maria D'Errico, Ettore Orlandi

Translated and revised by Rosemary Allpress

Printed in November 2017 by Faenza Printing Industries SpA
for Edi.Ermes - viale Enrico Forlanini, 65 - 20134 Milan, Italy
http://www.ediermes.com - Phone +39.02.70.21.121 - Fax +39.02.70.21.12.83

Foreword

The **Human Anatomy – Atlas** is in my opinion the finest Atlas of Human Anatomy that has ever been written. The main factors that make it so unique include the quality of both the anatomical and radiological images and the way they have been organized.

Artists and radiologists working in collaboration with Edi.Ermes in Milan have created a very high quality 3-D reconstructed images from CT scans and MRI's, used in the Atlas. This approach will give the student and the reader a very clear and accurate understanding of the three dimensional presentation of each structure covered in the Atlas.

All the images are accompanied by a very detailed information related to the anatomy and where appropriate clinical correlates have also been included. This approach will assist the student to relate each structure studied with a clinical condition.

In addition, the authorship of this Atlas has organized the images so that they present the flow of information needed by the student to build a clear image of the human anatomy.

An emphasis on cross sectional anatomy and lymphatic drainage has been made in this Atlas by including several illustrations and radiological images.

Each chapter of the Atlas covering both the anatomy and neuroanatomy contains an introduction, dissection movies and interactive slides used in building the anatomical regions with a stratigraphic approach.

It has been a great pleasure to collaborate with Edi.Ermes in preparing the English edition of this Atlas. I wish to thank in particular Raffaele Grandi the CEO of Edi.Ermes for allowing me to be part of the development team for this Atlas of Human Anatomy.

Estomih Mtui, MD
Editor English Edition

Professor of Clinical Anatomy in Radiology
Chief, Division of Anatomy
Department of Radiology
Weill Cornell Medicine
New York, USA

Contents Plan

Volume 1

GENERAL ANATOMY

MUSCULOSKELETAL SYSTEM

Volume 2

HEAD

NECK

THORAX

Volume 3

ABDOMEN

PELVIS

PERINEUM

UPPER LIMB

LOWER LIMB

NERVOUS SYSTEM

Table of Contents

HEAD AND NECK

Topographic Anatomy
Boundaries 2
Regions of the Head 4
Surface Anatomy 5
Regions of the Neck 6
Triangles of the Neck 8
Fasciae of the Neck 10
Compartments of the Neck 11
Compartments and Contents of the Head 12
Compartments and Contents of the Neck 14
Vessels
Arteries of the Head and Neck 16
Arteries of the Neck 18
Arteries of the Head 20
Subclavian Artery 22
Superficial Blood Supply 23
Deep Blood Supply 24
3D Reconstructions 26
Arterial Vascularization 32
Territories of Supply of the Arteries of the Head 34
Territories of Supply of the Arteries of the Neck 40
Veins of the Head and Neck 42
Veins of the Head 44
Veins of the Neck - Venous Sinuses 46
Superficial and Deep Venous Drainage 48
Deep Veins 50
3D Reconstructions 51
Venous Sinuses 52
3D Reconstructions 53
Cerebral Veins 56
Territories of Drainage of the Venous Sinuses 57
Territories of Drainage of the Veins of the Head 59
Territories of Drainage of the Veins of the Head and Neck 63
Lymphatic System
Lymphatic Ducts and Lymphatic Groups 65
Distribution of Lymphatic Vessels of the Head and Neck 72
Nerves
Cervical and Brachial Plexuses 75
Cervical Plexus 76
Brachial Plexus 77
Autonomic Division 78
Cutaneous Nerves 80
Cranial Nerves 82
Canals, Canaliculi and Fissures 83
Foramina, Hiatuses and Meatuses 84
Peripheral Nervous System - Trigeminal Nerve 85
Peripheral Nervous System - Facial Nerve 87
Distribution of the Nerves of the Head 89
Distribution of the Nerves of the Neck 94
Contents of the Head and Neck
Frontal View 96
3D Reconstruction 101
Neck - Frontal View 102
Lateral View 107
3D Reconstruction 117
Posterior View 118

HEAD

Mouth
Oral Cavity - Conformation and Structure 122
Tongue - Conformation and Structure 126
Topographic Relations 128
Vascularization and Innervation 129
Mucosa and Papillae 131
Innervation 132
Teeth - Conformation and Structure 134
Vascularization and Innervation 137
Pterygopalatine Ganglion 138
Parotid Space 139
Infratemporal Fossa 140
Pterygopalatine Fossa 143
Parotid Space 144
Isthmus of Fauces 145
Coronal Section 148

Nose
Conformation and Structure 149
Nasal Cavities and Paranasal Sinuses 150
Arteries 152
Veins 153
Lymphatic Drainage 154
Nerves 155
Vascularization, Innervation and Lymphatic Drainage 156
Nasal Cavity - Conformation and Structure 157

Eye
Position and Structure 158
Muscles 159
Arteries 161
Veins 163
Lymphatic Drainage 166
Nerves 167
Ciliary Ganglion 169
Cranial Nerves 170
Vascularization and Innervation 171
3D Reconstructions and Eye Muscles 175
Eyeball 176

Ear
Conformation 181
Auricle 182
Arteries 183
Veins 184
Lymphatic Drainage 185
Nerves 186
Vascularization and Innervation 187
Bone Structure 188
Auditory Ossicles 192
Bony Labyrinth 193
Membranous Labyrinth 195
Vestibulocochlear Nerve 197
Cochlea 198

NECK

Trachea
Position and Structure . . . 199
Pharynx
Muscles . . . 200
Larynx
Muscles and Structures . . . 201
Cartilages . . . 211
Tracheotomy . . . 213
Functional Aspects . . . 214
Esophagus
Structure . . . 216
Neck
Topographic Relations . . . 217
Arteries . . . 220
Veins . . . 222
Lymph Nodes . . . 224
Nerves . . . 225
Topography . . . 226
Cervical Plexus . . . 227
Posterior View . . . 228
Sections . . . 233
3D Reconstructions . . . 235

THORAX

Topographic Anatomy
Boundaries . . . 238
Thoracic Cavity . . . 240
Mediastinum . . . 241
Pleural Compartments . . . 243
Lateral Projections . . . 245
Vessels
Arteries . . . 246
Thoracic Aorta . . . 248
Parietal Blood Supply . . . 249
Intercostal Vessels . . . 250
Blood Supply of the Diaphragm . . . 252
3D Reconstructions . . . 253
Territories of Supply of the Arteries of the Thorax . . 255
Veins . . . 258
Parietal Cava-Caval Anastomoses . . . 260
Vertebral Venous Plexuses . . . 261
Territories of Drainage of the Veins of the Thorax . . 262
Lymphatic System
Lymphatic Ducts and Lymphatic Groups . . . 265
Distribution of the Lymphatic Vessels of the Thorax 267
Nerves
Cervical and Brachial Plexuses . . . 270
Intercostal Nerves . . . 271
Cervical Plexus . . . 272
Brachial Plexus . . . 273
Spinal Nerves and Ganglionic Chains . . . 274
Parietal Ganglia and Nerves . . . 275
Sympathetic and Parasympathetic Nervous Systems. 276
Distribution of the Nerves of the Thorax . . . 278
Breast
Conformation and Structure . . . 280
Arteries . . . 282
Veins . . . 283
Lymph nodes . . . 284
Nerves . . . 285
Contents of the Thorax
Frontal View . . . 286
3D Reconstructions . . . 298
Right Lateral View . . . 301
3D Reconstructions . . . 306
Left Lateral View . . . 308
Esophagus
Position . . . 313
Structure . . . 314
Topographic Relations . . . 315
Trachea
Conformation . . . 318
3D Reconstructions . . . 320
Great Vessels of the Mediastinum
Topographic Relations . . . 321
3D Reconstructions . . . 326
Heart
Topographic Relations . . . 328
3D Reconstructions . . . 334
Pericardium . . . 335
External Conformation . . . 336
Internal Configuration . . . 338
Fibrous Skeleton and Valves . . . 345
Cardiac Muscles . . . 347
Cardiac Vessels . . . 351
Coronary Arteries . . . 352
3D Reconstructions . . . 354
Cardiac Veins . . . 356
Conduction System . . . 357
Lymph Nodes
Chains of the Mediastinum . . . 358
Mediastinal Lymph Nodes . . . 359
Nerves
Heart - Innervation . . . 362
Heart and Esophagus - Innervation . . . 367
Heart - Innervation . . . 368
Vagus nerve . . . 369
Esophagus - Innervation . . . 370
Laryngeal and Phrenic Nerves . . . 371
Lungs
Pleural Compartments . . . 372
Conformation . . . 373
Tracheobronchial Tree . . . 374
3D Reconstructions . . . 376
Medial View . . . 378
3D Reconstructions . . . 379
Intrapulmonary Bronchi . . . 380
Pulmonary Segments . . . 381
Pleurae
Topography . . . 382
Cervical Pleura . . . 385
Biopsy, Thoracentesis and Drainage . . . 387
Respiratory Dynamics
Muscle Activity . . . 388
Bronchi
Structure of the Bronchial Tree . . . 390
Thorax - Transverse Sections
Thoracic Cavity . . . 392
Thorax - 3D Reconstructions
Lateral View . . . 394

INDEX . . . 397

HEAD AND NECK

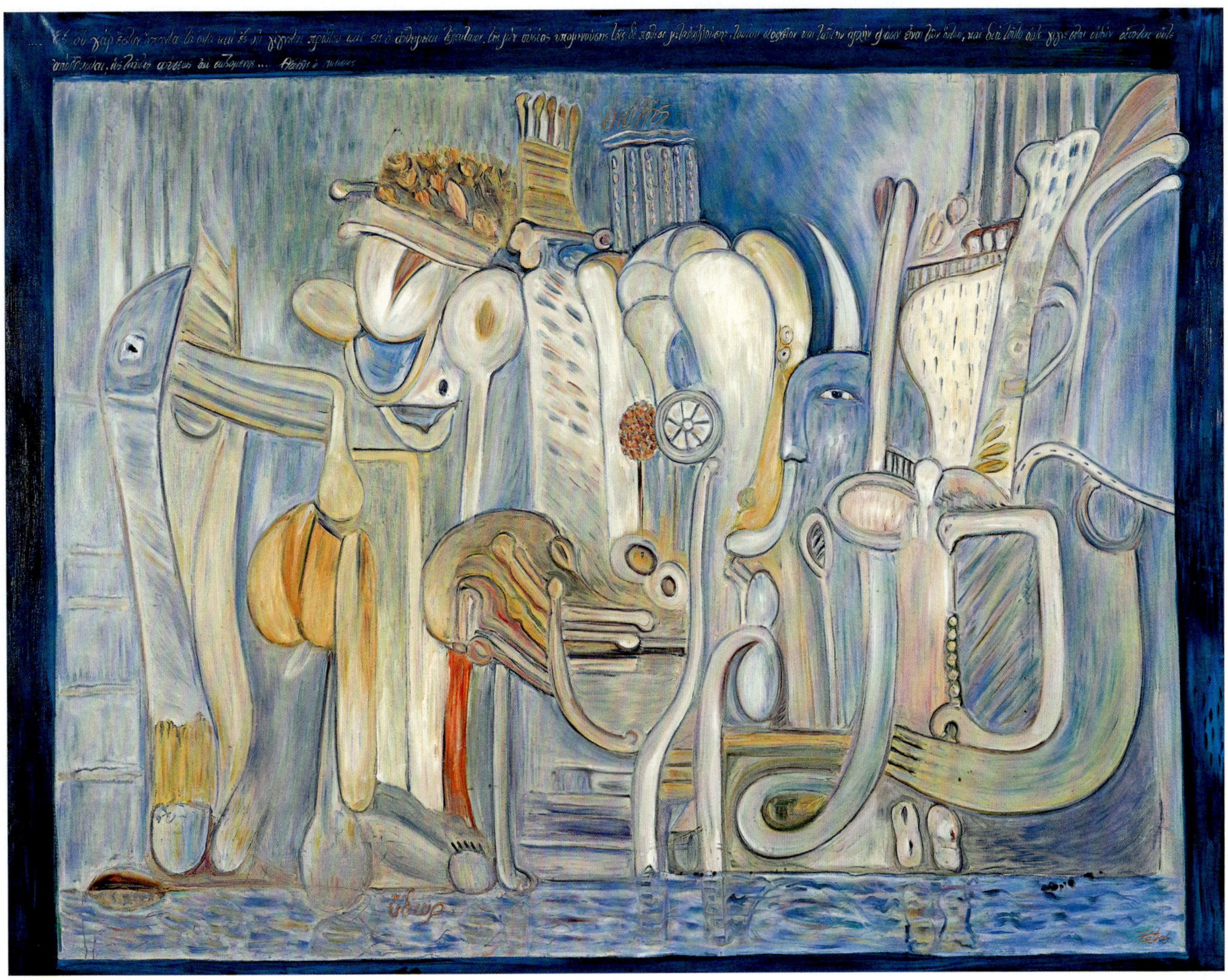

Petros (Athens, 1928 - Milan, 2014), *Talete*, oil on canvas, cm 150 × 200, 1990

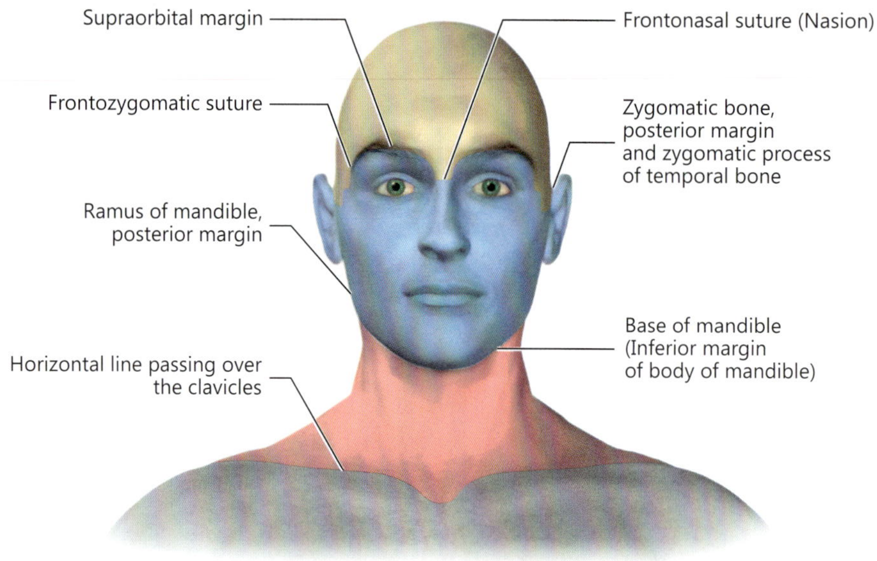

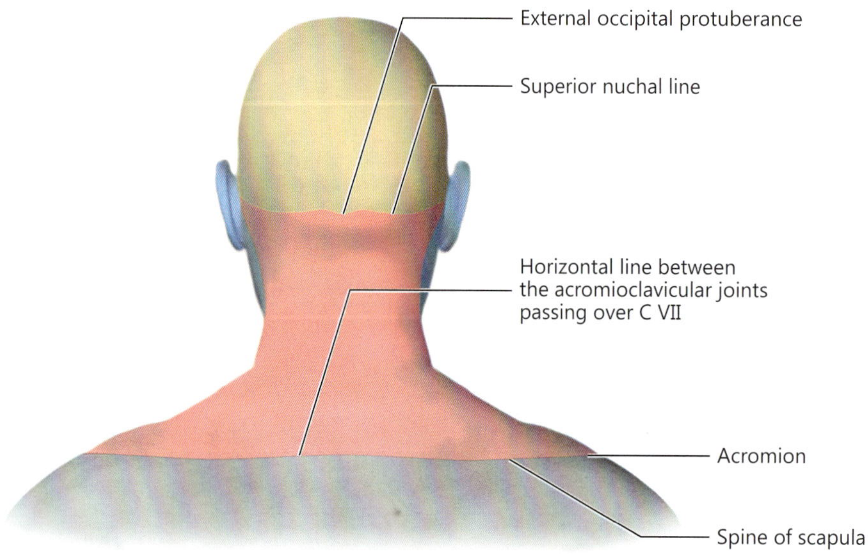

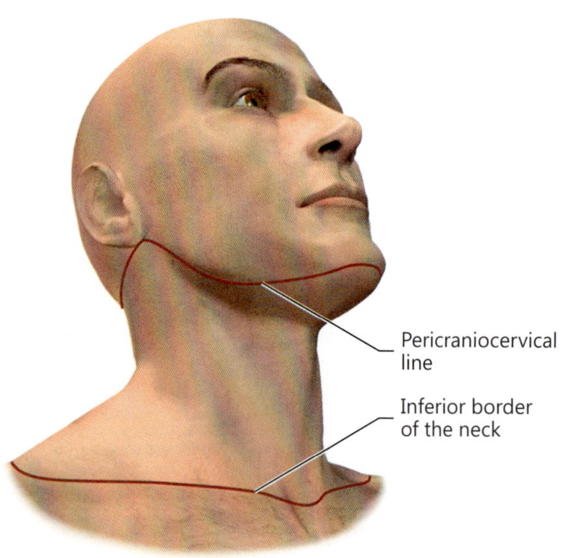

Superficial boundaries of the head and **neck**. The **head** is composed of the **cranium** (*yellow*) and **face** (*blue*), and is separated from the neck by the pericraniocervical line. This follows the inferior margin of the body of the mandible until its angle, then the posterior margin of the ramus, the temporomandibular joint, the edge of the mastoid process and the superior nuchal line, until it reaches the external occipital protuberance.
The **neck** (*pink*) lies between the pericraniocervical line (which separates it from the head) and the inferior border of the neck (which separates it from the thorax). The inferior border of the neck begins at the jugular notch of the sternum, and from there follows, on either side, a line that passes over the clavicles and acromion to reach the spinous process of the seventh cervical vertebra.

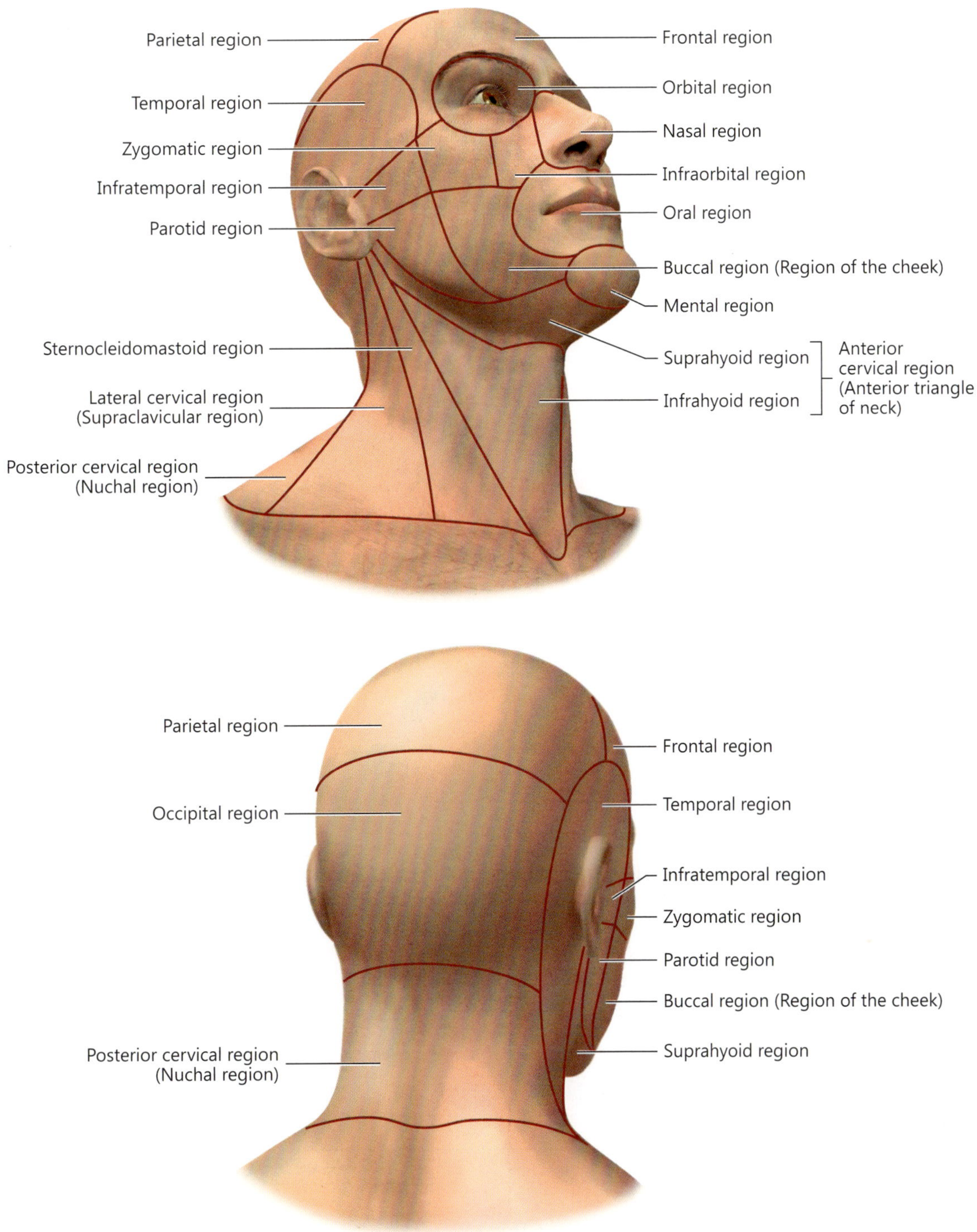

Regional subdivision of the head and the neck.

REGIONS OF THE HEAD	*REGIONS OF THE NECK*
Facial region – buccal region (cheek region) – infraorbital region – mental region (chin region) – nasal region – oral region (mouth region) – orbital region – parotid region – zygomatic region Frontal region ⎤ Occipital region ⎦ Occipitofrontal region Parietal region Temporal region Infratemporal region	Anterior cervical region (Anterior triangle of neck) – suprahyoid region – infrahyoid region – visceral space (Visceral compartment of neck) Sternocleidomastoid region or carotid region – vascular compartment (Carotid compartment) Lateral cervical region (Supraclavicular region) – supraclavicular compartment Posterior cervical region (Nuchal region)

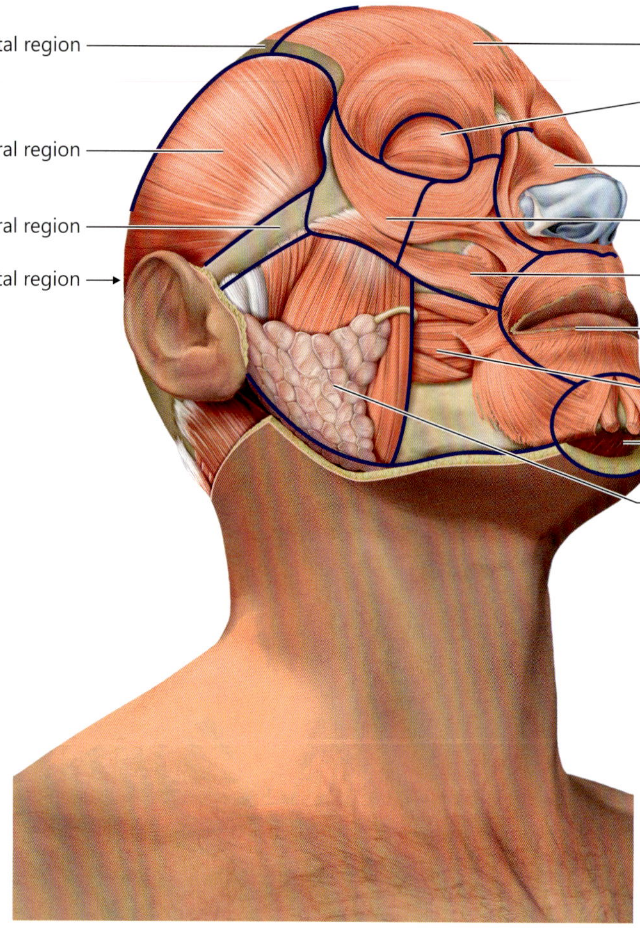

Regions of the head: right anterior oblique view. The frontal region corresponds to the area of the forehead that extends under the coronal suture. Adjacent to it is the parietal region, situated in correspondence to the parietal bone, while the temporal region is situated in correspondence to the squamous part of the temporal bone. The infratemporal region (or fossa) is covered by the zygomatic arch. Posteriorly, the occipital region (here not visible) lies over the occipital bone. The facial region is composed of the anterior fascial regions of the head: i.e. nasal, oral, mental, orbital (around the eye), infraorbital (to the side of the nose), buccal (to the side of the oral region), zygomatic (in correspondence to the zygomatic bone) and parotid (containing the masseter and the parotid gland).

Regions of the head: subdivision and boundaries

REGIONS OF THE HEAD	*BOUNDARIES OR LOCATION*
Facial	
– buccal (cheek region)	Zygomatic bone (superiorly), base of the mandible (inferiorly), nasolabial and nasogenian sulci (medially) and anterior border of the masseter (laterally). Corresponds to the outer surface of the buccinator
– infraorbital	Infraorbital margin (superiorly), sulcus delimiting the ala of nose (medially) and nasolabial sulcus (inferiorly)
– mental (chin region)	Mentolabial sulcus (superiorly) and base of the mandible (inferiorly)
– nasal	Root of nose (superiorly); line from medial angle of the eye to the ala of nose (laterally)
– oral (mouth region)	Nasolabial sulcus (superiorly) and mentolabial sulcus (inferiorly)
– orbital	Suprapalpebral sulcus (superiorly) and infrapalpebral sulcus (inferiorly)
– parotid (parotid-masseteric)	Zygomatic arch (superiorly), base of the mandible (inferiorly), anterior border of the masseter (anteriorly), anterior border of the sternocleidomastoid and external acoustic meatus (posteriorly)
– zygomatic	Corresponds to the zygomatic bone
Frontal	Edge of the frontal bone: coronal suture (superiorly), supraorbital margins of the frontal bone and frontonasal suture (inferiorly), sphenofrontal and frontozygomatic sutures (laterally)
Infratemporal	Corresponds to the zygomatic arch
Occipital	Edge of the occipital bone: lambdoid (superiorly) and occipitomastoid (inferiorly) sutures
Parietal	Edge of the parietal bone: sagittal suture (superiorly), coronal suture (anteriorly), squamous and parietomastoid sutures (inferiorly), lambdoid suture (posteriorly)
Temporal	Zygomatic bone, zygomatic process of the frontal bone and temporal crest (anteriorly), superior temporal line up to the asterion (superiorly and posteriorly); horizontal line passing through the zygomatic arch (inferiorly)

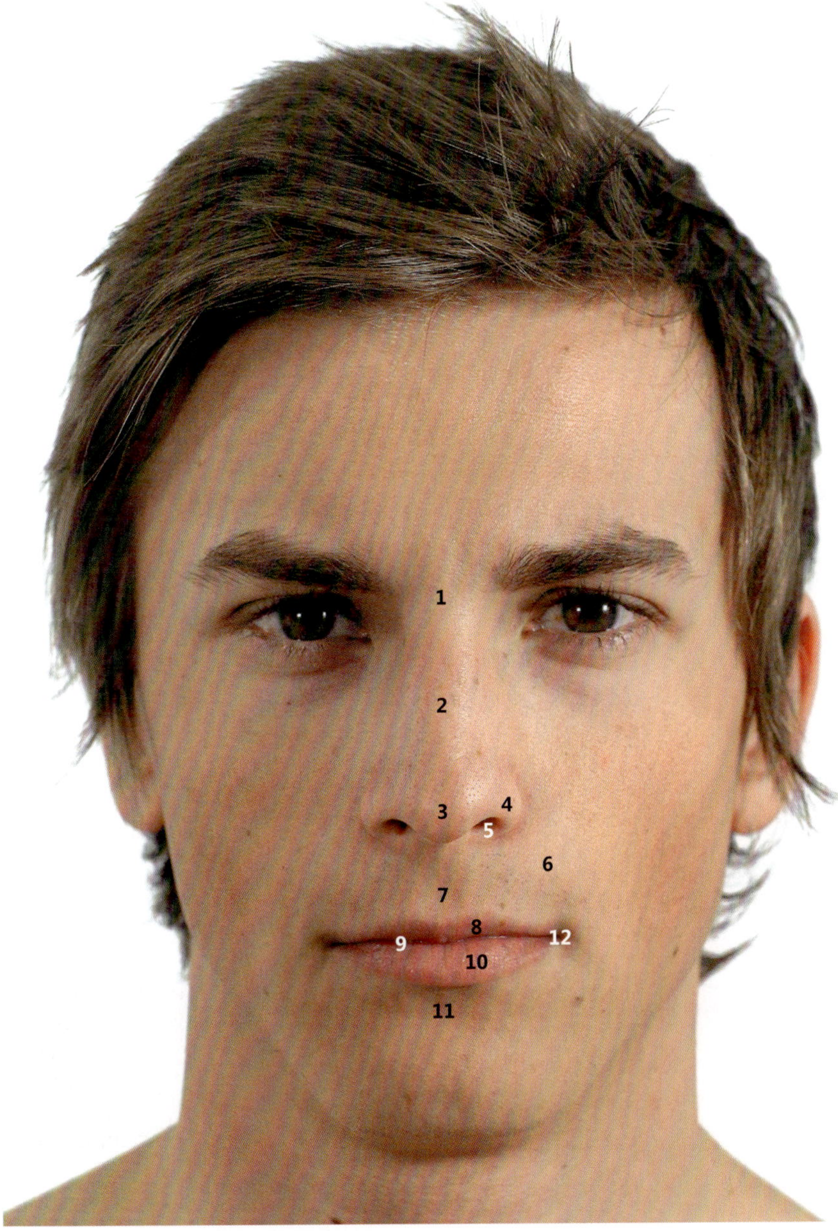

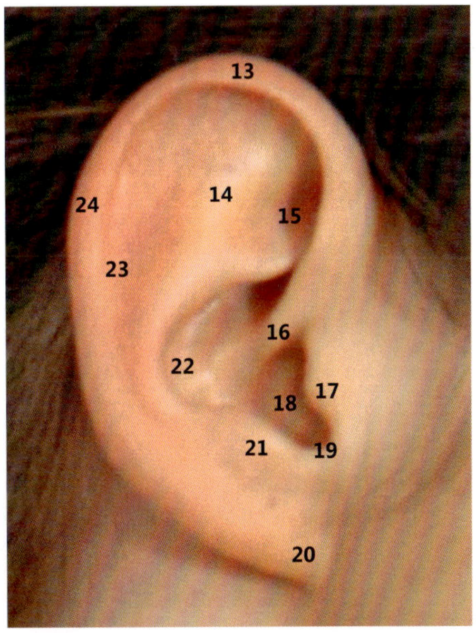

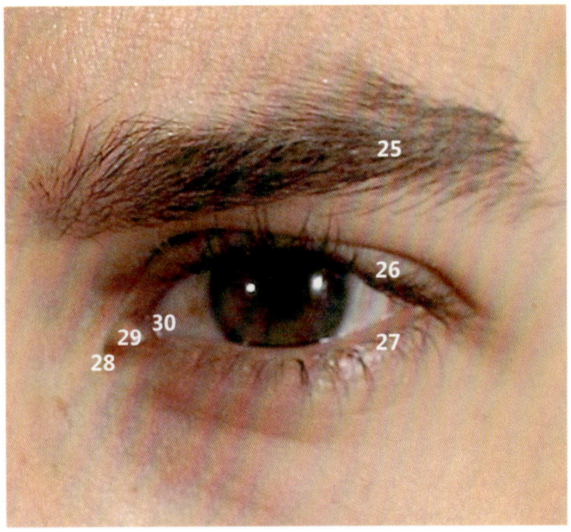

	Nose:
1	– root
2	– dorsum
3	– apex
4	– ala
5	– naris
	Lips:
6	– nasolabial sulcus
7	– philtrum
8	– upper lip
9	– oral fissure
10	– lower lip
11	– mentolabial sulcus
12	– angle of mouth

	Auricle (external ear):
13	– helix
14	– antihelix
15	– triangular fossa
16	– crus of helix
17	– tragus
18	– external acoustic meatus
19	– intertragic incisure
20	– lobule of auricle
21	– antitragus
22	– concha of auricle
23	– groove of helix
24	– auricular tubercle

	Eye:
25	– eyebrow (or superciliary arch)
26	– superior eyelid
27	– inferior eyelid
28	– lacrimal caruncle
29	– plica semilunaris
30	– lacus lacrimalis

General structure of the **external nose**, **eye**, **lips** and **external ear** in relation to the surrounding frontal regions.

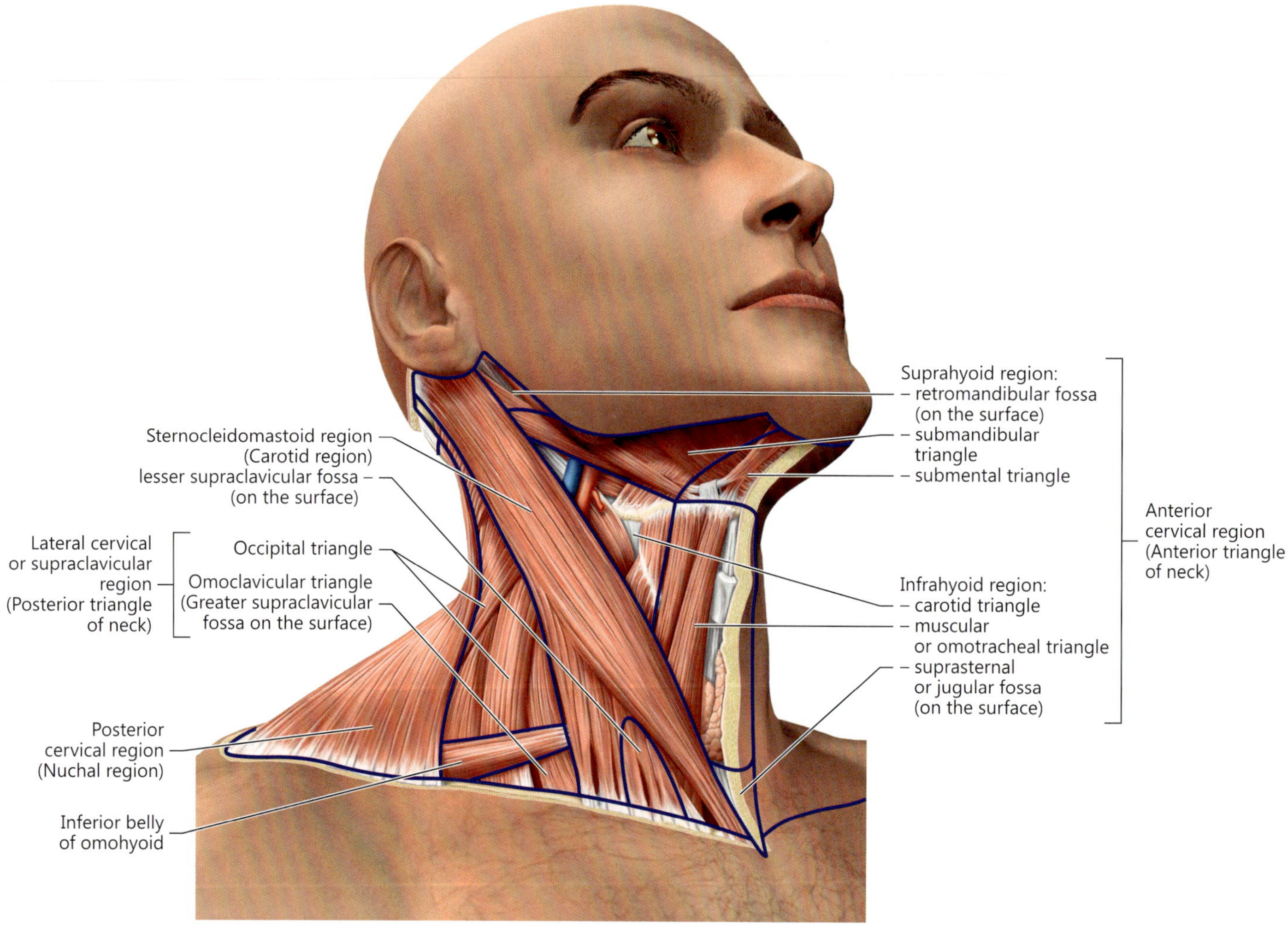

Regions of the neck: right lateral view. The sternocleidomastoid divides the anterior cervical region, or anterior triangle of the neck, with its base above (mandible) and apex below, from the lateral one, or posterior triangle of the neck, with its base below (clavicle) and apex above. The posterior cervical region lies within the anterior borders of the two trapezius muscles, which separate it from the posterior triangles of the neck. The anterior triangle of the neck is subdivided into smaller triangles: the submandibular, submental, carotid and muscular triangles. The posterior triangle is subdivided into the occipital and omoclavicular triangles.

Regions of the neck: subdivision and boundaries

REGIONS OF THE NECK	*BOUNDARIES OF THE REGIONS AND OF THE CORRESPONDING CONNECTIVE SPACES*	*TRIANGLES AND FOSSAE*	
Anterior cervical region:	*Superior*: base of the mandible *Lateral*: anterior border of the sternocleidomastoid *Medial*: anterior median line. The apex of the triangle corresponds to the jugular notch, the base to the inferior margin of the mandible and to a line that unites the angle of the mandible with the mastoid process	Anterior triangle of neck:	
Suprahyoid region	*Superior*: base of the mandible *Inferior*: horizontal line passing through the hyoid bone *Lateral*: anterior border of the sternocleidomastoid	– submandibular triangle	
		– retromandibular fossa	The retromandibular fossa, bordered by the ramus of the mandible, posterior belly of the digastric and by a split of the investing layer of cervical fascia between the angle of the mandible and anterior border of the sternocleidomastoid, contains the deep part of the parotid gland
		– submental triangle	

continued

Regions of the neck: subdivision and boundaries			*(continued)*
REGIONS OF THE NECK	***BOUNDARIES OF THE REGIONS AND OF THE CORRESPONDING CONNECTIVE SPACES***	***TRIANGLES AND FOSSAE***	
Infrahyoid region	*Superior*: horizontal line passing through the hyoid bone *Inferior*: jugular notch of the sternum *Lateral*: anterior border of the sternocleidomastoid. Deeply, it is bounded by the anterior fascia of the visceral sheath	– carotid triangle – muscular (or omotracheal) triangle – – suprasternal or jugular fossa	The suprasternal fossa is a superficial recess situated in correspondence to the jugular notch, bordered laterally by the sternal heads of the sternocleidomastoids
Visceral space (visceral compartment of neck)	*Anterior*: suprahyoid and infrahyoid regions *Posterior*: anterior surface of the cervical column covered by the prevertebral layer of cervical fascia *Lateral*: border with the vascular (carotid) compartment *Superior*: cranial base *Inferior*: mediastinum		
Sternocleidomastoid region or carotid region	Anterior and posterior borders of the sternocleidomastoid	Lesser supraclavicular fossa	The lesser supraclavicular fossa is a superficial recess situated between the clavicular and sternal heads of the sternocleidomastoid
Sternocleidomastoid compartment	Splitting of the investing layer of cervical fascia in which the sternocleidomastoid is enclosed		
Vascular compartment (carotid compartment)	*Anterolateral*: sternocleidomastoid region *Posterior*: prevertebral muscles and transverse processes of the cervical vertebrae *Medial*: border with the visceral space		
Lateral cervical region (supraclavicular region)	*Anterior*: posterior border of the sternocleidomastoid *Posterior*: anterior border of the trapezius *Superior*: intersection of the two sternocleidomastoids and the trapezius *Inferior*: tract of clavicle between the origin of the sternocleidomastoid and the insertion of the trapezius	Posterior triangle of neck: – occipital triangle – omoclavicular triangle (subclavian triangle) – – greater supraclavicular fossa	The greater supraclavicular fossa, situated between the posterior border of the sternocleidomastoid, the middle third of the clavicle and the inferior belly of the omohyoid, is the area of superficial recess corresponding to the omoclavicular triangle
Supraclavicular compartment	*Lateral*: skin, subcutaneous tissue, investing layer of cervical fascia and, in the lower part, pretracheal layer of cervical fascia and omohyoid *Anteromedial*: scalenus anterior *Posterior*: transverse processes of the cervical vertebrae covered, above, by the levator scapulae and splenius cervicis and, below, by the scalenus medius and scalenus posterior		
Posterior cervical region or nuchal region	*Inferior*: horizontal line that unites the acromion of the scapulae crossing the seventh cervical vertebra or vertebra prominens *Superior*: superior nuchal line and external occipital protuberance *Lateral*: anterior borders of the trapezius muscles		

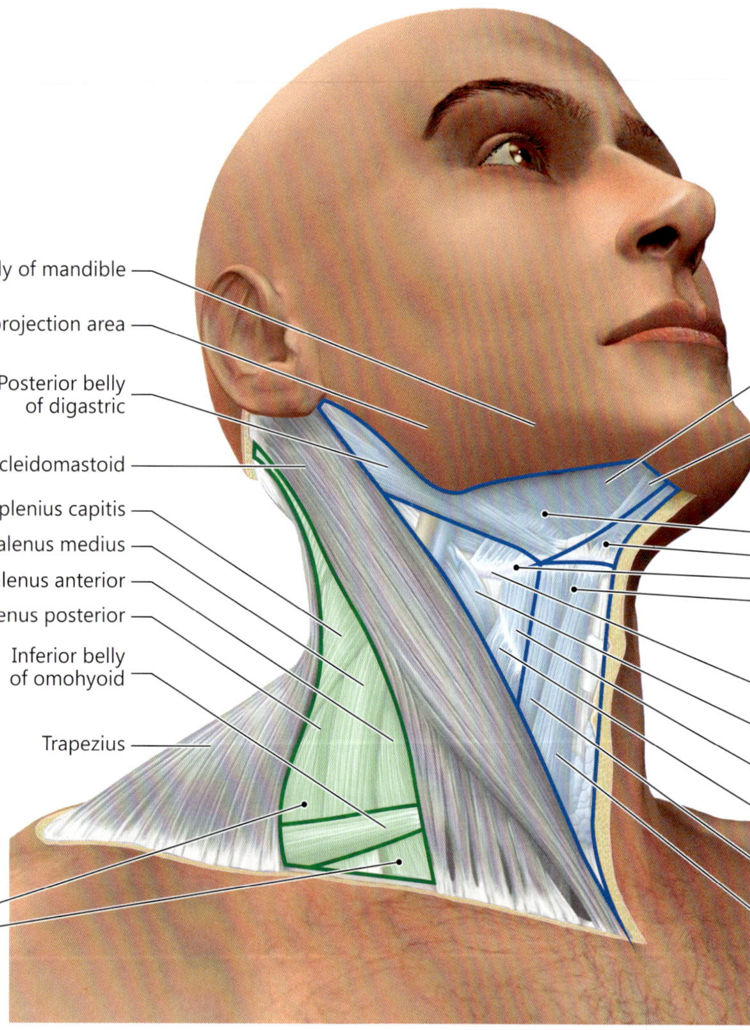

Anterior and **lateral cervical regions** and their respective **triangles**.

Triangles of the neck: subdivision, boundaries and contents

NAME	BOUNDARIES	SUBDIVISION	CONTENT
Anterior triangle (anterior cervical region)	*Anterior*: median line of the neck; *posterior*: anterior border of the sternocleidomastoid; *superior* (base of the triangle): inferior margin of the base of the mandible and its projection to the mastoid process; *apex*: manubrium of the sternum. Covered by: skin, subcutaneous tissue (superficial fascia of the skin), platysma and investing layer of cervical fascia	Divided by the anterior and posterior bellies of the digastric and by the superior belly of the omohyoid into the submental, submandibular, carotid and muscular triangles	*Bones*: hyoid bone *Muscles*: suprahyoid muscles: mylohyoid, geniohyoid, stylohyoid, digastric; infrahyoid muscles: sternohyoid, omohyoid, sternothyroid, thyrohyoid *Other formations*: ☞ submental triangle, submandibular triangle, carotid triangle and muscular triangle
– submental triangle	Single triangle between the anterior bellies of the digastric muscles; *apex*: chin; *base*: body of the hyoid bone; *floor*: both mylohyoid muscles		*Veins*: small veins uniting to form the anterior jugular vein *Lymph nodes*: submental

continued

Triangles of the neck: subdivision, boundaries and contents *(continued)*

NAME	BOUNDARIES	SUBDIVISION	CONTENT
– submandibular triangle (digastric triangle)	*Superior*: base of the mandible and its projection to the mastoid process; *posteroinferior*: posterior belly of the digastric and the stylohyoid; *anteroinferior*: anterior belly of the digastric; *floor*: mylohyoid and hyoglossus. Covered by: skin, subcutaneous tissue (superficial fascia of the skin), platysma and investing layer of cervical fascia		*Muscles*: styloglossus, stylopharyngeus *Arteries*: facial, submental, external carotid, internal carotid, mylohyoid branch of the inferior alveolar artery *Veins*: facial, internal jugular, small veins uniting to form the anterior jugular vein *Lymph nodes*: submandibular, submental *Nerves*: mylohyoid, glossopharyngeal [IX], vagus [X], branches of facial nerve and transverse cervical nerve *Organs*: inferior part of the parotid gland, submandibular gland
– carotid triangle	*Posterior*: sternocleidomastoid; *anteroinferior*: superior belly of the omohyoid; *superior*: stylohyoid and posterior belly of the digastric; anterior angle and adjacent floor of the hyoid bone; *floor*: parts of the thyrohyoid, hyoglossus, middle constrictor of pharynx and inferior constrictor of pharynx. Covered by: skin, subcutaneous tissue (superficial fascia of the skin), platysma and investing layer of cervical fascia		*Arteries*: superior part of the common carotid artery and its division into the external carotid and internal carotid arteries, branches of the external carotid artery (superior thyroid, lingual, facial, occipital, ascending pharyngeal arteries), sternocleidomastoid branches of the occipital artery *Veins*: internal jugular, superior thyroid, lingual, facial, ascending pharyngeal and, sometimes, occipital *Lymph nodes*: deep lateral cervical *Nerves*: vagus [X], accessory [XI], hypoglossal [XII], superior root of ansa cervicalis, external and internal branches of the superior laryngeal nerve, branches of the facial nerve and transverse cervical nerve (within the investing layer of cervical fascia)
– muscular triangle (omotracheal triangle)	*Anterior*: median line of the neck from the hyoid bone to the sternum; *inferoposterior*: anterior border of the sternocleidomastoid; *posterosuperior*: superior belly of the omohyoid		*Muscles*: infrahyoid muscles: omohyoid, sternohyoid, sternothyroid and thyrohyoid
Posterior triangle (lateral cervical or supraclavicular region)	*Anterior*: posterior border of the sternocleidomastoid; *posterior*: anterior border of the trapezius; *inferior*: middle third of the clavicle; *apex*: between insertions to the occipital bone of the sternocleidomastoid and the trapezius and, sometimes, also the semispinalis capitis; *roof*: investing layer of cervical fascia; *floor*: prevertebral layer of cervical fascia superimposing the splenius capitis, levator scapulae and scalene muscles. Covered by: skin, subcutaneous tissue (superficial fascia of the skin), platysma, and investing layer of cervical fascia	Divided by the inferior belly of the omohyoid into the occipital triangle, above, and the omoclavicular triangle, below	*Arteries*: transverse cervical, suprascapular, occipital, third part of the subclavian artery *Veins*: transverse cervical veins, suprascapular veins, external jugular, subclavian *Lymph nodes*: accessory (of the accessory nerve) *Nerves*: accessory [XI], phrenic, cervical and brachial plexuses, cutaneous branches of the cervical plexus (lesser occipital, great auricular, transverse cervical and supraclavicular nerves)
– occipital triangle	Same boundaries as the posterior triangle except for the *inferior border*: inferior belly of the omohyoid; *floor*: splenius capitis, levator scapulae, scalenus medius and scalenus posterior. Covered by: skin, subcutaneous tissue (superficial fascia of the skin), platysma (inferiorly), investing layer of cervical fascia		*Arteries*: transverse cervical, occipital *Veins*: transverse cervical *Lymph nodes*: accessory (of the accessory nerve) *Nerves*: accessory [XI], cutaneous and muscular branches of the cervical plexus (supraclavicular nerves, phrenic nerve), superior part of the brachial plexus
– omoclavicular triangle or subclavian triangle (supraclavicular triangle)	Same boundaries as the posterior triangle except for the *superior border*: omohyoid; *floor*: first rib, scalenus medius, first digitation of the serratus anterior. Covered by: skin, subcutaneous tissue (superficial fascia of the skin), platysma, investing layer of cervical fascia	Corresponds to the inferior part of the greater supraclavicular fossa	*Arteries*: suprascapular, transverse cervical, third part of the subclavian artery *Veins*: subclavian, suprascapular, transverse cervical, external jugular *Lymph nodes*: supraclavicular *Nerves*: supraclavicular nerves, subclavian nerve, trunks of the brachial plexus

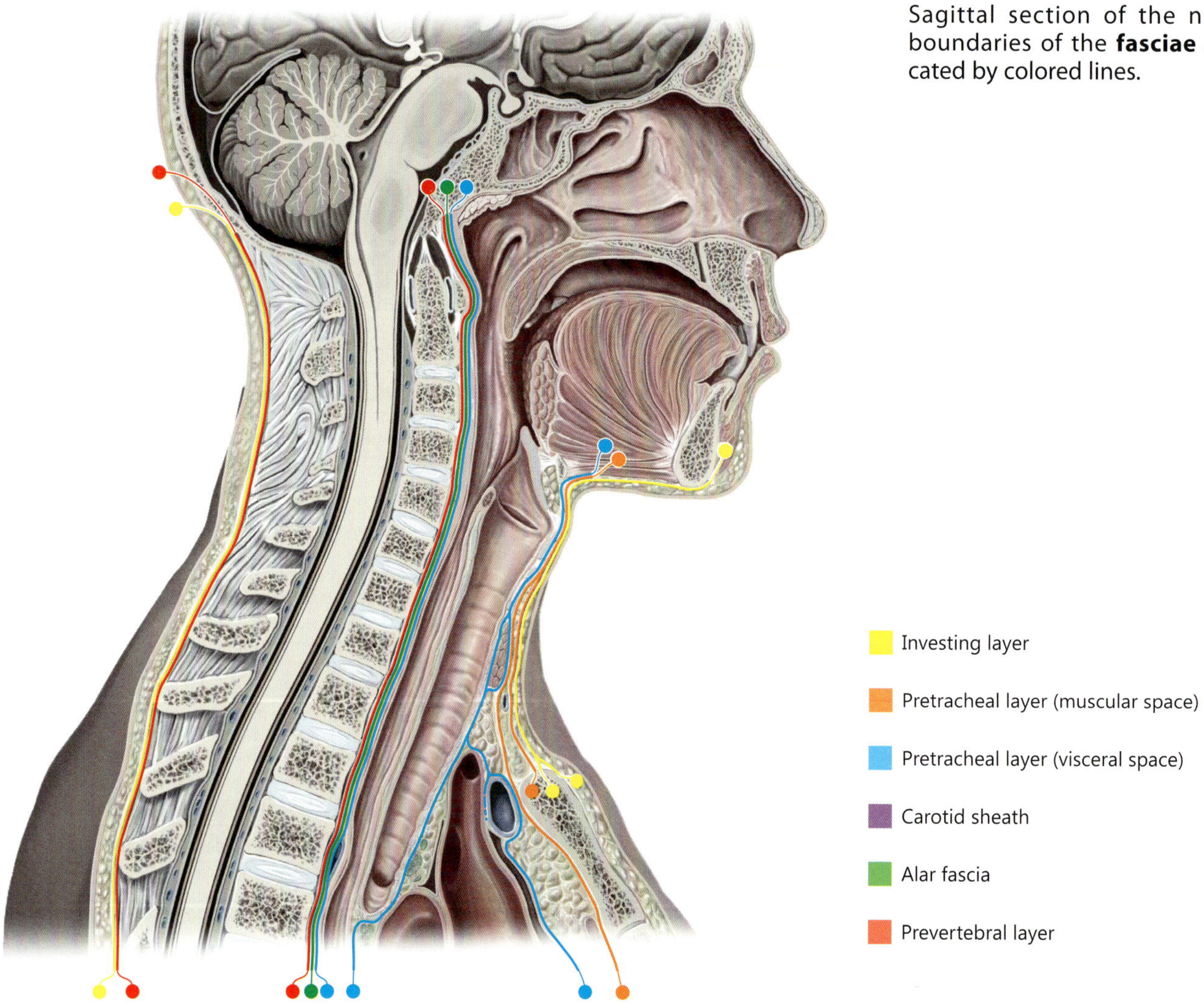

Sagittal section of the neck: the boundaries of the **fasciae** are indicated by colored lines.

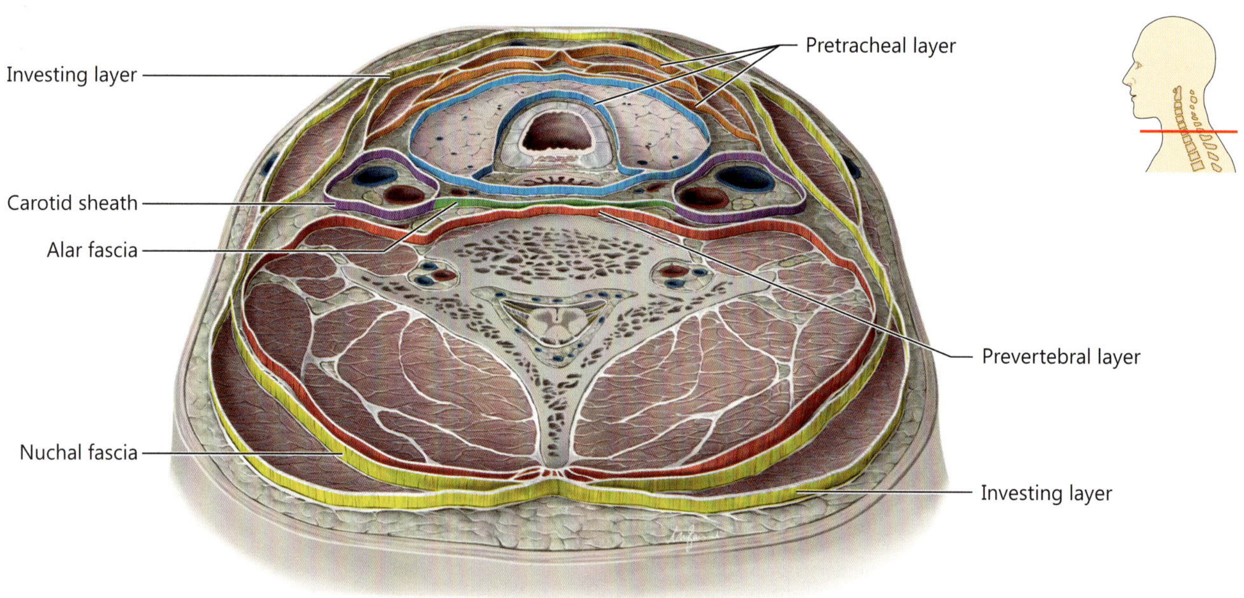

Transverse section of the neck through the 7th cervical vertebra, schematic representation showing its subdivisions by the **cervical** and **nuchal fasciae**.

Sagittal section of the neck: the **compartments** are indicated by different colors.

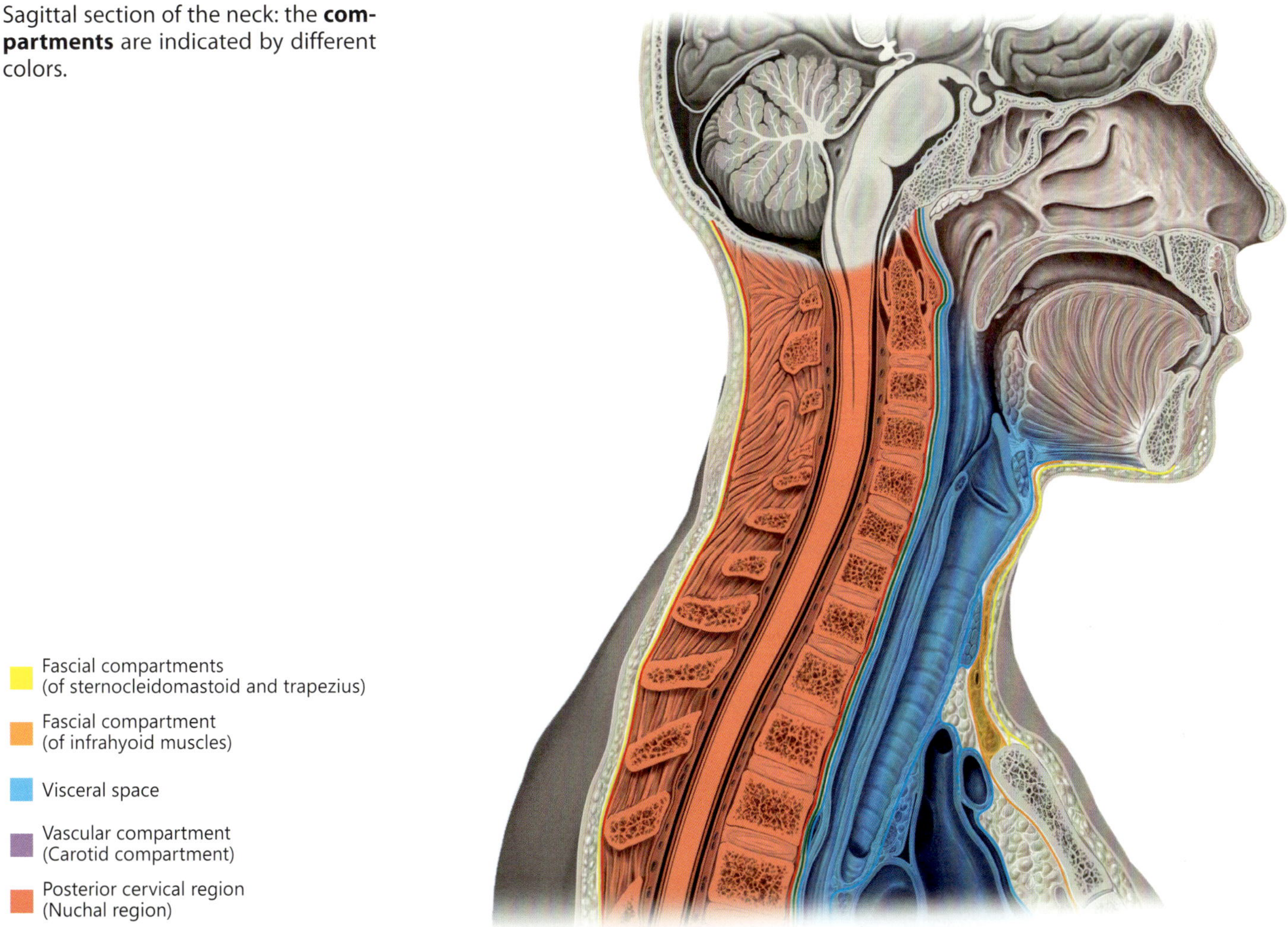

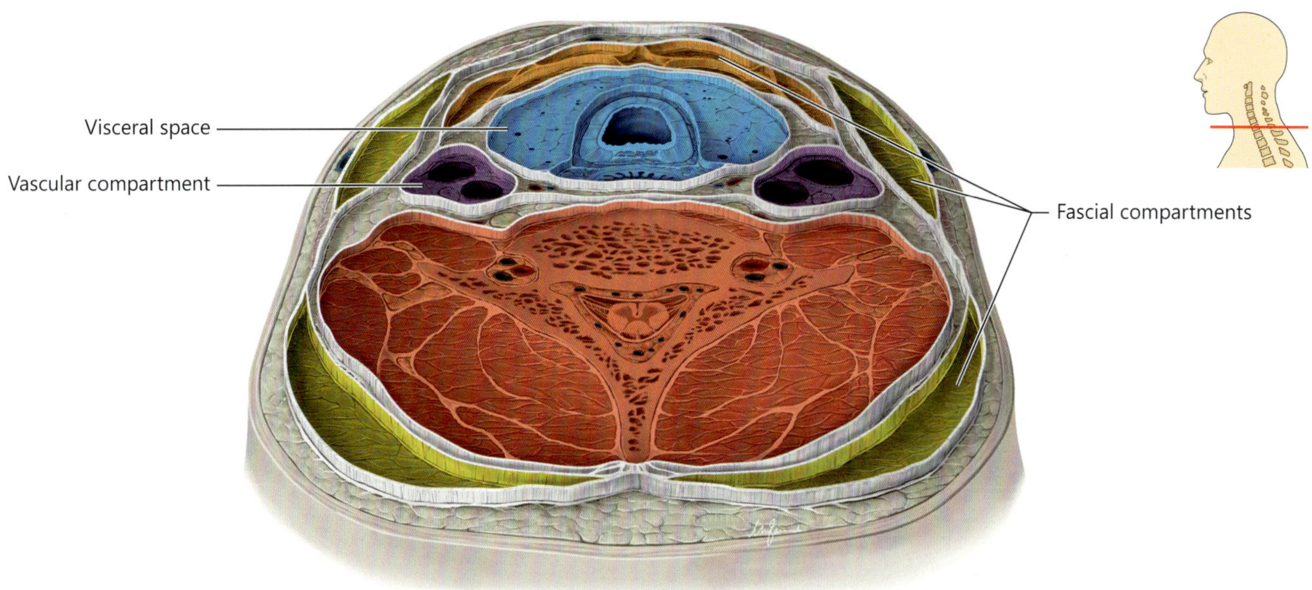

Transverse section of the neck through the seventh cervical vertebra, showing: the **visceral space** or **visceral compartment of the neck**, bounded, anteriorly, by the pretracheal layer of cervical fascia investing the infrahyoid muscles and, posteriorly, by the same layer on the posterior wall of the esophagus and around the trachea; the **vascular compartment** within the carotid sheath, which collects the neurovascular bundle of the neck; the **fascial compartments** formed by splits of the investing layer of cervical fascia to enclose the sternocleidomastoid and trapezius muscles; the **platysma**, which occupies the subcutaneous tissue, between the superficial fascia of skin and the investing layer of cervical fascia; the **fascial compartments** formed by splits of the pretracheal layer that envelop the infrahyoid muscles.

Compartments of the head: boundaries and contents			
NAME	***BOUNDARIES***	***SUBDIVISION***	***CONTENT***
Anterior subparotid space (paratonsillar space)	Between the medial pterygoid and lateral part of the pharynx		*Organs*: pharyngeal tonsil *Other formations*: adipose tissue
Cerebellar compartment	☞ Rhombencephalon cavity		
Cerebral compartment	*Superior and lateral*: calvaria *Inferior*: anterior and middle cranial fossae and tentorium cerebelli	Divided into two halves, right and left, by the falx cerebri	Cerebral hemispheres
Hypophyseal compartment	Between the diaphragma sellae and the sella turcica		*Organs*: pituitary gland
Lateral pharyngeal space	☞ Parapharyngeal space		
Lateropharyngeal space	☞ Parapharyngeal space		
Leptomeningeal spaces	Located between the arachnoid mater and the pia mater, they are described as cisterns: the cerebellomedullary cisterns, chiasmatic cistern, interpeduncular cistern, quadrigeminal cistern (or cistern of great cerebral vein), and the cistern of lateral cerebral fossa		
Masseteric compartment	*Lateral*: masseteric fascia *Medial*: ramus of the mandible		*Muscles*: masseter *Arteries*: masseteric *Nerves*: masseteric
Masticator space	Investing layer of cervical fascia surrounding, laterally, the masseter and, medially, the pterygoid muscles		*Bones*: mandible *Muscles*: temporalis, masseter, medial pterygoid and lateral pterygoid *Arteries*: maxillary *Veins and plexuses*: maxillary vein, pterygoid plexus *Nerves*: inferior alveolar and lingual *Other formations*: buccal fat pad
Maxillopharyngeal space	☞ Parapharyngeal space		
Meckel's cavity	Splitting of the dura mater that covers the trigeminal impression on the anterior surface of the petrous part of the temporal bone		*Nerves and ganglia*: trigeminal ganglion, trigeminal nerve [V], ophthalmic nerve [V_1], maxillary nerve [V_2] and mandibular nerve [V_3]
Parapharyngeal space (lateral pharyngeal, pharyngomaxillary or maxillopharyngeal space)	*Anterior*: pterygomandibular raphe *Posterior*: prevertebral layer of cervical fascia *Medial*: buccopharyngeal fascia and, above the mandible, investing (or superficial) layer of cervical fascia *Lateral*: medial pterygoid and parotid gland *Superior*: petrous part of the temporal bone and sphenoid *Inferior*: hyoid bone	Divided by the styloid process of the temporal bone into two parts: retrostyloid (retrostyloid space) and prestyloid (prestyloid space)	Retrostyloid part: *Arteries*: internal carotid, ascending pharyngeal and ascending palatine *Veins*: internal jugular *Nerves and trunks*: glossopharyngeal [IX], vagus [X], accessory [XI] and hypoglossal [XII] nerves, sympathetic trunk (within the prevertebral layer of cervical fascia) Prestyloid part: In addition to the formations already present in the retrostyloid part, with the exclusion of the sympathetic trunk, since the deep part of the parotid gland projects onto the lateral surface of the prestyloid space: *Arteries*: external carotid with its terminal branches, superficial temporal and maxillary *Veins*: retromandibular *Nerves*: facial [VII] and auriculotemporal
Paratonsillar space	☞ Anterior subparotid space		
Parotid compartment	Investing layer of cervical fascia through septa of connective tissue running from the parotid fascia into the parotid gland		*Arteries*: external carotid, superficial temporal, maxillary, posterior auricular, tympanic, transverse facial *Veins*: retromandibular *Lymph nodes*: deep parotid *Nerves and plexuses*: facial and auriculotemporal nerves, parotid plexus *Organs*: parotid gland and parotid duct
Peripharyngeal space	☞ Parapharyngeal space or Retropharyngeal space		
Pharyngomaxillary space	☞ Parapharyngeal space		
Prefascial compartment	Fascial sheath of the eyeball		Eyeball
Prestyloid space	☞ Parapharyngeal space		

continued

Compartments of the head: boundaries and contents			*(continued)*
NAME	***BOUNDARIES***	***SUBDIVISION***	***CONTENT***
Retrofascial compartment	Fascial sheath of the eyeball and walls of the orbit		*Muscles*: extraocular muscles *Arteries*: ophthalmic, lacrimal, central retinal, supraorbital, short and long posterior ciliary arteries, muscular arteries, anterior and posterior ethmoidal arteries, medial palpebral arteries, dorsal nasal, supratrochlear *Veins*: superior and inferior ophthalmic veins, central retinal *Nerves and ganglia*: optic [II], oculomotor [III], trochlear [IV], abducens [VI], lacrimal, nasociliary, frontal, zygomatic and zygomaticofacial and zygomaticotemporal branches of the zygomatic nerve, long ciliary nerves, anterior and posterior ethmoidal nerves, infratrochlear, supratrochlear, supraorbital, ciliary ganglion *Other formations*: retrobulbar fat
Retropharyngeal space (retrovisceral space)	*Anterior*: pretracheal layer of cervical fascia surrounding the pharynx (buccopharyngeal fascia) *Posterior*: alar fascia (part of the deep cervical fascia or prevertebral layer of cervical fascia)		*Lymph nodes*: retropharyngeal
Retrostyloid space	☞ Parapharyngeal space		
Retrovisceral space	☞ Retropharyngeal space		
Rhombencephalon cavity (cerebellar compartment)	*Superior*: tentorium cerebelli *Inferior*: cerebellar fossae *Anterior*: clivus and petrous part of the temporal bone		Rhombencephalon (cerebellum, pons and myelencephalon)
Subdural space	Virtual space between the dura mater and the arachnoid mater		
Sublingual compartment	*Superior*: mucous membrane of the mouth *Anterolateral*: internal surface of the body of the mandible *Posteromedial*: hyoglossus *Inferior*: mylohyoid In front: *Anterior*: mandibular symphysis *Posteroinferior*: genioglossus *Superior*: mucous membrane of the mouth		*Arteries*: sublingual *Veins*: sublingual *Nerves*: hypoglossal [XII] and lingual *Organs*: sublingual gland, prolongation of the submandibular gland and submandibular duct *Other formations*: adipose tissue
Temporal compartment	*Lateral*: investing layer of cervical fascia fixed to the infratemporal crest of the sphenoid, and zygomatic bone *Medial*: periosteum of the temporal bone		*Muscles*: temporalis *Arteries*: superficial temporal, middle temporal, anterior and posterior deep temporal arteries *Veins*: superficial temporal veins and deep temporal veins *Nerves*: auriculotemporal and deep temporal nerves *Other formations*: adipose tissue
Tonsillar compartment	*Superior*: soft palate *Inferior*: horizontal line prolonging the lateral border of the tongue *Anterior*: palatoglossal arch *Posterior*: palatopharyngeal arch *Lateral*: buccopharyngeal fascia		*Organs*: palatine tonsil

Compartments of the neck: boundaries and contents			
NAME	*BOUNDARIES*	*SUBDIVISION*	*CONTENT*
Carotid compartment	☞ Vascular compartment		
Carotid space	☞ Vascular compartment		
"Danger" space	Between the two layers of the prevertebral layer of cervical fascia (between the alar fascia and the prevertebral layer)		Areolar connective tissue
Lateral vascular space	☞ Vascular compartment		
Pre-epiglottic space	*Superior*: glossoepiglottic folds *Inferior*: insertion of the epiglottic cartilage on the thyroid cartilage *Anterior*: thyrohyoid membrane *Posterior*: epiglottic cartilage		Loose connective tissue
Prevertebral space	*Anterior*: prevertebral layer *Posterior*: vertebral column		*Muscles*: erector spinae, prevertebral, scalene muscles *Arteries*: vertebral *Veins*: vertebral *Nerves and plexuses*: phrenic nerve, brachial plexus
Previsceral space	☞ Visceral space		
Retroesophageal space (retrovisceral)	*Anterior*: posterior wall of the esophagus *Posterior*: prevertebral layer *Inferior*: at the level of the second-fourth thoracic vertebra (where the prevertebral layer fuses with the connective tissue on the posterior surface of the esophagus)		Areolar connective tissue
Retrovisceral space	☞ Retroesophageal space		
Sternocleidomastoid compartment	Splitting of the investing layer of cervical fascia		*Muscles*: sternocleidomastoid
Submandibular compartment	*Anterior and lateral*: mandible *Superior*: mucous membrane of the tongue *Posteroinferior*: hyoid bone *Inferior*: investing layer of cervical fascia		*Arteries*: facial, with its glandular branches, and submental *Veins*: facial and lingual *Nerves*: hypoglossal [XII], mylohyoid and lingual *Lymph nodes*: submental and submandibular *Organs*: submandibular gland and submandibular duct
Supraclavicular compartment	*Lateral*: skin, subcutaneous tissue and investing layer of cervical fascia; pretracheal layer of cervical fascia and omohyoid inferiorly *Anteromedial*: scalenus anterior *Posterior*: transverse processes of the cervical vertebrae covered, in the upper part, by the levator scapulae and splenius cervicis and, in the lower part, by the scalenus medius and scalenus posterior *Apex*: convergence towards the top of the sternocleidomastoid, trapezius, splenius cervicis and levator scapulae *Base*: clavicle and superior border of the scapula	The base of the compartment is subdivided into two portions, lateral and medial, by the superior surface of the first rib	*Arteries*: subclavian and origin of its branches: vertebral and internal thoracic artery, and thyrocervical and costocervical trunks *Veins*: subclavian *Lymph nodes and ducts*: supraclavicular nodes, thoracic duct and right lymphatic duct *Nerves, plexuses and ganglia*: accessory [XI] and phrenic nerves, brachial plexus, cervicothoracic (stellate) ganglion *Other formations*: cervical pleura
Suprasternal space	Splitting of the investing layer of cervical fascia		*Veins*: anterior jugular veins with jugular venous arch
Vascular compartment (carotid compartment, carotid space or lateral vascular space)	Located within the carotid sheath, to whose formation all three layers of the cervical fascia (investing, pretracheal and prevertebral) contribute		*Arteries*: common carotid, external carotid and internal carotid *Veins*: internal jugular *Lymph nodes*: deep lateral cervical *Nerves, branches and plexuses*: vagus nerve [X], carotid branch of glossopharyngeal nerve [IX], common carotid plexus and internal carotid plexus, hypoglossal nerve [XII] *Other formations*: adipose tissue

continued

Compartments of the neck: boundaries and contents			(*continued*)
NAME	***BOUNDARIES***	***SUBDIVISION***	***CONTENT***
Visceral compartment of neck	☞ Visceral space		
Visceral space (previsceral space or visceral compartment of neck)	*Anterior*: pretracheal layer of cervical fascia and infrahyoid muscles *Posterior*: pretracheal layer around the trachea and adhering to the posterior wall of the esophagus *Superior*: insertions of the infrahyoid muscles on the thyroid cartilage of the larynx	Anterior cervical space: space lying between the fascia covering the infrahyoid muscles and the perithyroid fascia, with the posterolateral border consisting of the carotid sheath and sternocleidomastoid fascia Perithyroid "danger" space: interstitium between the internal surface of the perithyroid sheath and the thyroid gland capsule	*Organs*: pharynx, esophagus, larynx, trachea, thyroid and parathyroid glands

Schematic representation of the branches of the **aorta**, showing the arch and its branches involved in the vascularization of the superior part of the thoracic cage, neck and head.

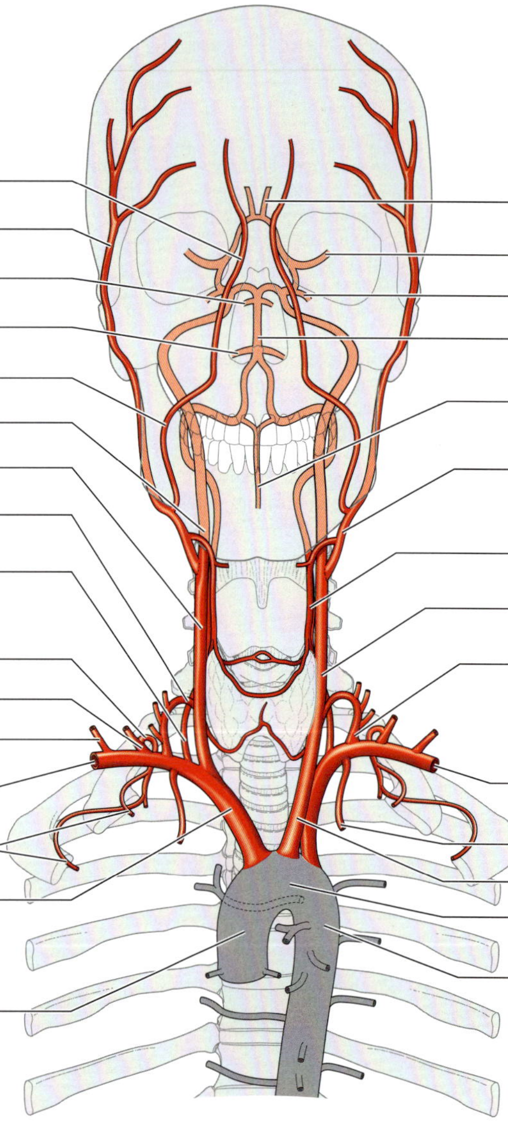

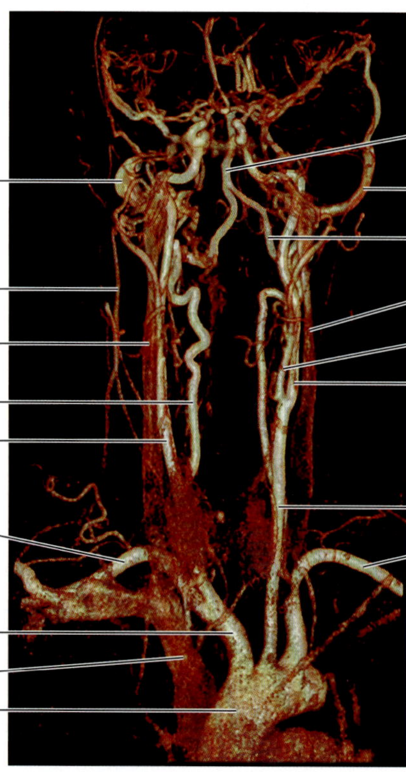

Three-dimensional image of a living human body, obtained by contrast-enhanced NMR using a 3D volume rendering technique, showing the **arteries** and **veins of the head** and **neck**.

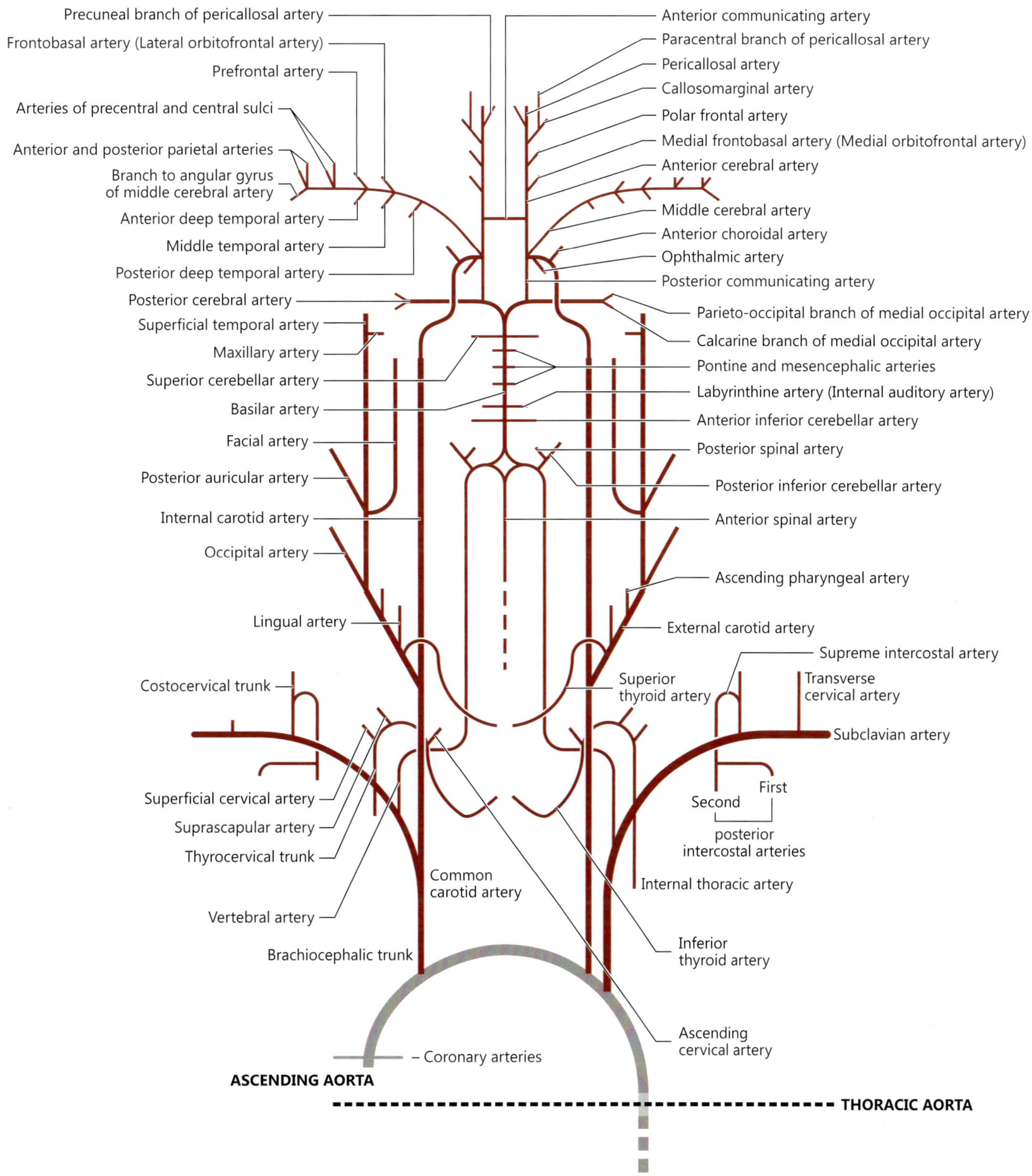

Schematic representation of the arterial blood supply to the head and neck highlighting, in particular, the ramifications of the external carotid, internal carotid, vertebral and basilar arteries.
The **external carotid artery** has as its collateral branches the superior thyroid, ascending pharyngeal, lingual, facial, occipital and posterior auricular arteries; its terminal branches are the superficial temporal and internal maxillary arteries.
The **internal carotid artery** has as its collateral branches the caroticotympanic arteries, the artery of pterygoid canal, the cavernous branches (not indicated here) in the carotid canal, and the ophthalmic artery in the cranial cavity; its main terminal branches are the anterior choroidal, anterior cerebral, middle cerebral and posterior communicating arteries.
The **vertebral artery** has as its collateral branches the spinal and muscular branches in the cervical part and meningeal and medullary branches in the intracranial part (not indicated here), and the posterior inferior cerebellar artery and anterior and posterior spinal arteries. At the point of confluence of the two vertebral arteries begins the **basilar artery**, which has as its collateral branches the pontine and mesencephalic arteries, the labyrinthine artery, the anterior inferior cerebellar and superior cerebellar arteries, and as its terminal branches the posterior cerebral arteries. Details of the blood supply to the brain are reported in the chapter on the nervous system.

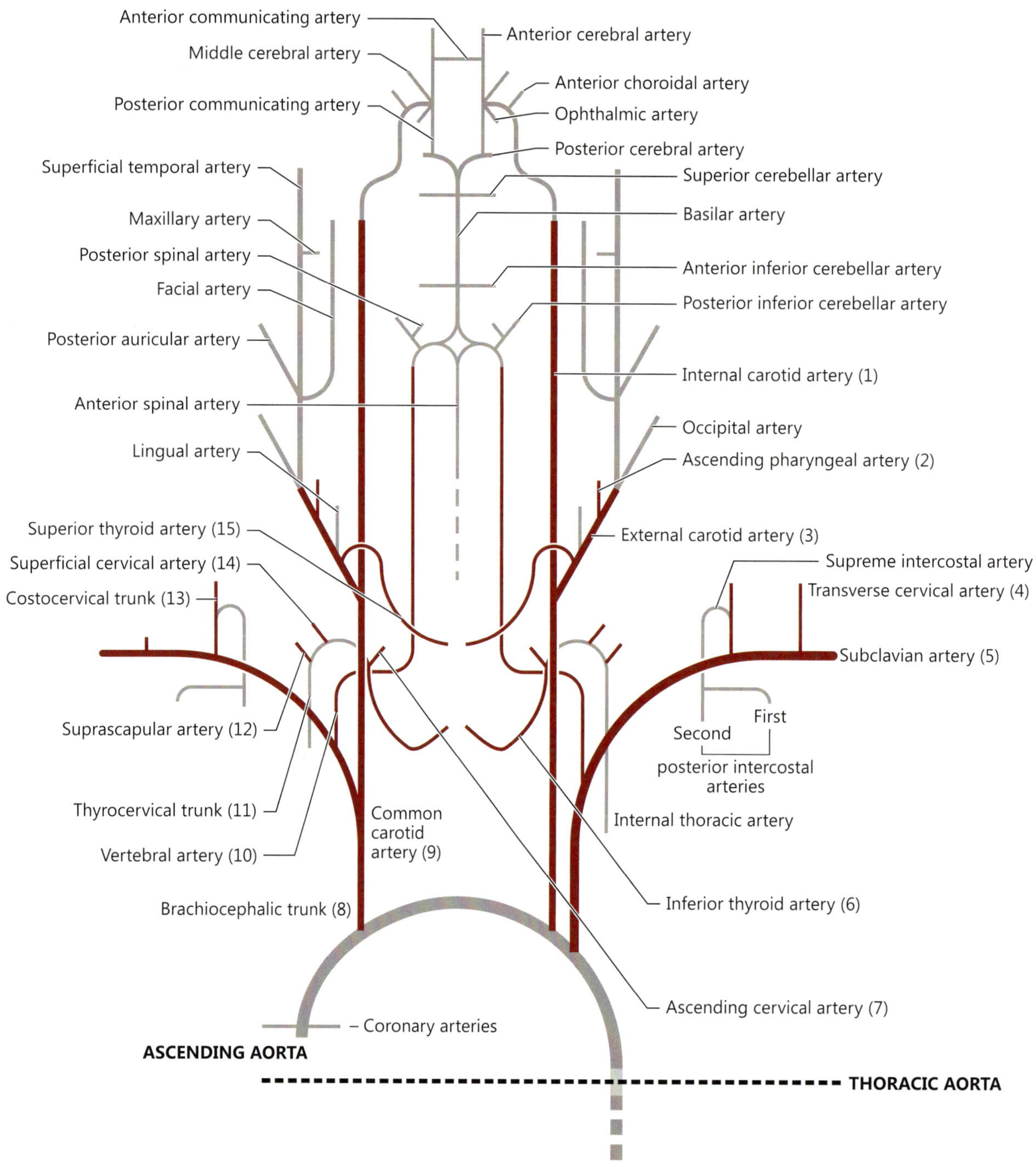

Schematic representation of the arterial blood supply to the head and neck.
This page focuses on the role of the subclavian arteries involved together with some of their collateral branches: the **vertebral arteries**, from whose confluence originates the **basilar artery**, the internal thoracic artery, the **thyrocervical** and **costocervical trunks**, and the **transverse cervical artery**. The relative territories of supply (indicated numerically) are described in the table alongside. In general, the **vertebral artery** supplies the semispinalis and suboccipital muscles, the cervical spinal cord, myelencephalon (or medulla oblongata or bulb), cerebellum and dura mater of the cerebellar fossa, while the **basilar artery** supplies the pons, internal ear, cerebellum, cortex of the temporal and occipital lobes, third ventricle, thalamus, hypothalamus and mesencephalon.

Main arteries of the neck: territories of blood supply		
	ARTERIES OF THE NECK	TERRITORIES OF SUPPLY
1	Internal carotid artery (cervical part)	Middle ear, orbital cavity, nasal cavity, brain, pituitary gland, trigeminal ganglion, meninges
2	Ascending pharyngeal artery	Pharynx, soft palate, longus capitis and longus colli, sympathetic trunk, palatine tonsil, pharyngotympanic tube, tympanic cavity, dura mater of the cerebellar fossa
3	External carotid artery	Anterior part of the face and neck, lateral part of the head, walls of the cranial cavity, dura mater, posterior part of the scalp
4	Transverse cervical artery	Posterior cervical, shoulder and back muscles
5	Subclavian artery	Territory of supply of the vertebral artery (☞ 10), anterior and superior thoracic wall, upper limb
6	Inferior thyroid artery	Infrahyoid muscles, longus colli, scalenus anterior and inferior constrictor of pharynx, cervical part of the esophagus, muscles and mucosa of the larynx, inferior part of the pharynx, trachea, posteroinferior part of the thyroid gland
7	Ascending cervical artery	Sternocleidomastoid, omohyoid, trapezius, longus capitis, phrenic nerve, spinal cord
8	Brachiocephalic trunk (at the level of the superior border of the right sternoclavicular joint where it divides into the right common carotid and subclavian arteries)	Head and neck, upper limb, superior part of the thorax
9	Common carotid artery	Head and neck
10	Vertebral artery	Semispinalis capitis, suboccipital muscles, prevertebral muscles and muscles of back proper, vertebral canal, meninges and spinal cord of the cervical tract, myelencephalon, cerebellum, dura mater of the cerebellar fossa, pons, mesencephalon, thalamus, hypothalamus, third ventricle, temporal and occipital lobes, internal ear
11	Thyrocervical trunk	Territories of supply of the inferior thyroid artery (☞ 6), ascending cervical artery (☞ 7), suprascapular artery (☞ 12) and transverse cervical artery (☞ 4)
12	Suprascapular artery	Clavicle, scapula, sternocleidomastoid, subclavius, supraspinatus and subscapularis, acromioclavicular and glenohumeral joints, suprascapular region, skin over the acromion
13	Costocervical trunk	First two intercostal spaces, semispinalis capitis and semispinalis cervicis, spinal cord
14	Superficial cervical artery	Trapezius
15	Superior thyroid artery	Thyroid gland, infrahyoid muscles and sternocleidomastoid, muscles and mucosa of the larynx

N.B.: for a general overview of the arteries and their territories of supply, see the table summarizing the arteries of the neck.

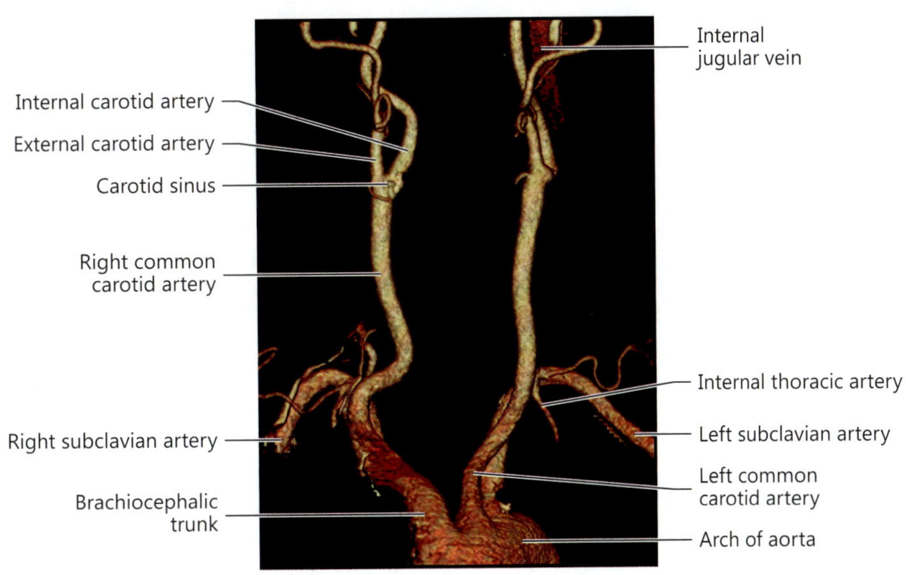

Three-dimensional image of a living human body, obtained by CT scan using a 3D volume rendering technique, showing the ramification and distribution of the **vessels that originate from the arch of the aorta**. The convex face of the arch gives rise to the brachiocephalic trunk, the left common carotid artery and left subclavian artery. The brachiocephalic trunk subdivides into the right common carotid and the right subclavian arteries. The common carotid arteries are the main arteries supplying blood to the head and neck and terminate with subdivision into the external carotid and internal carotid arteries.

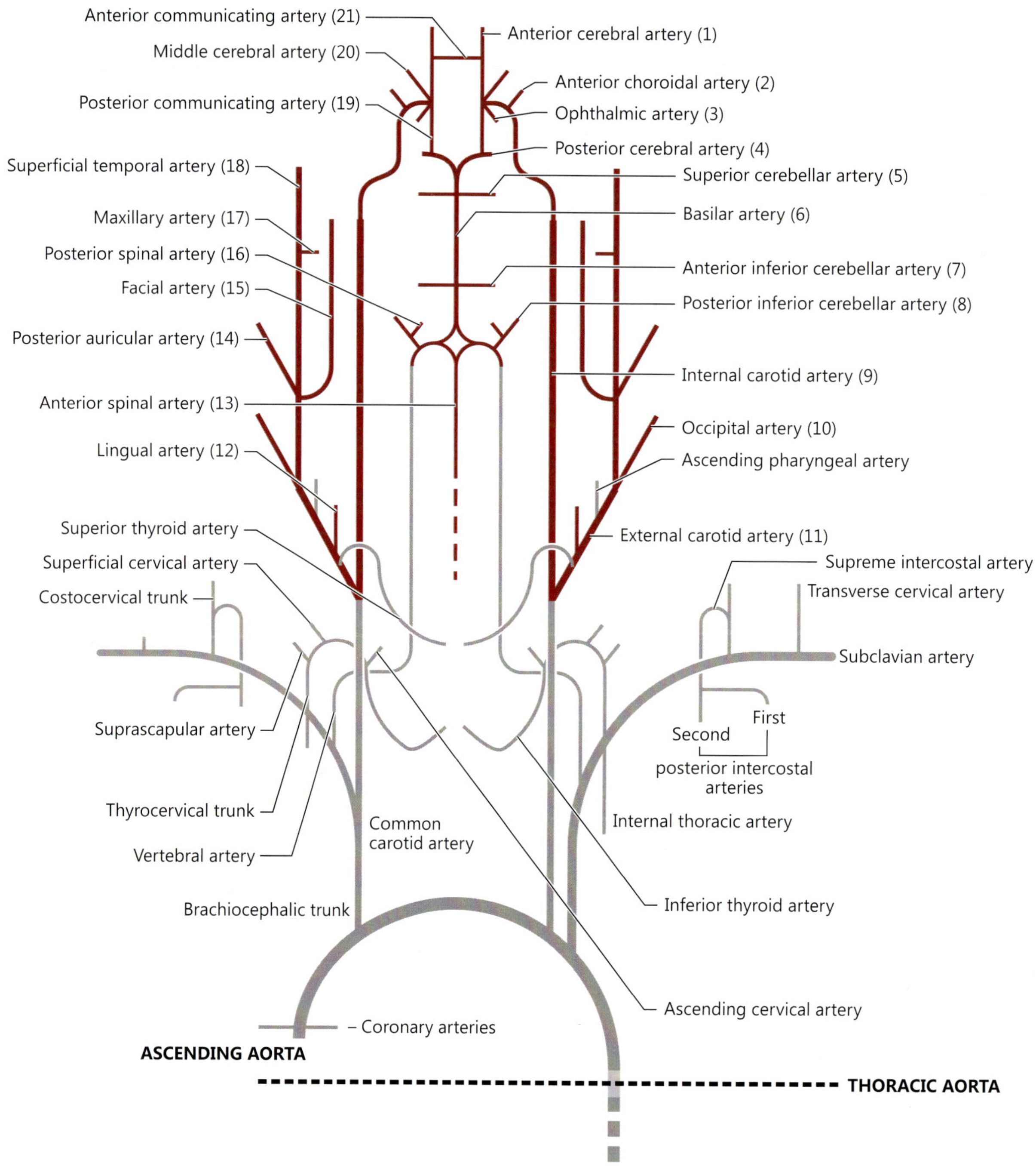

Schematic representation of the arterial blood supply to the head.
This page focuses on the role of the external and internal carotid arteries involved. The relative territories of blood supply (indicated numerically) are described in the table alongside. In general, the **external carotid artery** supplies the neck, face and the walls of the cranium, while the **internal carotid artery** supplies the brain and intracranial formations of the orbital cavity and nasal cavities. The circulation upstream of the cerebral arterial circle, or circle of Willis, is described in the chapter on the nervous system.

Main arteries of the head: territories of blood supply		
	ARTERIES OF THE HEAD	***TERRITORIES OF SUPPLY***
1	Anterior cerebral artery	Hypothalamus, lamina terminalis, anterior perforated substance, anterior commissure, column of the fornix, caudate nucleus, putamen, pallidum, internal capsule, choroid plexuses, lateral ventricle, corpus striatum, corpus callosum, medial part of the frontal and parietal lobes, straight gyrus, olfactory bulb
2	Anterior choroidal artery	Choroid plexus of the lateral ventricle, optic tract, optic radiation, cerebral peduncle, hippocampus, fimbria of hippocampus, lateral geniculate body, caudate nucleus, red nucleus, pallidum, amygdaloid body, hypothalamus, tuber cinereum, substantia nigra, posterior limb of the internal capsule
3	Ophthalmic artery	Orbital cavity, eyeball, extraocular muscles, eyelids, dura mater of the anterior cranial fossa, vault and lateral walls of the nasal cavities
4	Posterior cerebral artery	Thalamus, walls of the third ventricle, hypothalamus, globus pallidus, cerebral peduncle, mesencephalon, tectal plate, epiphysis, medial and lateral geniculate bodies, uncus, parahippocampal gyrus, medial occipitotemporal gyrus, lateral occipitotemporal gyrus, temporal and occipital lobes, choroid plexus of the lateral ventricle and choroid plexus of the third ventricle
5	Superior cerebellar artery	Superior surface of the cerebellum, vermis of cerebellum [I-X], pons, epiphysis, superior medullary velum, choroid membrane of the third ventricle
6	Basilar artery	Internal ear, pons, cerebellum, mesencephalon, thalamus, hypothalamus, epiphysis, third ventricle, cerebral ventricles, cortex of the temporal and occipital lobes
7	Anterior inferior cerebellar artery	Anterolateral region of the inferior surface of the hemisphere of cerebellum, choroid plexus of the fourth ventricle
8	Posterior inferior cerebellar artery	Hemisphere of cerebellum [H II - H X], vermis of cerebellum [I-X], choroid plexus of the fourth ventricle
9	Internal carotid artery	Brain, pituitary gland, orbit, nasal cavity, trigeminal ganglion, meninges, middle ear
10	Occipital artery	Lateral and posterior cervical muscles, auricle, mastoid cells, dura mater of the posterior cranial fossa, diploë, muscles and skin of the occipital region, scalp
11	External carotid artery	Anterior parts of the face and neck and lateral part of the head, walls of the cranial cavity, dura mater, posterior part of the scalp
12	Lingual artery	Muscles and mucous membrane of the tongue, sublingual gland, gingivae, lingual and palatine tonsils, epiglottis, suprahyoid muscles
13	Anterior spinal artery	Anterior two-thirds of the spinal cord
14	Posterior auricular artery	Middle ear, mastoid cells, auricle, digastric, stylohyoid, sternocleidomastoid, skin of the occipital region, parotid gland
15	Facial artery	Soft palate, palatine tonsil, submandibular gland and labial glands, skin and muscles of the chin, lips and external nose, ala and dorsum of the nose
16	Posterior spinal artery	Myelencephalon, spinal cord, pia mater
17	Maxillary artery	Tympanic cavity, external acoustic meatus, dental arcades, upper lip, chin, dura mater of the middle cranial fossa, of the walls and the calvaria, trigeminal ganglion, temporalis, masseter, buccinator, extraocular muscles, lacrimal sac, lacrimal gland, palatine tonsil, palate, nasopharynx, pharyngotympanic tube, nasal cavity and paranasal sinuses
18	Superficial temporal artery	Masseter and temporalis, frontal belly of occipitofrontalis, orbicularis oculi, external acoustic meatus, auricle, skin of the face, scalp, parotid gland, temporomandibular joint
19	Posterior communicating artery	Base of the telencephalon between the infundibulum and optic tract, optic chiasm, hippocampus, cerebral peduncle, internal capsule, anterior third of the thalamus, third ventricle, anterior perforated substance
20	Middle cerebral artery	Lentiform nucleus, internal capsule, caudate nucleus, corpus striatum, insula, frontal lobe, parietal lobe, temporal lobe, precentral gyrus, postcentral gyrus, inferior frontal gyrus, superior temporal gyrus, middle temporal gyrus, supramarginal gyrus and angular gyrus
21	Anterior communicating artery	Cerebral cortex, orbitomesial giri

N.B.: for a general overview of the arteries and their territories of supply, see the table summarizing the arteries of the head.

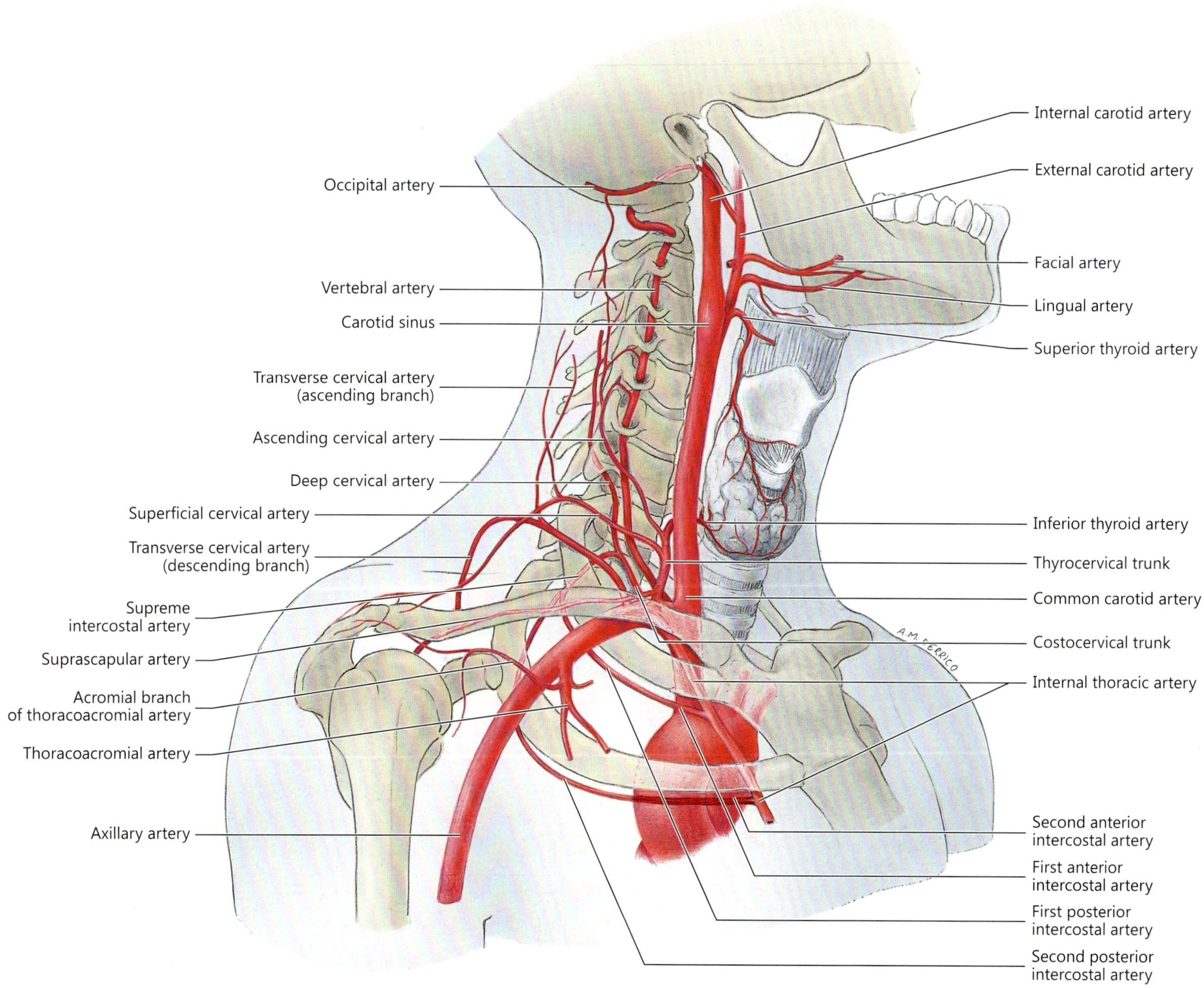

Right subclavian artery and its branches. Note the course of the **vertebral artery** that, on reaching the 6th cervical vertebra, ascends the neck passing through the foramina transversaria; inferiorly, the **supreme intercostal artery** supplies branches for the 1st and 2nd intercostal spaces, and further on anastomoses with the **internal thoracic artery**.

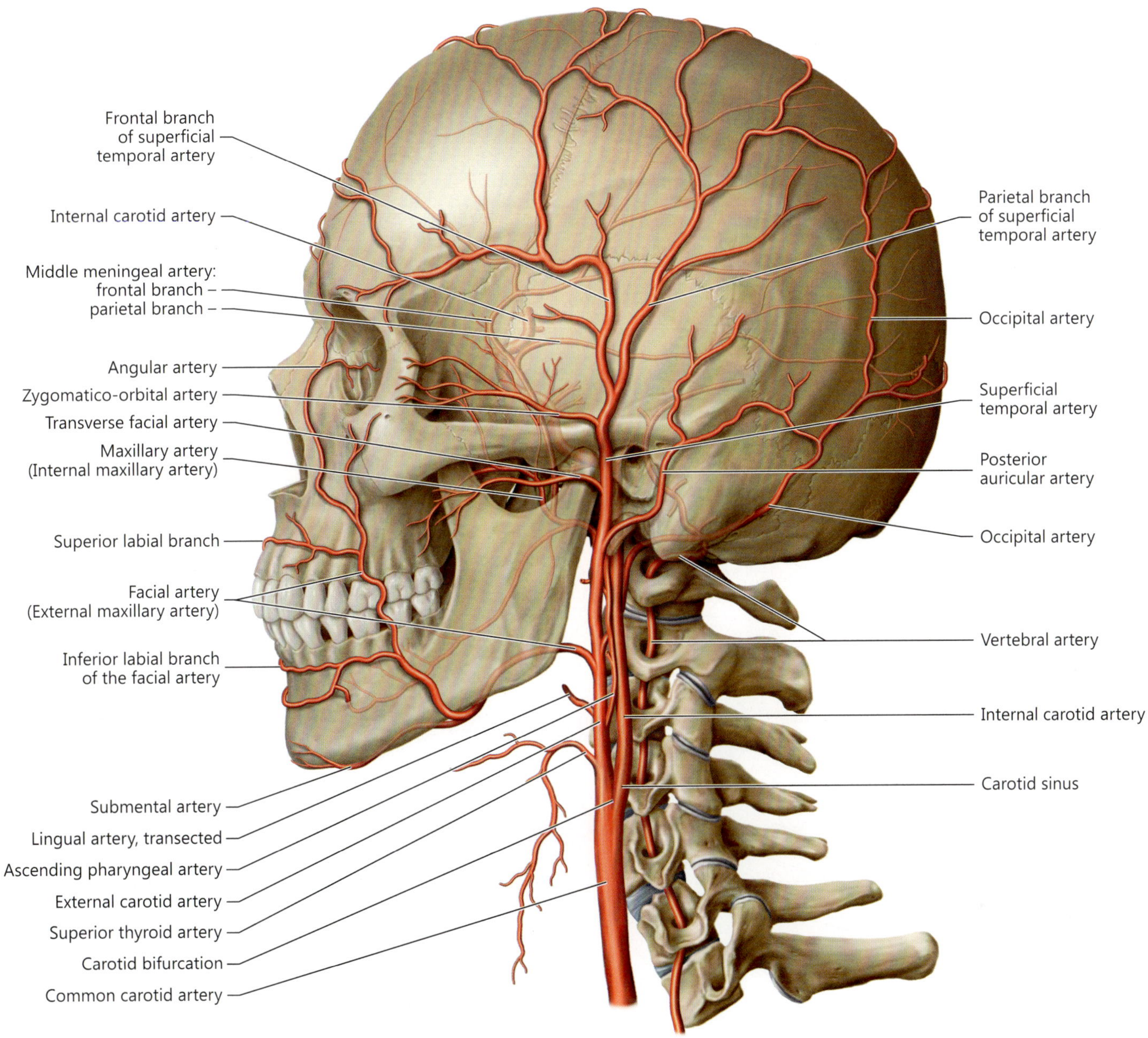

Course of the **external carotid artery** and relative collateral and terminal branches. Also visible are the internal carotid artery and vertebral artery and, in transparency, some of their intracranial branches.

Deep Blood Supply

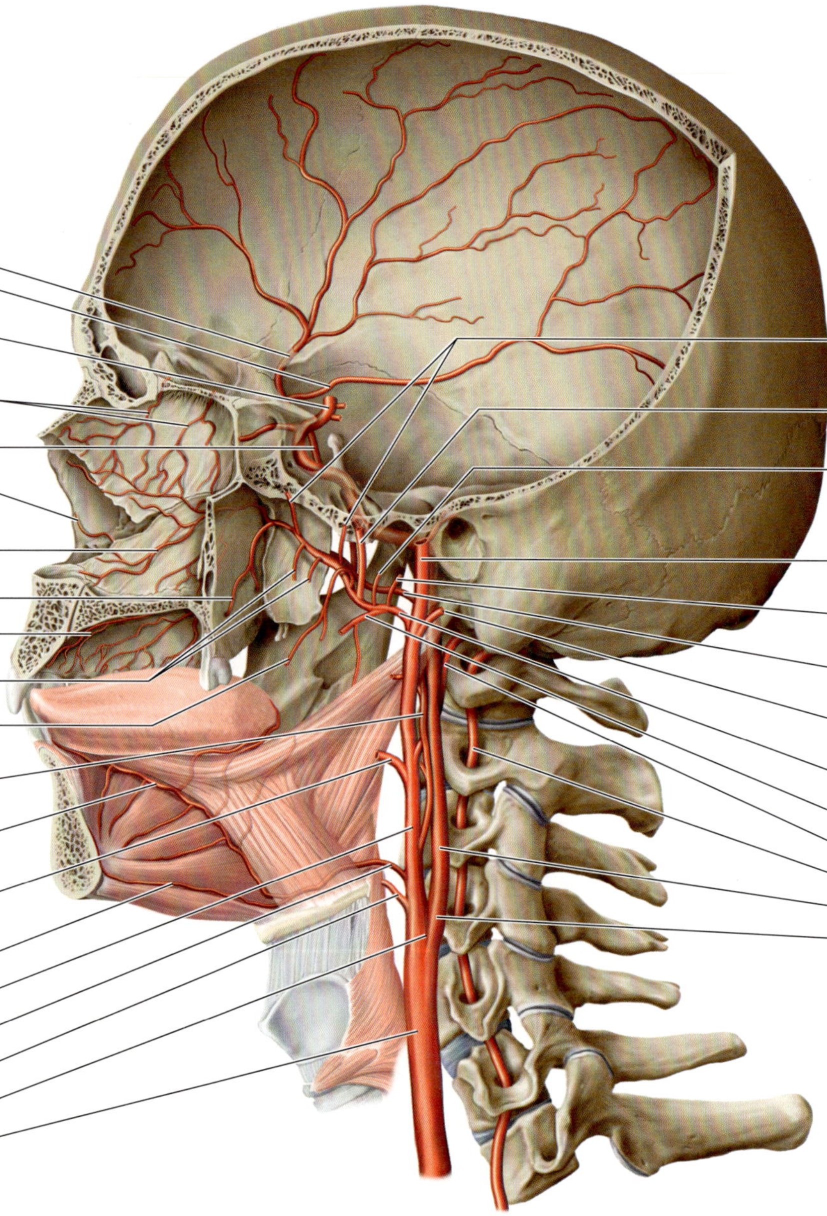

The collateral and terminal branches of the **external carotid artery** have important relations with the cranium and with the muscles of the mouth and tongue.

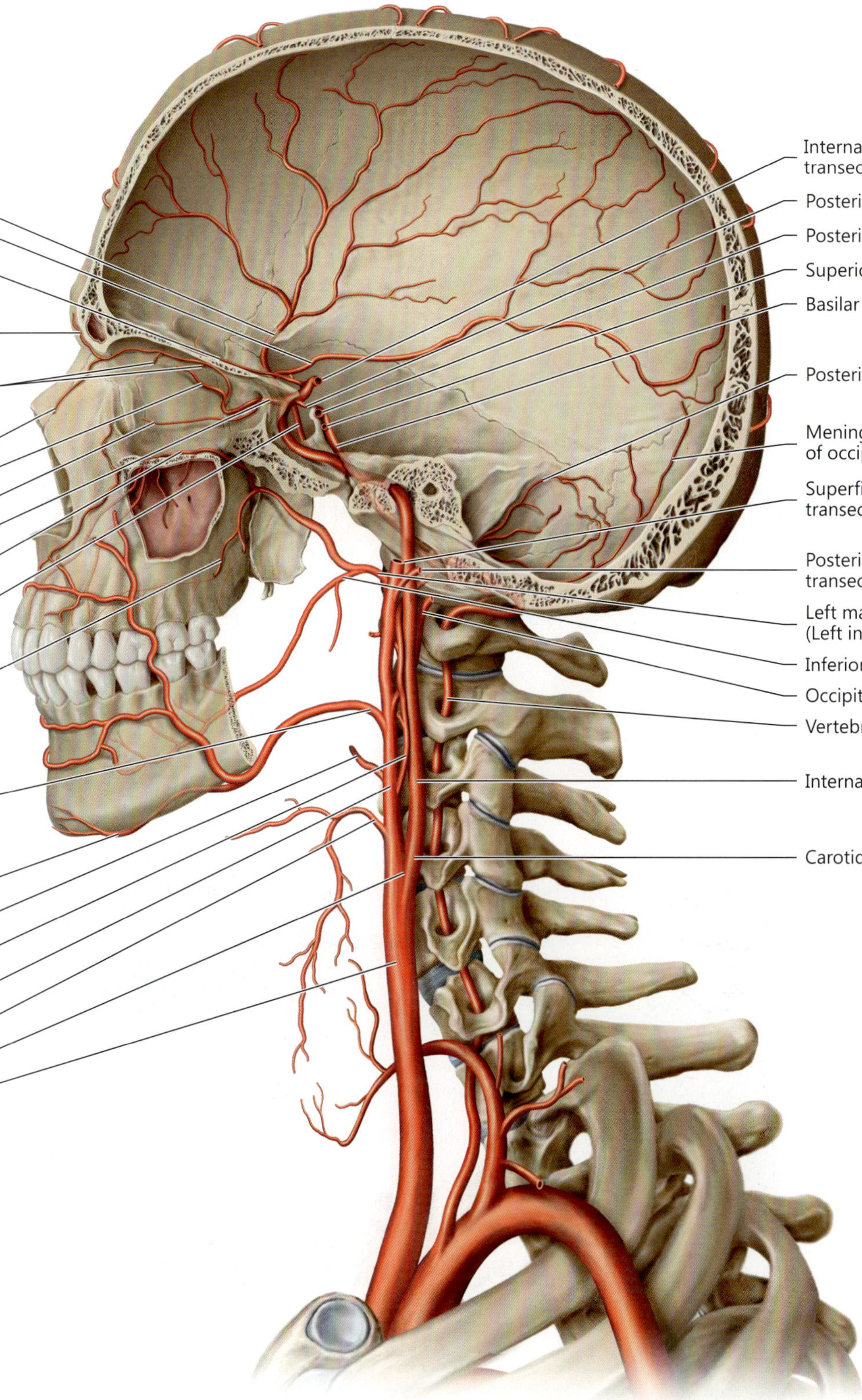

Course and branches of the **external carotid artery** and **maxillary artery** (in the three portions: mandibular, pterygoid and pterygopalatine). With respect to the previous figure, large parts of the soft tissues, facial skeleton and calvaria have been resected and removed. Highlighted are the right middle meningeal artery, with its intracranial course, and the meningeal branches of the posterior cranial fossa: the posterior meningeal artery, branch of the ascending pharyngeal artery, and the meningeal branch of the occipital artery. Further detail on the course of the maxillary (or internal maxillary) artery can be found on page 141.

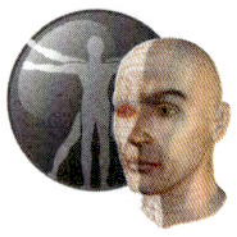

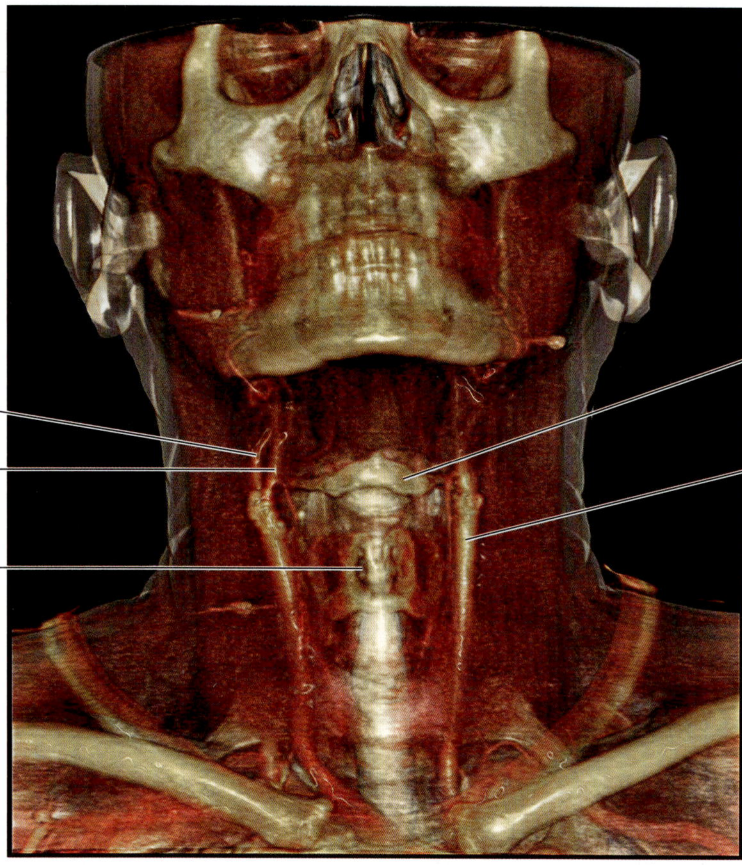

Three-dimensional image of a living human body, obtained by CT scan using a 3D volume rendering technique, showing in transparency the bifurcation of the **common carotid artery** into the **internal carotid artery** and **external carotid artery** in relation to the hyoid bone and the thyroid cartilage of the larynx, in frontal view.

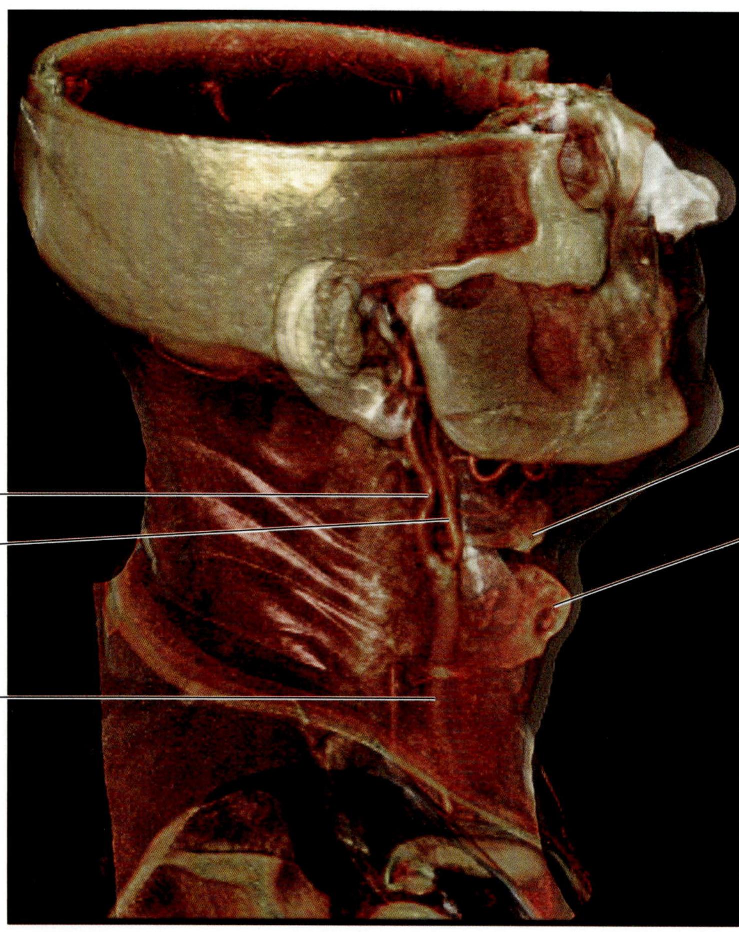

Three-dimensional image of a living human body, obtained by CT scan using a 3D volume rendering technique, showing in transparency the bifurcation of the **common carotid artery** into the **internal carotid artery** and **external carotid artery** in relation to the hyoid bone and the thyroid cartilage of the larynx, in right posterolateral view.

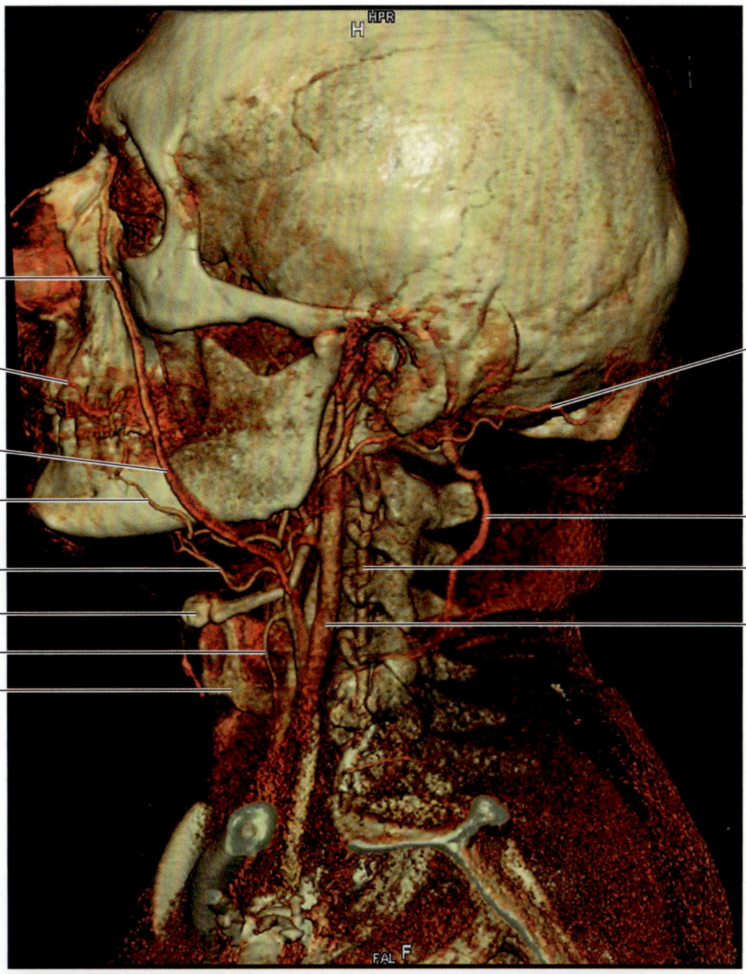

Three-dimensional images of a living human body, obtained by CT scan using a 3D volume rendering technique. Above: **collateral branches of the external carotid artery** and course of the **vertebral artery**. Below: **arteries of the neck** in relation to the skeleton of the neck and head, viewed on a deeper plane with respect to the image above, for which reason the external maxillary artery in its tangential course to the mandible is not visible, thus making it possible to see the internal maxillary artery.

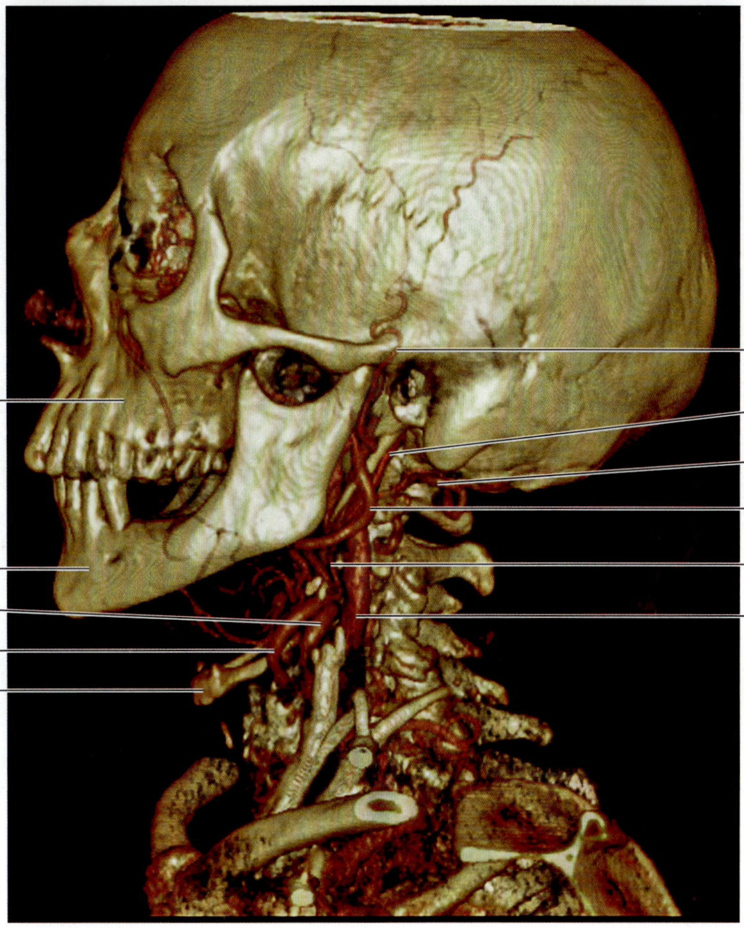

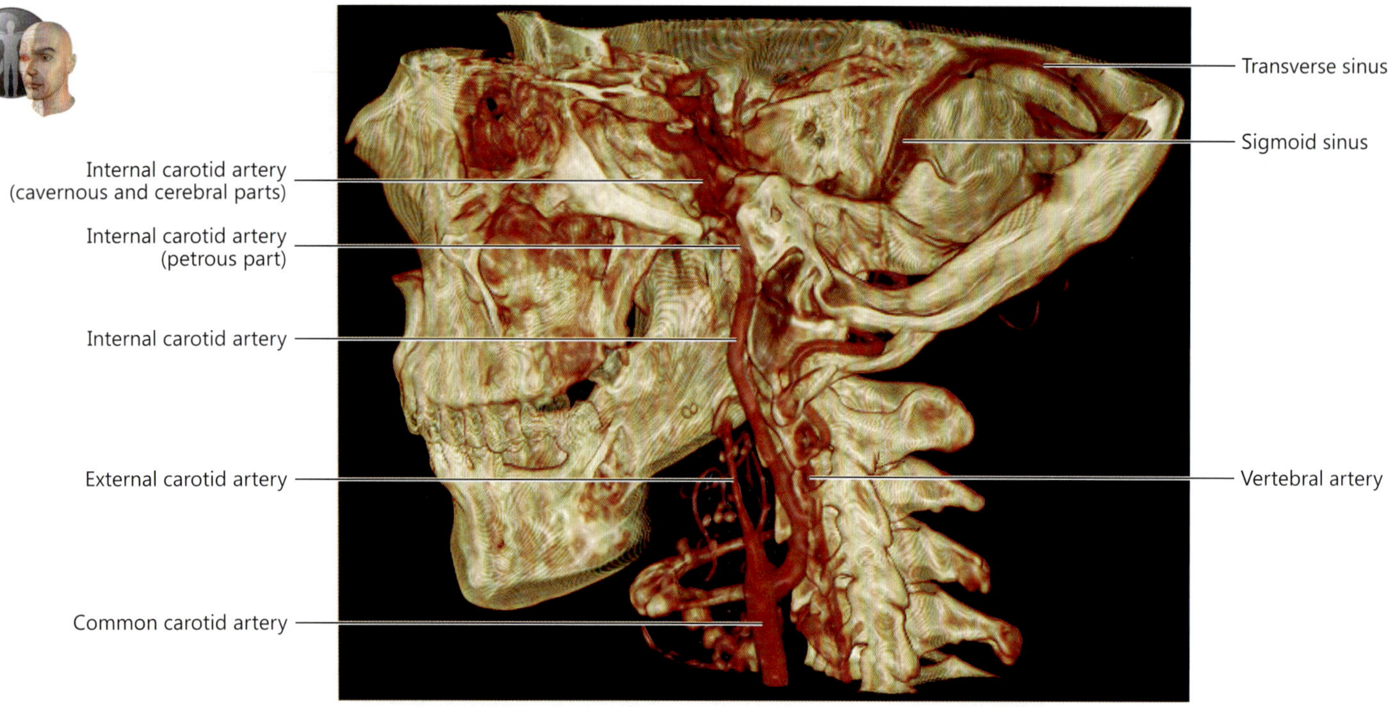

Three-dimensional image of a living human body, obtained by contrast-enhanced CT scan using a 3D volume rendering technique, showing the course of the **internal carotid artery**, in relation to the skeleton, from the bifurcation to the intracranial part.

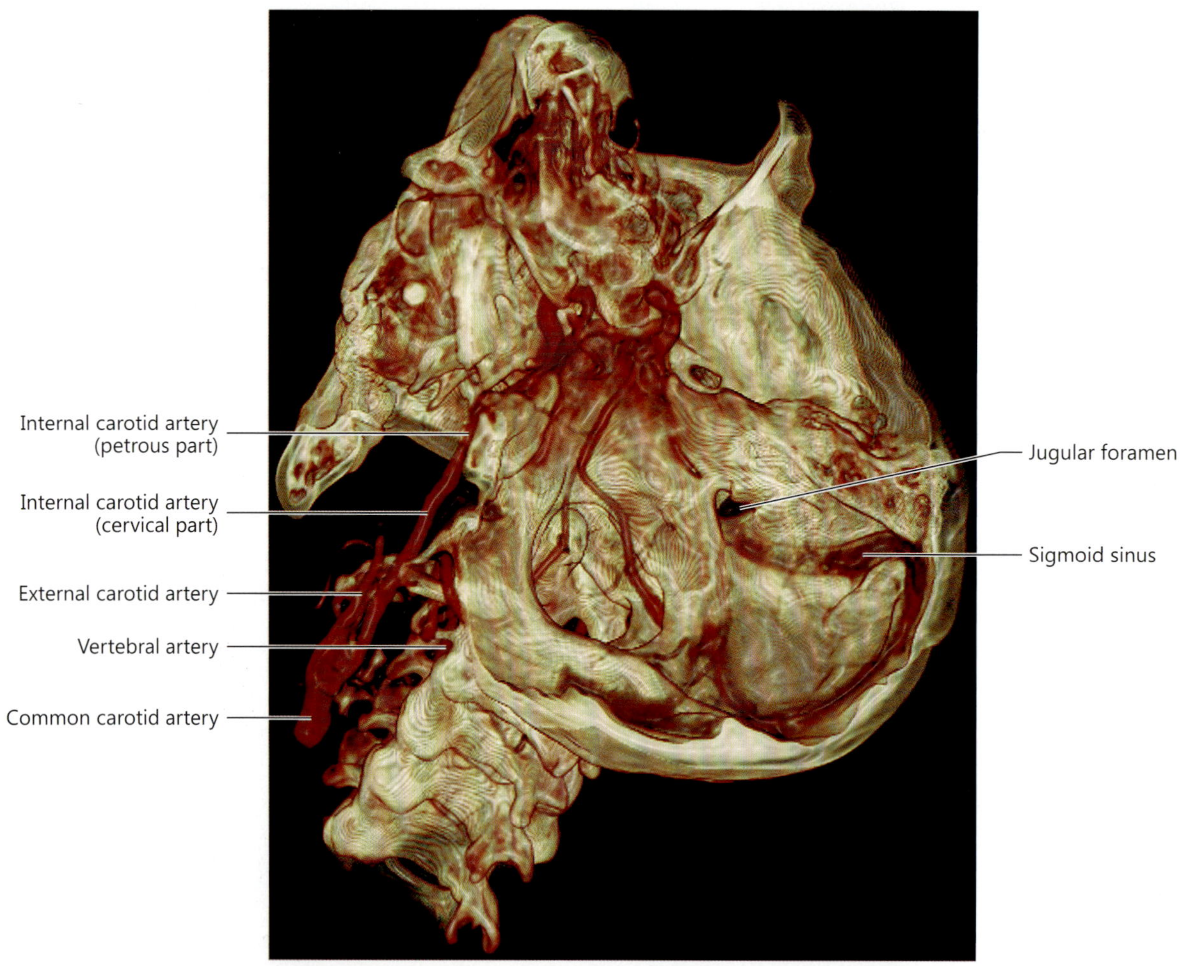

Three-dimensional image of a living human body, obtained by contrast-enhanced CT scan using a 3D volume rendering technique, showing the course of the **internal carotid artery**, in relation to the skeleton, from the bifurcation to the intracranial part, viewed from above and posterolaterally.

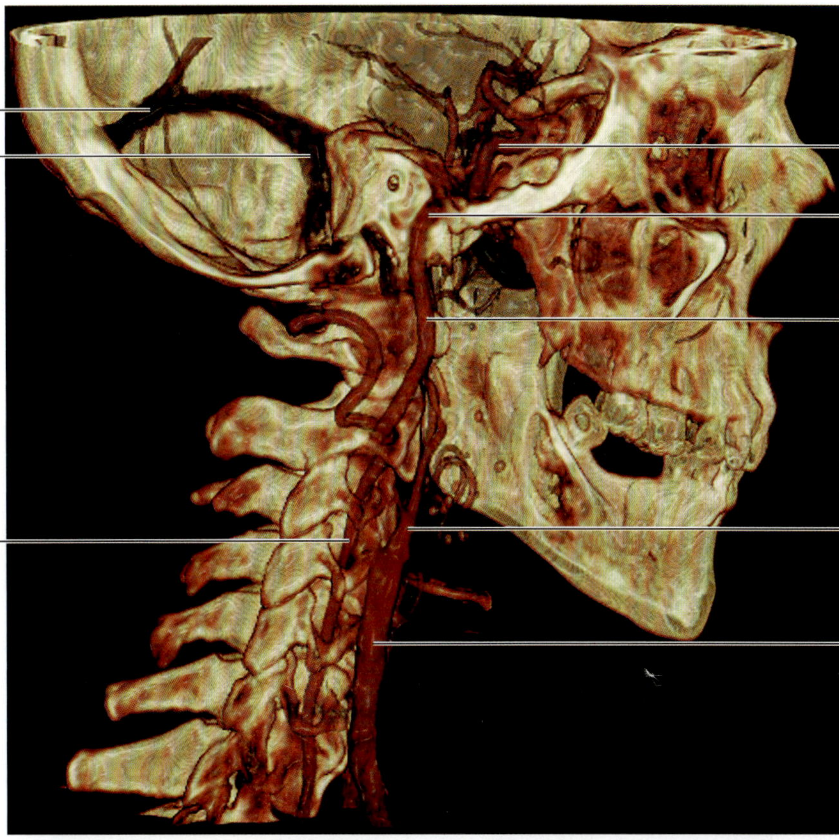

Three-dimensional image of a living human body, obtained by contrast-enhanced CT scan using a 3D volume rendering technique, showing the course of the **internal carotid artery**, in relation to the skeleton, from the point proximal to the entrance into the carotid canal to its end.

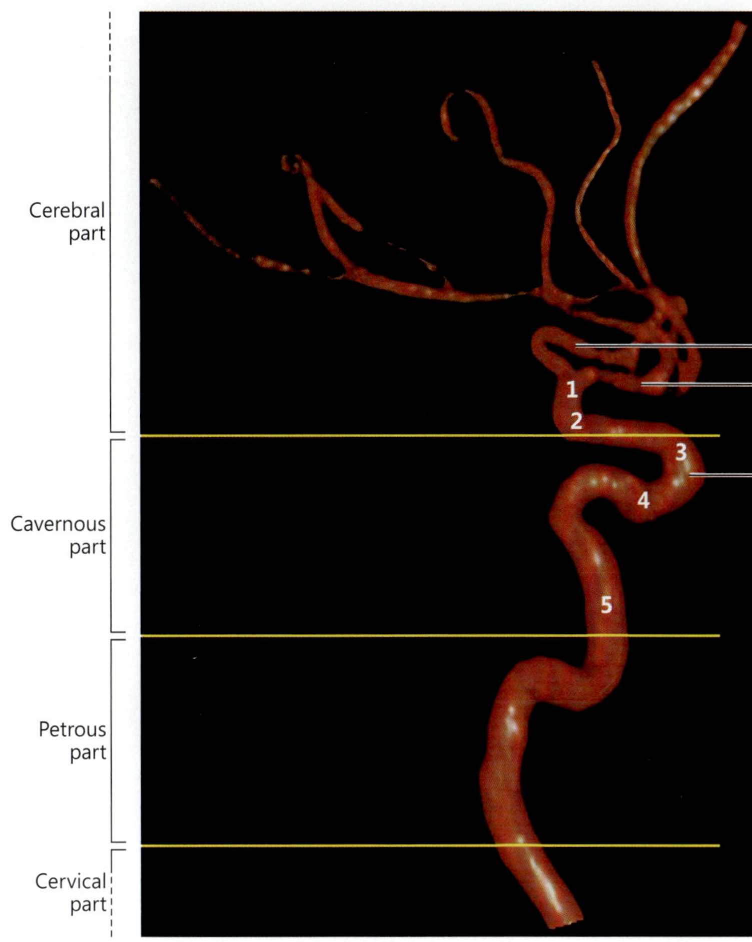

Three-dimensional image of a living human body, obtained by contrast-enhanced CT scan using a 3D volume rendering technique, showing the course of the **internal carotid artery**. The intracranial part subdivides into the cavernous part and cerebral part and, successively, the two parts further subdivide into five segments, according to Fisher's scheme:

1. communicating or distal supraclinoid tract
2. ophthalmic or proximal supraclinoid tract
3. clinoid tract
4. cavernous tract
5. precavernous tract

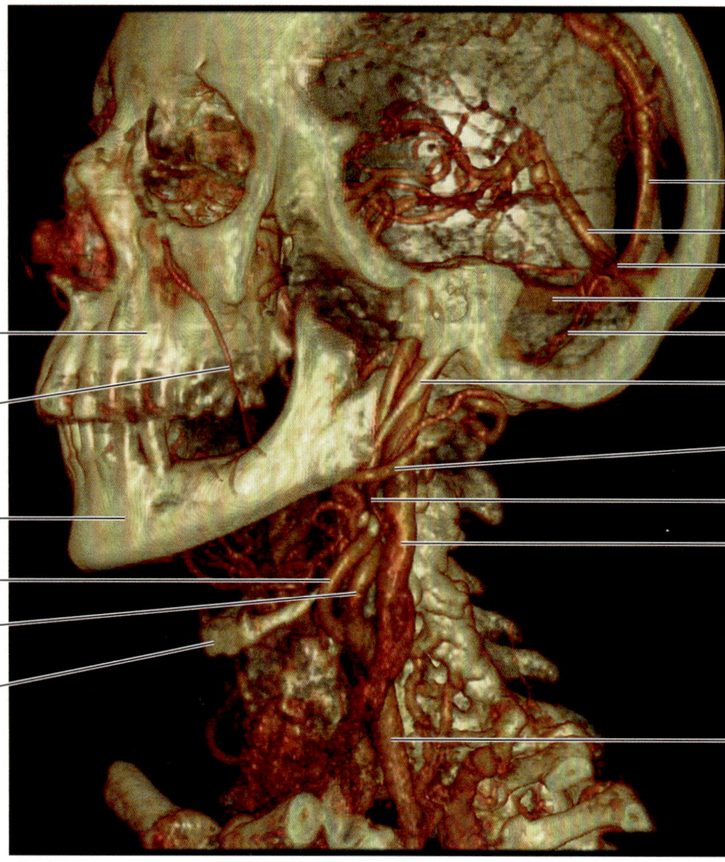

Three-dimensional image of a living human body, obtained by CT scan using a 3D volume rendering technique, showing the vessels passing through the neck in relation to the bone structures, in left anterolateral view. With the left cranial wall removed, one can observe the principal **venous sinuses** within the **cranial cavity**.

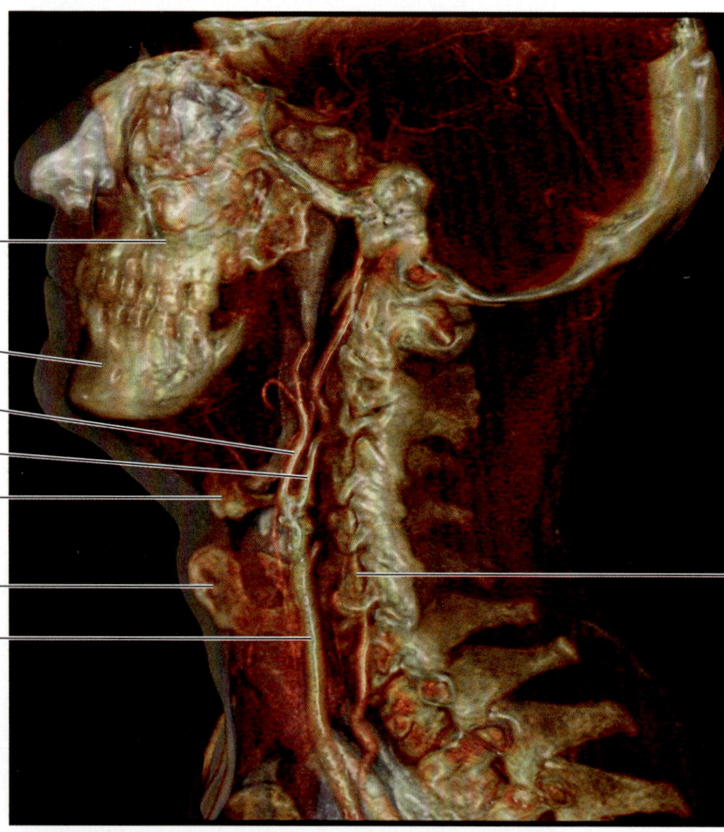

Three-dimensional image of a living human body, obtained by CT scan using a 3D volume rendering technique, showing the passage of the **vessels within the neck** in relation to the bone structures, in left lateral view.

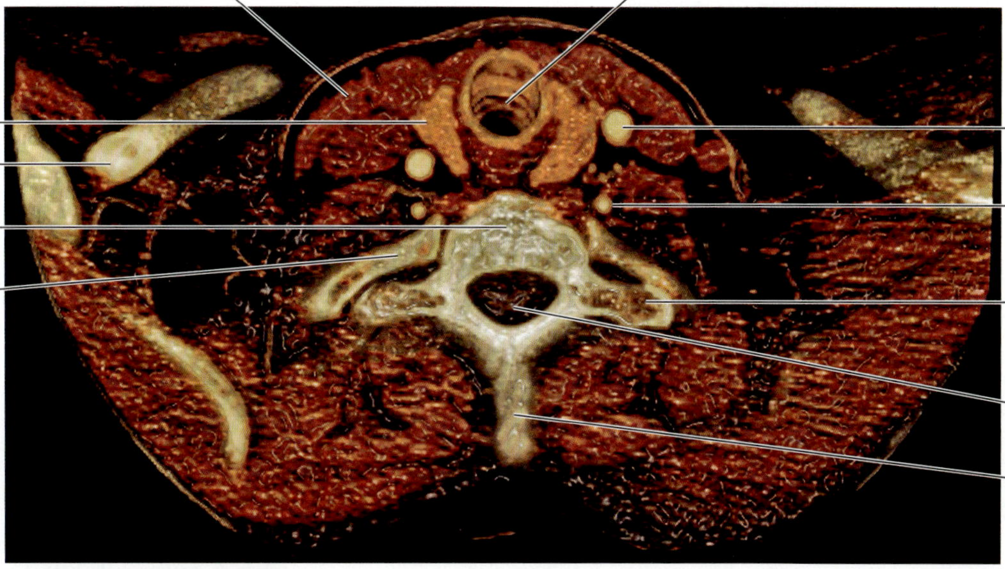

Three-dimensional image of a living human body, obtained by CT scan using a 3D volume rendering technique, showing a transverse section of the **neck** at the **level of the first thoracic vertebra**.

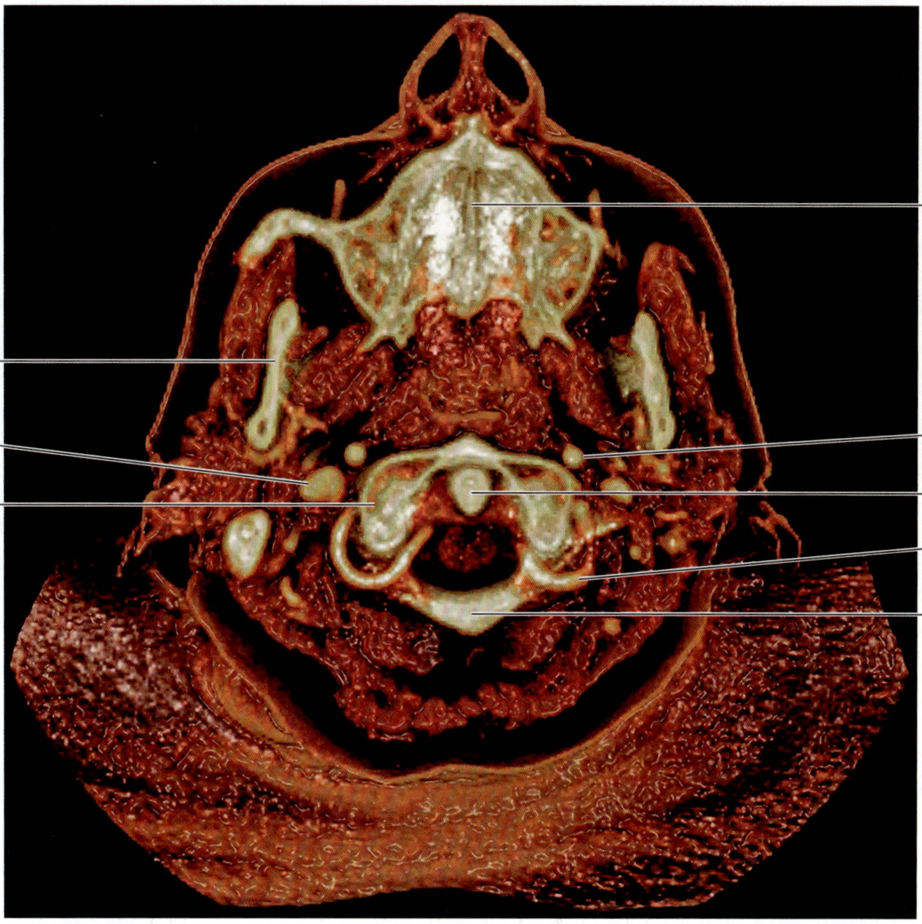

Three-dimensional image of a living human body, obtained by CT scan using a 3D volume rendering technique, showing a transverse section of the **neck** at the **level of the atlas-axis joint**.

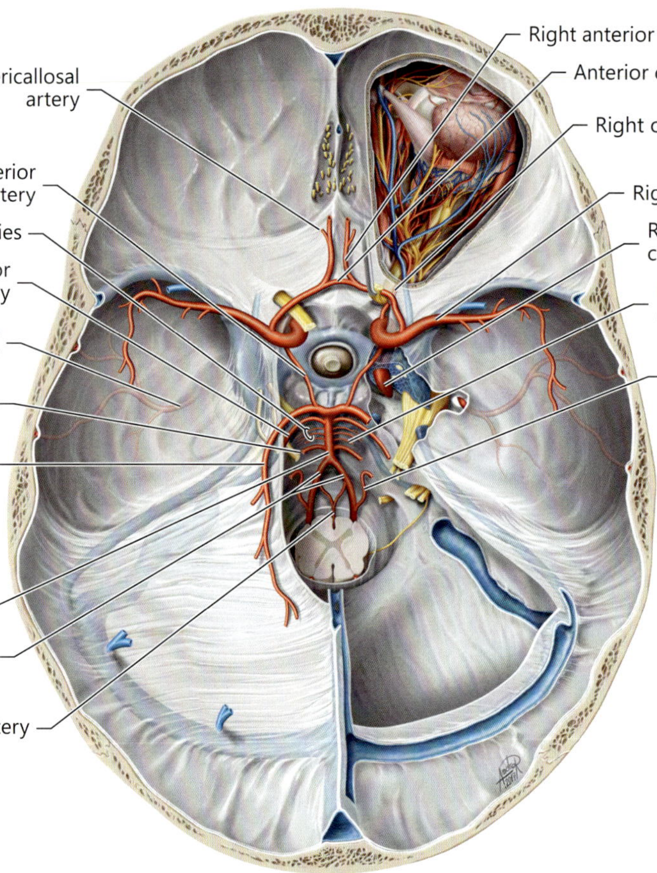

The **circle of Willis** (cerebral arterial circle) and intracranial branches of the **internal carotid artery**, **vertebral artery** and **basilar artery**.
Below: the circle of Willis is shown as it looks in a three-dimensional image of a living human body, obtained by CT scan using a 3D volume rendering technique.

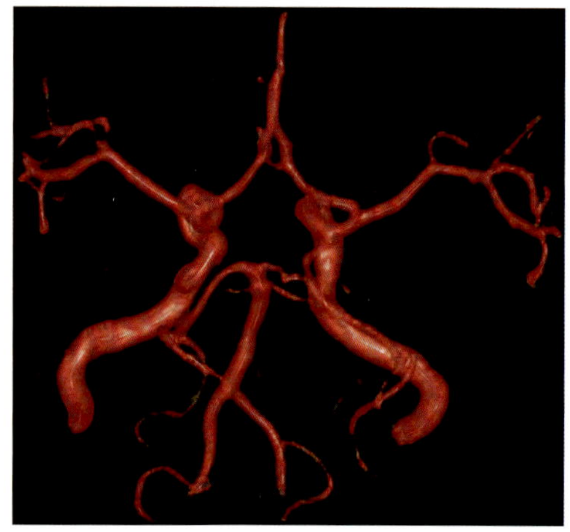

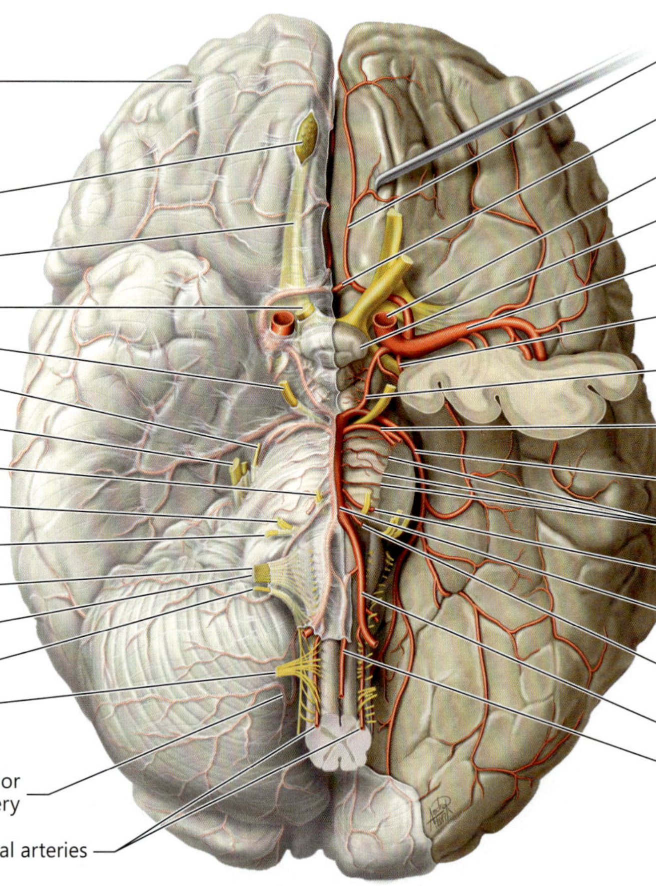

Arteries of the base of the brain: the left cerebellar hemisphere and part of the left temporal lobe have been removed to show the middle and posterior cerebral arteries. On the left side of the figure, the apparent origins of the cranial nerves are indicated.

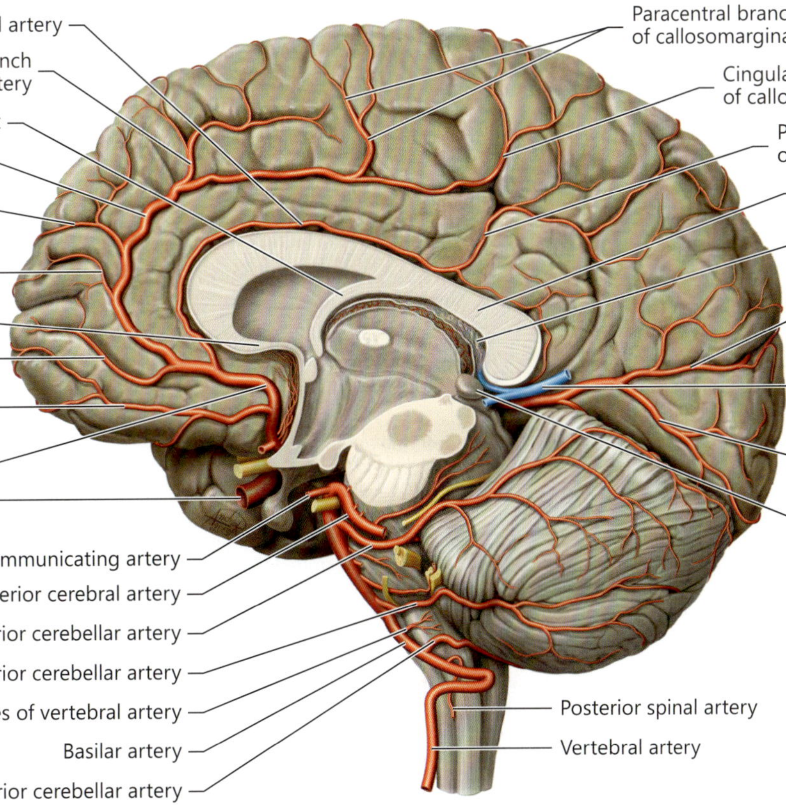

Anterior and **posterior cerebral arteries**. Medial view of the right cerebral hemisphere.

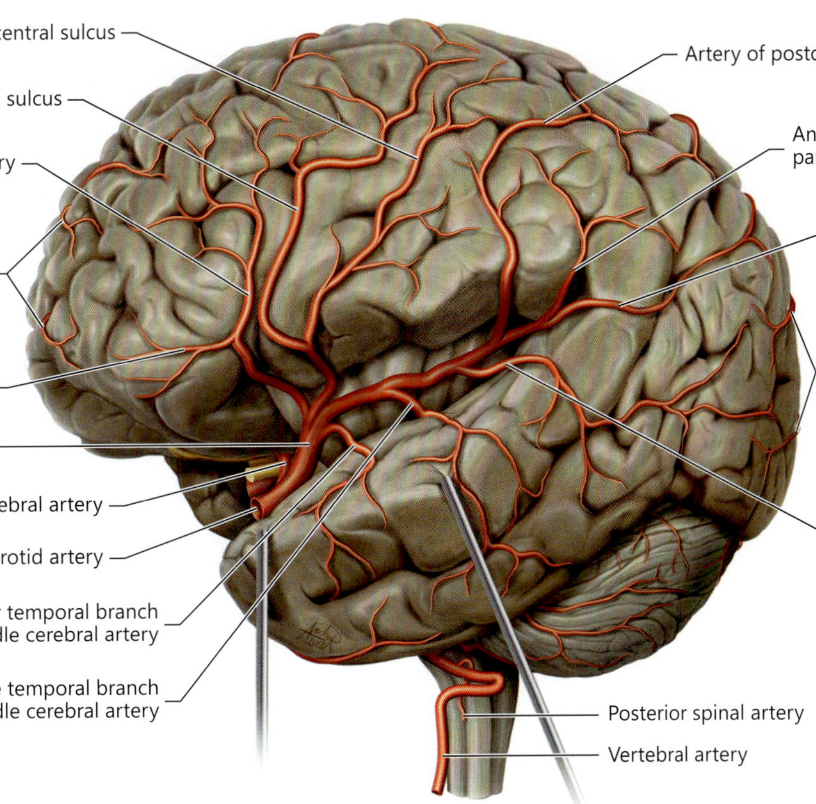

Middle cerebral artery. Lateral view of the left cerebral hemisphere. The lips of the lateral sulcus on the superolateral face of the hemisphere have been parted to show the insular part of the middle cerebral artery.

Summary table of the arteries of the head

ARTERY	ORIGIN	BRANCHES	TERRITORIES OF SUPPLY
angular	Facial		Ala of nose, lacrimal sac
anterior cerebral	Internal carotid (at the medial end of the lateral sulcus of telencephalon)	*Precommunicating part (A1 segment)*: anteromedial central arteries; anterior communicating artery; *postcommunicating part (A2 segment)*: distal medial striate, medial frontobasal (orbitofrontal), polar frontal, callosomarginal and pericallosal arteries	Hypothalamus, lamina terminalis, anterior perforated substance, anterior commissure, column of the fornix, caudate nucleus, putamen, pallidum, internal capsule, choroid plexuses, lateral ventricle, corpus striatum, corpus callosum, medial part of the frontal and parietal lobes, straight gyrus, olfactory bulb
anterior choroidal	Internal carotid (cerebral part)	Choroidal branches to the lateral ventricle, choroidal branches to the third ventricle, branches to the anterior perforated substance, to the optic chiasm, to the optic tract, to the lateral geniculate body, to the genu of the internal capsule, to the posterior limb of the internal capsule, to the retrolentiform limb of the internal capsule, to the globus pallidus, to the tail of the caudate nucleus, to the hippocampus, to the uncus, to the amygdaloid body, to the tuber cinereum, to the hypothalamic nuclei, to the thalamic nuclei, to the substantia nigra, to the red nucleus, to the crus cerebri	Choroid plexus of the lateral ventricle, optic tract, optic radiation, cerebral peduncle, hippocampus, fimbria of hippocampus, lateral geniculate body, caudate nucleus, red nucleus, pallidum, amygdaloid body, hypothalamus, tuber cinereum, substantia nigra, posterior limb of the internal capsule
anterior ciliary	Ophthalmic or lacrimal (muscular branches)		Conjunctiva, iris
anterior communicating	Anterior cerebral (anastomosis between the anterior cerebral arteries)	Anteromedial central arteries	Anterior perforated substance
anterior conjunctival	Ophthalmic (muscular branches or anterior ciliary arteries)		Conjunctiva
anterior deep temporal	Maxillary		Temporalis
anterior ethmoidal	Ophthalmic	Anterior meningeal, anterior septal, anterior lateral nasal	Anterior and middle ethmoidal cells, frontal sinus, dura mater, nasal cavity
anterior inferior cerebellar	Basilar	Labyrinthine artery	Anterolateral region of the posterior surface of the hemisphere of cerebellum, choroid plexus of the fourth ventricle
anterior parietal	Middle cerebral (superior terminal branches)		Parietal lobe
anterior perforating	Precommunicating part of the anterior cerebral artery (anteromedial central branches)		Anterior perforated substance
anterior spinal	Vertebral (intracranial part)		Anterior two-thirds of the spinal cord
anterior superior alveolar (anterior dental)	Infraorbital		Incisor and canine teeth of the maxillary dental arcade, mucosa of the maxillary sinus
anterior temporal	Middle cerebral (sphenoid part)		Temporal gyri
anterior tympanic	Maxillary		Tympanic membrane, tympanic cavity, auditory ossicles
anterolateral central	Middle cerebral (sphenoid part)	Proximal and distal lateral striate arteries	Corpus striatum, lentiform nucleus
anteromedial central	Anterior cerebral (precommunicating part)	Proximal medial striate arteries, supraoptic artery, anterior perforating arteries, preoptic arteries	Anteromedial part of the corpus striatum and part of the thalamus
	Anterior communicating	Suprachiasmatic, median commissural and median callosal arteries	Anteromedial part of the corpus striatum and part of the thalamus

continued

Summary table of the arteries of the head			*(continued)*
ARTERY	***ORIGIN***	***BRANCHES***	***TERRITORIES OF SUPPLY***
ascending palatine	Facial		Soft palate, palatine glands, pharyngotympanic tube
ascending pharyngeal	External carotid	Posterior meningeal artery; pharyngeal branches; inferior tympanic artery	Wall of the pharynx, soft palate, tonsils, ear, meninges, posterior cervical and head muscles
basilar	From the union of the two vertebral arteries	Anterior inferior cerebellar artery, pontine arteries, mesencephalic arteries, superior cerebellar artery, posterior cerebral artery	Internal ear, pons, cerebellum, mesencephalon, thalamus, hypothalamus, epiphysis, third ventricle, cerebral ventricles, cortex of the temporal and occipital lobes
buccal (buccinator)	Maxillary		Buccinator, mucosa of the maxillary gingivae, mucosa and skin of the cheeks
callosomarginal	Anterior cerebral (postcommunicating part)	Anteromedial frontal, intermediomedial frontal, posteromedial frontal, cingular, paracentral branches	Paracentral lobule, parts of the cingulate gyrus
caroticotympanic	Internal carotid (petrous part)		Tympanic cavity
central retinal	Ophthalmic	Extraocular part; intraocular part	Retina
collicular (quadrigeminal)	Posterior cerebral (precommunicating part)		Tectal plate
deep auricular	Maxillary		Skin of the external acoustic meatus, external surface of the tympanic membrane, temporomandibular joint
deep lingual (or ranine)	Lingual (terminal part)		Mucosa and intrinsic muscles of the tongue
descending palatine	Maxillary	Greater palatine artery and lesser palatine arteries; pharyngeal branch	Soft palate, hard palate, palatine tonsil, gingivae
distal medial striate	Anterior cerebral (postcommunicating part)		Anterior part of the caudate nucleus, putamen, anterior limb of the internal capsule
dorsal lingual	Lingual		Mucosa of the posterior part of the tongue; palatoglossal arch, lingual tonsil, epiglottis
dorsal nasal (external nasal)	Ophthalmic		Skin of the nose, lacrimal sac
episcleral	Ophthalmic (muscular branches or anterior ciliary arteries)		Iris, ciliary body
external carotid	Common carotid	*Anterior tract*: superior thyroid, lingual and facial arteries; *posterior tract*: occipital and posterior auricular arteries; *medial tract*: ascending pharyngeal artery; *terminal tract*: superficial temporal and maxillary (or internal maxillary) arteries	Anterior parts of the face and neck and lateral part of the head, walls of the cranial cavity, dura mater, posterior part of the scalp
facial (external maxillary)	External carotid	*Cervical part*: ascending palatine artery, tonsillar branch; glandular branches; submental artery; *facial part*: inferior and superior labial branches	Soft palate, palatine tonsil, submandibular gland and labial glands, skin and muscles of the chin, of the lips and external nose, ala and dorsum of the nose
greater palatine	Descending palatine		Hard palate, gingivae, palatine glands
hyaloid (generally disappears in the ninth month of intrauterine life)	Central retinal		Vitreous body, lens
inferior alveolar (inferior dental or mandibular)	Maxillary	Dental, peridental, mental, mylohyoid	Mandible, mandibular dental arcade, gingiva, mucous membrane of the mouth, of the lower lip and cheek, mylohyoid
inferior hypophysial	Internal carotid (cavernous part)		Neurohypophysis
inferior labial	Facial		Labial glands, mucosa and muscles of the lower lip

continued

Summary table of the arteries of the head *(continued)*

ARTERY	*ORIGIN*	*BRANCHES*	*TERRITORIES OF SUPPLY*
inferior tympanic	Ascending pharyngeal		Medial wall of the tympanic cavity
infraorbital	Maxillary	Anterior superior alveolar arteries; dental branches, peridental branches	Orbit, maxilla, maxillary sinus, maxillary dental arcade, inferior eyelid, extraocular muscles, cheeks, ala of nose
insular	Middle cerebral (insular part)		Insula
internal carotid	Common carotid	*Cervical part*: carotid sinus; *petrous part*: caroticotympanic arteries, artery of the pterygoid canal (vidian artery); *cavernous part*: tentorial basal, tentorial marginal, meningeal, cavernous, inferior hypophysial artery; branches to the trigeminal ganglion, branches to nerves of the internal carotid artery; *cerebral part*: ophthalmic, superior hypophysial, anterior cerebral, middle cerebral, posterior communicating, anterior choroidal and uncal arteries; clivus branches, meningeal branch; carotid syphon	Brain, pituitary gland, orbit, nasal cavity, trigeminal ganglion, meninges, middle ear
labyrinthine (internal auditory)	Anterior inferior cerebellar (or from the basilar artery)		Internal ear
lacrimal	Ophthalmic (near the optic canal)	Lateral palpebral arteries; anastomotic branch with the middle meningeal artery	Lacrimal gland, conjunctiva, superior rectus and lateral rectus (extraocular muscles), cheeks, ciliary processes, eyelids
lateral frontobasal (orbitofrontal)	Middle cerebral (superior terminal branches)		Lateral half of the inferior surface of the frontal lobe
lateral nasal (of the ala of nose)	Facial		Ala of nose
lateral occipital (P3 segment of posterior cerebral artery)	Posterior cerebral	Anterior temporal, intermediate (middle) temporal, posterior temporal	Anterior, medial, intermediate and posterior parts of the temporal lobe
lateral palpebral	Lacrimal		Eyelids, conjunctiva
lesser palatine	Descending palatine		Soft palate, palatine tonsil
lingual	External carotid	Suprahyoid branch; dorsal lingual branches; sublingual and deep lingual arteries	Muscles and mucous membrane of the tongue, sublingual gland, gingivae, lingual and palatine tonsils, epiglottis, suprahyoid muscles
long posterior ciliary (2 in number)	Ophthalmic		Iris, ciliary body
mammillary	Posterior communicating		Mammillary bodies
masseteric	Maxillary (or internal maxillary)		Masseter
maxillary (internal maxillary or deep facial)	External carotid	*Mandibular part*: deep auricular, anterior tympanic, inferior alveolar and middle meningeal arteries; *pterygoid part*: pterygomeningeal, masseteric, anterior deep temporal, posterior deep temporal and buccal arteries; *pterygopalatine part*: posterior superior alveolar artery, infraorbital artery, descending palatine artery, artery of pterygoid canal, sphenopalatine artery	Tympanic cavity, external acoustic meatus, dental arcades, upper lip, chin, dura mater of the middle cranial fossa, of the walls and the calvaria, trigeminal ganglion, temporalis, masseter, buccinator, extraocular muscles, lacrimal sac, lacrimal gland, palatine tonsil, palate, nasopharynx, pharyngotympanic tube, nasal cavity and paranasal sinuses
medial frontobasal (orbitofrontal)	Anterior cerebral (postcommunicating part)		Medial half of the inferior surface of the frontal lobe
medial occipital (P4 segment of posterior cerebral artery)	Posterior cerebral	Dorsal branch to the corpus callosum, parietal, parieto-occipital, calcarine, occipitotemporal	Dorsum of the corpus callosum, precuneus, cuneus, lingual gyrus, posterior part of the lateral surface of the occipital lobe
medial palpebral	Ophthalmic (near the trochlea of the superior oblique)	Posterior conjunctival arteries; inferior palpebral arch, superior palpebral arch	Eyelids, conjunctiva, nasolacrimal duct

continued

Summary table of the arteries of the head			(continued)
ARTERY	**ORIGIN**	**BRANCHES**	**TERRITORIES OF SUPPLY**
median callosal	Anterior communicating (anteromedial central branches)		Lamina terminalis and rostrum of corpus callosum
median commissural	Anterior communicating (anteromedial central branches)		Supraoptic commissure and optic chiasm
mesencephalic	Basilar		Area of the mesencephalon located medially to the reticular part of the substantia nigra
middle cerebral	Internal carotid	*Sphenoid part (horizontal part or M1 segment)*: anterolateral central arteries; uncal, polar temporal and anterior temporal arteries; *insular part (M2 segment)*: insular arteries; *inferior terminal branches (inferior cortical or M2 segment)*: anterior temporal, intermediate temporal, posterior temporal, temporo-occipital, branch to the angular gyrus; *superior terminal branches (superior cortical or M2 segment)*: lateral frontobasal (orbitofrontal) artery, prefrontal artery, artery of precentral sulcus, artery of central sulcus, artery of postcentral sulcus, anterior parietal artery, posterior parietal artery	Lentiform nucleus, internal capsule, caudate nucleus, corpus striatum, insula, frontal lobe, parietal lobe, temporal lobe, precentral gyrus, postcentral gyrus, inferior frontal gyrus, superior temporal gyrus, middle temporal gyrus, supramarginal gyrus and angular gyrus
middle meningeal (sphenospinous or pterygomeningeal)	Maxillary (or internal maxillary)	Accessory, frontal, orbital, parietal, petrosal; superior tympanic artery; anastomotic branch with the lacrimal artery	Cranium, dura mater, tensor tympani, trigeminal ganglion, orbit
middle temporal	Superficial temporal (immediately above the zygomatic arch)		Temporalis
muscular	Ophthalmic	Anterior ciliary, anterior conjunctival and episcleral arteries	Extraocular muscles
occipital	External carotid	Mastoid, auricular, sternocleidomastoid, occipital, meningeal, descending	Lateral and posterior cervical muscles, auricle, mastoid cells, dura mater of the posterior cranial fossa, diploë, muscles and skin of the occipital region, scalp
of central sulcus	Middle cerebral (superior terminal branches)		Central sulcus
of postcentral sulcus	Middle cerebral (superior terminal branches)		Postcentral gyrus
of precentral sulcus	Middle cerebral (superior terminal branches)		Precentral gyrus
of pterygoid canal (vidian)	Maxillary Internal carotid (petrous part)	Pharyngeal	Sphenoidal sinus Mucosa of the superior part of the nasopharynx, pharyngotympanic tube and tympanic cavity
of tuber cinereum	Posterior communicating	Medial, lateral	Tuber cinereum
ophthalmic	Internal carotid	*Orbital part*: lacrimal artery; recurrent meningeal; supraorbital, posterior ethmoidal, anterior ethmoidal, supratrochlear, medial palpebral and dorsal nasal arteries; *ocular part*: central retinal, short posterior ciliary, long posterior ciliary and muscular arteries	Orbital cavity, eyeball, extraocular muscles, eyelids, dura mater of the anterior cranial fossa, vault and lateral walls of the nasal cavities
pericallosal	Anterior cerebral (postcommunicating part)	Precuneal, parieto-occipital	Corpus callosum, precuneus, medial and superolateral surfaces of the posterior parietal lobe up to the paracentral lobule
polar frontal	Anterior cerebral (postcommunicating part)		Frontal lobe
polar temporal	Middle cerebral (sphenoid part)		Temporal lobe
pontine	Basilar	Medial, lateral	Pons and adjacent areas

continued

Summary table of the arteries of the head *(continued)*

ARTERY	*ORIGIN*	*BRANCHES*	*TERRITORIES OF SUPPLY*
posterior auricular	External carotid	Stylomastoid, posterior tympanic, auricular and occipital arteries; parotid branch	Middle ear, mastoid cells, auricle, digastric, stylohyoid, sternocleidomastoid, skin of the occipital region, parotid gland
posterior cerebral	Terminal bifurcation of the basilar artery	*Precommunicating part (P1 segment)*: posteromedial central, short circumferential arteries; thalamoperforating and collicular arteries; *postcommunicating part (P2 segment)*: posterolateral central; thalamogeniculate artery; posterior medial choroidal, posterior lateral choroidal, peduncular; *lateral occipital (P3 segment)*: anterior temporal, intermediate temporal, posterior temporal; *medial occipital (P4 segment)*: dorsal branch to the corpus callosum, parietal, parieto-occipital, calcarine, occipitotemporal	Thalamus, walls of third ventricle, hypothalamus, globus pallidus, cerebral peduncle, mesencephalon, tectal plate, epiphysis, medial and lateral geniculate bodies, uncus, parahippocampal gyrus, medial occipitotemporal gyrus, lateral occipitotemporal gyrus, temporal and occipital lobes, choroid plexus of the lateral ventricle and choroid plexus of the third ventricle
posterior communicating	Internal carotid (cerebral part); links the internal carotid artery with the posterior cerebral artery	Posteromedial central arteries; chiasmatic; arteries of tuber cinereum, thalamotuberal artery; hypothalamic; mammillary arteries; branch to the oculomotor nerve	Base of the telencephalon between the infundibulum and optic tract, optic chiasm, hippocampus, cerebral peduncle, internal capsule, anterior third of the thalamus, third ventricle
posterior conjunctival	Medial palpebral arteries		Conjunctiva
posterior deep temporal	Maxillary	Pterygoid	Temporalis, medial pterygoid and lateral pterygoid
posterior ethmoidal	Ophthalmic		Posterior ethmoidal cells, dura mater, nasal cavity
posterior inferior cerebellar	Vertebral (intracranial part) or basilar	Posterior spinal artery (can originate from the vertebral artery); cerebellar tonsillar branch, choroidal branch to the fourth ventricle	Hemisphere of cerebellum [H II - H X], vermis of cerebellum [I-X], choroid plexus of the fourth ventricle
posterior lateral nasal	Sphenopalatine		Posterior part of the nasal conchae and lateral wall of the nose
posterior meningeal	Ascending pharyngeal		Bones and dura mater of the posterior cranial fossa
posterior parietal	Middle cerebral (superior terminal branches)		Parietal lobe
posterior spinal	Posterior inferior cerebellar or vertebral (intracranial part)		Myelencephalon, spinal cord, pia mater
posterior superior alveolar (posterior dental)	Maxillary	Dental, peridental	Premolar and molar teeth of the maxillary dental arcade, mucosa of the maxillary sinus, gingivae
posterior tympanic	Posterior auricular	Mastoid, stapedial branch	Tympanic cavity, posterior part of the tympanic membrane
posterolateral central	Posterior cerebral (postcommunicating part)		Posterolateral part of the mesencephalon
posteromedial central	Posterior communicating Posterior cerebral (precommunicating part)	Anterior and posterior branches Anterior and posterior branches	Posteromedial part of the mesencephalon Posteromedial part of the mesencephalon
prefrontal	Middle cerebral (superior terminal branches)		Frontal lobe
preoptic	Precommunicating part of the anterior cerebral artery (anteromedial central branches)		Preoptic area
proximal medial striate	Precommunicating part of the anterior cerebral artery (anteromedial central branches)		Inferior part of the frontal lobe, thalamus, corpus striatum
pterygomeningeal	Maxillary		Trigeminal ganglion, dura mater, internal table of the calvaria
short circumferential	Posterior cerebral (precommunicating part)		Posterior part of the thalamus

continued

Summary table of the arteries of the head *(continued)*

ARTERY	*ORIGIN*	*BRANCHES*	*TERRITORIES OF SUPPLY*
short posterior ciliary (from 6 to 12 in number)	Ophthalmic or one of its branches		Choroid and ciliary processes of the eyeball
sphenopalatine (nasopalatine)	Maxillary	Posterior lateral nasal arteries; posterior septal branches	Frontal sinus, maxillary sinus, sphenoidal sinus, ethmoidal cells, nasal septum
stylomastoid	Posterior auricular		Tympanic cavity, stapes, stapedius, mastoid cells, semicircular canals
sublingual	Lingual		Sublingual gland, mylohyoid, geniohyoid and genioglossus, mucous membrane of the mouth and of the gingivae
submental	Facial		Mylohyoid, digastric and platysma, sublingual gland, skin of the chin, lips
superficial temporal	External carotid	Parotid; transverse facial artery; anterior auricular; zygomatico-orbital and middle temporal arteries; frontal, parietal	Masseter and temporalis, frontal belly of the occipitofrontalis, orbicularis oculi, external acoustic meatus, auricle, skin of the face, scalp, parotid gland, temporomandibular joint
superior cerebellar	Basilar (near its termination)	Medial: superior vermian, lateral	Superior surface of cerebellum, vermis of cerebellum [I-X], pons, epiphysis, superior medullary velum, choroid membrane of the third ventricle
superior hypophysial	Internal carotid (cerebral part)		Pars tuberalis of the adenohypophysis and infundibulum of the neurohypophysis, median eminence
superior labial	Facial	Nasal septal branch	Upper lip, nasal septum, ala of nose
superior tympanic	Middle meningeal		Tympanic cavity, tensor tympani
suprachiasmatic	Anterior communicating (anteromedial central branches)		Supraoptic recess and hypothalamic area
supraoptic	Precommunicating part of the anterior cerebral artery (anteromedial central branches)		Superior part of the optic nerve and of the optic chiasm
supraorbital	Ophthalmic (where it crosses the optic nerve)	Diploic	Skin, muscles and pericranium of the forehead, superior rectus of the eyeball, levator palpebrae, diploë
supratrochlear (frontal)	Ophthalmic		Skin, muscles and pericranium of the forehead
thalamogeniculate	Posterior cerebral (postcommunicating part)		Thalamus, geniculate bodies
thalamoperforating	Posterior cerebral (precommunicating part)		Thalamic nuclei
thalamotuberal	Posterior communicating		Thalamus and adjacent structures
transverse facial	Superficial temporal (in the tract that runs in the parotid gland)		Parotid gland and parotid duct, masseter, skin of the face
uncal	Internal carotid (cerebral part) or, sometimes, middle cerebral (sphenoid part)		Uncus
vertebral	Subclavian	*Intracranial part*: meningeal; posterior inferior cerebellar and anterior spinal arteries; medial medullary, lateral medullary	Bodies of the vertebrae, deep muscles of the neck, falx cerebelli, spinal cord, cerebellum, brainstem
zygomatico-orbital	Superficial temporal (occasionally middle temporal)		Lateral part of the orbit, orbicularis oculi

Arteries of the brain
- anterior choroidal
- anterior cerebral
- middle cerebral
- posterior communicating
- cerebral arterial circle
- posterior cerebral

Cerebral arterial circle
– internal carotid
– – anterior cerebral
– – – anterior communicating
– – middle cerebral
– – posterior communicating
– basilar
– – posterior cerebral

Summary table of the arteries of the neck			
ARTERY	*ORIGIN*	*BRANCHES*	*TERRITORIES OF SUPPLY*
anterior spinal	Vertebral		Anterior two-thirds of the spinal cord
ascending cervical	Thyrocervical trunk (or superior thyroid artery)	Spinal	Sternocleidomastoid, omohyoid, trapezius, longus capitis, phrenic nerve, spinal cord
ascending palatine	Facial		Muscles and mucosa of the soft palate
ascending pharyngeal (pharyngomeningeal)	External carotid	Pharyngeal branches; inferior tympanic artery, posterior meningeal artery	Pharynx, soft palate, longus capitis and longus colli, sympathetic trunk, palatine tonsil, pharyngotympanic tube, tympanic cavity, dura mater of the cerebellar fossa
brachiocephalic trunk	Arch of aorta	Thyroid ima artery (inconstant)	Head and neck, upper limb, superior part of the thorax
common carotid	*To the right*: bifurcation of the brachiocephalic trunk; *to the left*: most elevated part of the arch of aorta	External carotid and internal carotid arteries	Head and neck
costocervical trunk	Subclavian	Supreme intercostal and deep cervical arteries	First two intercostal spaces, semispinalis capitis and semispinalis cervicis, spinal cord
cricothyroid	Superior thyroid		Median cricothyroid ligament
deep cervical	Costocervical trunk		Spinal cord, semispinalis capitis and semispinalis cervicis
descending palatine	Maxillary	Greater palatine artery, lesser palatine arteries; pharyngeal branch	Soft palate, palatine tonsil
– pharyngeal branch	Descending palatine		Mucosa of the vault of the nasal cavities and pharynx, sphenoidal sinus, pharyngotympanic tube
dorsal scapular (deep branch)	Trasversa del collo (o tronco tireocervicale)		Muscles of the shoulder and the back
esophageal (esophageal branches, from 4 to 5 in number)	Thoracic aorta; inferior thyroid artery; left gastric artery		Esophagus
external carotid	Common carotid	*Anterior tract*: superior thyroid artery, lingual artery, facial artery; *posterior tract*: occipital artery, posterior auricular artery; *medial tract*: ascending pharyngeal artery; *terminal tract*: superficial temporal artery, maxillary artery	Anterior part of the face and neck, lateral part of the head, walls of the cranial cavity, dura mater, posterior part of the scalp
inferior laryngeal	Inferior thyroid		Muscles and mucosa of the larynx
inferior thyroid	Thyrocervical trunk	Inferior laryngeal artery; tracheal, esophageal, pharyngeal and glandular branches	Infrahyoid muscles, longus colli, scalenus anterior and inferior constrictor of pharynx, cervical part of the esophagus, muscles and mucosa of the larynx, inferior part of the pharynx, trachea, posteroinferior part of the thyroid gland
infrahyoid	Superior thyroid		Thyrohyoid
internal carotid	Common carotid	*Cervical part*: carotid sinus; *petrous part*: caroticotympanic arteries, artery of the pterygoid canal; *cavernous part*: inferior hypophysial artery; tentorial basal, tentorial marginal, meningeal, cavernous branches, branch to the trigeminal ganglion, branches to nerves of the internal carotid artery; *cerebral part*: ophthalmic, superior hypophysial, posterior communicating, anterior choroidal and uncal arteries; clivus branches, meningeal branch; anterior cerebral and middle cerebral arteries	Middle ear, orbital cavity, nasal cavity, brain, pituitary gland, trigeminal ganglion, meninges

continued

Summary table of the arteries of the neck *(continued)*

ARTERY	ORIGIN	BRANCHES	TERRITORIES OF SUPPLY
internal thoracic (internal mammary)	First part of the subclavian artery	Musculophrenic, superior epigastric and pericardiacophrenic arteries; mediastinal, thymic, bronchial, tracheal, sternal, perforating, lateral costal, anterior intercostal	Thoracic wall (the internal thoracic artery is listed in this table as it begins in the neck, but it belongs to the thorax in terms of the branches it gives rise to and its area of supply)
mylohyoid	Inferior alveolar		Mylohyoid
occipital	External carotid	Mastoid, sternocleidomastoid, auricular, meningeal, descending, occipital	Dura mater, diploë, mastoid cells, muscles of neck and scalp
posterior spinal	Posterior inferior cerebellar (or vertebral)		Myelencephalon, spinal cord, pia mater
sternocleidomastoid	Superior thyroid		Sternocleidomastoid
subclavian	*To the right*: brachiocephalic trunk; *to the left*: arch of aorta	Vertebral artery; thyrocervical trunk; internal thoracic artery; costocervical trunk; becomes the axillary artery in correspondence to the external margin of the first rib	Same territory of supply as the vertebral artery, anterior and superior thoracic wall, upper limb
submental	Facial		Skin and muscles of the chin and the lower lip
superficial cervical	Transverse cervical (or thyrocervical trunk)	Ascending, descending	Trapezius
superior laryngeal	Superior thyroid (or external carotid)		Muscles, mucosa and cartilages of the larynx
superior thyroid	External carotid	Infrahyoid arteries, sternocleidomastoid, superior laryngeal and cricothyroid arteries; anterior, posterior and lateral glandular branches	Thyroid gland, infrahyoid muscles and sternocleidomastoid, muscles and mucosa of the larynx
suprahyoid	Lingual		Genioglossus and geniohyoid
suprascapular (transverse scapular)	Thyrocervical	Acromial	Clavicle, scapula, sternocleidomastoid, subclavius, supraspinatus and subscapularis, acromioclavicular and glenohumeral joints, suprascapular region, skin over the acromion
supreme intercostal (at its origin from the costocervical trunk)	Costocervical trunk	First and second posterior intercostal arteries	Thoracic wall, first and second intercostal spaces
thyrocervical trunk	First part of the subclavian artery	Inferior thyroid, ascending cervical, suprascapular, transverse cervical and dorsal scapular arteries	Same areas of supply as the inferior thyroid, ascending cervical, suprascapular and transverse cervical arteries
thyroid ima (inconstant)	Arch of aorta or brachiocephalic trunk		Thyroid gland, thymus
tonsillar	Facial or ascending palatine		Pharyngeal tonsil and posterior part of the tongue
transverse cervical	Thyrocervical trunk (or from the third part of the subclavian artery)	Superficial (superficial cervical artery), deep (dorsal scapular artery)	Posterior cervical, shoulder and back muscles
vertebral (prevertebral, cervical and atlantic part)	Subclavian	Spinal (radicular and segmental medullary artery) and muscular branches, meningeal, medial and lateral medullary branches; posterior inferior cerebellar artery (cerebellar tonsillar branch and choroidal branch to the fourth ventricle; posterior spinal artery); anterior spinal artery	Semispinalis capitis, suboccipital muscles, prevertebral muscles and muscles of back proper, vertebral canal, meninges and spinal cord of the cervical tract, myelencephalon, cerebellum, dura mater of the cerebellar fossa, pons, mesencephalon, thalamus, hypothalamus, third ventricle, temporal and occipital lobes, internal ear
– muscular branches	Vertebral		Prevertebral muscles and muscles of back proper
– spinal branches (spinal or vertebromedullary arteries)	Vertebral	Radicular, segmental medullary	Vertebral canal, meninges and spinal cord of the cervical tract

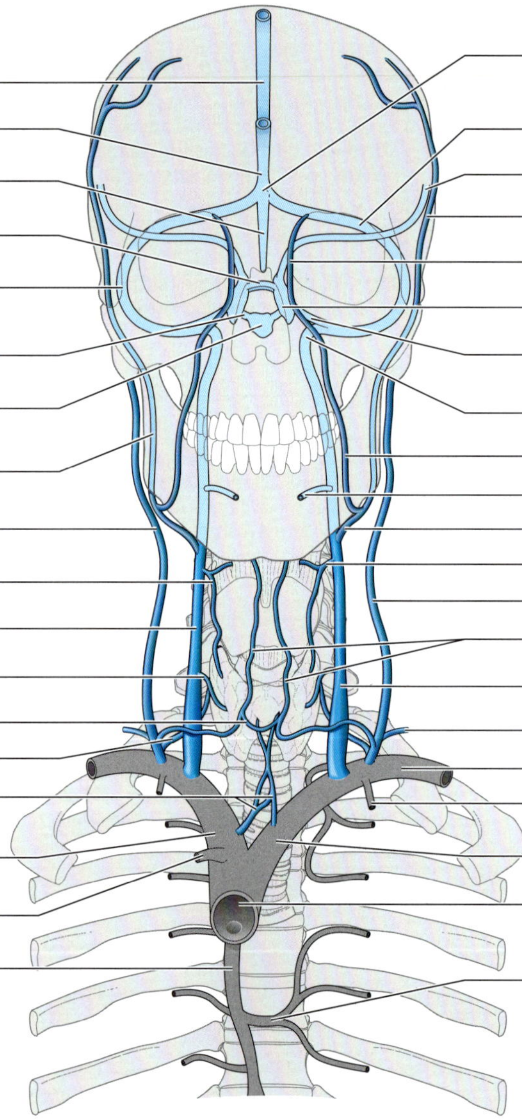

Schematic representation of the **dural venous sinuses** and **veins of the neck** in anterior projection. The right and left transverse sinuses continue with the sigmoid sinuses and then with the internal jugular veins, through jugular foramina of the external surface of the cranial base. Tributaries of the internal jugular vein in the cervical tract are: the common facial vein, which originates at the angle of the mandible from the confluence of the (anterior) facial vein and anterior division of the retromandibular vein; the lingual and pharyngeal veins, and the superior and middle thyroid veins. The external jugular vein originates at the level of the angle of the mandible from the posterior auricular vein and the posterior division of the retromandibular vein. The anterior jugular veins, which originate at the level of the hyoid bone from the confluence of the veins that drain the submandibular region, anastomose under the thyroid gland through the jugular venous arch, then continue in a lateral direction opening into the external jugular veins.

Veins of the Head and Neck

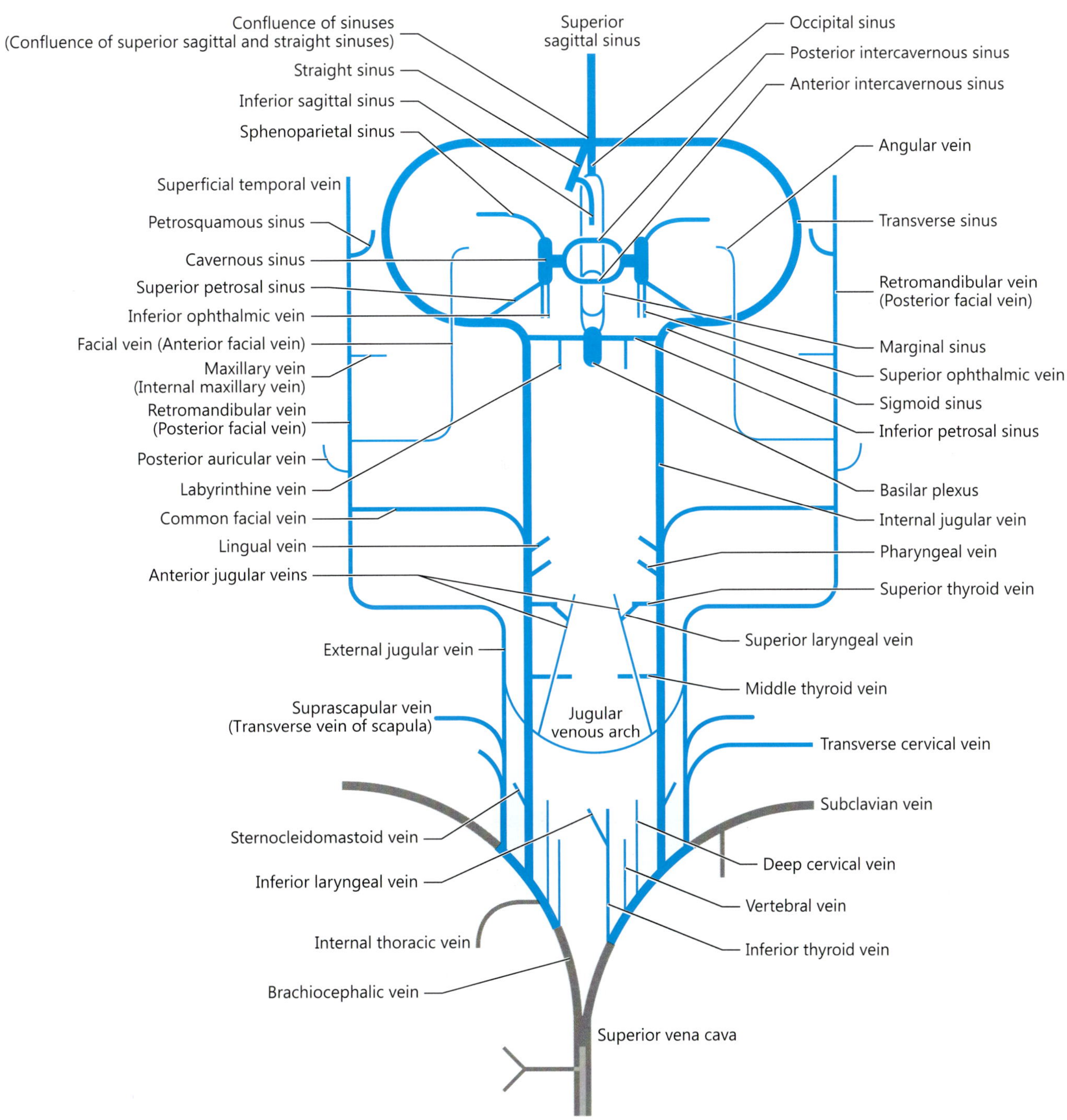

Schematic representation of the **external** and **internal jugular vein tributaries** in the neck. The suprascapular and anterior jugular veins are tributaries of the external jugular vein. Branches that enter the cervical tract of the internal jugular vein are: the common facial, lingual, sternocleidomastoid, pharyngeal, superior thyroid and middle thyroid veins. From the confluence of the internal jugular and subclavian veins originate the brachiocephalic veins. The inferior thyroid veins and the vertebral veins terminate in the brachiocephalic veins (or innominate veins). The external jugular vein terminates in the subclavian vein, which receives also the transverse cervical vein. The latter can, however, unite with the suprascapular vein in a common trunk terminating in correspondence to the terminal tract of the external jugular vein. The jugular venous arch is an anastomotic trunk that unites the two anterior jugular veins.

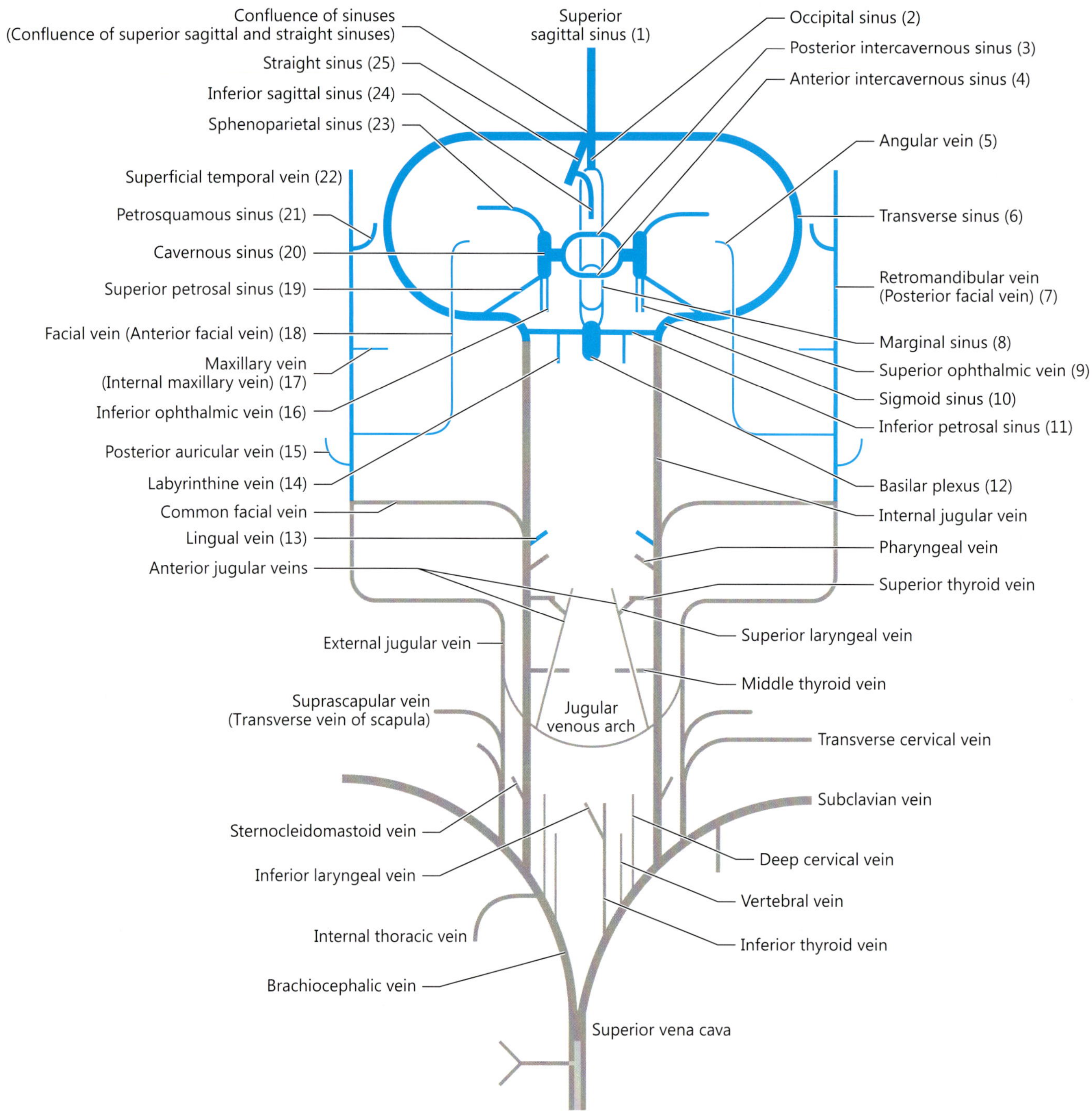

Schematic representation of the **roots of the internal jugular vein**. The roots of the internal jugular vein are composed of the **dural venous sinuses** and the veins that enter it. The internal jugular vein originates at the level of the posterolateral part of the jugular foramen as a continuation of the sigmoid sinus in which the transverse sinus continues, into which drain the diploic, meningeal, cerebral veins and those of the visual and auditory organs. The branches that open into the cranial tract of the internal jugular vein are the inferior petrosal sinus, the vein of the cochlear aqueduct and the emissary veins of the internal carotid venous plexus. The sequence of graphic representations follows the course of blood flow.

➤

Three-dimensional image of a living human body, obtained by contrast-enhanced CT scan using a 3D volume rendering technique, showing the **dural venous sinuses** viewed from above after almost complete removal of the superior sagittal sinus.

Venous sinuses and main veins of the head: territories of drainage		
	VENOUS SINUSES AND VEINS OF THE HEAD	***TERRITORIES OF DRAINAGE***
1	Superior sagittal sinus	Medial and superolateral surfaces of the cerebral hemispheres, diploë, meninges
2	Occipital sinus	Dura mater, diploë, cerebellum
3	Posterior intercavernous sinus	Pituitary gland
4	Anterior intercavernous sinus	Pituitary gland
5	Angular vein	Frontal region
6	Transverse sinus	Inferior surfaces, medial surfaces and inferior halves of the lateral surfaces of the cerebral hemispheres, cerebellum, labyrinth
7	Retromandibular vein (Posterior facial vein)	Parotid gland, temporomandibular joint, masseter, temporalis, medial pterygoid, lateral pterygoid and frontal belly of occipitofrontalis, skin of the face, of the auricle, of the external acoustic meatus and of the frontal and occipital regions
8	Marginal sinus	Posterior cranial fossa
9	Superior ophthalmic vein	Eyeball, extraocular muscles and eyelids
10	Sigmoid sinus	Inferior surfaces, medial surfaces and inferior halves of the lateral surfaces of the cerebral hemispheres, cerebellum, labyrinth
11	Inferior petrosal sinus	Meninges, cerebellum, pons, myelencephalon, labyrinth
12	Basilar plexus	Occipital bone, pons and myelencephalon
13	Lingual vein	Tongue
14	Labyrinthine vein	Internal ear
15	Posterior auricular vein	Posterior part of the ear
16	Inferior ophthalmic vein	Inferior rectus and inferior oblique (extraocular muscles), lacrimal sac, eyelids
17	Maxillary vein (Internal maxillary vein)	Pterygoid plexus (structures of the infratemporal fossa)
18	Facial vein (Anterior facial vein)	Superficial structures of the face
19	Superior petrosal sinus	Inferior surfaces, parts of the medial surfaces inferior and posterior to the inferior frontal sulcus, and inferior halves of the lateral surfaces of the cerebral hemispheres, cerebellum, pons, tympanic cavity, vestibular labyrinth
20	Cavernous sinus	Eyeball and organs contained within the orbital cavity, cerebral hemispheres
21	Petrosquamous sinus	Meninges
22	Superficial temporal vein	Forehead and scalp
23	Sphenoparietal sinus	Diploë, meninges, inferior, medial surfaces and inferior half of the lateral surfaces of the cerebral hemispheres, corpus callosum
24	Inferior sagittal sinus	Falx cerebri (or cerebral falx), corpus callosum
25	Straight sinus	Basal nuclei, walls of the lateral ventricles, central part of the cerebral hemispheres, tentorium cerebelli

N.B.: for veins of the brain and a general overview of the veins of the head and their territories of drainage, see the table summarizing the veins of the head.

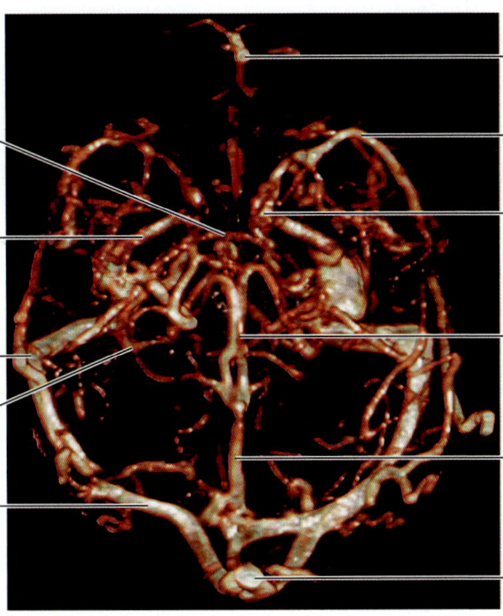

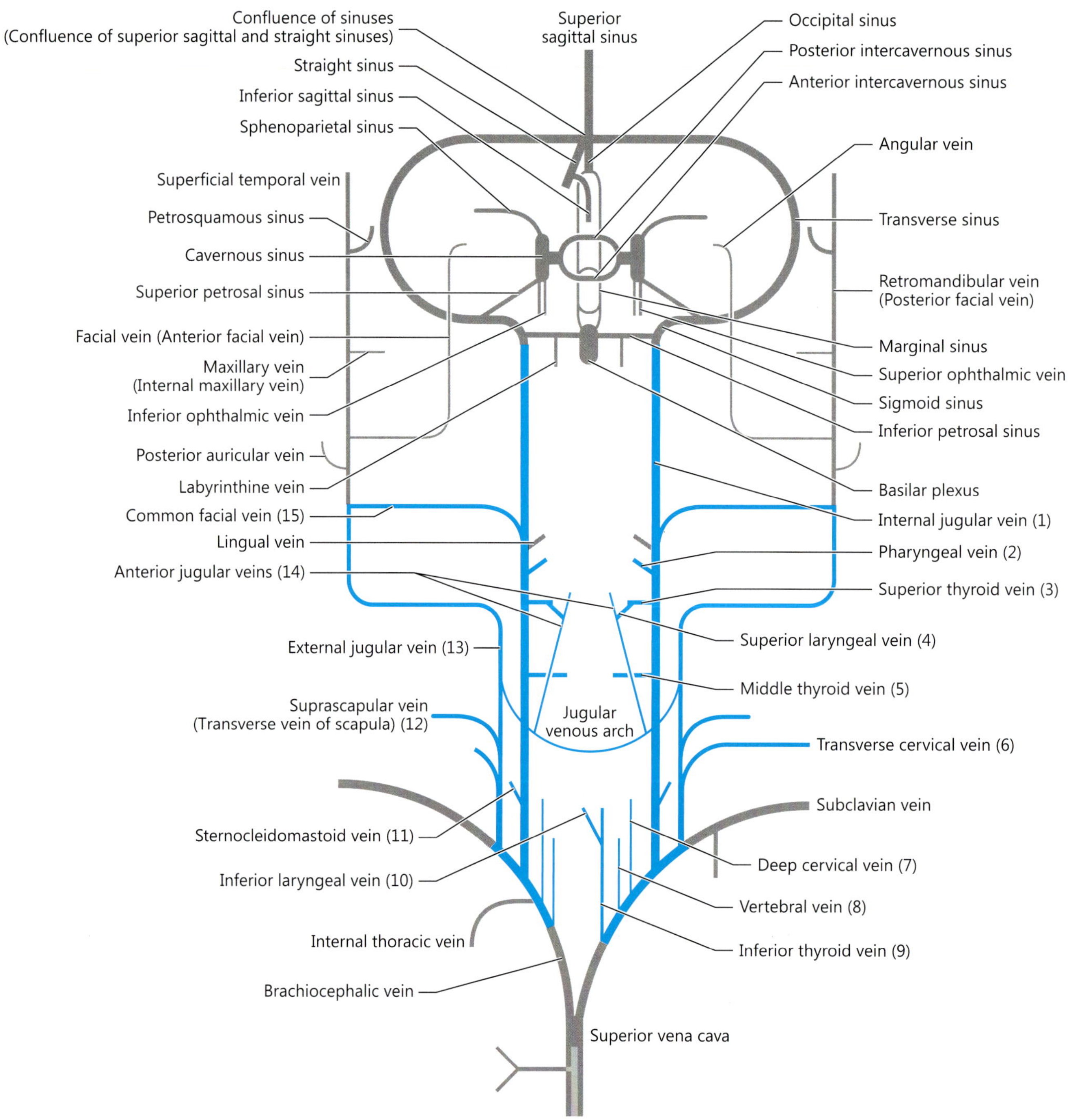

Schematic representation of the **internal jugular** and **external jugular venous trees**. The internal jugular vein originates as a continuation of the sigmoid sinus, which is a continuation at full caliber of the transverse sinus, into which drain the diploic, meningeal, cerebral veins and those of the visual and auditory organs. Tributary branches of the internal jugular vein are the inferior petrosal sinus, the vein of the cochlear aqueduct, and the emissary veins of the internal carotid venous plexus in the cranial tract, and the common facial, lingual, pharyngeal, superior thyroid and middle thyroid veins in the cervical tract. The external jugular vein originates from the confluence of the retromandibular (posterior facial) vein and posterior auricular vein, and has as its main tributaries the suprascapular, transverse cervical and anterior jugular veins. The external jugular vein flows into the subclavian vein within a short distance of the confluence of the internal jugular vein with the subclavian vein.

Main veins of the neck: territories of drainage		
	VEINS OF THE NECK	TERRITORIES OF DRAINAGE
1	Internal jugular vein	Cranium, cranial dura mater, brain, organs of sight and hearing, structures of the face and of the deep regions of the neck
2	Pharyngeal vein	Pharyngeal plexus
3	Superior thyroid vein	Superior part of the thyroid gland, larynx
4	Superior laryngeal vein	Glands, muscles and mucosa of the larynx
5	Middle thyroid vein	Inferior part of the thyroid gland
6	Transverse cervical vein	Trapezius and posterior cervical muscles
7	Deep cervical vein	Deep posterior cervical muscles
8	Vertebral vein	Internal and external vertebral venous plexuses
9	Inferior thyroid vein	Unpaired thyroid plexus
10	Inferior laryngeal vein	Muscles and mucosa of the larynx
11	Sternocleidomastoid vein	Sternocleidomastoid
12	Suprascapular vein (Transverse vein of scapula)	Clavicle, scapula, sternocleidomastoid, subclavius, supraspinatus and subscapularis, acromioclavicular and glenohumeral joints, suprascapular region, skin over the acromion
13	External jugular vein	Superficial territories of the posterior region of the neck, teguments and superficial muscles of the anterior region of the neck, teguments and superficial muscles of the occipital region and the nuchal region
14	Anterior jugular vein	Teguments and superficial muscles of the anterior region of the neck
15	Common facial vein	Territories of drainage of the facial and retromandibular veins

N.B.: for a general overview of the veins of the neck and their territories of drainage, see the table summarizing the veins of the neck.

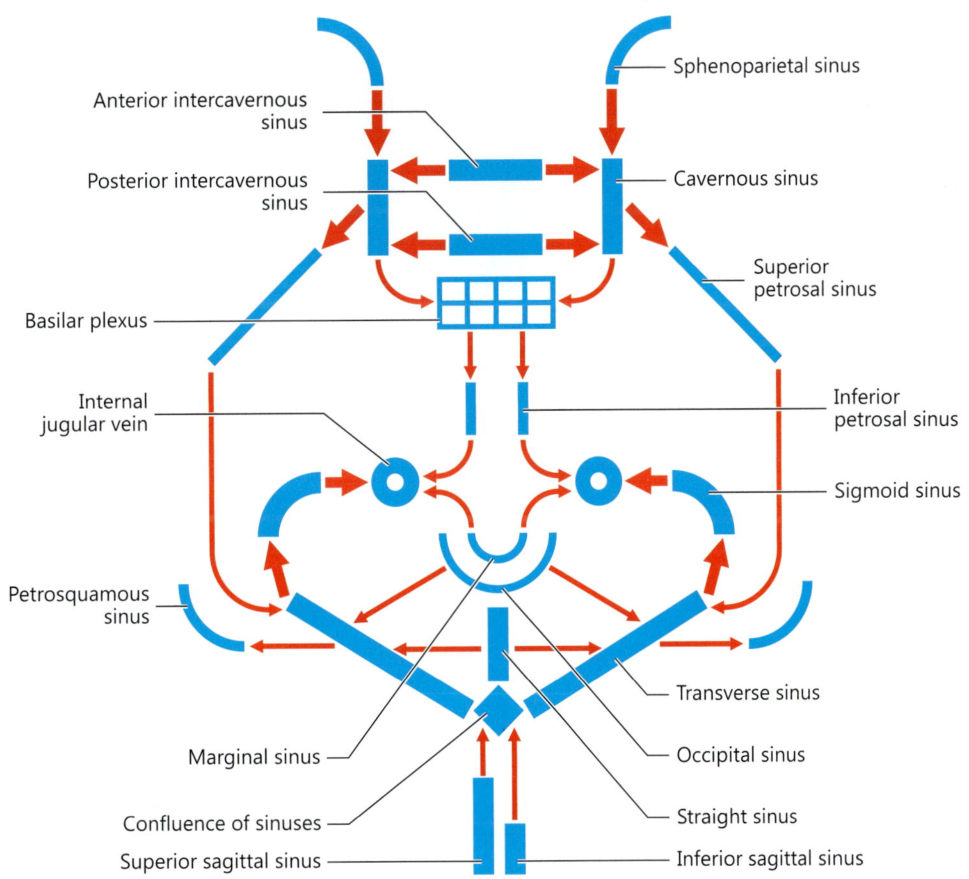

Schematic representation showing the origins and terminations of the **dural venous sinuses**. Arrows indicate the direction of drainage. The sphenoparietal sinus originates from the superior sagittal sinus, though actually today it is considered to be formed by the sinus of the lesser wing of the sphenoid and the parietal part of the anterior branch of the middle meningeal vein. The superior sagittal sinus originates from the confluence of veins in the foramen cecum. The inferior sagittal sinus begins in a blind end. The petrosquamous sinus has two drainage canals, into the retromandibular vein and into the pterygoid plexus, and it generally disappears in the last three months of intrauterine life.

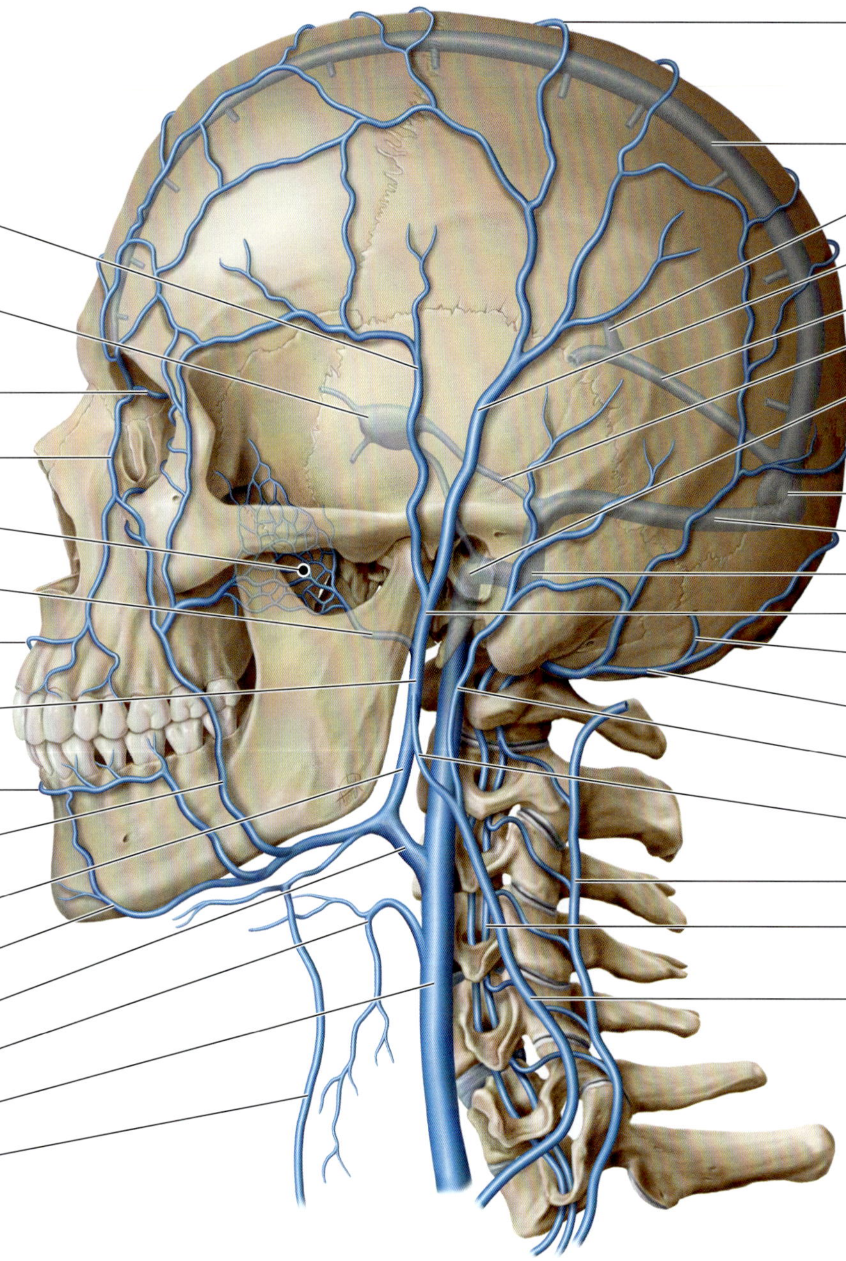

Superficial and **deep circulation** of the veins of the head and neck, in left lateral view. Looking through into the interior of the cranium, some dural venous sinuses are visible.

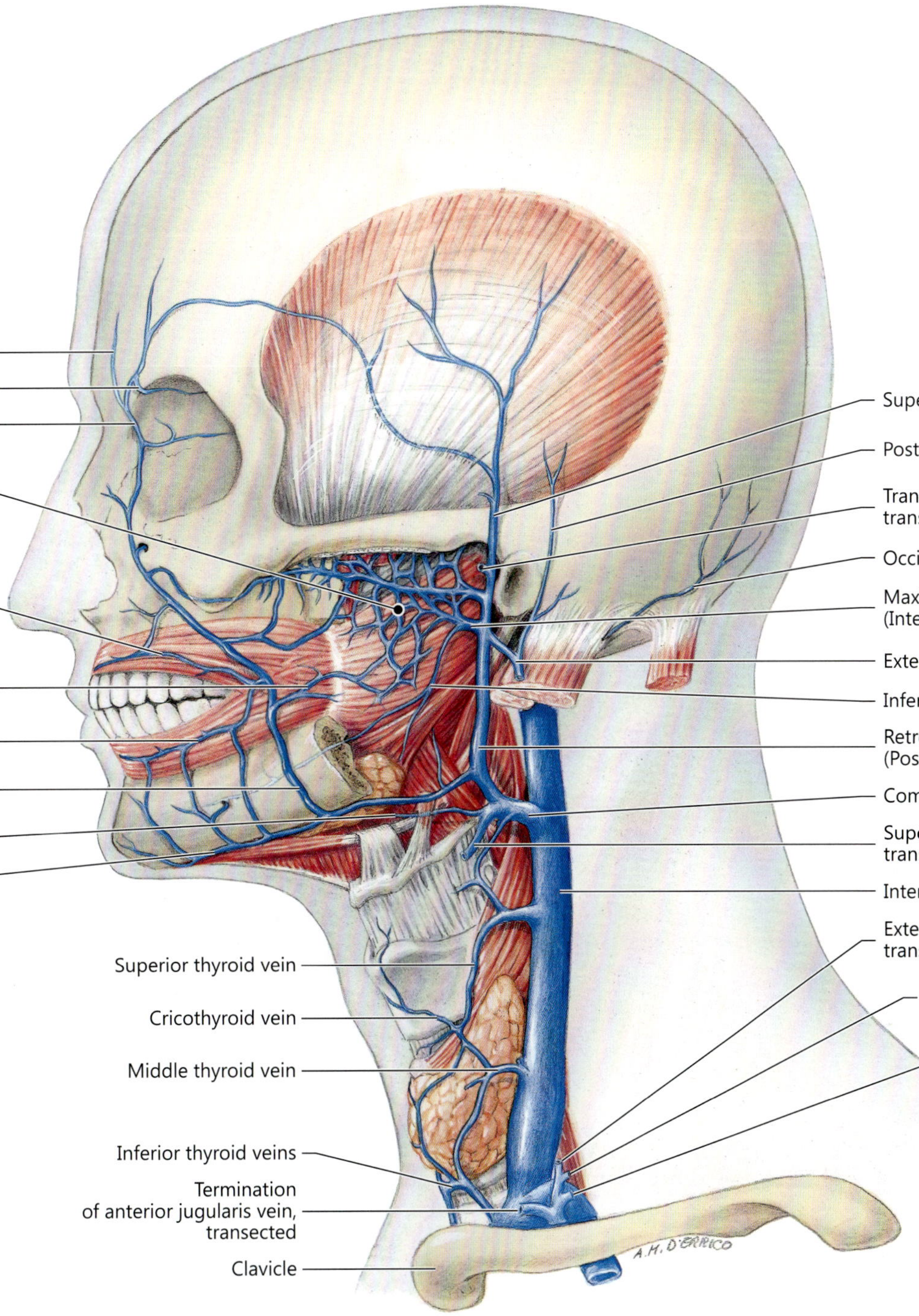

Illustration of the **internal jugular vein**, left side, in the cervical region, and its venous tributaries. The pterygoid venous plexus, drained by the internal maxillary vein, can be seen.

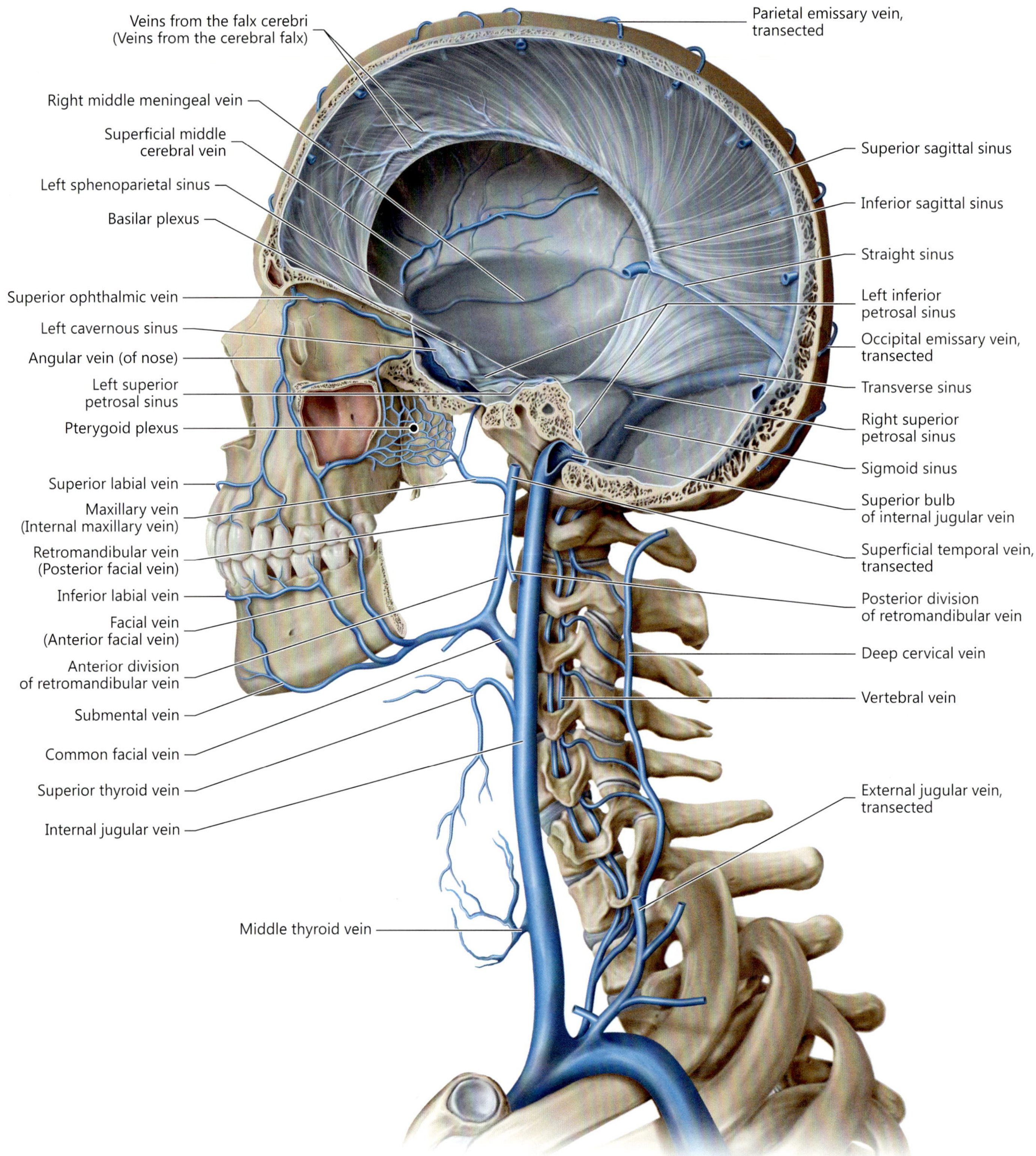

Internal jugular vein showing in detail its facial and head tributaries. Inside the cranium are the principal **dural venous sinuses** from whose confluence it originates.

Three-dimensional image of a living human body, obtained by CT scan using a 3D volume rendering technique, showing the **internal jugular vein** and **dural venous sinuses** in relation to the skeleton and contiguous vascular structures, in lateral view.

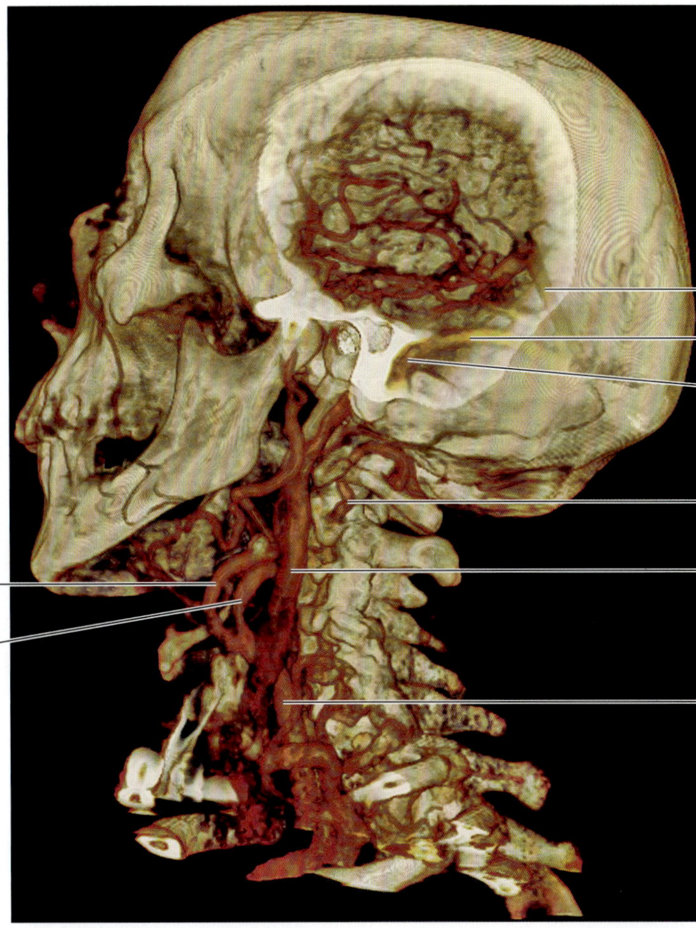

Three-dimensional image of a living human body, obtained by CT scan using a 3D volume rendering technique, showing the **internal jugular vein** and **carotid arteries** in relation to the skeleton, in posterolateral view.

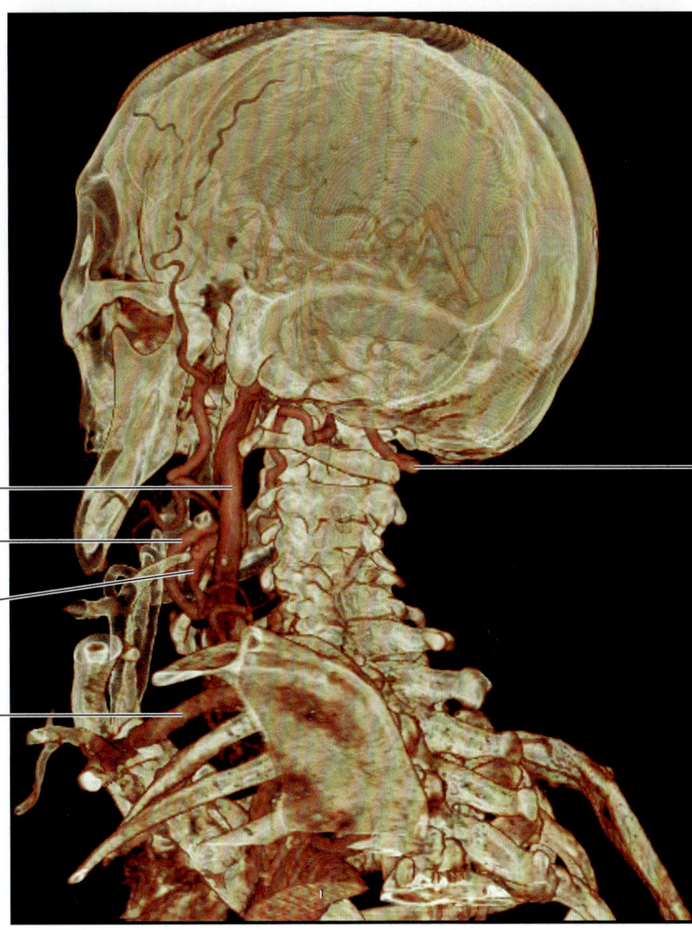

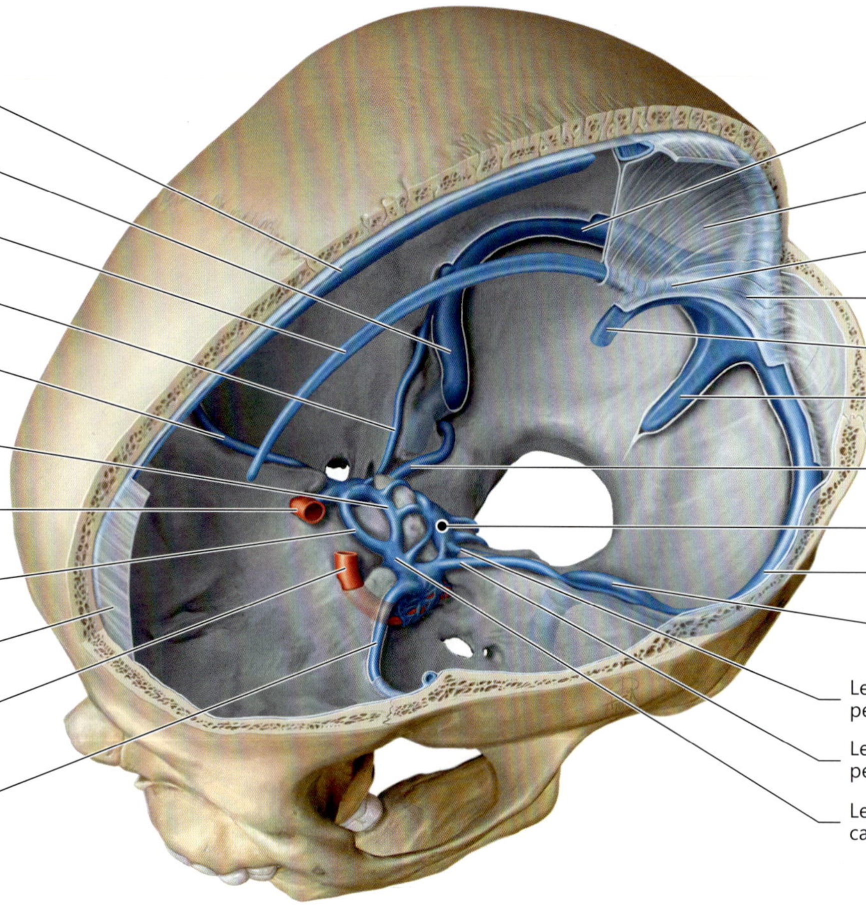

Schematic representation showing the structure and course of the **dural venous sinuses** also in relation to the bones forming the cranium.

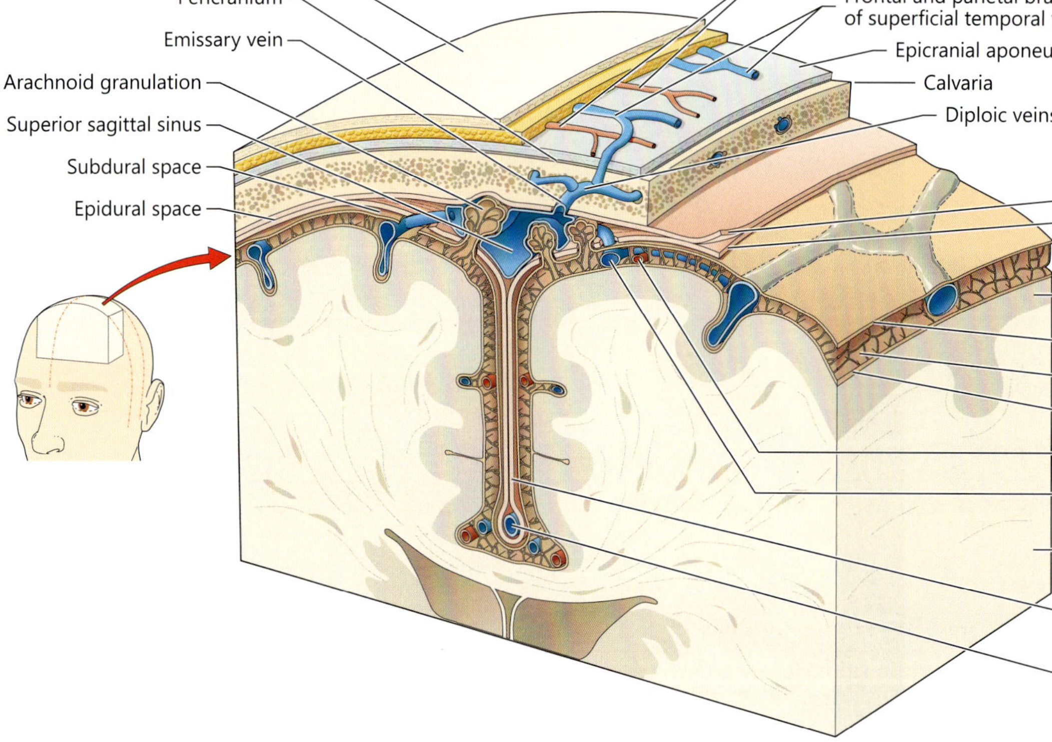

Position of the **superior sagittal sinus** in a frontal section of the cranium. Note the triangular form of the sinus, which receives, on the left, a cerebral vein and, on the right, diploic veins, in the venous lake that it forms.

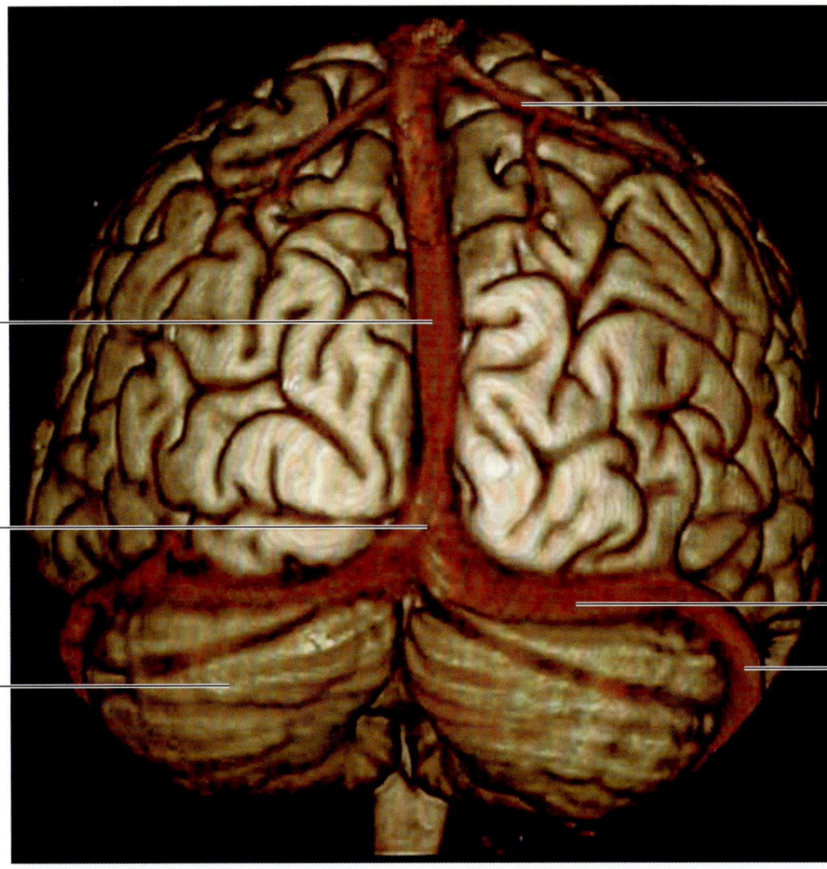

Three-dimensional image of a living human body, posterior view, obtained by CT scan using a 3D volume rendering technique, showing some **vessels** and **venous sinuses** inside the cranium, in relation to the brain hemispheres and cerebellum.

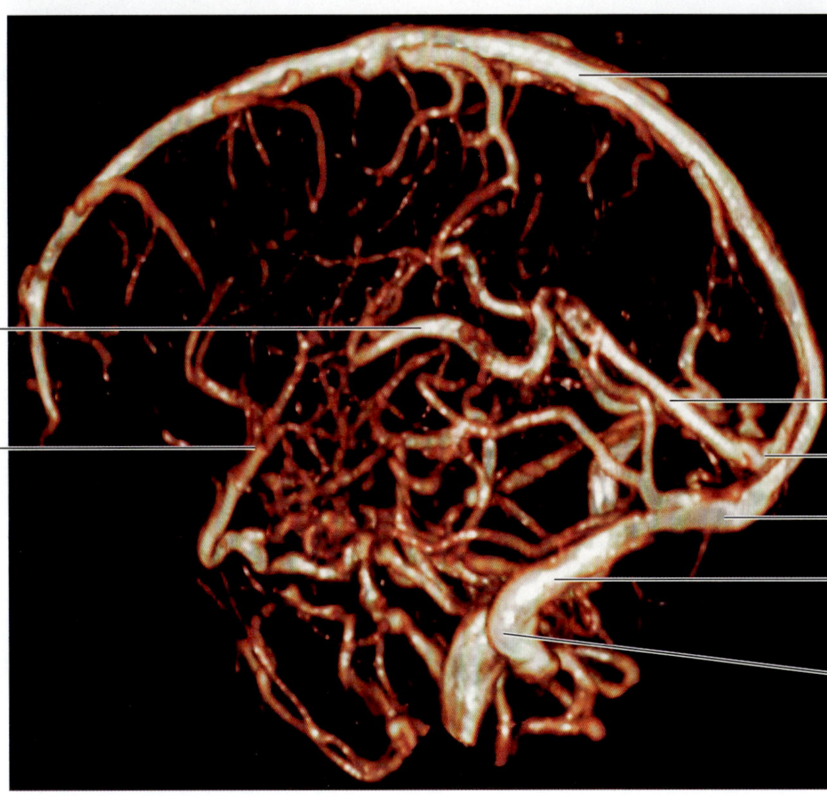

Three-dimensional image of a living human body, sagittal view, obtained by CT scan using a 3D volume rendering technique, showing the **dural venous sinuses** in left lateral view.

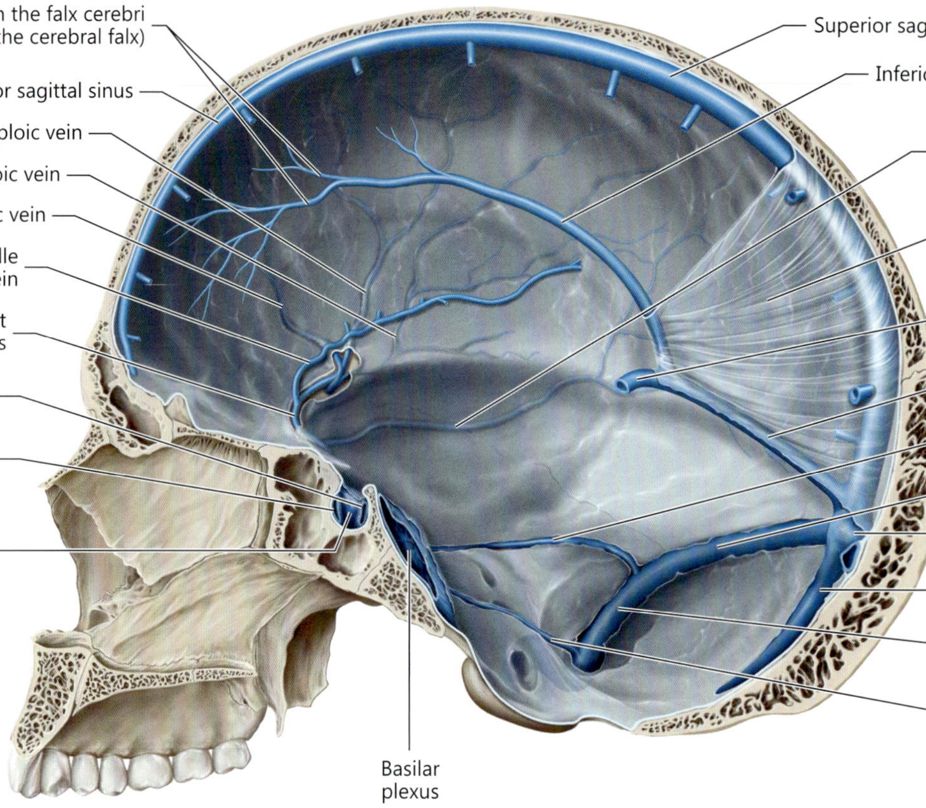

Schematic representation of the **dural venous sinuses** in a sagittal section of the cranium immediately to the right of the median plane; the cranial cavity has been emptied leaving visible part (the left surface) of the falx cerebri (cerebral falx).

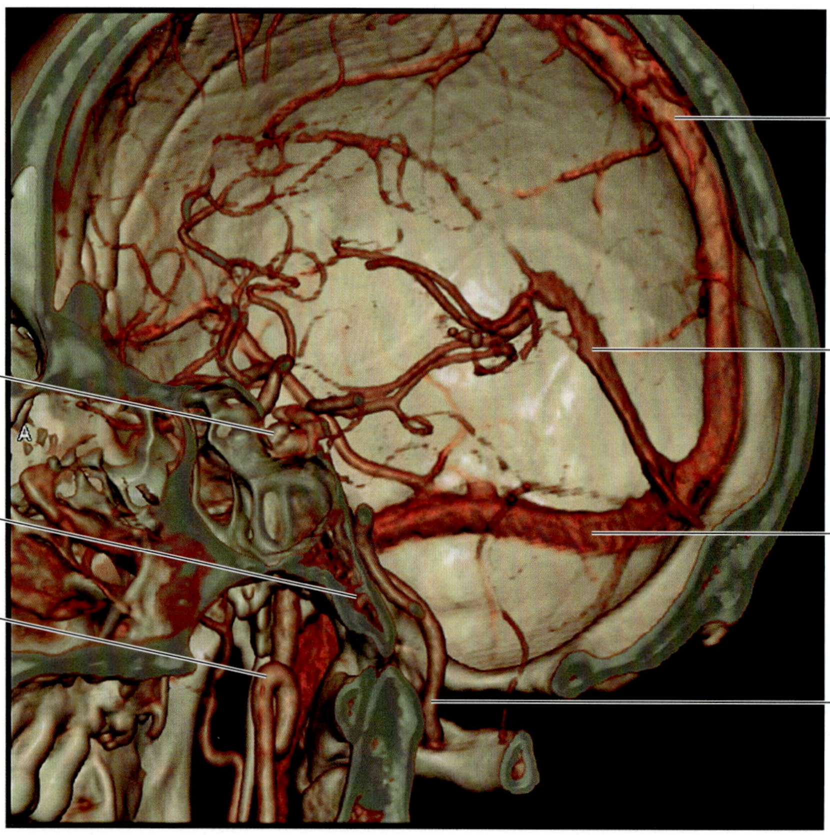

Three-dimensional image of a living human body, obtained by CT scan using a 3D volume rendering technique, showing in left posterolateral view two of the three **arterial sources of the neurocranium** and some **venous sinuses**.

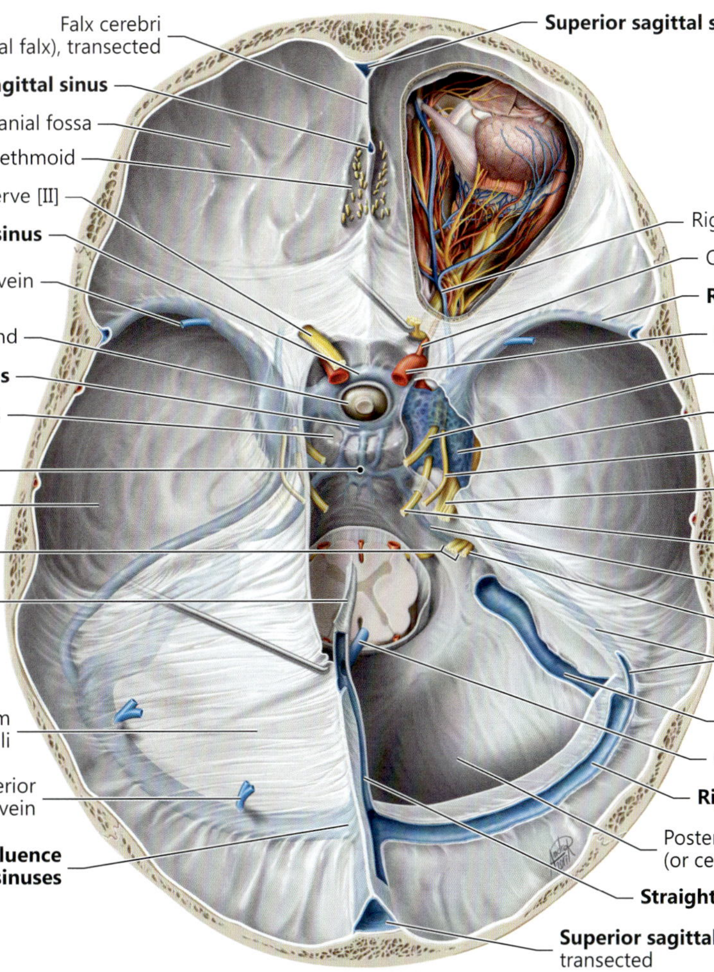

View, looking down from above, of some **dural venous sinuses** on the cranial base. With the aid of resection and demolition, one can see directly the left cavernous sinus and left superior ophthalmic vein.

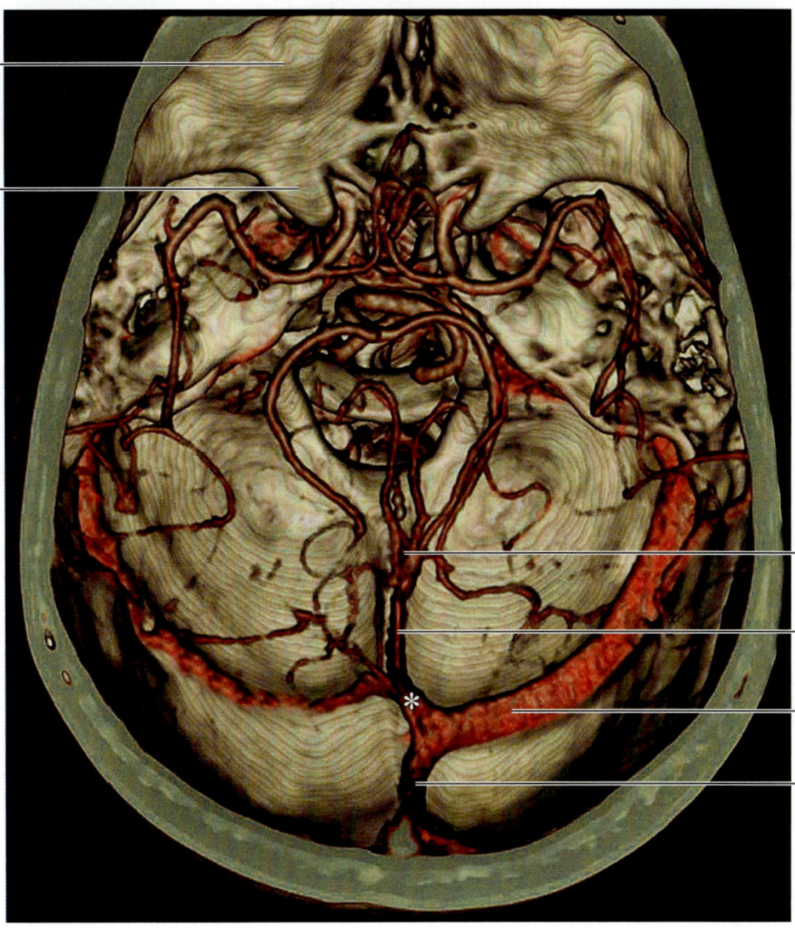

Three-dimensional image of a living human body, obtained by CT scan using a 3D volume rendering technique, showing some **vessels** and **venous sinuses** located principally in the posterior cranial fossa. In particular, an anatomic variant can be observed; in contrast to what is seen in the image above, the superior sagittal sinus drains first and predominantly into the right transverse sinus and only secondarily, through a communicating tract (*), into the left transverse sinus. It is important to remember that this variant does not correspond to any pathology.

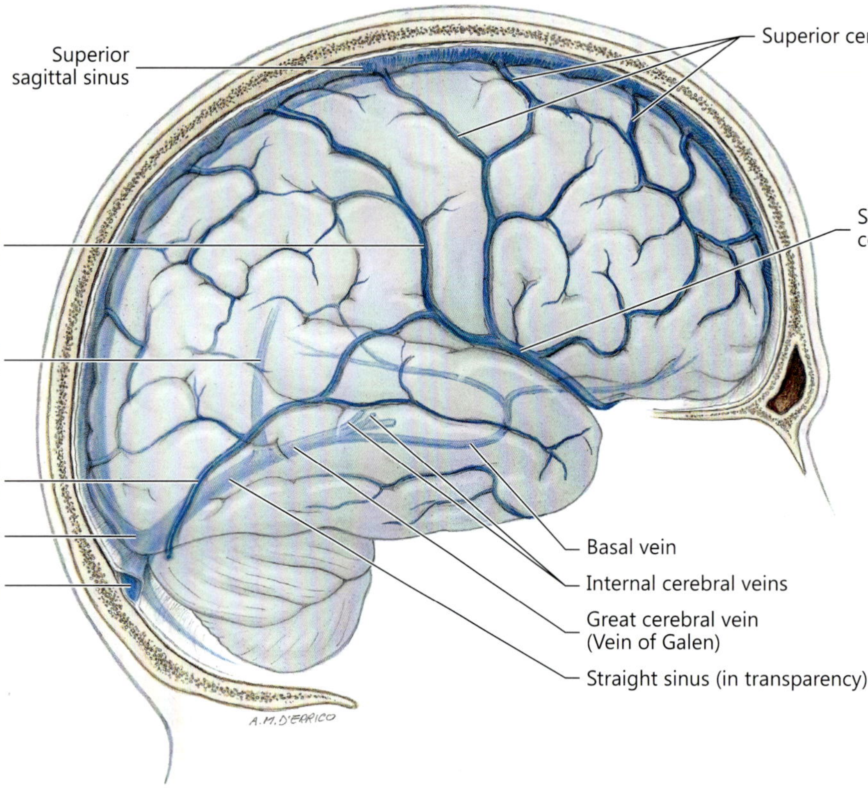

Illustration showing the **cerebral veins** after resection and removal of the right half of the cranium. One can see, on the surface of the right hemisphere of the telencephalon, the superior cerebral veins and, in the lateral sulcus, the middle cerebral vein. This vein, in its continuation as the superior anastomotic vein, connects the superior sagittal sinus, the sphenoparietal sinus and the cavernous sinus. In transparency, the internal cerebral veins.

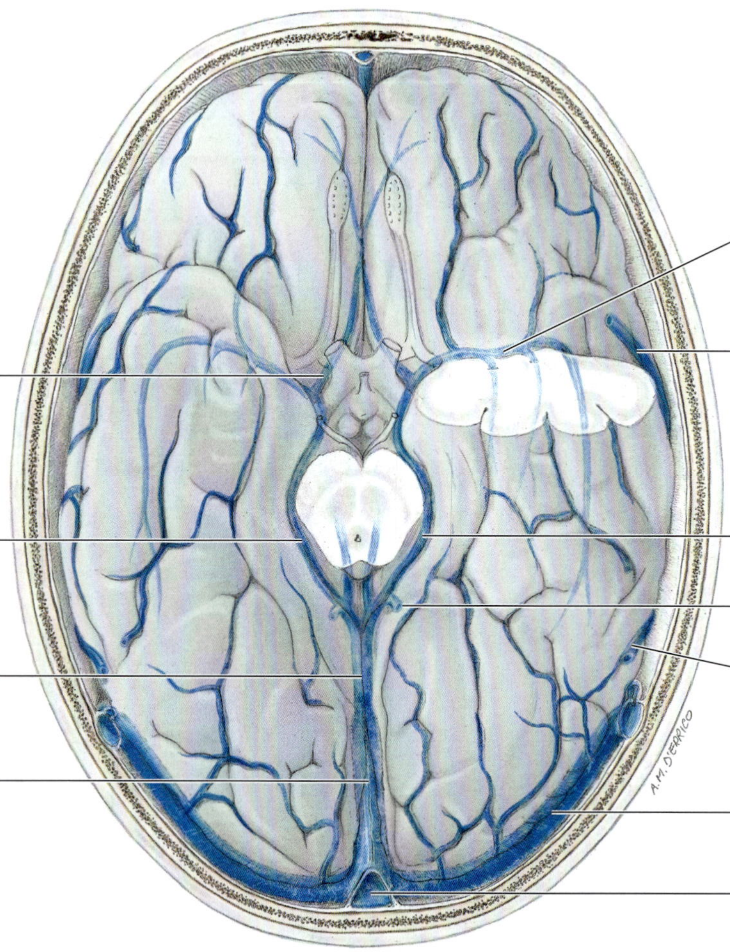

Cerebral veins on the basal surface of the brain. Resection and removal of part of the left temporal lobe permits one to see directly the insular vein. Note the great cerebral vein (vein of Galen), formed by the union of the two internal cerebral veins, into which drain the deep cerebral veins.

Summary table of the dural venous sinuses

NAME	ORIGIN	LOCATION OR COURSE	DRAINAGE AND TRIBUTARIES	CONTINUATION OR TERMINATION	CONNECTIONS
Anterior intercavernous sinus (anterior coronary sinus)		Between the cavernous sinuses of the two sides	Pituitary gland; small sinuses from the pituitary gland		
Basilar plexus (unpaired)	Clivus of the occipital bone (between the internal and external layers of the dura mater)		Occipital veins, pontine veins, veins of the medulla oblongata		Intracranial: cavernous, inferior and, sometimes, superior petrosal sinuses Extracranial: internal vertebral venous plexuses
Cavernous sinus (paired)		Laterally to the sella turcica of the sphenoid, from the medial extremity of the superior orbital fissure at the apex of the petrous part of the temporal bone	Eyeball and organs contained in the orbital cavity, cerebral hemispheres; superior and inferior ophthalmic veins, central retinal vein, inferior cerebral veins and superficial middle cerebral vein, sphenoparietal sinus, superior anastomotic vein	Drainage into the superior and inferior petrosal sinuses, into the basilar, internal carotid and pterygoid plexuses, into the facial vein through the superior ophthalmic vein	Anterior and posterior intercavernous sinuses (between the cavernous sinuses of the two sides), into which drain small sinuses from the pituitary gland, and basilar plexus
Confluence of sinuses (torcula Herophili, sometimes missing)	Confluence of the superior sagittal and straight sinuses	Internal occipital protuberance	Superior and occipital sagittal sinuses	Gives origin to the transverse sinuses	
Inferior petrosal sinus (paired)	Posterior extremity of the cavernous sinus	Groove for the inferior petrosal sinus of the temporal bone, medial part of the petro-occipital synchondrosis up to the jugular foramen	Meninges, cerebellum, pons, myelencephalon, labyrinth; meningeal, cerebellar, pontine veins, veins of medulla oblongata, labyrinthine vein and, at times, condylar emissary veins, petro-occipital sinus and pharyngeal veins	Superior bulb of the internal jugular vein or, sometimes, in the suboccipital venous plexus through a vein in the hypoglossal canal	Intracranial: basilar plexus
Inferior sagittal sinus (unpaired)	In a blind end	Posterior half or two-thirds of the free margin of the falx cerebri (cerebral falx)	Falx cerebri (cerebral falx), corpus callosum; posterior vein of the corpus callosum and small veins from the falx cerebri	Ends in the straight sinus	
Marginal sinus (unpaired)		Surrounds the foramen magnum	Posterior cranial fossa	Sigmoid sinus or superior bulb of the internal jugular vein	Intracranial: basilar plexus and occipital sinus Extracranial: internal vertebral venous plexuses and deep cervical vein
Occipital sinus (usually unpaired, sometimes paired or missing)	Near the foramen magnum, from many small canals, one of which is a joint canal with the termination of the sigmoid sinus	Adherent margin of the falx cerebelli (cerebellar falx), bifurcation into two branches that follow the margins of the foramen magnum	Dura mater, diploë, cerebellum; veins from the tentorium cerebelli, diploic veins and cerebellar veins	Ends in the confluence of sinuses or in one of the transverse sinuses or in the straight sinus	Intracranial: superior sagittal and sigmoid sinuses Extracranial: internal vertebral venous plexuses
Petrosquamous sinus		In a sulcus or canal along the junction between the squamous and petrous parts of the temporal bone	Meninges	Transverse sinus or retromandibular vein	Extracranial: retromandibular vein
Posterior intercavernous sinus (posterior coronary sinus)		Between the cavernous sinuses of the two sides	Pituitary gland; small sinuses from the pituitary gland		

continued

Summary table of the dural venous sinuses *(continued)*

NAME	ORIGIN	LOCATION OR COURSE	DRAINAGE AND TRIBUTARIES	CONTINUATION OR TERMINATION	CONNECTIONS
Sigmoid sinus (paired)	Continuation of the transverse sinus	Sulcus on the mastoid process of the temporal bone, jugular process of the occipital bone, jugular foramen	Inferior and medial surfaces, and inferior halves of the lateral surfaces of the cerebral hemispheres, cerebellum, labyrinth	Internal jugular vein	Mastoid and condylar emissary veins, occipital sinus
Sphenoparietal sinus (paired)	Superior sagittal sinus	Sulcus or canal in the parietal bone, along the posterior side of the coronal suture, sulcus on the lesser wing of the sphenoid, along its posterior margin	Diploë, meninges, inferior and medial surfaces, and inferior halves of the lateral surfaces of the cerebral hemispheres, corpus callosum; diploic veins, in particular, the anterior temporal diploic vein, middle meningeal veins, anterior cerebral veins and superficial middle cerebral vein, and vein from the temporal lobe	Anterior part of the cavernous sinus	
Straight sinus (unpaired)	Continuation of the inferior sagittal sinus	Attachment of the falx cerebri to the tentorium cerebelli	Basal nuclei, walls of the lateral ventricles, central part of the cerebral hemispheres, tentorium cerebelli; great cerebral vein, superior veins of cerebellar hemisphere and veins from the tentorium cerebelli, occipital sinus	Ends in the confluence of sinuses or in the transverse sinus	
Superior petrosal sinus (paired)	Posterior part of the cavernous sinus	Groove for the superior petrosal sinus of the temporal bone, adherent margin of the tentorium cerebelli	Inferior surfaces, parts of the medial surfaces inferiorly and posteriorly to the inferior frontal sulcus, and inferior halves of the lateral surfaces of the cerebral hemispheres, cerebellum, pons, tympanic cavity, vestibular labyrinth; inferior cerebral, cerebellar, pontine, tympanic veins, vein of the vestibular aqueduct and, sometimes, superior anastomotic vein	Ends in the transverse sinus in the tract where this continues in the sigmoid sinus	Intracranial: at times, inferior petrosal sinus and basilar plexus
Superior sagittal sinus (unpaired)	Near the crista galli, immediately behind the foramen cecum of the frontal bone, through confluence of the veins of the foramen cecum	Adherent convex margin of the falx cerebri, sulcus on the internal surface of the frontal bone, adjacent margins of the parietal bones, squamous part of the occipital bone, internal occipital protuberance	Medial and superolateral surfaces of the cerebral hemispheres, diploë, meninges; superior cerebral veins	Ends in the confluence of sinuses or in the right transverse sinus	Intracranial: lateral lacunae in the dura mater, which drain the meningeal and diploic veins, left transverse and occipital sinuses Extracranial: parietal emissary vein
Transverse sinus (paired)	Conjunction of the bifurcating branches of the superior sagittal and straight sinuses or confluence of sinuses At times, right transverse sinus: direct continuation of the superior sagittal sinus; left transverse sinus: direct continuation of the straight sinus	Internal occipital protuberance, groove for the transverse sinus of the parietal bone (squamous part) and the occipital bone (squamous part) in the adherent margin of the tentorium cerebelli, groove for the transverse sinus of the occipital bone (lateral part), posterior part of the jugular foramen	Inferior and medial surfaces, and inferior halves of the lateral surfaces of the cerebral hemispheres, cerebellum, labyrinth; inferior cerebral veins, inferior veins of cerebellar hemisphere, labyrinthine, diploic and inferior anastomotic veins, superior petrosal sinus and occipital sinus	Continuation in the sigmoid sinus	Intracranial: mastoid and occipital emissary veins

Summary table of the veins of the head			
VEIN	***ORIGIN***	***DRAINAGE***	***CONFLUENCE***
angular	From the union of the supratrochlear and supraorbital veins in correspondence to the medial angle of the eye and root of nose	Frontal region; receives the superior and inferior palpebral veins and external nasal veins	Facial vein
anterior auricular	Anteriorly to the external ear	Anterior surface of the external ear	Pterygoid plexus or superficial temporal veins
anterior cerebral	Superior surface of the corpus callosum	Anterior perforated substance, lamina terminalis, rostrum of corpus callosum, septum pellucidum	Basal vein
anterior ciliary	Ciliary body	External part of the ciliary muscle; receive the scleral venous sinus and the scleral veins	Superior ophthalmic vein
anterior temporal diploic	Diploë of the lateral part of the frontal bone	Frontal bone	Sphenoparietal sinus, deep temporal vein or middle meningeal vein
basal (of Rosenthal)	Anterior perforated substance	Rostral parts of the cingulate gyrus, corpus callosum, orbital surface of the frontal lobe, insula, part of the ventral striatum; receives the anterior cerebral veins; the deep middle cerebral vein, of which the insular veins are tributaries; the inferior thalamostriate veins; the vein of the olfactory gyrus; the inferior ventricular vein; the inferior choroid vein and the peduncular veins	Internal cerebral veins
central retinal	Capillaries of the retina	Retina	Superior ophthalmic vein or cavernous sinus
cerebellar (include the superior and inferior veins of cerebellar hemisphere and precentral cerebellar vein, superior and inferior veins of vermis, petrosal vein)	Cerebellum	Cerebellum	Transverse, superior petrosal, occipital and straight sinuses, great cerebral vein
ciliary	Ciliary body	Sclera	Superior ophthalmic vein
cochlear	Osseous spiral lamina and basal lamina	Cochlea	Labyrinthine veins
common facial	Formal term for the inferior trunk of the facial vein (sometimes united with the retromandibular vein) that empties into the internal jugular vein		
common modiolar	Modiolus	Cochlea	Vein of the cochlear aqueduct
condylar emissary	Condylar canal	Sigmoid sinus	Suboccipital venous plexus
conjunctival	Eye	Bulbar conjunctiva	Episcleral veins
deep cerebral (two in number; include the basal vein and the great cerebral vein)	Corpus callosum	Lateral ventricle, third ventricle, basal nuclei, semioval center (white matter between the cortex and subcortical nuclei), thalamus	Straight sinus
deep facial	Between the buccinator and masseter	Buccinator, zygomaticus major and zygomaticus minor, masseter	Facial vein
deep lingual vein (ranine)	Tongue	Apex and deep part of the tongue	Lingual vein
deep middle cerebral (deep Sylvian)	Inferior part of the lateral sulcus	Insula and insular gyri	Basal vein
deep temporal	Deep to the anterior part of the temporalis	Temporal region	Pterygoid plexus
dorsal lingual	Tongue	Posterior parte of the tongue	Lingual vein
emissary of foramen lacerum (two or three in number)	Foramen lacerum	Cavernous sinus	Pterygoid plexus
emissary of foramen of Vesalius	Foramen of Vesalius (when present)	Cavernous sinus	Pterygoid plexus
episcleral	Sclera, near the corneoscleral junction	Medial angle of the eye, sclera, conjunctiva; receive the palpebral and conjunctival veins	Superior ophthalmic vein or anterior ciliary veins

continued

Summary table of the veins of the head *(continued)*

VEIN	ORIGIN	DRAINAGE	CONFLUENCE
ethmoidal	Ethmoidal cells	Ethmoidal cells, frontal sinus, dura mater, walls of the nasal cavity, nasal septum	Superior ophthalmic vein
external jugular	Angle of the mandible through confluence of the retromandibular and posterior auricular veins	Superficial territories of the posterior region of the neck, integuments and superficial muscles of the anterior region of the neck, integuments and superficial muscles of the occipital region and the nuchal region; receives the anterior jugular, suprascapular, transverse cervical and, sometimes, occipital veins	Internal jugular vein or subclavian vein
external nasal (several in number)	Ala of nose	External part of the nose	Angular vein or facial vein
external palatine	Palate	Soft palate and palatine tonsil	Facial vein
facial (anterior facial)	Continuation of the angular vein	Superficial structures of the face; receives the superior and inferior labial veins, deep facial, parotid, external palatine and submental veins	Common facial vein or internal jugular vein
frontal diploic	Diploë of the median part of the frontal bone	Frontal bone	Supraorbital vein and superior sagittal sinus
great cerebral (of Galen)	Around the posterior part of the corpus callosum	Thalamus, hypothalamus, basal nuclei and mesencephalon; receives the internal cerebral veins, of which the superior choroid vein is a tributary; superior thalamostriate vein, of which the anterior and posterior veins of the septum pellucidum are tributaries, medial vein of the lateral ventricle, lateral vein of the lateral ventricle, of which the veins of the caudate nucleus are tributaries; lateral direct veins and posterior vein of the corpus callosum	Anterior extremity of the straight sinus
inferior alveolar (inferior dental)	Mandibular canal	Mandible and mandibular dental arcade	Pterygoid plexus
inferior anastomotic (Labbé's vein)	Temporal lobe	Superficial middle cerebral vein	Transverse sinus
inferior cerebral	Inferior surface of the cerebral hemispheres	Inferior surface of the cerebral hemispheres; receive the vein of the uncus and the orbital and temporal veins	Superior sagittal, cavernous, superior petrosal, transverse and straight sinuses
inferior choroid	Lateral ventricle	Inferior part of the choroid plexus of the lateral ventricle	Basal vein
inferior labial	Lower lip	Labial glands, mucosa and muscles of the lower lip	Facial vein
inferior ophthalmic	Anterior part of the floor and medial wall of the orbit	Inferior rectus and inferior oblique (extraocular muscles), lacrimal sac, eyelids	Pterygoid plexus and cavernous sinus
inferior palpebral	Inferior eyelid	Inferior eyelid	Facial vein
inferior thalamostriate (inferior striate)	Corpus striatum	Perforated substance	Basal vein
inferior vein of vermis	Behind the cerebellar tonsil	Vermis and cerebral hemispheres	Transverse sinus or straight sinus
inferior veins of cerebellar hemisphere	Inferior surface of the cerebellum	Inferior surface of the cerebellum	Transverse, superior petrosal and occipital sinuses
internal cerebral (deep cerebral veins of Galen; two in number)	Interventricular foramen	Deep parts of the cerebral hemispheres; receive the superior choroid vein	Great cerebral vein
internal jugular	At the level of the posterolateral part of the jugular foramen as a continuation of the sigmoid sinus which is the continuation of the transverse sinus	Cranium, cranial dura mater, brain, organs of sight and hearing, facial and deep neck structures; in the cranial tract: receives the inferior petrosal sinus, the vein of the cochlear aqueduct and the emissary veins of the internal carotid venous plexus; in the cervical tract: receives the facial, sternocleidomastoid, lingual, pharyngeal from the pharyngeal plexus, superior thyroid, middle thyroid and superior laryngeal veins	Unites with the subclavian vein to form the brachiocephalic vein (innominate vein)

continued

Summary table of the veins of the head			(continued)
VEIN	*ORIGIN*	*DRAINAGE*	*CONFLUENCE*
labyrinthine (internal auditory)	Internal ear	Internal ear	Inferior petrosal sinus or transverse sinus
lacrimal	Orbit	Lacrimal gland, eyelids, conjunctiva	Superior ophthalmic vein
lingual	Tongue	Tongue; receives the dorsal lingual veins, vena comitans of hypoglossal nerve, sublingual vein and deep lingual vein	Internal jugular vein or inferior part of the facial vein
mastoid emissary (mastoid)	Mastoid foramen	Transverse sinus	Posterior auricular vein or occipital vein
maxillary	Between the head of the mandible and the sphenomandibular ligament	Pterygoid plexus	Retromandibular vein
meningeal	Plexiform vessels In the dura mater	Cranial dura mater	Efferent vessels in the external layer of the dura mater that link with the lacunae of the dura mater sinuses
middle meningeal	Lateral lacunae of the superior sagittal sinus	Dura mater, internal surface of the cranium, trigeminal ganglion	Pterygoid plexus
middle temporal	Lateral angle of the eye	Temporalis	Retromandibular vein
nasofrontal	Anterior medial part of the orbit	Frontal belly of the occipitofrontalis, medial angle of the eye and root of nose	Superior ophthalmic vein
occipital	Plexus on the posterior part of the cranium	Occipital region	Vertebral vein and deep cervical vein or external jugular vein through the posterior auricular vein or internal jugular vein (following the course of the occipital artery)
occipital diploic (largest of the four diploic veins)	Diploë of the occipital bone	Occipital bone	Occipital vein, transverse sinus or occipital emissary vein
occipital emissary	Occipital protuberance	Confluence of sinuses and occipital diploic vein	Occipital vein
of brainstem (include the pontomesencephalic, interpeduncular, intercollicular, lateral mesencephalic, and pontine veins, and veins of the medulla oblongata, of the lateral recess of the fourth ventricle, and of the cerebellomedullary cistern)	Brainstem	Brainstem	Basal and petrosal veins, inferior petrosal sinus and marginal sinus
of cochlear aqueduct (of cochlear canaliculus)	Perilymphatic space	Cochlea	Internal jugular vein
of medulla oblongata (of the myelencephalon; includes the anteromedian, anterolateral, transverse, dorsal and posteromedian medullary veins)	Myelencephalon	Myelencephalon	Anterior spinal vein and petrosal vein
of pterygoid canal (vidian)	Pterygoid canal	Sphenoidal sinus	Pterygoid plexus
of vestibular aqueduct	Vestibular aqueduct	Internal ear	Superior petrosal sinus
parietal emissary	Parietal foramen	Scalp	Superior sagittal sinus
parotid (anterior and posterior)	Parotid gland	Superficial and deep parts of the parotid gland, parotid duct	Pterygoid plexus (anterior veins), facial vein (posterior veins)
petrosal	Pons	Myelencephalon, pons and cerebellum	Superior petrosal sinus

continued

Summary table of the veins of the head *(continued)*

VEIN	*ORIGIN*	*DRAINAGE*	*CONFLUENCE*
pontine (include the anteromedian, anterolateral, transverse and lateral pontine veins)	Pons	Pons	Petrosal vein
posterior auricular	Plexus behind the ear	Posterior part of the ear	Forms the external jugular vein In connection with the posterior division of the retromandibular vein
posterior temporal diploic	Diploë of the parietal bone	Parietal bone	Transverse sinus, posterior auricular vein or mastoid emissary vein
precentral cerebellar	Precentral fissure	Vermis and superior part of the hemisphere of the cerebellum	Great cerebral vein
pterygoid plexus	Infratemporal fossa	Structures of the infratemporal fossa; receives the middle meningeal veins, deep temporal veins, vein of the pterygoid canal, anterior auricular veins, parotid veins, articular veins, tympanic veins, stylomastoid vein, superior and inferior alveolar veins	Retromandibular vein or maxillary veins
retromandibular (posterior facial vein)	Anteriorly to the auricle	Parotid gland, temporomandibular joint, masseter, temporalis, medial pterygoid, lateral pterygoid and frontal belly of occipitofrontalis, skin of the face, of the auricle, of the external acoustic meatus and the frontal and occipital regions; receives the superficial and middle temporal veins, transverse facial vein and maxillary veins and drains the pterygoid plexus	Common facial vein through the anterior division that unites with the facial vein; external jugular vein through the posterior division that unites with the posterior auricular vein
stylomastoid	Stylomastoid foramen	Mastoid cells, tympanic cavity, semicircular canals	Pterygoid plexus
sublingual	Under the tongue	Sublingual gland, mylohyoid, mucous membrane of the mouth, gingivae, alveolar process of the mandible	Lingual vein
submental	Under the base of the mandible	Submandibular gland; mylohyoid, digastric and platysma	Facial vein
superficial cerebral (include the superior and inferior cerebral veins and the superficial middle cerebral vein)	Surface of the cerebral hemispheres	Superior, lateral, medial and inferior surfaces of the cerebral hemispheres	Superior sagittal, cavernous, superior petrosal, transverse, straight and sphenoparietal sinuses
superficial middle cerebral (superficial Sylvian)	Lateral surface of the cerebral hemisphere	Lateral surface of the cerebral hemisphere; receives the superior anastomotic vein and inferior anastomotic vein	Superior petrosal and sphenoparietal sinuses
superficial temporal	Plexus at the apex and on the lateral surface of the cranium	Forehead and scalp	Retromandibular vein
superior anastomotic (of Trolard)	Lateral sulcus	Superficial middle cerebral vein	Superior sagittal sinus
superior cerebral (8-12 in number)	Cerebral cortex	Superior, lateral, medial surfaces of the cerebral hemispheres; receive the prefrontal, frontal, parietal, temporal and occipital veins	Superior sagittal sinus
superior choroid	Lateral ventricle	Lateral ventricle and choroid plexus of the lateral ventricle, corpus callosum	Internal cerebral veins
superior labial	Upper lip	Upper lip, nose, nasal septum	Facial vein
superior ophthalmic	Internal angle of the orbit	Eyeball, extraocular muscles and eyelids; receives the nasofrontal vein; ethmoidal veins; lacrimal vein; vorticose veins; ciliary veins; anterior ciliary veins, of which the scleral venous sinus and the scleral veins are tributaries; central retinal vein; episcleral veins, of which the palpebral and conjunctival veins are tributaries	Cavernous sinus

continued

Summary table of the veins of the head *(continued)*

VEIN	ORIGIN	DRAINAGE	CONFLUENCE
superior palpebral	Superior eyelid	Superior eyelid	Facial vein or angular vein and superior ophthalmic vein
superior thalamostriate (superior or terminal striate)	Deep part of the telencephalon	Corpus striatum, thalamus and corpus callosum; receives the anterior and posterior veins of the septum pellucidum, medial and lateral veins of the lateral ventricle	Great cerebral vein or internal cerebral vein
superior vein of vermis	Culmen	Culmen	Great cerebral vein
superior veins of cerebellar hemisphere	Superior surface of the vermis	Superior surface of the cerebellum	Straight sinus and internal cerebral veins
supraorbital	Forehead	Frontal belly of occipitofrontalis	Angular vein
supratrochlear (generally two in number)	Forehead	Forehead, near the median line	Angular vein
transverse facial	Cheek	Zygomatic region	Retromandibular vein or superficial temporal veins
tympanic	Middle ear	Tympanic cavity, tympanic membrane, mastoid cells, pharyngotympanic tube	Pterygoid plexus
vestibular	Internal ear	Saccule and utricle	Labyrinthine veins and vein of the vestibular aqueduct
vorticose (generally 4 or 5 in number)	Eyeball, halfway between the lamina cribrosa of the sclera and the corneoscleral junction	Choroid	Superior ophthalmic vein or inferior ophthalmic vein

N.B.: for dural venous sinuses, see the table summarizing the venous sinuses.

Cerebral veins
- superficial cerebral
- deep cerebral
- of brainstem
- cerebellar

Summary table of the veins of the neck

VEIN	ORIGIN	DRAINAGE	CONFLUENCE
anterior jugular	At the level of the hyoid bone (inferiorly anastomoses with the contralateral vein through the jugular venous arch)	Integuments and superficial muscles of the anterior region of the neck	External jugular vein
ascending cervical (anterior vertebral)	Anteriorly to the bodies and transverse processes of the cervical vertebrae, from the anterior external vertebral venous plexus	Anterior external vertebral venous plexus, prevertebral and scalene muscles	Vertebral vein
brachiocephalic (brachiocephalic venous trunk or innominate vein)	Behind the sternoclavicular joint through confluence of the internal jugular vein and subclavian vein	Head, neck, upper limb, parts of the thoracic walls and some thoracic organs	The two right and left brachiocephalic veins unite to form the superior vena cava
common facial (formal term for the inferior trunk of the facial vein that empties into the internal jugular vein)	At the level of the angle of the mandible through confluence of the facial and retromandibular veins	Territories of drainage of the facial and retromandibular veins	Internal jugular vein
deep cervical (posterior jugular)	Superior part of the posterior cervical region	Deep posterior cervical muscles; drains the suboccipital venous plexus	Brachiocephalic vein, at the point of union between the internal jugular vein and subclavian vein

continued

Summary table of the veins of the neck *(continued)*

VEIN	ORIGIN	DRAINAGE	CONFLUENCE
external jugular	Angle of the mandible through confluence of the retromandibular and posterior auricular veins	Superficial territories of the posterior region of the neck, integuments and superficial muscles of the anterior region of the neck, integuments and superficial muscles of the occipital region and the nuchal region; receives the anterior jugular, suprascapular, transverse cervical and, sometimes, occipital veins	Internal jugular vein or subclavian vein
inferior laryngeal	Posterior part of the larynx	Muscles and mucosa of the larynx	Brachiocephalic vein
inferior thyroid	Anterior surface of the isthmus of thyroid gland	Unpaired thyroid plexus	Brachiocephalic vein
internal jugular	At the level of the posterolateral part of the jugular foramen as a continuation of the transverse sinus	Cranium, cranial dura mater, brain, organs of sight and hearing, facial and deep neck structures; in the cranial tract: receives the inferior petrosal sinus, the vein of the cochlear aqueduct and the emissary veins of the internal carotid venous plexus; in the cervical tract: receives the facial, sternocleidomastoid, lingual, pharyngeal from the pharyngeal plexus, superior thyroid, middle thyroid and superior laryngeal veins	Unites with the subclavian vein to form the brachiocephalic vein
middle thyroid	Lateral surface of the thyroid gland	Inferior part of the thyroid gland; receives tributary veins from the trachea and larynx	Internal jugular vein
occipital	Posterior venous plexus of the scalp	Integuments and superficial muscles of the occipital region and the nuchal region	External jugular vein or vertebral vein
pharyngeal (several in number)	External surface of the pharynx	Pharyngeal plexus	Internal jugular vein
posterior external jugular (posterior subcutaneous vein of neck)	Occipital region	Superficial territories of the posterior region of the neck	External jugular vein
retromandibular (posterior facial)	Anterior and posterior dividing branches that unite, respectively, with the facial vein to form the common facial vein, and with the posterior auricular vein to form the external jugular vein	Territory of drainage corresponding to the territory of supply of the superficial temporal artery and part of that of the maxillary artery	Internal and external jugular veins
sternocleidomastoid	Sternocleidomastoid	Sternocleidomastoid	Internal jugular vein or superior thyroid vein
subclavian	Medial point of the clavicle	Superior regions of the thorax, upper limb, some structures of the head and neck; receives the external jugular vein	At the level of the sternoclavicular joint unites with the internal jugular vein to form the brachiocephalic vein
superior laryngeal	Larynx	Glands, muscles and mucosa of the larynx	Superior thyroid vein or internal jugular vein
superior thyroid	Superior part of the lobe of the thyroid gland	Superior part of the thyroid gland; receives the superior laryngeal and cricothyroid veins and, sometimes, sternocleidomastoid vein	Internal jugular vein
suprascapular (transverse vein of scapula)	Superior border of the scapula; often unites in a common trunk with the transverse cervical veins	Clavicle, scapula, sternocleidomastoid, subclavius, supraspinatus and subscapularis, acromioclavicular and glenohumeral joints, suprascapular region, skin over the acromion	External jugular vein
transverse cervical	Lateral cervical region; they often unite in a common trunk with the suprascapular vein	Trapezius and posterior cervical muscles	External jugular vein or, sometimes, subclavian vein
vertebral	Between the occipital bone and the atlas, from the internal vertebral venous plexuses	Internal and external vertebral venous plexuses; receives the intervertebral vein	Brachiocephalic vein

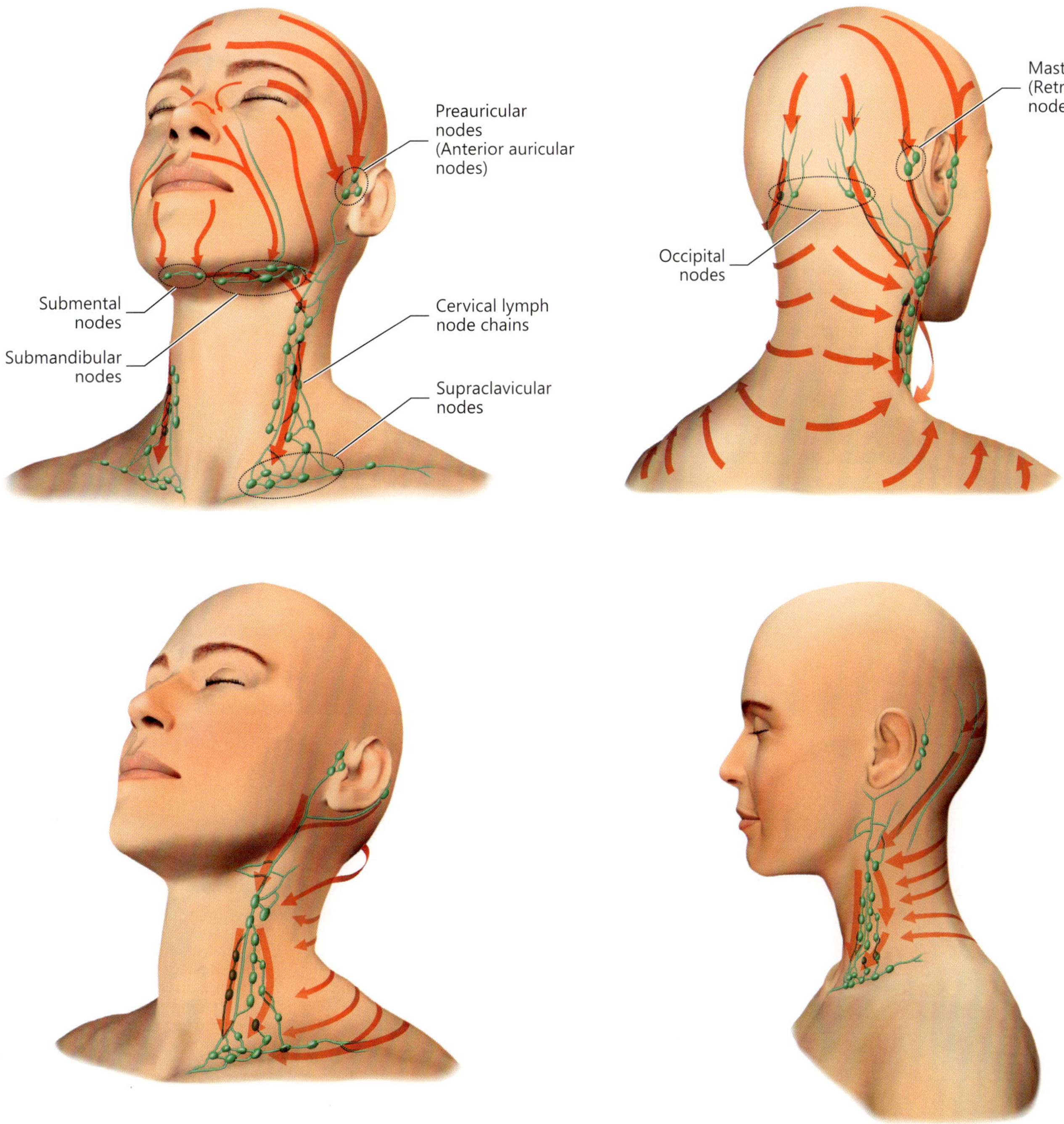

a

b

c

Lymph nodes and **lymphatic drainage of the head** and **neck**. Frontal (**a**), posterior (**b**) and lateral (**c**) views.

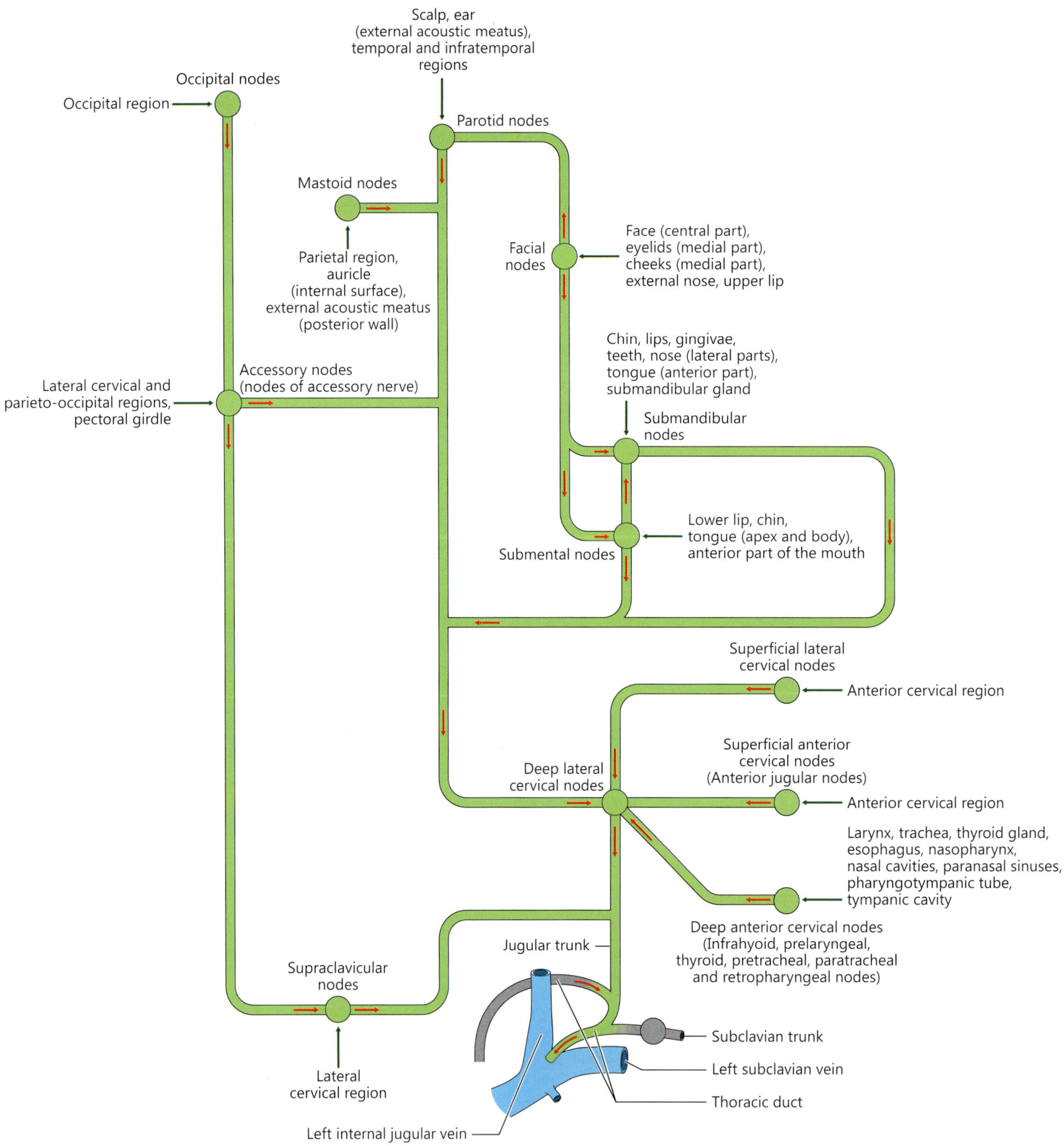

Schematic representation of the **lymphatic groups** of the **head**. Arrows indicate the direction of lymphatic flow. The principal lymphatic ducts (jugular, subclavian, bronchomediastinal, thoracic) reach the homolateral union of the subclavian and internal jugular veins into which they discharge either directly or through a common lymphatic duct.

Distribution of **lymphatic groups of the head** and **neck** in horizontal and vertical chains (dotted lines). There are two horizontal chains, superior and inferior, and four vertical chains, situated at superficial and deep levels.

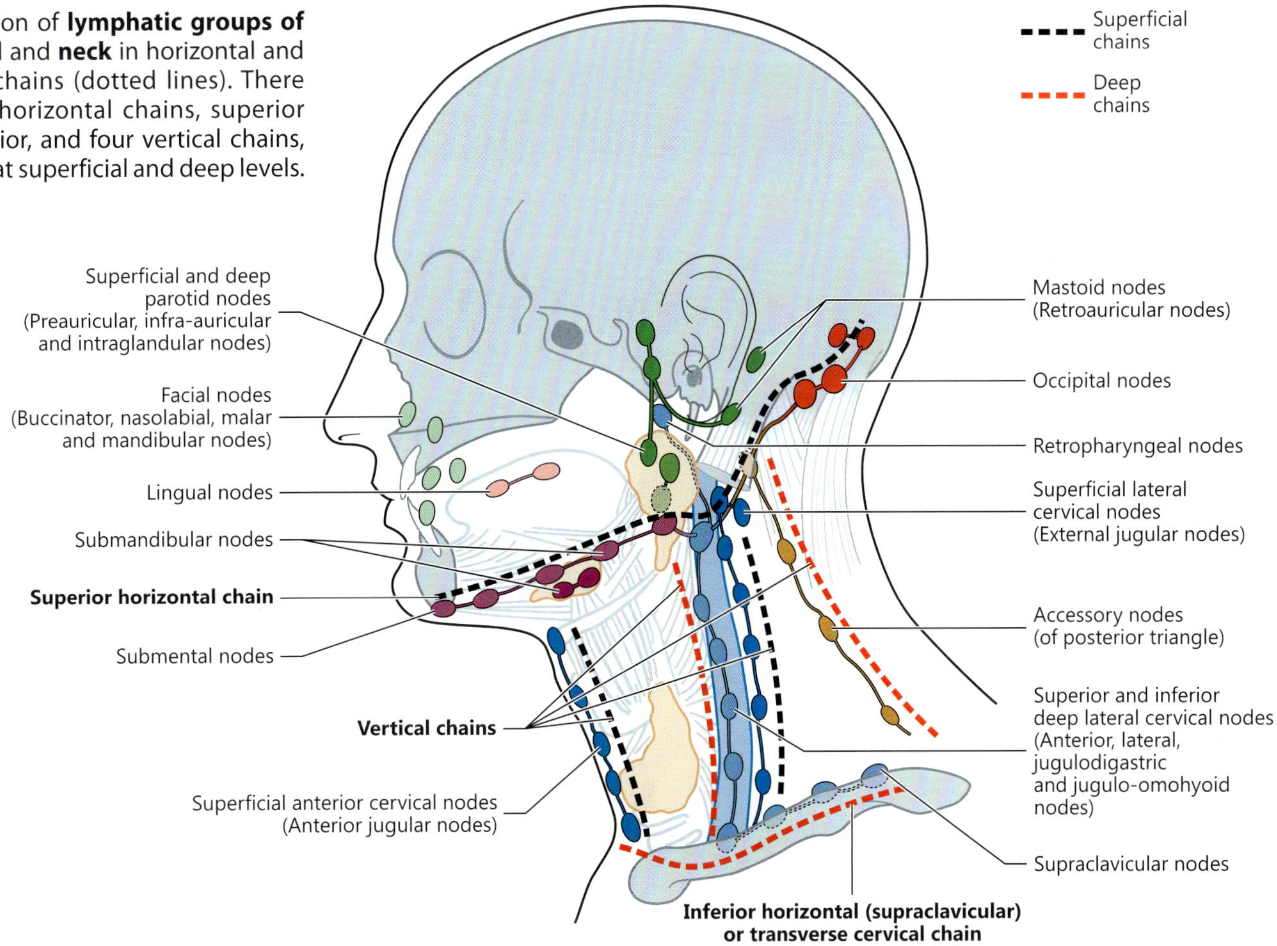

Schematic representation of **deep lymphatic groups of the head** and **neck**. The different groups, with their relative tributaries and flow pathways, are differentiated by color. Arrows indicate the direction of lymphatic flow. All lymph nodes in the region lead to the deep cervical nodes, from where the jugular trunk originates.

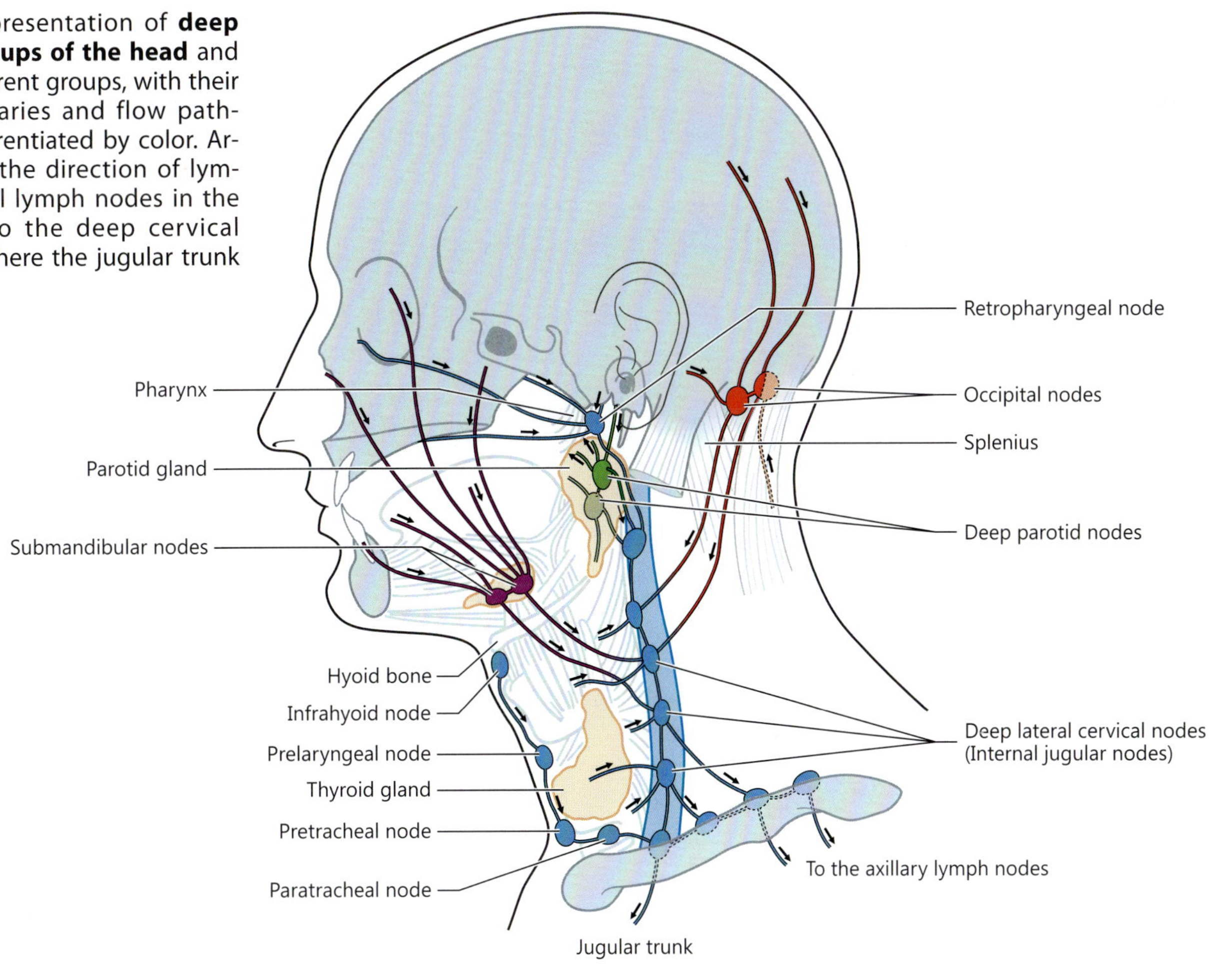

Schematic representation of **lymph node chains of** the **head** and **neck**, anterior view. The cervical nodes can be subdivided into horizontal and vertical chains consisting of diverse groups of lymph nodes. The *superior horizontal chain* includes the submental, submandibular, parotid, mastoid and occipital groups (the latter two visible in posterior view). The *vertical chains* include the superficial anterior, superficial lateral, and deep lateral cervical groups, and the accessory group (not visible here). The *inferior horizontal chain* consists of the supraclavicular, or transverse cervical, group.

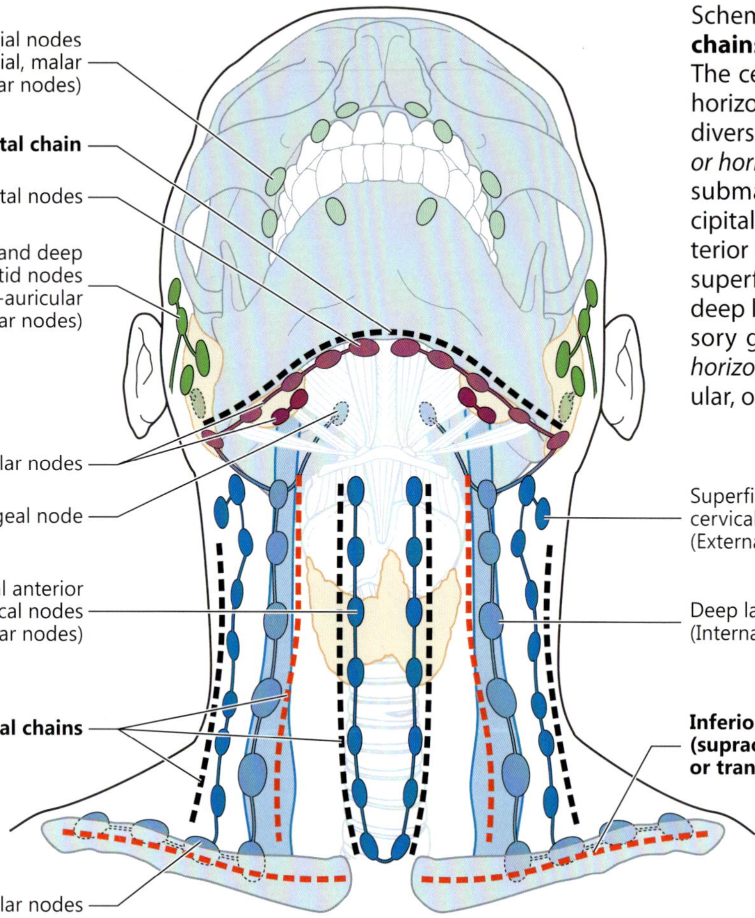

Schematic representation of the **lymph node chains of** the **head** and **neck**, posterior view. The *superior horizontal chain* includes the submental, submandibular, parotid, mastoid and occipital groups (the first three visible in anterior view). The *posterior deep vertical chain* is composed of the accessory nodes (of posterior triangle); the other chains (not visible here) are formed by the superficial anterior and superficial lateral cervical nodes, and by the deep lateral cervical nodes.

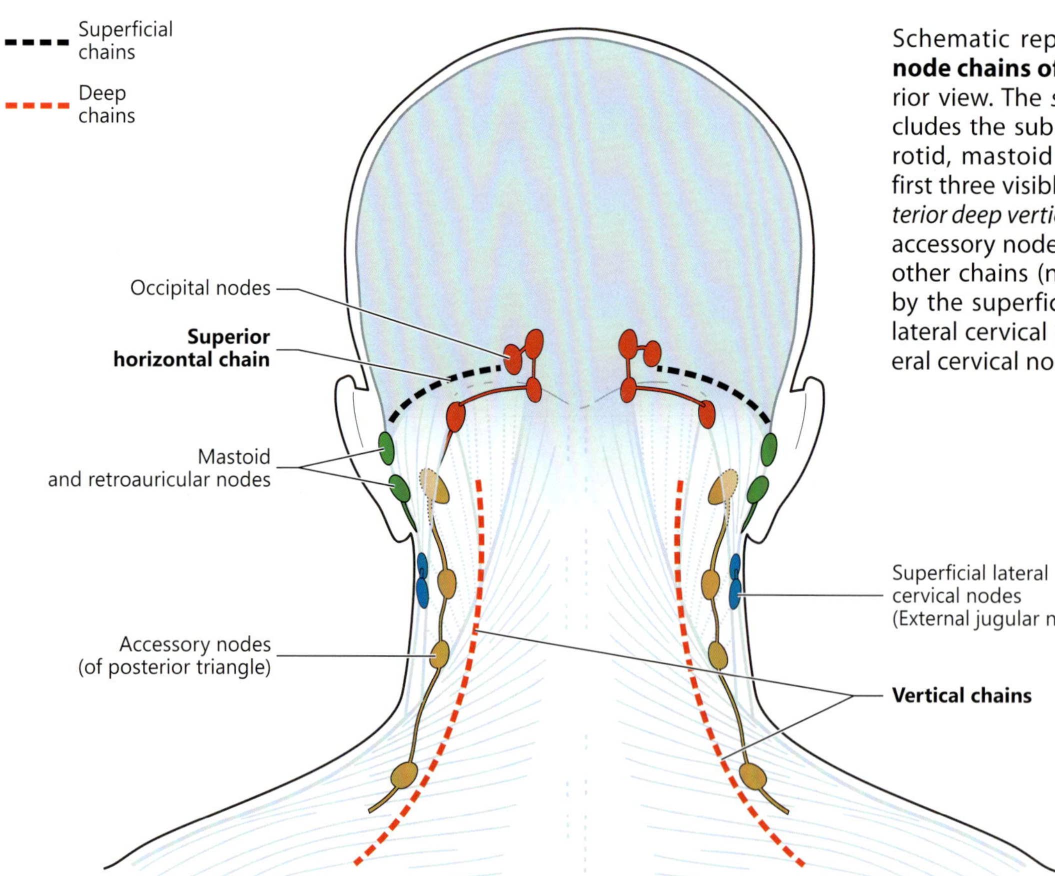

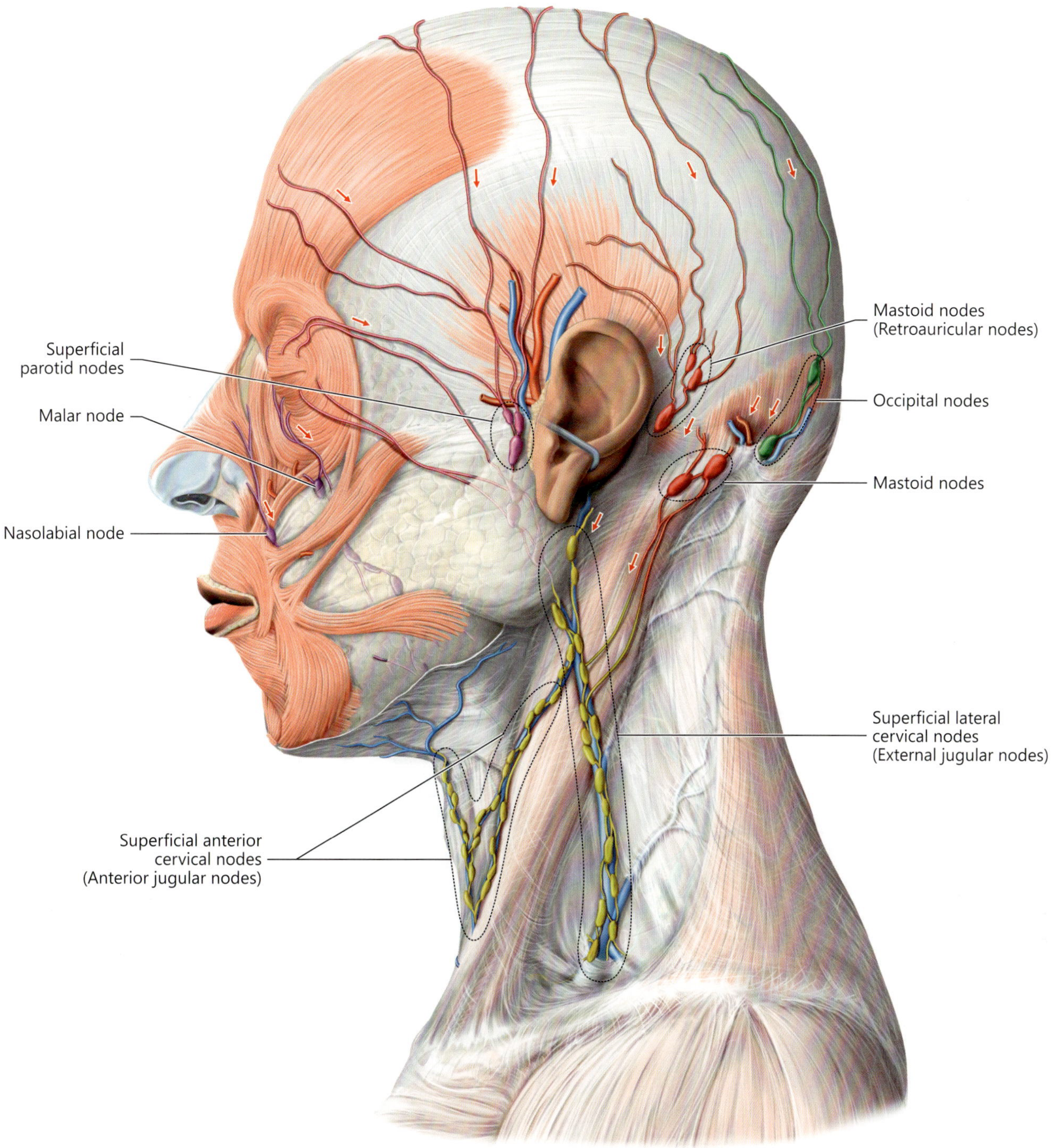

Lymph nodes of the **head** and **neck**. The cervicocephalic nodes are situated at superficial and deep levels. The **superficial parotid nodes** are located anteriorly to the tragus, above the parotid fascia. The **mastoid nodes**, which include also the **retroauricular nodes**, are located superficially to the origin of the sternocleidomastoid. The **occipital nodes** are situated superficially to the origin of the descending part of the trapezius. **Cervical nodes** are found also along the external jugular vein, superficially with respect to the sternocleidomastoid (**external jugular nodes**), and along the anterior jugular vein (**anterior jugular nodes**). The **malar node**, located superficially near the zygomaticus minor, and the **nasolabial node**, also superficial, located deep to the nasolabial sulcus, belong to the lymph nodes of the face (**facial nodes**).

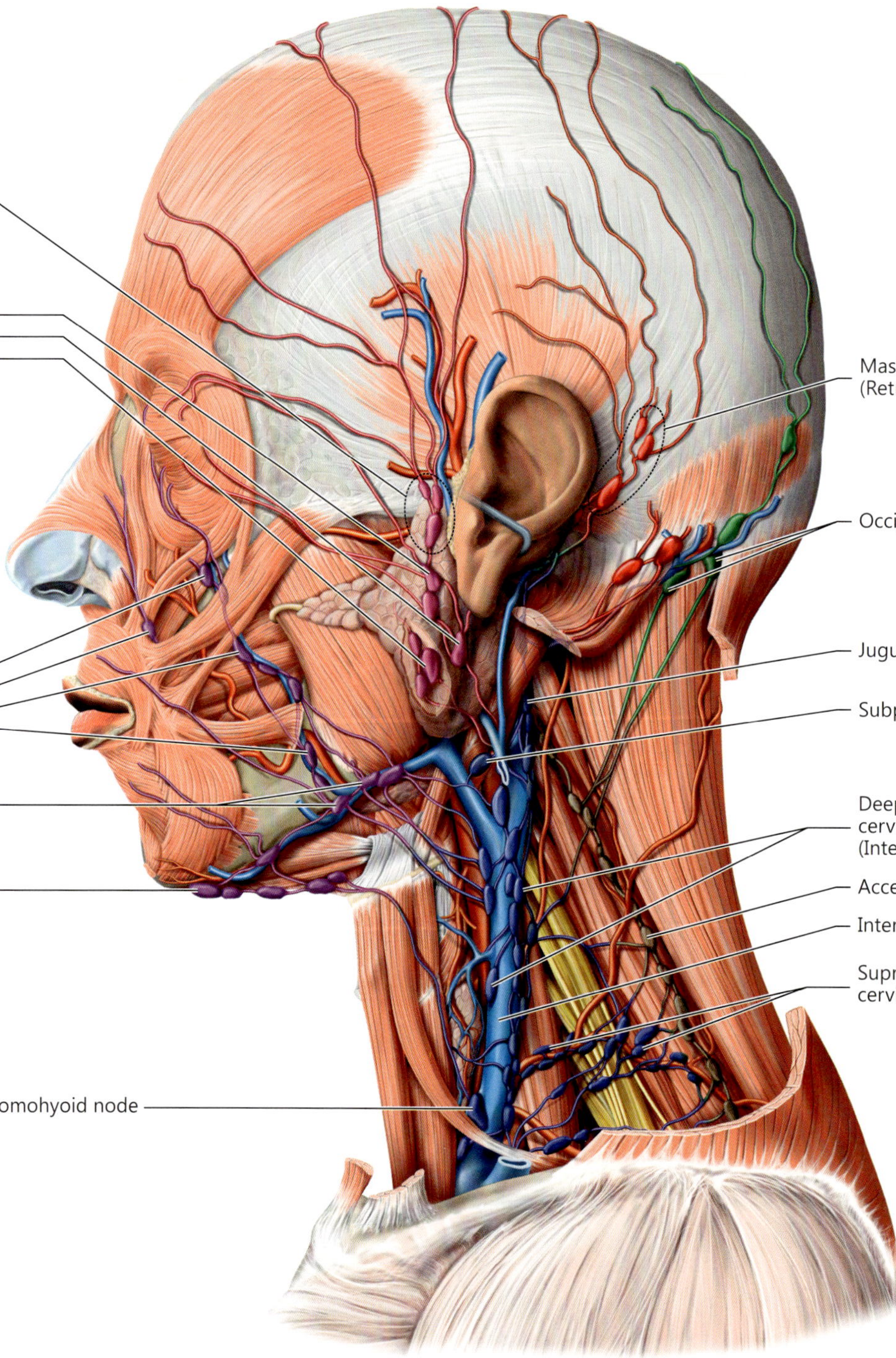

Lymph nodes of the **head** and **neck**. The **deep parotid nodes** are located beneath the parotid fascia at the preauricular and infra-auricular sites and inside the parotid gland (**intraglandular nodes**). The lymph nodes of the face (**facial nodes**) include, besides the **malar** and **nasolabial nodes**, also the **buccinator node**, on the surface of the buccinator, and **mandibular node**, situated in front of the masseter. In the submandibular triangle, at a deeper level with respect to the investing layer of cervical fascia, are the **submandibular nodes**, located on the superior face of the submandibular gland. The **submental nodes** are located on the inferior surface of the mylohyoid, between the anterior bellies of the digastric muscles. Located along the course of the internal jugular vein are the **deep lateral cervical nodes** (**internal jugular nodes**), as well as the **jugulodigastric node**, in the triangle bounded by the posterior belly of the digastric, the internal jugular vein and the facial vein, and **jugulo-omohyoid node**, situated at the level of the intermediate tendon of the omohyoid. The **accessory nodes**, along the anterior border of the trapezius, follow the path of the accessory nerve and from the upper extremity of the internal jugular nodal chain travel downward and posteriorly until they are below the trapezius. The **supraclavicular nodes** or **transverse cervical artery nodes** follow the path of the transverse cervical artery.

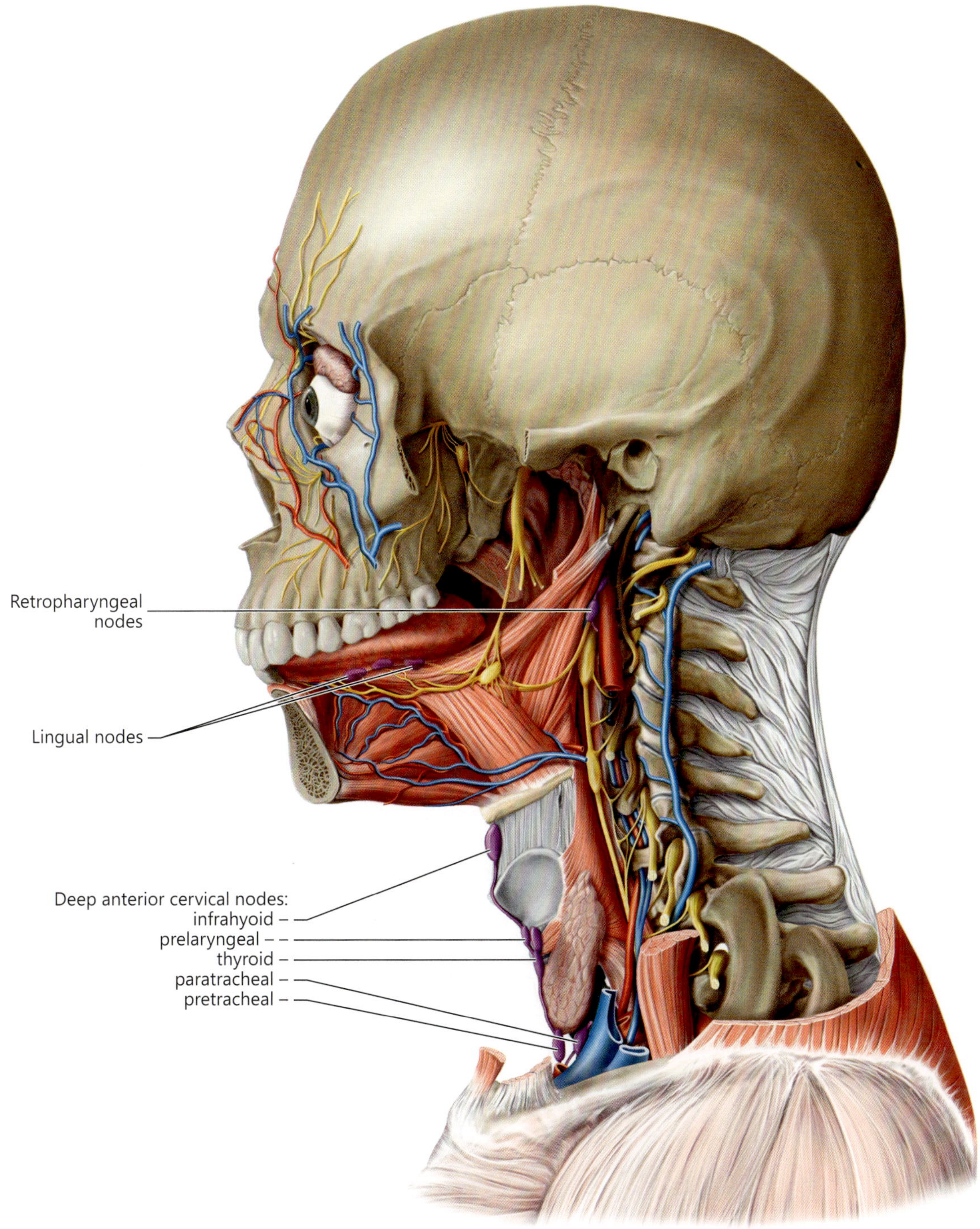

Lymph nodes of the **head** and **neck**. The deep anterior cervical nodes comprise the **infrahyoid nodes**, which include the **prelaryngeal nodes**, and the **thyroid**, **pretracheal** and **paratracheal nodes**, together defined also as anterior visceral nodes. The **retropharyngeal nodes** (these, too, are deep anterior cervical nodes) are situated above, between the posterolateral wall of the pharynx and the prevertebral layer of cervical fascia, on the adventitia that covers the posterior part of the nasopharynx. The **lingual nodes**, when present, lie on the external surface of the hyoglossus and between the two genioglossus muscles or along the lingual vein.

Summary table of the lymph nodes of the head

LYMPH NODE	*GROUP*	*SITE*	*AFFERENTS*	*EFFERENTS*
Deep parotid	Superior horizontal chain	Deep	Scalp, external acoustic meatus, temporal and infratemporal regions	Nodes of the internal jugular vein
– infra-auricular				
– intraglandular				
– preauricular (anterior auricular)	Superior horizontal chain	Deep	Anterior part of the auricle and anterior wall of the external acoustic meatus	Nodes of the internal jugular vein
Facial		Superficial	Cheeks, lips	Superficial parotid nodes
– buccinator				
– malar				
– mandibular (supramandibular)				
– nasolabial				
Lingual (inconstant)		Deep	Inferior surface and lateral margin of the tongue, medial anterior two-thirds of the dorsum of the tongue	Superior deep cervical nodes
Mastoid (retroauricular)	Superior horizontal chain	Superficial	Parietal region, internal surface of the auricle, posterior wall of the external acoustic meatus	Nodes of the internal jugular vein
Occipital	Superior horizontal chain	Superficial	Nuchal region	Nodes of the spinal accessory nerve
Submandibular	Superior horizontal chain and level I	Superficial	Chin, lips, gingivae, teeth, lateral parts of the nose, middle third of the tongue, submandibular gland, periocular area	Nodes of the internal jugular vein and contralateral submandibular nodes
Submental	Superior horizontal chain and level I	Superficial	Lower lip, chin, apex and body of the tongue, anterior part of the mouth	Retromandibular and jugulo-omohyoid nodes
Subparotid		Deep	Scalp, external acoustic meatus, temporal and infratemporal regions	Nodes of the internal jugular vein
Superficial parotid	Superior horizontal chain	Superficial	Scalp, external acoustic meatus, periocular area, nasal, upper frontal, temporal and anterior auricular regions	Nodes of the internal jugular vein

Summary table of the lymph nodes of the neck

LYMPH NODE	GROUP	SITE	AFFERENTS	EFFERENTS
Accessory (nodes of posterior triangle or nodes of spinal accessory nerve)	Vertical chain, level V and posterior triangle	Deep	Lateral region of the neck and parieto-occipital region, pectoral girdle, posterior third of the tongue	Anastomosis with the deep cervical nodes and inferior horizontal chain
Anterior cervical		Superficial and deep		
– deep		Deep	Larynx, trachea, thyroid gland, esophagus	Nodes of the internal jugular vein
– – infrahyoid				
– – – prelaryngeal	Anterior visceral and level VI			
– – paratracheal	Anterior visceral			
– – pretracheal	Anterior visceral and level VI			
– – thyroid	Anterior visceral and level VI			
– superficial (anterior jugular or of anterior jugular vein)	Vertical chain	Superficial	Anterior region of the neck	Transverse cervical artery nodes and nodes of the internal jugular vein
Lateral cervical	Vertical chain	Superficial and deep		
– deep (of internal jugular vein or internal, anterior and posterolateral jugular)	Posterior triangle	Deep	Nodes of the external jugular vein and retropharyngeal nodes, nasal cavities, pharynx, esophagus, larynx, trachea, submental region, mandible, middle third of the tongue, nuchal region	Jugular trunk
– – superior	Superior cervical chain and level II			
– – – lateral				
– – – anterior				
– – – jugulodigastric (subdigastric)		Deep	Palatine tonsil, retromolar triangle, posterior third of the tongue	Jugular trunk
– – middle	Middle cervical chain and level III			
– – inferior	Inferior cervical chain and level IV			
– – – laterale				
– – – anteriori				
– – – jugulo-omohyoid		Deep	Anterior part of the tongue	Jugular trunk
– superficial (of external jugular vein or external jugular)		Superficial	Lateral region of the neck, periocular area, nasal regions	Transverse cervical artery nodes and nodes of the internal jugular vein
Retropharyngeal		Deep	Nasopharynx, nasal cavities, paranasal sinuses, pharyngotympanic tube, tympanic cavity	Transverse cervical artery nodes and nodes of the internal jugular vein
Supraclavicular (transverse cervical artery nodes or nodes of transverse cervical chain)	Inferior horizontal (supraclavicular) chain, level V and posterior triangle	Deep	Collectors from the paraspinal and subclavicular nodes, lymph of the mammary region and of the upper limb	Subclavian nodes (apical axillary)

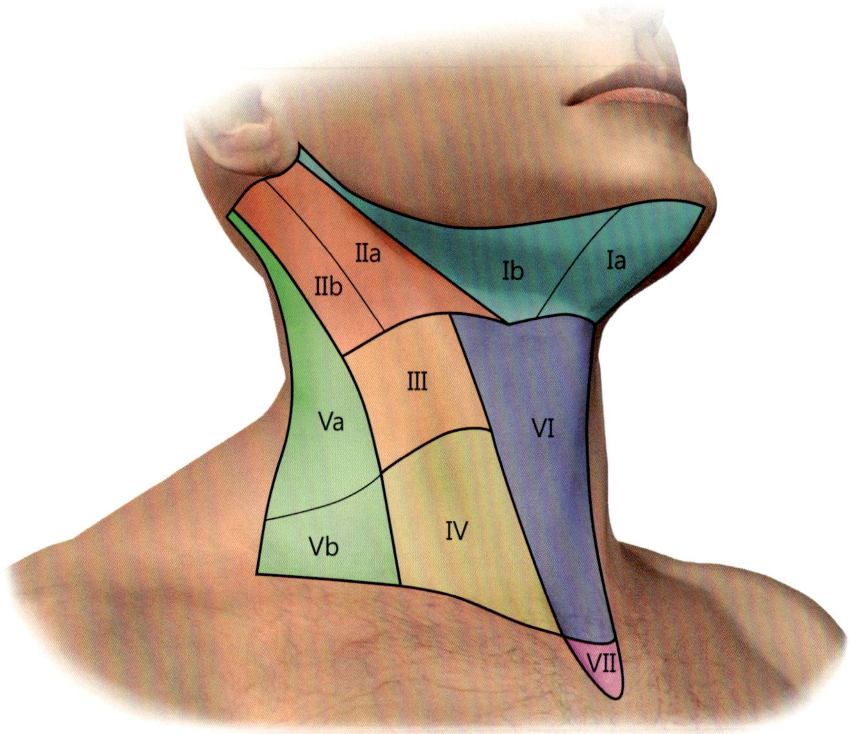

Simplified classification of the clinically palpable **lymphatic groups** of **head** and **neck**. The seven levels of subdivision identified are listed in the table below.

Levels of subdivision of the lymphatic groups of the head and neck

LEVEL	*GROUP*	*CHAIN*
I	Submental and submandibular	Superior horizontal
a	submental	
b	submandibular	
II	Superior deep lateral cervical, including the jugulodigastric node	Superior cervical (upper part of the internal jugular chain or vertical chain of superficial and deep lateral cervical nodes)
a	superior deep lateral cervical	
b	jugulodigastric	
III	Middle deep lateral cervical, including the jugulo-omohyoid node	Middle cervical (middle part of the internal jugular chain or vertical chain of superficial and deep lateral cervical nodes)
IV	Inferior deep lateral cervical	Inferior cervical (lower part of the internal jugular chain or vertical chain of superficial and deep lateral cervical nodes)
V	Accessory (or of posterior triangle), supraclavicular (or transverse cervical artery)	Vertical of the accessory nodes and inferior horizontal supraclavicular or transverse cervical
a	accessory (or of posterior triangle)	
b	supraclavicular (or transverse cervical artery)	
VI	Deep anterior cervical: thyroid, prelaryngeal and pretracheal nodes	
VII	Paratracheal and juxtaesophageal	

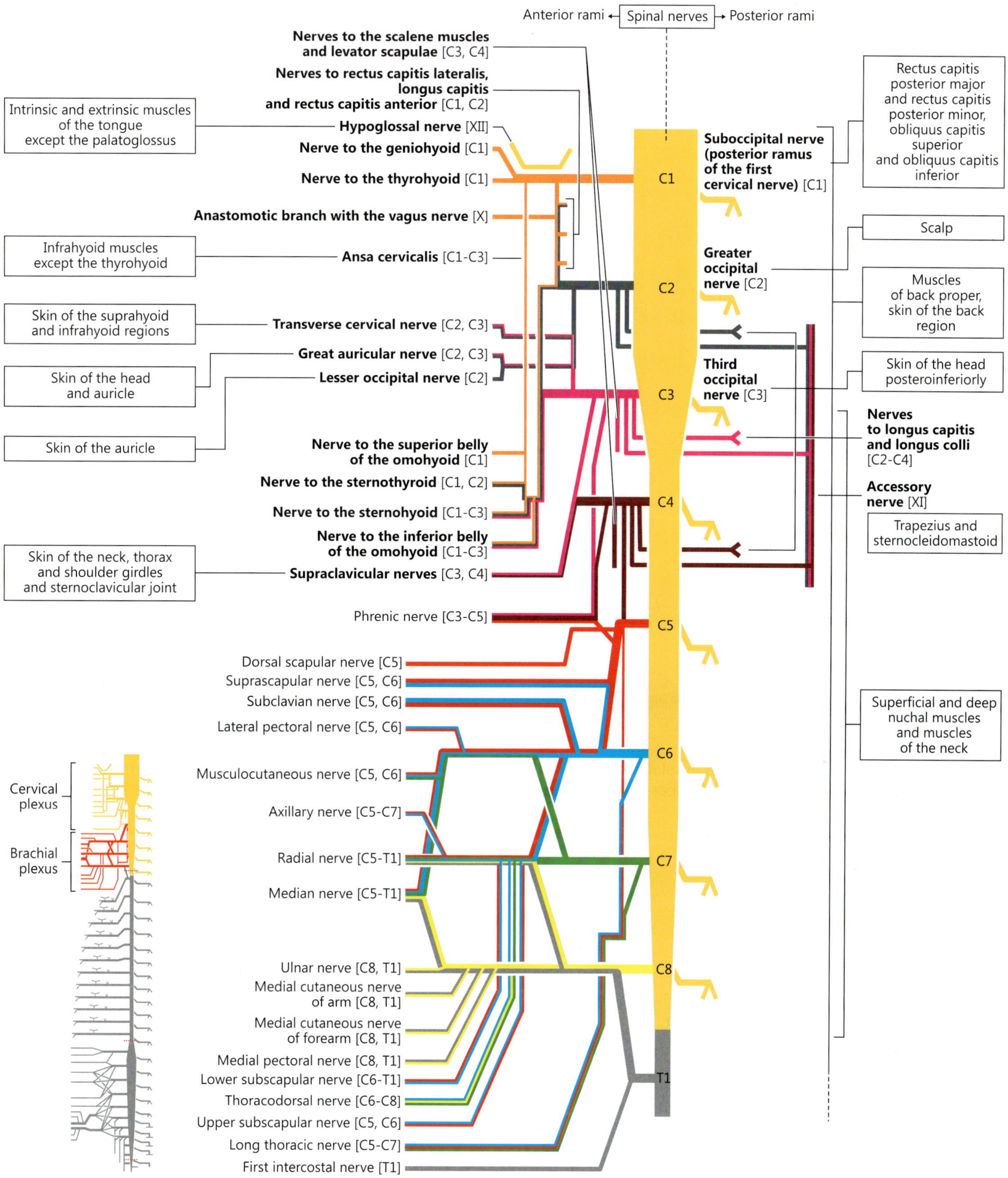

Schematic representation of the **cervical** and **brachial plexuses**. On the left-hand side of the image, at the top, the cervical plexus is represented. It is formed by the anterior rami of the first four cervical nerves. Note that each anterior ramus, with the exception of the first cervical nerve [C1], divides into an ascending and descending branch, which unite with the corresponding branches of contiguous nerves to constitute the cervical loops; the descending branch of the fourth cervical nerve [C4] anastomoses with the anterior ramus of the fifth cervical nerve [C5], which is part of the brachial plexus. The lower part of the diagram, on the left, shows the brachial plexus. It is composed of the anterior rami of the fifth, sixth, seventh and eighth cervical nerves [C5, C6, C7, C8] and of the first thoracic nerve [T1] (whose anterior ramus, which unites with the anterior ramus of C8, is indicated here in *gray* since it originates in the thorax). On the right-hand side of the diagram, the dorsal branches of the cervical nerves are represented.

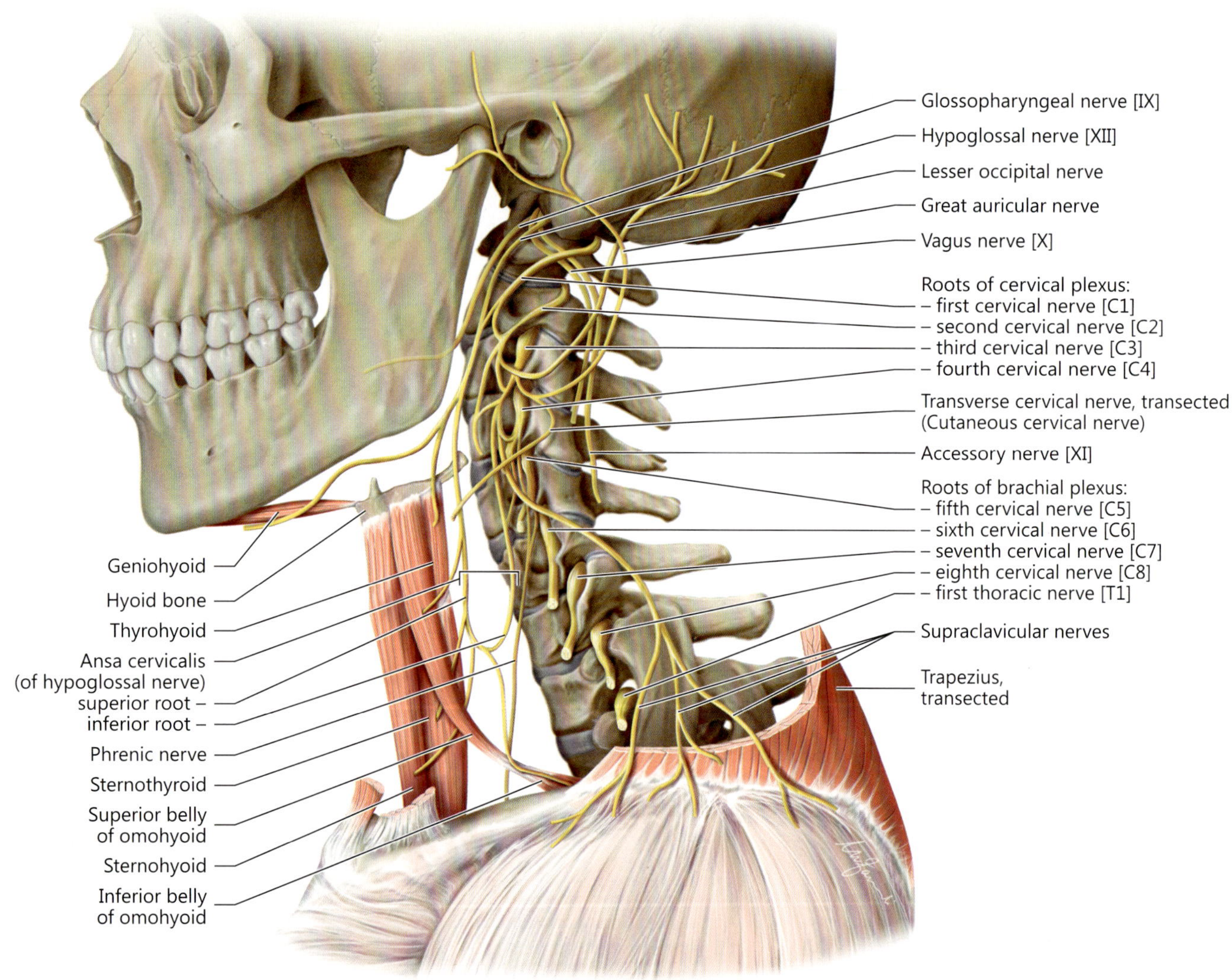

Figure showing the **cervical plexus** in relation to the skeleton of the cervical column. The relationship of the cervical plexus to the glossopharyngeal [IX], vagus [X], accessory [XI] and hypoglossal [XII] nerves can also be seen.

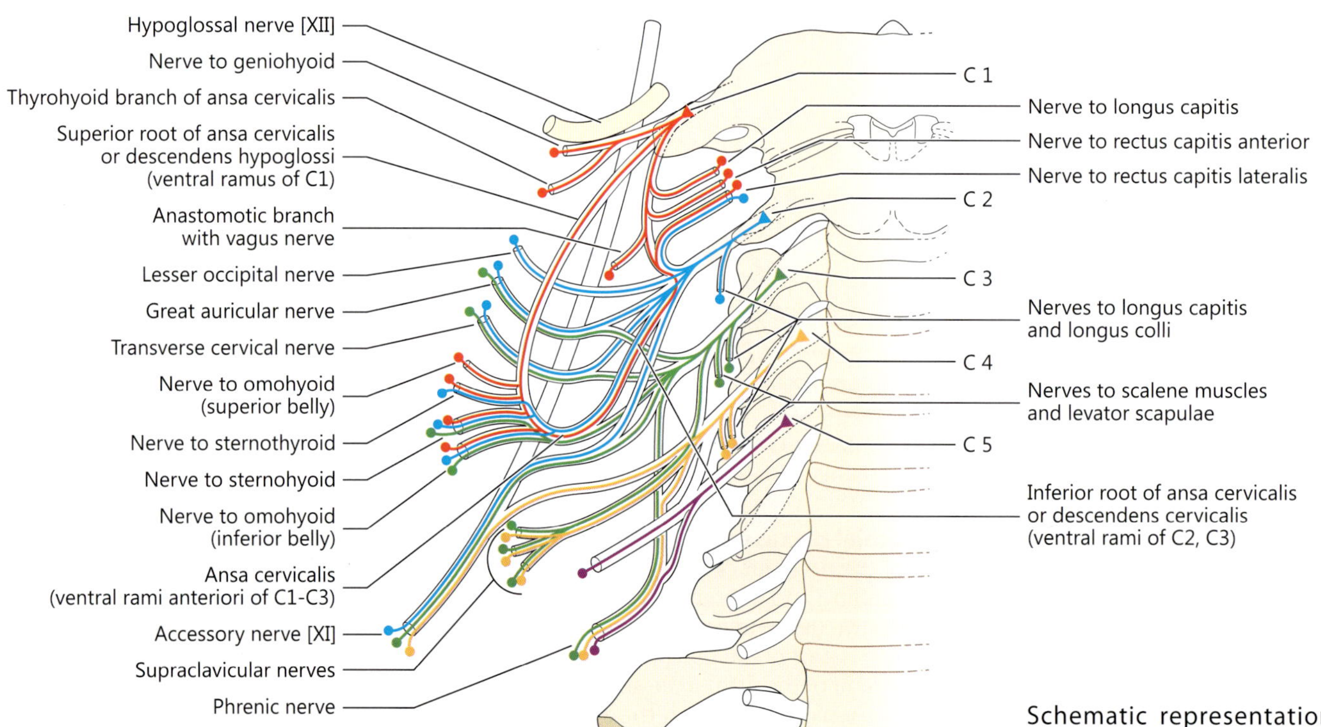

Schematic representation of the structure of the **cervical plexus**.

Figure showing the **brachial plexus** in relation to the skeleton of the vertebral column.

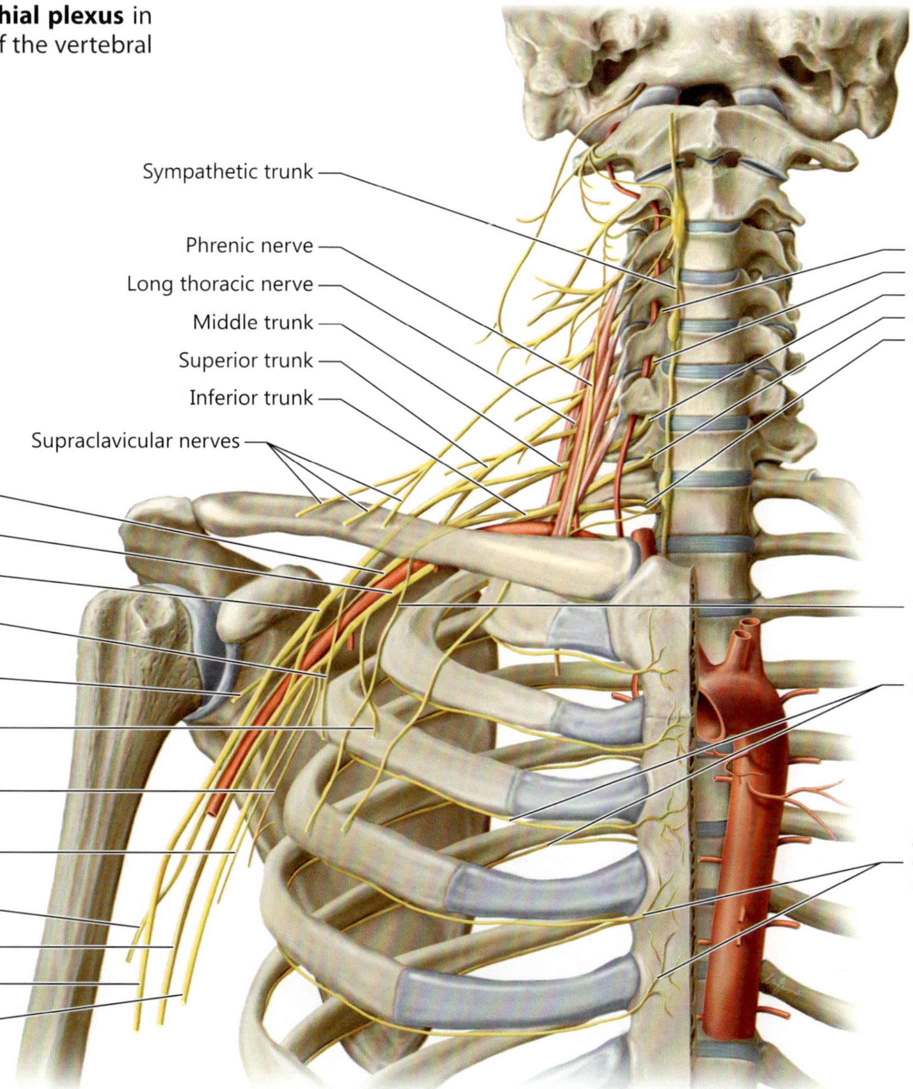

Schematic representation of the structure of the **brachial plexus**. One can see the position of the anterior branches (ant. b.), with the formation of the trunks (superior, middle and inferior) and cords, and of the posterior branches (post. b.) and terminal branches (term. b.). The phrenic nerve [C3, C4, C5] belongs to the cervical plexus; the first intercostal nerve to the thoracic nerves (anterior ramus of first thoracic nerve).

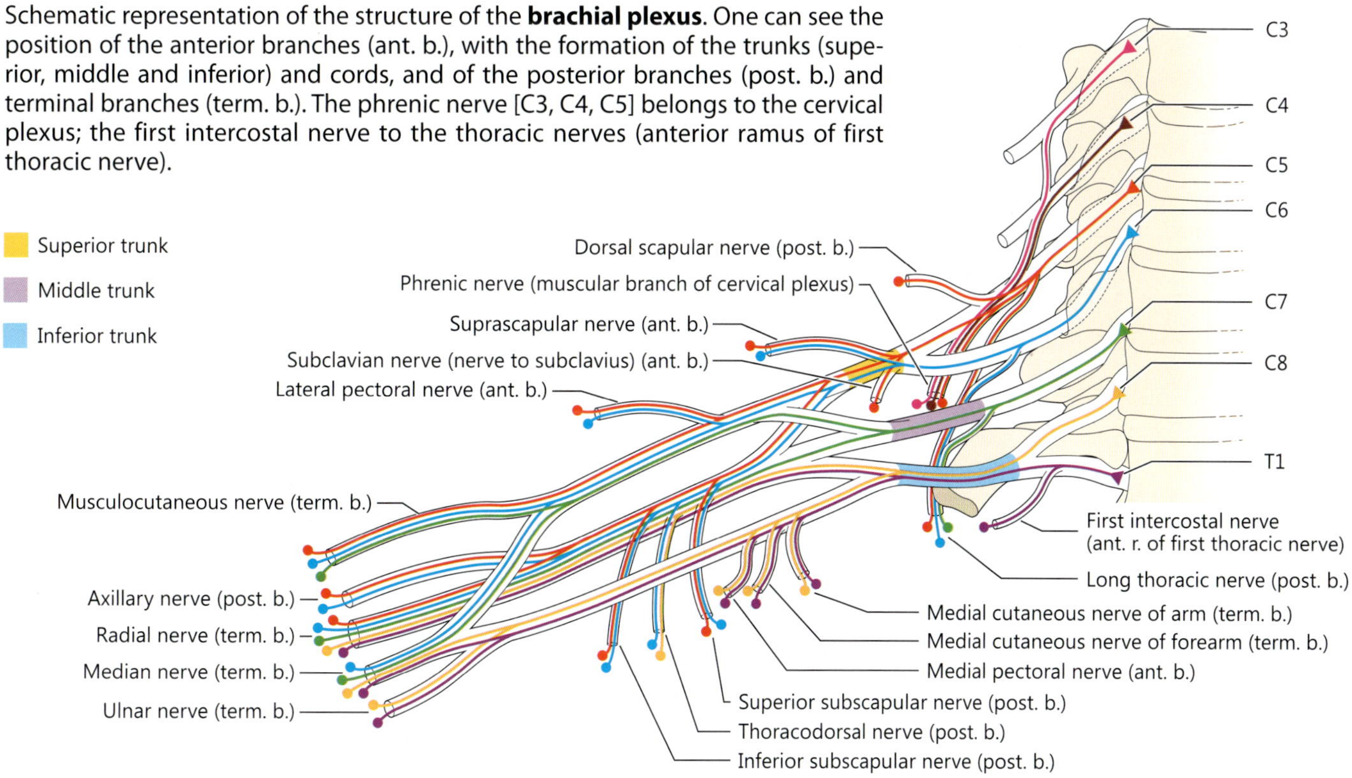

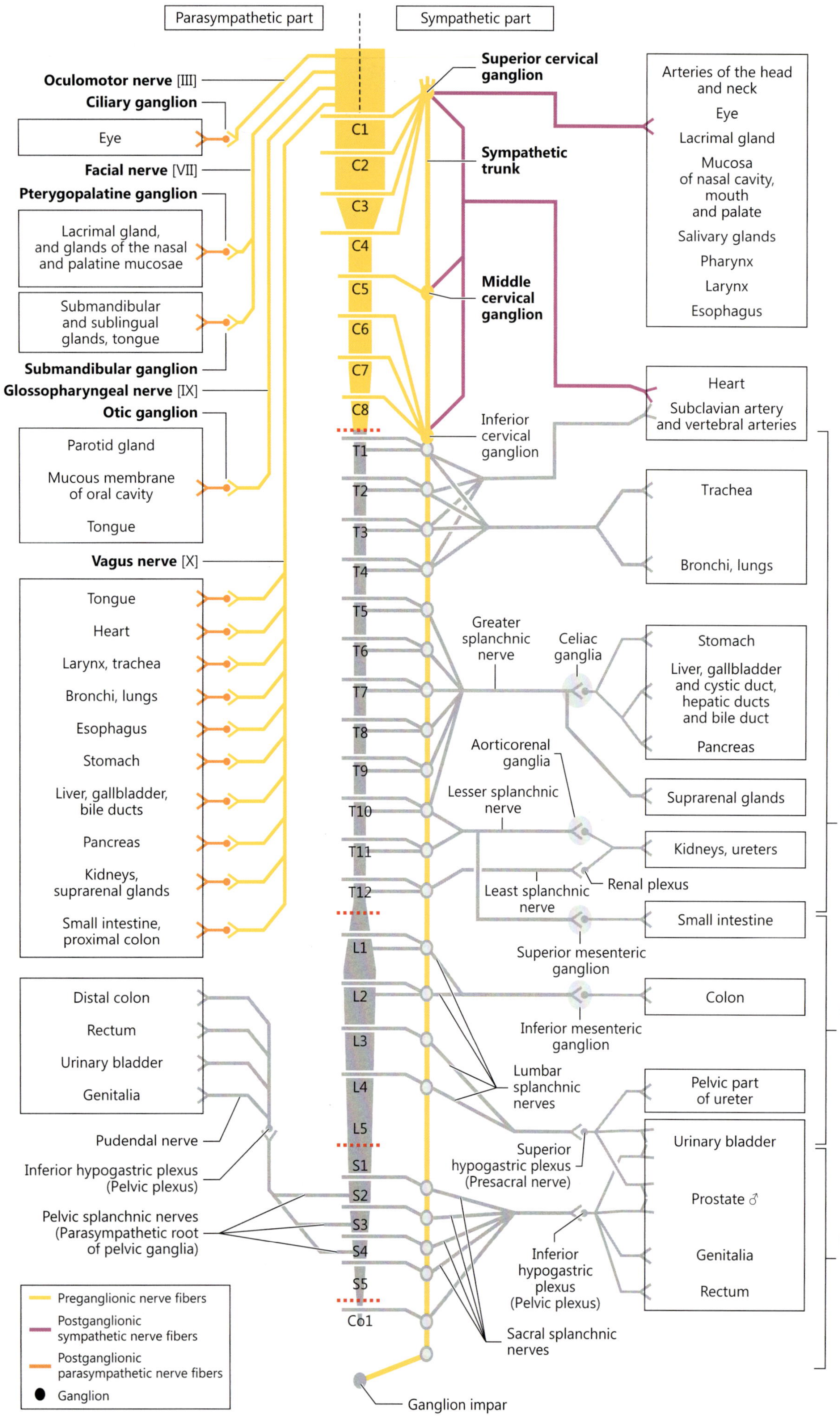

Schematic representation of the **autonomic division** composed of the sympathetic nervous system (on the right) and parasympathetic nervous system (on the left). The autonomic division is the part of the central nervous system that controls the secretory functions of glands and wall motility of internal organs and vessels, thus regulating the vital functions of the organs and all body systems. The organs that are innervated by nerve fibers of the autonomic division are listed, in detail, in the boxes. The preganglionic nerve fibers are represented in *yellow*; in *purple*, the postganglionic fibers of the sympathetic nervous system, and in *orange* those of the parasympathetic nervous system. The parasympathetic (cranial and sacral) nervous system comprises the neuraxial visceral centers situated, respectively, in the brainstem and sacral segment of the spinal cord. Note, in particular, the elevated number of visceral efferent (motor) fibers of the parasympathetic part of the vagus nerve.

Organization of the **autonomic division** in the head region. While the parasympathetic fibers travel inside the cranial nerves III, VII, IX and X, the sympathetic fibers penetrate into the cranium as plexuses that accompany the vertebral and carotid (internal and external) arteries. They can link to cranial nerves and cross parasympathetic ganglia without being interrupted.

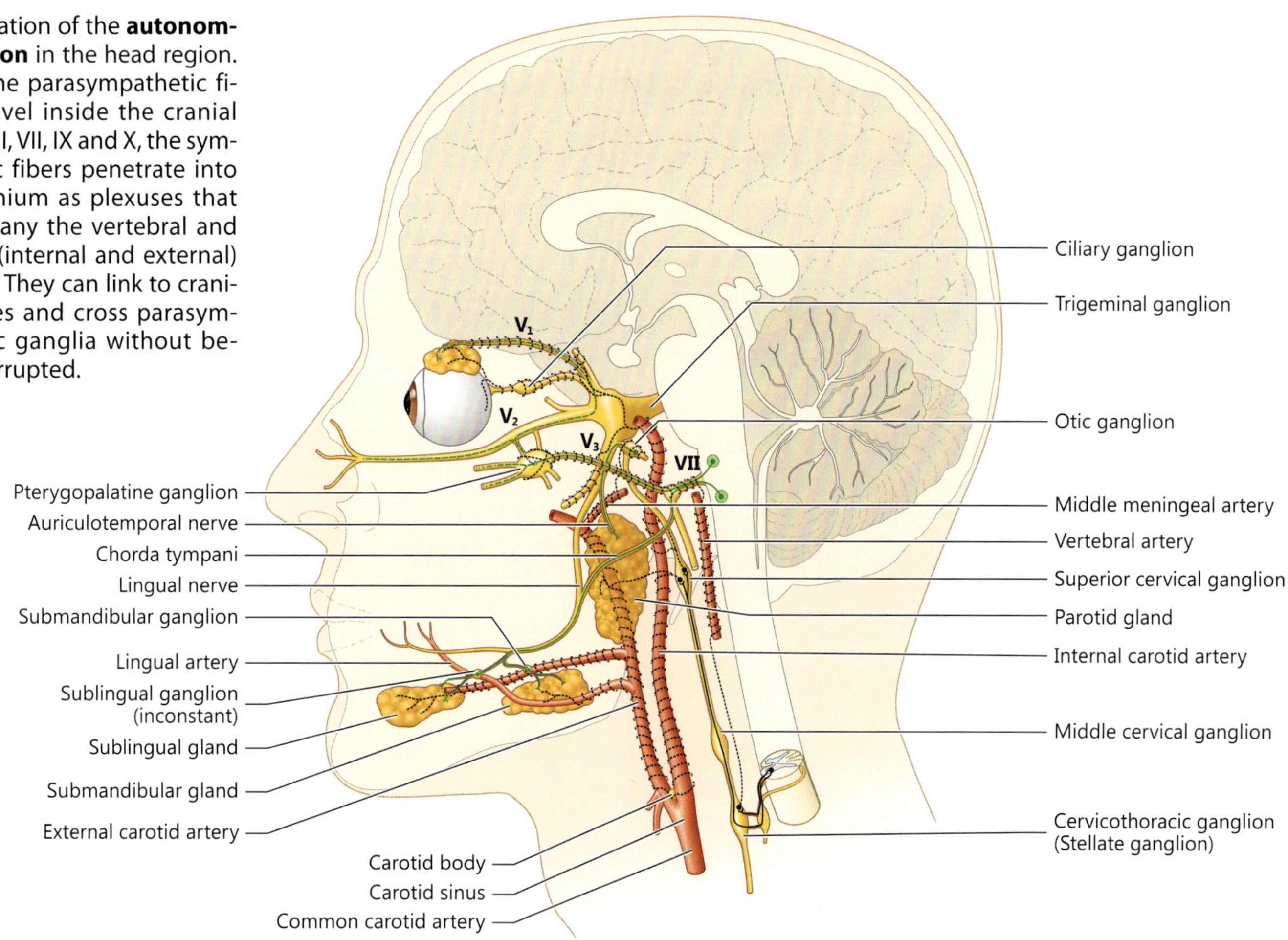

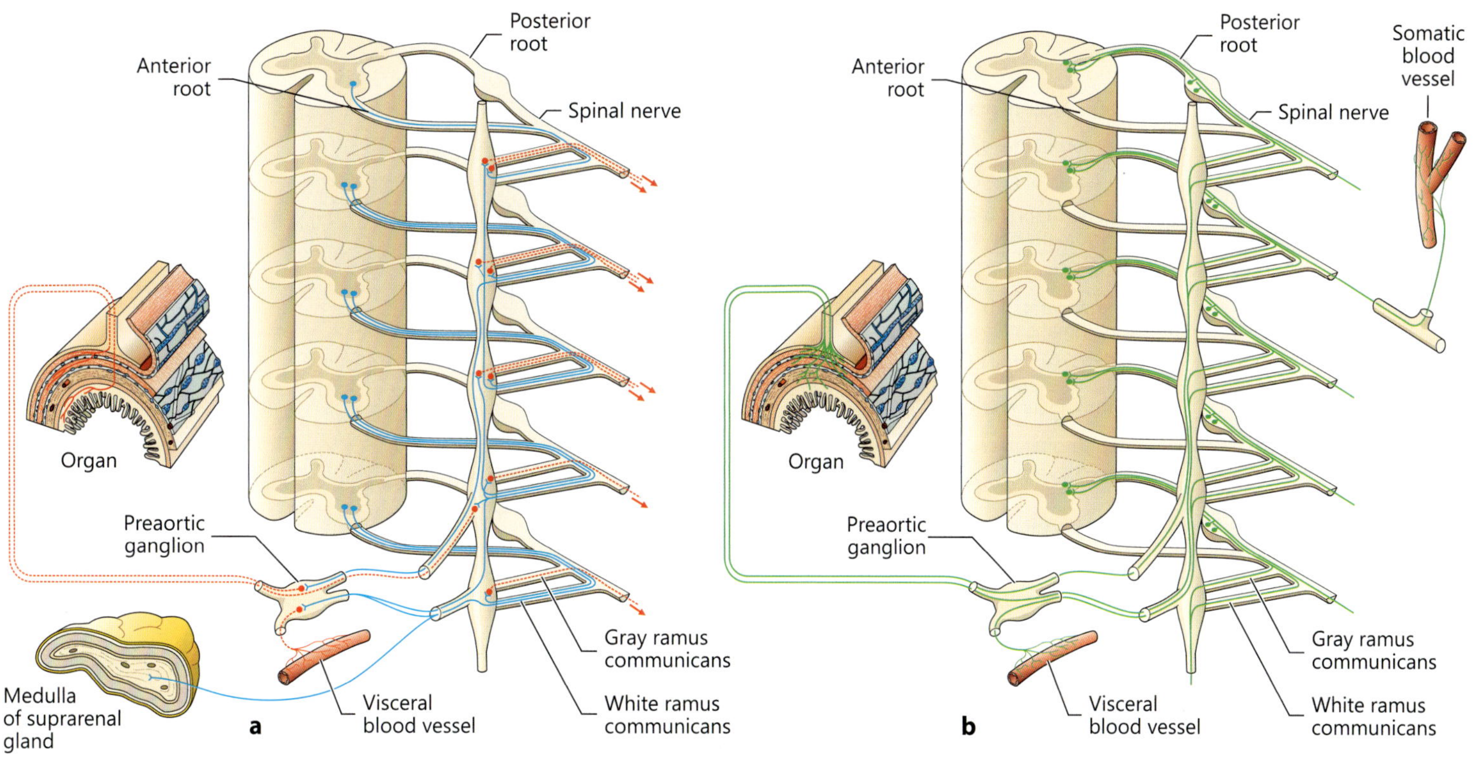

a, Peripheral distribution of the **sympathetic visceral motor fibers**. The different pathways that the preganglionic fibers (*blue*) of medullary origin can follow are indicated, as well as the possible peripheral paths of the postganglionic fibers (*red*) towards vessels and organs. **b**, Peripheral distribution of the **sympathetic visceral sensory fibers**. Localized in the spinal ganglion, together with the somatic sensory neurons, visceral sensory neurons (*green*) are distributed to the periphery with the spinal nerves or, through the trunk of the sympathetic system, with the autonomic nerves.

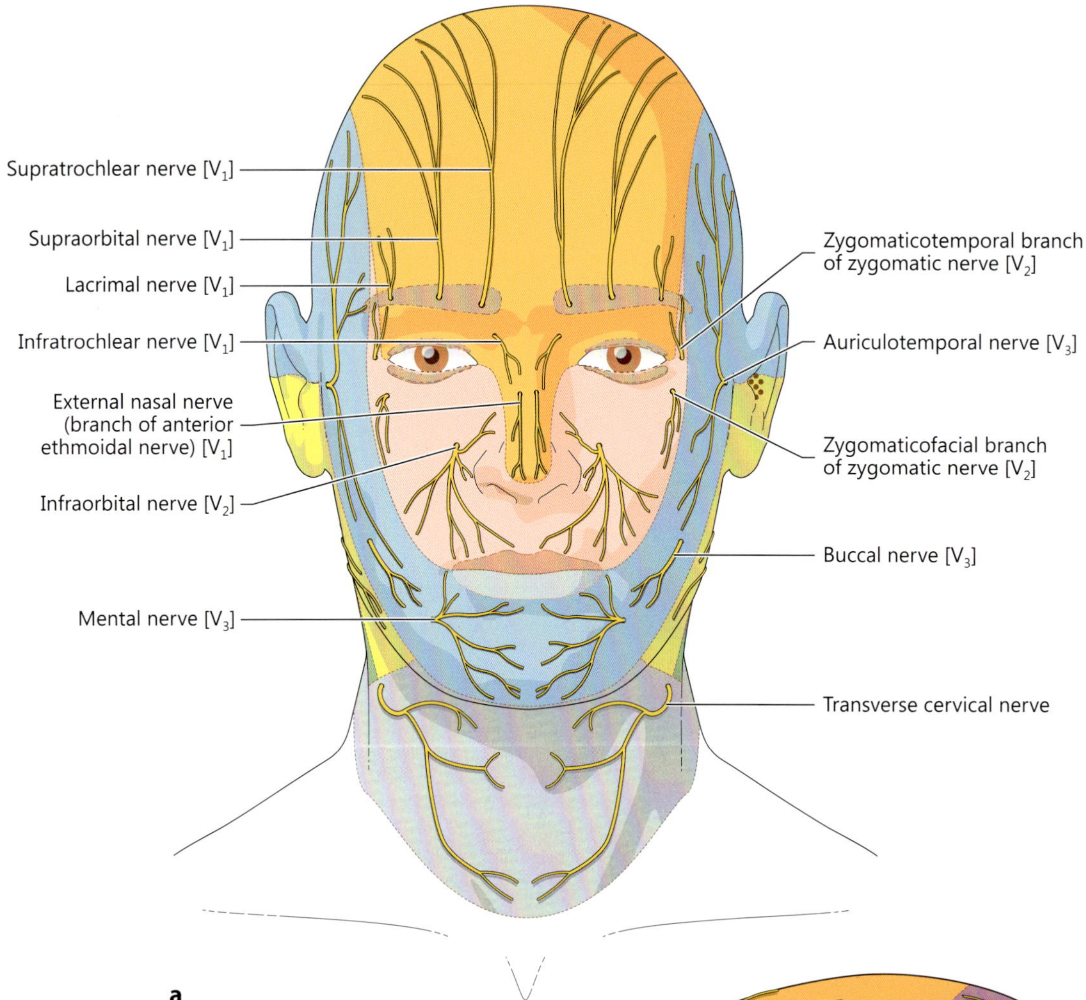

Supratrochlear nerve [V1]
Supraorbital nerve [V1]
Lacrimal nerve [V1]
Infratrochlear nerve [V1]
External nasal nerve (branch of anterior ethmoidal nerve) [V1]
Infraorbital nerve [V2]
Mental nerve [V3]
Zygomaticotemporal branch of zygomatic nerve [V2]
Auriculotemporal nerve [V3]
Zygomaticofacial branch of zygomatic nerve [V2]
Buccal nerve [V3]
Transverse cervical nerve

a

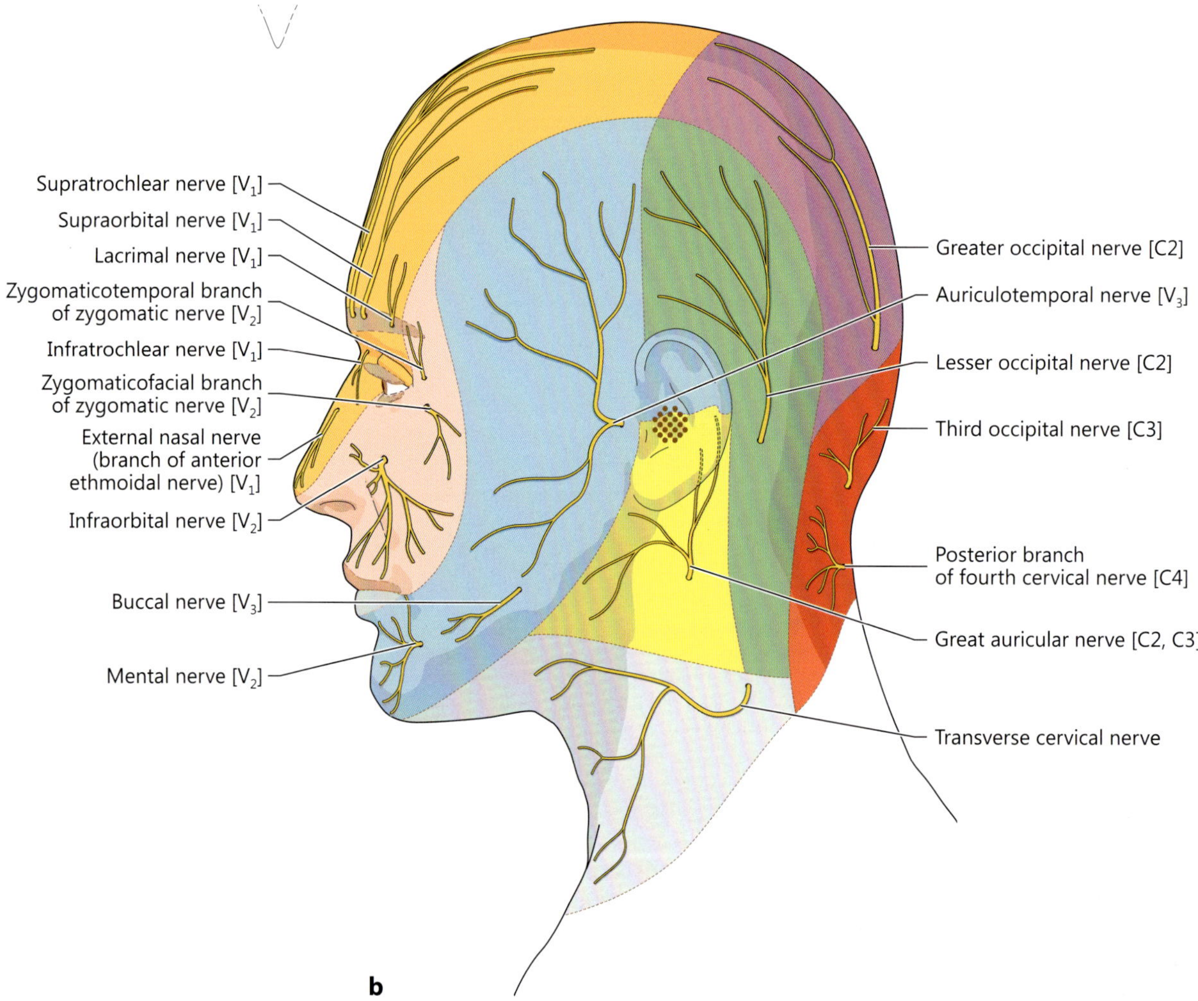

Supratrochlear nerve [V1]
Supraorbital nerve [V1]
Lacrimal nerve [V1]
Zygomaticotemporal branch of zygomatic nerve [V2]
Infratrochlear nerve [V1]
Zygomaticofacial branch of zygomatic nerve [V2]
External nasal nerve (branch of anterior ethmoidal nerve) [V1]
Infraorbital nerve [V2]
Buccal nerve [V3]
Mental nerve [V2]
Greater occipital nerve [C2]
Auriculotemporal nerve [V3]
Lesser occipital nerve [C2]
Third occipital nerve [C3]
Posterior branch of fourth cervical nerve [C4]
Great auricular nerve [C2, C3]
Transverse cervical nerve

b

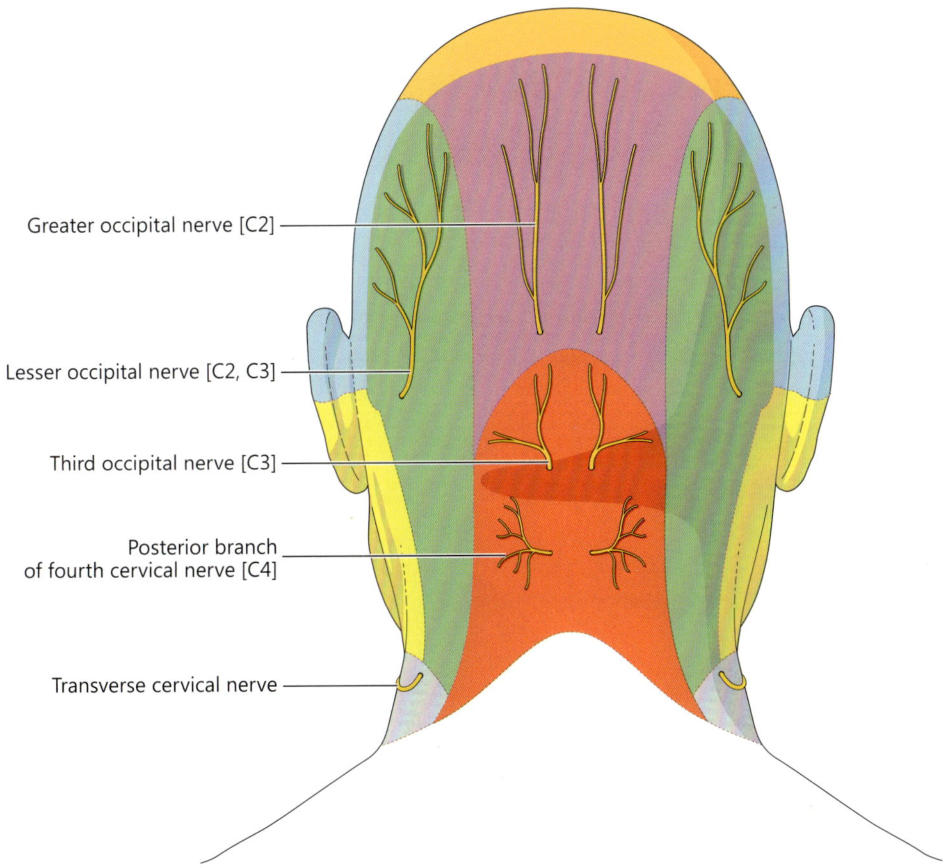

a, **Cutaneous territories of innervation of the head** and **neck**, anterior view. Indicated in *orange*, *pink* and *blue* are the areas supplied, respectively, by the ophthalmic, maxillary and mandibular nerves. In *yellow*, is the territory of distribution of the great auricular nerve (anterior rami of C2 and C3 via the cervical plexus). The dotted area, representing the skin of the concha of auricle, receives sensory fibers from the facial [VII], glossopharyngeal [IX] and vagus [X] nerves. The transverse cervical nerve innervates the skin in the suprahyoid and infrahyoid regions and lateral cervical region (in *gray*).

b, **Cutaneous territories of innervation of the head** and **neck**, left lateral view. The trigeminal nerve supplies, with its three branches, the whole face and the anterior half of the cranium. Indicated in *orange*, *pink* and *blue* are the areas supplied, respectively, by the ophthalmic, maxillary and mandibular nerves. In *yellow* is the territory of distribution of the great auricular nerve (anterior rami of C2 and C3 via the cervical plexus). The dotted area, representing the skin of the concha of auricle, receives sensory fibers from the facial [VII], glossopharyngeal [IX] and vagus [X] nerves. The transverse cervical nerve innervates the skin in the suprahyoid and infrahyoid regions and in the lateral cervical region (in *gray*).

c, **Cutaneous territories of innervation of the head** and **neck**, posterior view. Indicated in *purple*, *green* and *red* are the areas supplied by the posterior and anterior rami of the cervical nerves: respectively, the greater occipital nerve (posterior ramus of C2); the lesser occipital nerve (anterior ramus of C2 via the cervical plexus); and the third occipital nerve (posterior ramus of C3) and the posterior ramus of C4. Indicated in *yellow* is the territory of distribution of the great auricular nerve (anterior rami of C2 and C3 via the cervical plexus). The transverse cervical nerve innervates the skin in the suprahyoid and infrahyoid regions and in the lateral cervical region (in *gray*). Indicated in *orange* is the area supplied by the ophthalmic nerve via the supratrochlear and supraorbital nerves.

External surface of the cranial base, showing **the passage of vessels** and **nerves through the foramina**.

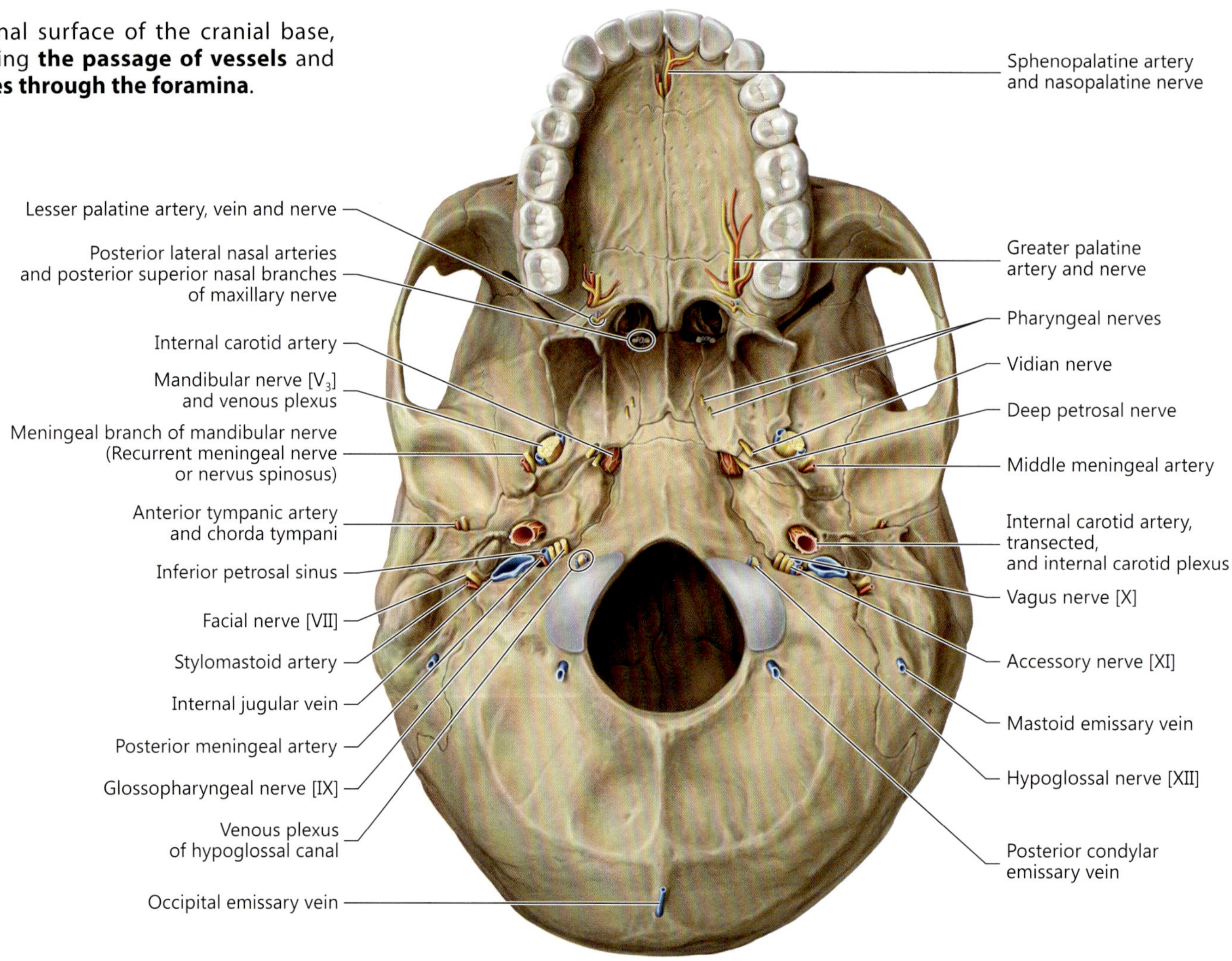

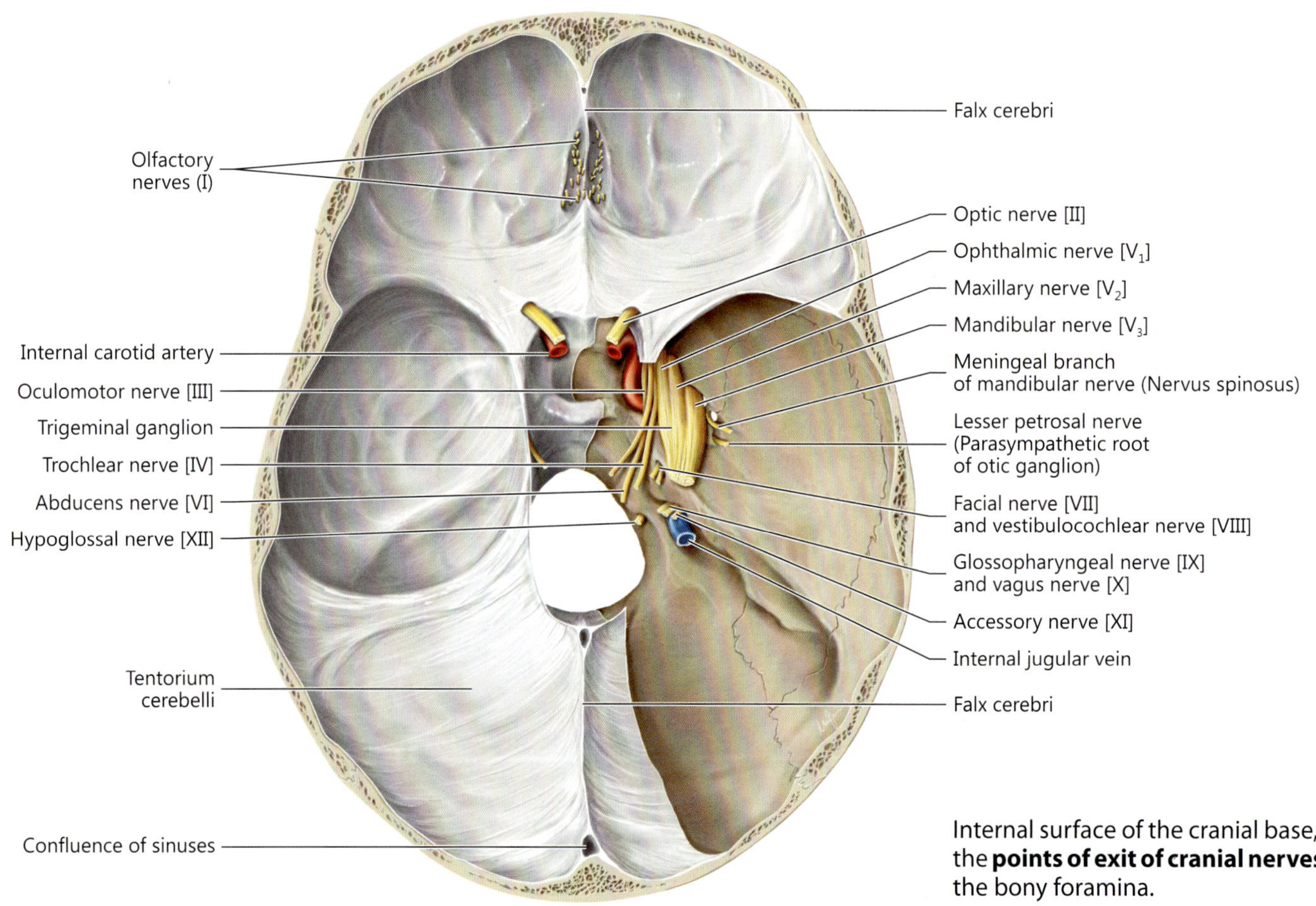

Internal surface of the cranial base, showing the **points of exit of cranial nerves** through the bony foramina.

Canals and canaliculi

CANAL OR CANALICULUS	BONE	FORMATIONS THAT PASS THROUGH IT
Alveolar canals	Maxilla	Posterior superior alveolar artery and vein; posterior superior alveolar branches of the superior alveolar nerves
Canal for auditory tube	Temporal bone	Pharyngotympanic tube (auditory tube)
Canal for tensor tympani	Temporal bone	Tensor tympani
Canaliculus for chorda tympani (petrotympanic fissure)	Temporal bone	Chorda tympani
Caroticotympanic canaliculi	Temporal bone	Caroticotympanic arteries and nerves
Carotid canal	Temporal bone	Internal carotid artery; internal carotid venous plexus; internal carotid nerve plexus
Cochlear canaliculus	Temporal bone	Perilymph
Condylar canal	Occipital bone	Condylar emissary vein
Diploic canals	Diploë	Diploic veins
Facial canal	Temporal bone	Facial nerve [VII]
Greater palatine or pterygopalatine canal	Maxilla and palatine bone	Greater palatine and lesser palatine arteries and veins, greater palatine nerve and lesser palatine nerves
Hypoglossal canal	Occipital bone	Meningeal branch of the ascending pharyngeal artery; emissary vein from the sigmoid sinus to the internal jugular vein; hypoglossal nerve [XII]; meningeal branch of the hypoglossal nerve
Incisive canals	Maxilla	Sphenopalatine artery and veins; nasopalatine nerve
Infraorbital canal	Maxilla	Infraorbital and anterior superior alveolar arteries; infraorbital nerve and middle superior and anterior superior alveolar branches of the superior alveolar nerves
Lesser palatine canals	Palatine bone	Lesser palatine arteries, veins and nerves
Mandibular canal	Mandible	Inferior alveolar artery, vein and nerve
Mastoid canaliculus	Temporal bone	Auricular branch of the vagus nerve (at entry)
Musculotubal canal	Temporal bone	Septum of musculotubal canal; canal for auditory tube and canal for tensor tympani
Nasolacrimal canal	Inferior nasal concha, maxilla and lacrimal bone	Nasolacrimal duct
Optic canal	Sphenoid	Ophthalmic artery, central retinal vein; optic nerve [II], autonomic nerve fibers
Palatovaginal or pharyngeal canal	Sphenoid and palatine bone	Pharyngeal branch of the artery of pterygoid canal and of the descending palatine artery; branches of pterygopalatine ganglion and pharyngeal nerve
Pterygoid or vidian canal	Sphenoid	Artery, vein and nerve of the pterygoid canal (mixed sympathetic and parasympathetic nerve)
Tympanic canaliculus	Temporal bone	Tympanic nerve (from the glossopharyngeal nerve [IX])
Vestibular canaliculus	Temporal bone	Vestibular aqueduct containing the endolymphatic sac
Vomerorostral or vomerobasilar canal	Sphenoid and vomer	Small veins
Vomerovaginal canal	Sphenoid and, at times, vomer	Branch of the sphenopalatine artery; branches of the pterygopalatine ganglion

Fissures

FISSURE	BONE	FORMATIONS THAT PASS THROUGH IT
Inferior orbital fissure	Sphenoid and maxilla	Infraorbital artery and vein; inferior ophthalmic vein; infraorbital and zygomatic nerves from the maxillary nerve [V_2]; branches of pterygopalatine ganglion
Petrotympanic fissure	Temporal bone	Chorda tympani through a small patent portion, the canaliculus for chorda tympani
Superior orbital fissure	Sphenoid	Superior ophthalmic vein; oculomotor nerve [III], trochlear nerve [IV], lacrimal, frontal and nasociliary nerves (from the ophthalmic nerve, V_1), abducens nerve [VI]
Tympanomastoid fissure	Temporal bone	Auricular branch of vagus nerve (at exit)

Foramina

FORAMEN	BONE	FORMATIONS THAT PASS THROUGH IT
Anterior and posterior incisive foramina	Maxilla	Sphenopalatine artery and vein; left and right nasopalatine nerves
Anterior ethmoidal foramen	Ethmoid	Anterior ethmoidal artery; ethmoidal veins; anterior ethmoidal nerve
Cribriform foramina	Ethmoid	Olfactory nerves [I] (from the nasal cavity to the anterior cranial fossa)
Foramen cecum	Frontal bone	Pharyngeal veins, pterygoid venous plexus, vein from the mucosa of the nasal cavity to the superior sagittal sinus
Foramen lacerum anterior	Sphenoid and temporal bone	Meningeal branch of the ascending pharyngeal artery; artery, vein and nerve of the pterygoid canal; internal carotid artery and greater petrosal nerve (they pass through it only in part)
Foramen magnum or great occipital foramen	Occipital bone	Continuation of the spinal cord in the myelencephalon; vertebral arteries and veins, and anterior and posterior spinal arteries and veins; spinal root of the accessory nerve
Foramen ovale	Sphenoid	Accessory and (sometimes) frontal branches of the middle meningeal artery; emissary vein from the cavernous sinus to the pterygoid plexus; mandibular nerve [V_3]; accessory meningeal nerve; lesser petrosal nerve (sometimes)
Foramen petrosum (not always present)	Temporal bone	Lesser petrosal nerve
Foramen rotundum	Sphenoid	Maxillary nerve [V_2]
Foramen spinosum	Sphenoid	Parietal branch of the middle meningeal artery; middle meningeal veins; nervus spinosus (meningeal branch of the mandibular nerve)
Frontal notch/foramen	Frontal bone	Supratrochlear artery and veins; medial branch of the supraorbital nerve
Greater palatine foramen	Palatine bone	Greater palatine artery, vein and nerve
Infraorbital foramen	Maxilla	Infraorbital artery, vein and nerve
Jugular foramen or foramen lacerum posterior	Temporal bone	Inferior petrosal sinus (anteriorly); meningeal branch of the ascending pharyngeal artery and glossopharyngeal [IX], vagus [X], accessory [XI] nerves (in the center); occipital artery and veins, sigmoid sinus which continues in the internal jugular vein and occipital emissary vein (posteriorly)
Lesser palatine foramina	Palatine bone and maxilla	Lesser palatine arteries, veins and nerves
Mandibular foramen	Mandible	Inferior alveolar artery, vein and nerve
Mastoid foramen	Temporal bone	Mastoid emissary vein
Mental foramen	Mandible	Mental branches of the inferior alveolar artery and vein; mental nerve
Optic foramen	Sphenoid	Optic nerve [II] and ophthalmic artery
Parietal foramen	Parietal bone	Parietal emissary vein
Posterior ethmoidal foramen	Ethmoid	Posterior ethmoidal artery; ethmoidal veins; posterior ethmoidal nerve
Sphenoidal emissary foramen (not always present)	Sphenoid	Emissary vein from the pterygoid plexus to the cavernous sinus (vein of Vesalius)
Sphenopalatine foramen	Palatine bone	Branches of the maxillary nerve to the pterygopalatine ganglion (sphenopalatine nerves); sphenopalatine artery and vein
Stylomastoid foramen	Temporal bone	Stylomastoid branch of the posterior auricular artery and stylomastoid vein; facial nerve [VII]
Supraorbital notch/foramen	Frontal bone	Supraorbital artery, vein and nerve
Zygomatico-orbital foramen	Zygomatic bone	Zygomaticofacial and zygomaticotemporal branches of the zygomatic nerve
Zygomaticofacial foramen	Zygomatic bone	Zygomaticofacial branch of the zygomatic nerve
Zygomaticotemporal foramen	Zygomatic bone	Zygomaticotemporal branch of the zygomatic nerve

Hiatuses

HIATUS	BONE	FORMATIONS THAT PASS THROUGH IT
Hiatus for greater petrosal nerve	Temporal bone	Petrosal branch of the middle meningeal artery; greater petrosal nerve
Hiatus for lesser petrosal nerve	Temporal bone	Lesser petrosal nerve

Meatuses

MEATUS	BONE	FORMATIONS THAT PASS THROUGH IT
External acoustic meatus	Temporal bone	–
Internal acoustic meatus	Temporal bone	Labyrinthine arteries and veins; facial [VII], vestibulocochlear [VIII] and intermediate nerves

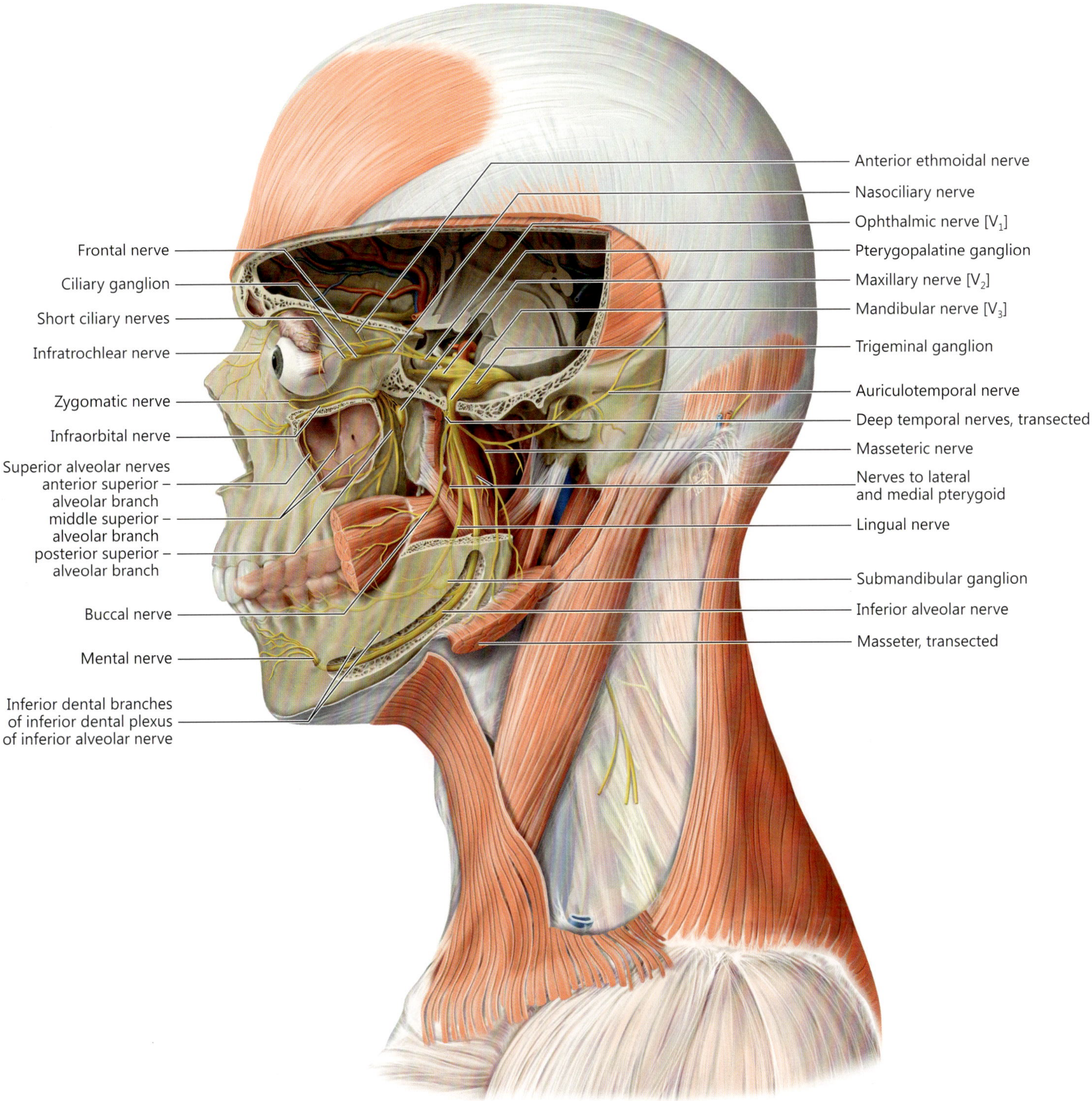

The **trigeminal nerve** [V] divides into three branches: the ophthalmic [V_1], maxillary [V_2] and mandibular [V_3] nerves. The first, a somatic sensory branch, innervates the forehead, calvaria and part of the nose, the eyeball, conjunctiva and part of the mucosa of the nasal cavity. The second branch, also somatic sensory, innervates an extended area of the face and mucosa of the nasal cavities; in addition, it supplies the mucosa of the superior part of the oral cavity and of the superior dento-alveolar arch. The third, a somatic motor and somatic sensory branch, innervates, with its somatic motor component, the masticatory muscles, tensor tympani, tensor veli palatini, anterior belly of the digastric, and mylohyoid, and, with its somatic sensory component, the inferior part of the face, part of the oral mucosa, the inferior dento-alveolar arch, most of the temporal region, part of the auricle, the tympanic membrane, and the masticatory muscles for proprioceptive sensitivity. The three branches, with the exception of the somatic motor component of the mandibular nerve, originate from the convex margin of the trigeminal ganglion or semilunar ganglion.

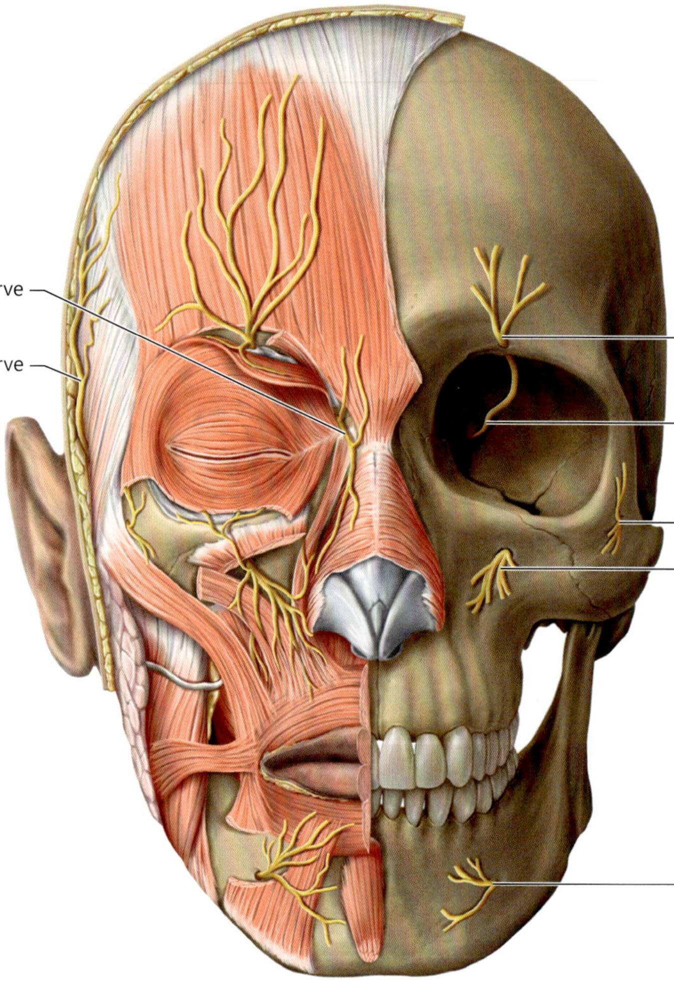

In the left hemicranium, one can see the supraorbital nerve, a branch of the frontal nerve which in turn is a terminal branch of the ophthalmic nerve (**first branch of the trigeminal nerve**), the zygomatic and infraorbital nerves, branches of the maxillary nerve (**second branch of the trigeminal nerve**), and the mental nerve, a branch of the inferior alveolar nerve, in its turn a dividing branch of the mandibular nerve (**third branch of the trigeminal nerve**). They emerge, respectively, from the supraorbital, zygomaticofacial, infraorbital and mental foramina. In the right hemicranium, one can see, in addition to the auriculotemporal nerve, the muscular and, hence also, cutaneous territories pertaining to these nerves. Also seen is the infratrochlear nerve, one of the terminal branches of the nasociliary nerve, which is the medial branch of division of the ophthalmic nerve.

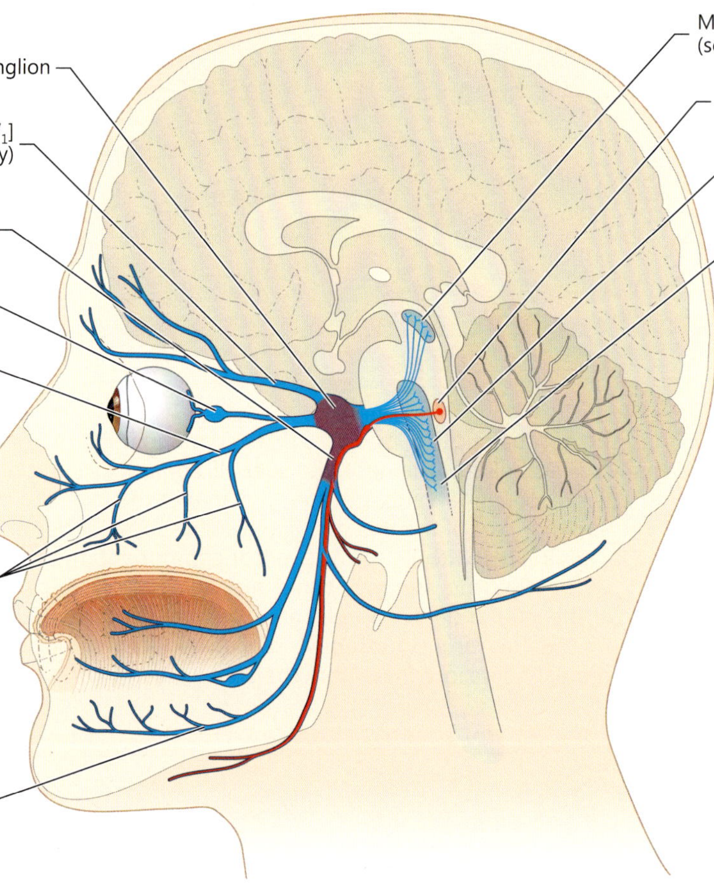

The somatic sensory fibers of the **trigeminal nerve** originate in the trigeminal ganglion. The ganglionic protoneurons send their central projection to the principal and spinal nuclei, and in small part also to the mesencephalic nucleus, and their peripheral projection to the three nerve branches: ophthalmic, maxillary and mandibular. The mesencephalic nucleus receives central projections of ganglionic protoneurons that gather principally the proprioceptive sensitivity of muscles. The mesencephalic nucleus is also composed of protoneurons that receive the mechanoreceptive sensitivity from the desmodentium of the superior and inferior dental arcades. The somatic motor component originates from the motor neurons of the motor nucleus, also known as the masticatory nucleus.

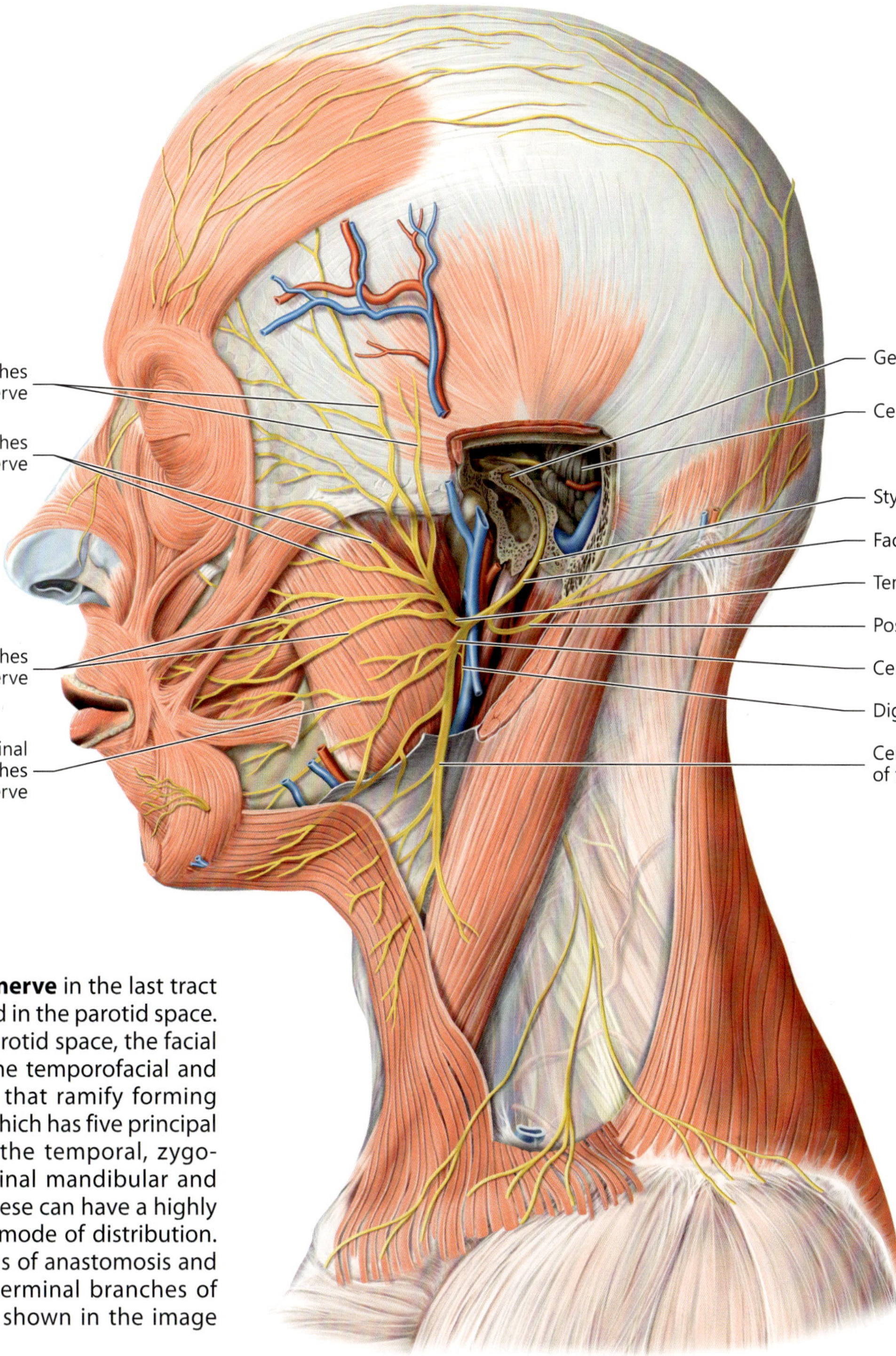

Course of the **facial nerve** in the last tract of the facial canal and in the parotid space. At the level of the parotid space, the facial nerve divides into the temporofacial and cervicofacial trunks that ramify forming the parotid plexus, which has five principal terminal branches: the temporal, zygomatic, buccal, marginal mandibular and cervical branches. These can have a highly variable course and mode of distribution. The different patterns of anastomosis and subdivision of the terminal branches of the facial nerve are shown in the image below.

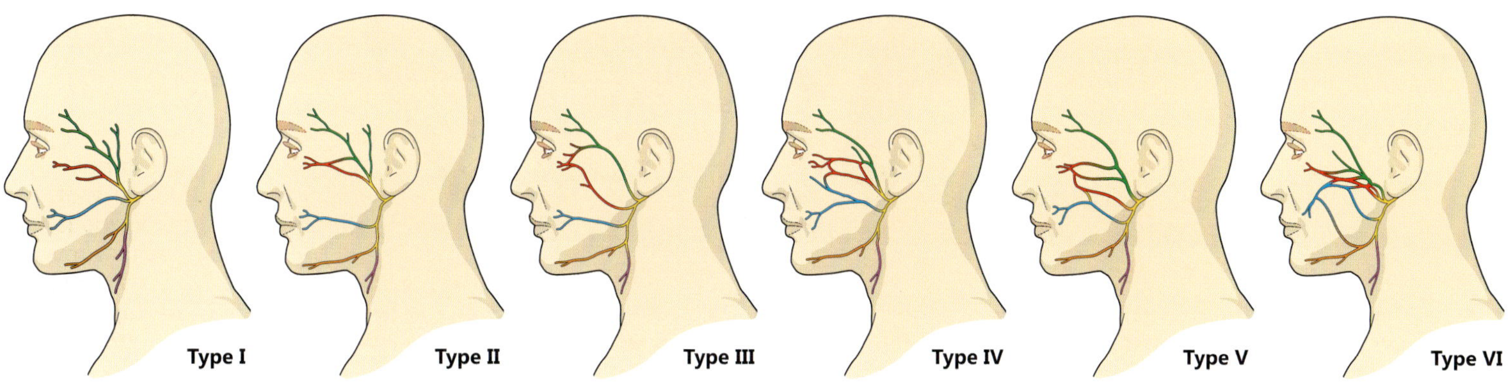

Modified from Berkovits BKB, Moxham BJ 2002, Head and Neck Anatomy. London: Martin Dunitz.

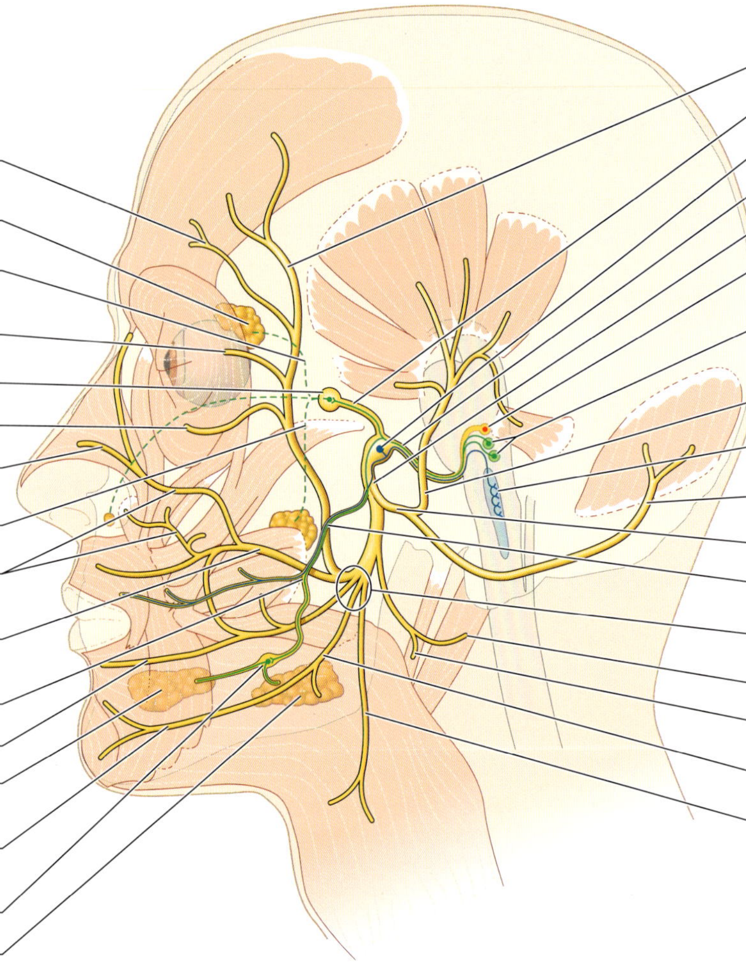

Schematic representation of the **facial nerve** and its branches. The somatic motor component appears clearly predominant with respect to the visceral motor (in *green*) and special visceral sensory (gustatory, in *blue*) components.

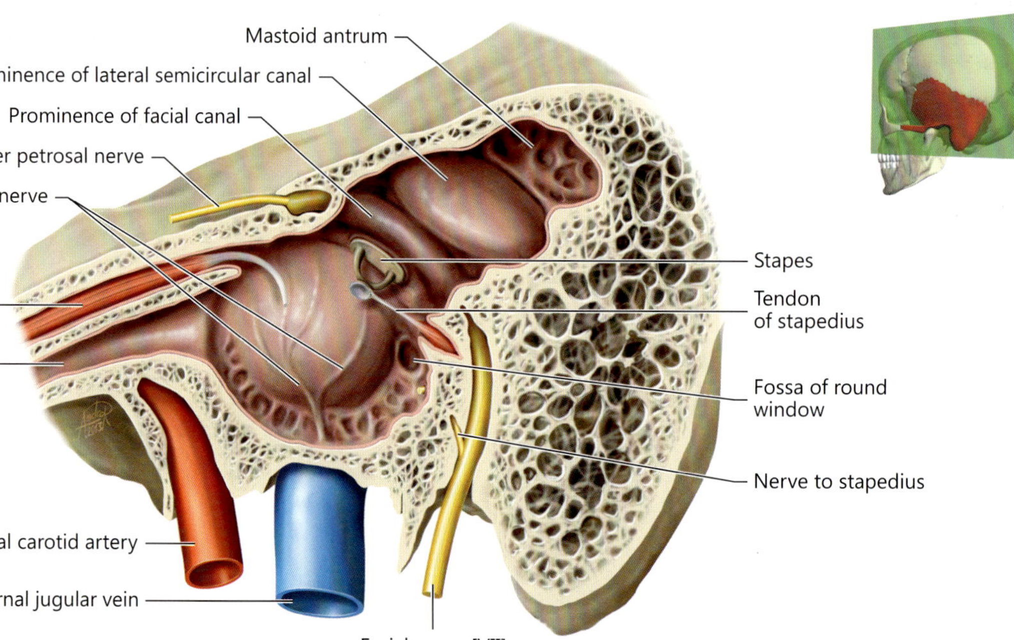

Tympanic cavity, opened, and viewed from the exterior; one can see the **intrapetrous course of the facial nerve** and the facial canal in relation to the internal carotid artery and internal jugular vein. The facial nerve exits from the cranium in front of the mastoid process, passing through the stylomastoid foramen, which, in this diagram, has been partially removed. One can also see the relationship of the facial nerve, in its intrapetrous journey and near the point where it emerges from the cranium, with the bone cavities of the mastoid antrum.

Summary table of the nerves of the head

NERVE	ORIGIN	RAMIFICATIONS	DISTRIBUTION
abducens, VI cranial nerve	Emerges from the brainstem in correspondence to inferior border of the pons	Filaments	Lateral rectus of the eyeball
anterior ampullary (superior ampullary)	Vestibular nerve [VIII]	Filaments	Ampulla of the anterior semicircular duct
anterior auricular (generally two in number)	Auriculotemporal nerve	Filaments	Skin of the anterosuperior part of the external ear (principally of the helix and tragus)
anterior ethmoidal	Nasociliary nerve	Internal, lateral and medial nasal branches, and external nasal branch	Mucosa of the anterior ethmoidal cells and the nasal cavities
– **internal nasal branches**	Anterior ethmoidal nerve	Filaments	Mucosa of the vault of the nasal cavities
– **external nasal nerve**	Anterior ethmoidal nerve	Filaments	Skin of the ala of nose, vestibule and dorsum of the nose, including the apex of the nose
auriculotemporal	Mandibular nerve [V_3]	Parotid and superficial temporal branches, branches to the tympanic membrane, communicating branches with the facial nerve; nerve to external acoustic meatus and anterior auricular nerves	Skin anterior to the auricle and of the posterior two-thirds of the temporal region; skin of the tragus and adjacent to the helix; skin of the roof of the external acoustic meatus and of the superior part of the tympanic membrane; temporomandibular joint
buccal (buccinator)	Mandibular nerve [V_3]	Collateral branches and anastomotic branches with the buccal branches of the facial nerve	Skin and oral mucosa of the cheek (above and deep to the anterior part of the buccinator); vestibular gingiva adjacent to second and third molar teeth
caroticotympanic	Superior cervical ganglion and tympanic plexus	Filaments	Internal ear, pharyngotympanic tube
chorda tympani	Intermediate nerve [VII] and lingual nerve	Filaments	Anterior two-thirds of the tongue, submandibular and sublingual glands
cochlear [VIII] (acoustic)	Vestibulocochlear nerve [VIII]	Filaments	Spiral organ (of Corti)
cranial (encephalic)	12 nerve pairs: olfactory [I]; optic [II]; oculomotor [III]; trochlear [IV]; trigeminal [V]; abducens [VI]; facial [VII]; vestibulocochlear [VIII]; glossopharyngeal [IX]; vagus [X]; accessory [XI]; hypoglossal [XII]		
deep petrosal	Internal carotid plexus	Unites with the greater petrosal nerve to form the nerve of pterygoid canal	Glands of the nasal and palatine mucosae, lacrimal gland
deep temporal (generally two in number)	Mandibular nerve [V_3]	Filaments	Temporalis
external carotid	Superior cervical ganglion	Filaments	External carotid artery and its branches, sublingual and submandibular glands
facial, VII cranial nerve (facial nerve proper)	Emerges from the brainstem in correspondence to the inferior border of the pons	Nerve to stapedius and posterior auricular nerve: occipital and auricular branches; digastric branch, stylohyoid branch, communicating branch with the hypoglossal nerve; parotid plexus: temporal, zygomatic, buccal, marginal mandibular and cervical branches	Facial muscles, muscles of the scalp and auricle; buccinator, platysma, stapedius, stylohyoid and posterior belly of the digastric
frontal	Ophthalmic nerve [V_1]	Supraorbital and supratrochlear nerves	Conjunctiva, skin of the superior eyelid and the forehead, corrugator supercilii and frontal belly of the occipitofrontalis, scalp and frontal sinus
glossopharyngeal, IX cranial nerve	Emerges from the superior part of the myelencephalon	Tympanic nerve: tympanic plexus, tubal branch and caroticotympanic nerves; pharyngeal, tonsillar and lingual branches, stylopharyngeal branch and carotid branch; communicating branches with the auricular branch of vagus nerve, with the meningeal branch, with the auriculotemporal nerve and with the chorda tympani; lesser petrosal nerve	Mucosa of the middle ear and pharyngotympanic tube, tongue, pharynx, fauces, palatine tonsil, baroreceptors of the carotid sinus, stylopharyngeus, parotid gland

continued

Summary table of the nerves of the head *(continued)*

NERVE	*ORIGIN*	*RAMIFICATIONS*	*DISTRIBUTION*
great auricular	Cervical plexus (from the anterior rami of C2 and C3)	Posterior and anterior rami and anastomotic branches with the facial nerve	Skin above the angle of the mandible and inferior to the lobule of the auricle; skin of the auricle; parotid fascia
greater occipital	Posterior ramus of C2	Terminal branches and anastomotic branches with the posterior rami of C1 and C3	Scalp of the occipital region; obliquus capitis inferior, semispinalis capitis, longissimus capitis, splenius capitis, splenius cervicis and trapezius
greater palatine (anterior palatine)	Maxillary nerve [V_2]	Posterior inferior nasal nerves	Gingivae, mucosa, glands and taste buds of the palate
– **posterior inferior nasal nerves**	Greater palatine nerve	Filaments	Mucosa of the nasal conchae
greater petrosal (greater superficial petrosal)	Intermediate nerve [VII]	Unites with the sympathetic root of pterygopalatine ganglion to form the nerve of pterygoid canal	Nasal and palatine glands, lacrimal gland
hypoglossal, XII cranial nerve	Emerges from the anterolateral sulcus of the myelencephalon, between the pyramid and inferior olive	Lingual and anastomotic branches with the cervical plexus	Intrinsic and extrinsic muscles of the tongue
inferior alveolar (inferior dental)	Mandibular nerve [V_3]	Nerve to mylohyoid, inferior dental plexus: inferior dental branches and inferior gingival branches, mental nerve	Mylohyoid and anterior belly of the digastric, periodontium and pulp of the mandibular teeth, gingiva of the alveolar arch of the mandible, skin of the chin, mucosa of the lower lip
infraorbital	Maxillary nerve [V_2]	Middle and anterior branches of the superior alveolar nerves, palpebral branches, nasal branches and superior labial branches	Maxillary sinus; premolar teeth, canine teeth and maxillary incisors; skin and palpebral conjunctiva of the inferior eyelid; skin of the cheek, lateral part of the nose and anteroinferior to the nasal septum; skin and oral mucosa of the upper lip
– **inferior palpebral branches**	Infraorbital	Filaments	Inferior eyelid
infratrochlear	Nasociliary nerve	Palpebral branches	Skin lateral to the root of the nose; skin and palpebral conjunctiva adjacent to the medial angle of the eye, to the lacrimal sac and to the lacrimal caruncle
– **palpebral branches**	Infratrochlear	Filaments	Superior eyelid
intermediate [VII] (glossopalatine or of Wrisberg)	Emerges from the brainstem in correspondence to the inferior border of the pons	Greater petrosal nerve and chorda tympani; communicating branches with the tympanic plexus and the vagus nerve	Gustatory papillae of the anterior two-thirds of the tongue, nasal and soft palate glands, submandibular, sublingual and lacrimal glands, skin of the external acoustic meatus and the mastoid process
internal carotid	Superior cervical ganglion	Filaments	Internal carotid artery and its branches, dilator pupillae, salivary, lacrimal and pineal glands
lacrimal	Ophthalmic nerve [VI]	Terminal branches	Lacrimal gland (postganglionic secretory fibers originating in the pterygopalatine ganglion that reach the lacrimal nerve via the zygomaticotemporal branch of the zygomatic nerve); small area of the skin and palpebral conjunctiva of the lateral third of the superior eyelid
lateral ampullary	Vestibular nerve [VIII]	Filaments	Ampulla of the lateral semicircular duct
lesser occipital	Cervical plexus (from the anterior rami of C2 and C3)	Filaments	Scalp posterior to the auricle; skin of the occipital and mastoid regions

continued

Summary table of the nerves of the head *(continued)*

NERVE	ORIGIN	RAMIFICATIONS	DISTRIBUTION
lesser palatine	Maxillary nerve [V_2]	Tonsillar branches	Soft palate, uvula, palatine tonsil
lesser petrosal	Glossopharyngeal nerve [IX]	Ganglionic, filaments	Parotid and minor salivary glands
lingual (small hypoglossal)	Mandibular nerve [V_3]	Branches to the isthmus of fauces, communicating branches with the hypoglossal nerve, lingual and ganglionic branches (to the submandibular ganglion and sublingual ganglion); chorda tympani and sublingual nerve	Mucosa of anterior two-thirds of the tongue, floor of the mouth, gingivae and submandibular and sublingual glands
long ciliary (2 or 3 in number)	Nasociliary nerve	Filaments	Iris and cornea
mandibular [V_3] (inferior maxillary)	Trigeminal nerve [V]	Nerve to medial pterygoid and nerve to lateral pterygoid, nerve to tensor veli palatini and nerve to tensor tympani, masseteric nerve; deep temporal, auriculotemporal, buccal, lingual, inferior alveolar and mental nerves; meningeal branch and branch to otic ganglion	Masticatory muscles, tensor tympani, tensor veli palatini, mylohyoid and anterior belly of the digastric; mandible, gingiva and mandibular teeth; anterior two-thirds of the tongue, cheek, inferior part of the face; meninges, temporomandibular joint, skin of the temporal region, external ear
– **meningeal branch** (nervus spinosus)	Mandibular nerve [V_3]	Filaments	Meninges
masseteric	Mandibular nerve [V_3]	Filaments	Masseter, temporomandibular joint
maxillary [V_2] (superior maxillary)	Trigeminal nerve [V]	Nasopalatine, pharyngeal, greater palatine, lesser palatine, superior alveolar, zygomatic and infraorbital nerves; meningeal, ganglionic (to pterygopalatine ganglion), orbital, and lateral and medial posterior superior nasal branches	Skin of the middle part of the face, nose, inferior eyelids and upper lip; gingiva and maxillary teeth; tonsils and floor of the mouth, soft palate, maxillary sinus, mucosa of the nasopharynx
– **meningeal branch** (middle meningeal branch)	Maxillary nerve [V_2]	Filaments	Dura mater of the middle cranial fossa
– **ganglionic branches** (to pterygopalatine ganglion) (pterygopalatine or sphenopalatine nerves or nerves of Bock)	Maxillary nerve [V_2]	Postganglionic nerve fibers	Glands of the nasal and palatine mucosae, lacrimal gland
– **posterior superior nasal branches**	Maxillary nerve [V_2]	Filaments	Vault of the pharynx, lateral wall of the nasal cavities, mucosa of the nasal septum, glands of the nasal mucosa
mental	Mandibular nerve [V_3]	Mental, labial and gingival branches	Skin of the chin; skin and oral mucosa of the lower lip
nasociliary (nasal)	Ophthalmic nerve [V_1]	Communicating branches with the ciliary ganglion, long ciliary nerves	Mucosa of the nasal cavity, frontal sinus; iris, cornea, conjunctiva, lacrimal sac, skin of the eyelids and ala of nose
nasopalatine (of Scarpa)	Maxillary nerve [V_2]	Filaments	Anterior part of the hard palate
oculomotor, III cranial nerve (common oculomotor)	Mesencephalon in correspondence to the medial surface of the cerebral peduncle	Superior, inferior and ganglionic branches (to the ciliary ganglion)	Extraocular muscles: superior rectus, levator palpebrae superioris, medial rectus, inferior rectus and inferior oblique; intrinsic muscles of the eyeball: sphincter pupillae, ciliary muscle
of pterygoid canal (vidian)	Formed by the union of the greater petrosal and deep petrosal nerves	Filaments	Glands of the nasal and palatine mucosae, lacrimal gland

continued

Summary table of the nerves of the head *(continued)*

NERVE	ORIGIN	RAMIFICATIONS	DISTRIBUTION
olfactory, I cranial nerve	Olfactory part of the nasal mucosa	Filaments	Olfactory bulb
ophthalmic [V_1]	Trigeminal nerve [V]	Lacrimal, frontal, nasociliary, anterior and posterior ethmoidal and infratrochlear nerves; recurrent meningeal branch or tentorial nerve	Dura mater, eyeball, conjunctiva, lacrimal gland; mucous membrane of the nose and the paranasal sinuses; skin of the forehead, the eyelids and the nose
– **recurrent meningeal branch** (tentorial nerve or of Arnold)	Ophthalmic nerve [V_1]	Filaments	Dura mater bordering the cavernous sinus and forming the tentorium cerebelli
optic, II cranial nerve	Ganglionic layer of the retina	Filaments	Lateral geniculate body
posterior ampullary (inferior ampullary)	Vestibular nerve [VIII]	Filaments	Ampulla of the posterior semicircular duct
posterior auricular	Facial nerve [VII]	Auricular and occipital branches	Auricularis posterior and occipital belly of the occipitofrontalis, skin of the external ear
posterior ethmoidal	Nasociliary nerve	Anterior meningeal branch	Mucosa of the posterior ethmoidal cells and the paranasal sinuses; meninges
– **anterior meningeal branch**	Posterior ethmoidal nerve	Filaments	Meninges
saccular	Vestibular nerve [VIII]	Filaments	Saccule
short ciliary (from 6 to 10 in number)	Ciliary ganglion	Filaments	Ciliary body, iris and cornea
sublingual	Lingual nerve	Filaments	Sublingual gland and mucosa of the floor of the mouth
superior alveolar (superior dental)	Maxillary nerve [V_2]	Anterior and posterior superior alveolar branches, middle superior alveolar branch	Maxillary sinus, periodontium and pulp of the maxillary teeth, gingiva of the alveolar arch of the maxilla
– **anterior superior alveolar branches** (anterior superior dental)	Superior alveolar nerves	Superior dental plexus: superior dental branches and superior gingival branches	Maxillary sinus, periodontium and pulp of the maxillary teeth, gingiva of the alveolar arch of the maxilla, floor of the nose
– **posterior superior alveolar branches** (posterior superior dental)	Superior alveolar nerves	Filaments	Maxillary sinus, periodontium and pulp of the maxillary teeth, gingiva of the alveolar arch of the maxilla
– **middle superior alveolar branch** (middle superior dental)	Superior alveolar nerves	Filaments	Maxillary sinus, periodontium and pulp of the maxillary teeth, gingiva of the alveolar arch of the maxilla
supraorbital	Frontal nerve	Medial and lateral branches	Skin and palpebral conjunctiva of the middle third of the superior eyelid; skin and periosteum of the anterolateral part of the forehead and scalp up to the vertex of the calvaria
supratrochlear	Frontal nerve	Lateral and medial descending branches	Skin and palpebral conjunctiva of the medial third of the superior eyelid; skin and periosteum of the anterolateral part of the forehead
terminal	Associated to the olfactory nerve [I]	Filaments	Inferior and anterior parts of the nasal septum
third occipital	Posterior ramus of C3	Filaments	Scalp of the inferior occipital and suboccipital regions
to external acoustic meatus	Auriculotemporal nerve	Filaments	External acoustic meatus

continued

Summary table of the nerves of the head			*(continued)*
NERVE	***ORIGIN***	***RAMIFICATIONS***	***DISTRIBUTION***
to lateral pterygoid	Mandibular nerve [V_3]	Filaments	Lateral pterygoid
to medial pterygoid	Mandibular nerve [V_3]	Filaments	Medial pterygoid
to stapedius	Facial nerve [VII]	Filaments	Stapedius
to tensor tympani	Mandibular nerve [V_3]	Filaments	Tensor tympani
to tensor veli palatini	Mandibular nerve [V_3]	Filaments	Tensor veli palatini
trigeminal, V cranial nerve (largest of the cranial nerves)	Emerges from the brainstem in correspondence to the inferior surface of the pons	Two roots (motor and sensory) that reach the trigeminal ganglion near the apex of the petrous part of the temporal bone, from which arise the ophthalmic [V_1], maxillary [V_2] and mandibular [V_3] branches or nerves	Skin of the face, masticatory muscles, teeth, mouth and nasal cavity
trochlear, IV cranial nerve (smallest of the cranial nerves)	Emerges from the mesencephalon immediately behind the inferior colliculus	Filaments	Superior oblique of the eyeball
tympanic (Jacobson's nerve)	Glossopharyngeal nerve [IX]	Tympanic plexus: tubal branch and caroticotympanic nerves	Tympanic cavity and membrane, mastoid cells, pharyngotympanic tube, parotid gland
utricular	Vestibular nerve [VIII]	Filaments	Utricle
utriculoampullary	Vestibular nerve [VIII]	Filaments	Macula of utricle and ampulla of the lateral and anterior semicircular ducts
vagus, X cranial nerve (pneumogastric)	Emerges from the posterior lateral sulcus of the myelencephalon	Meningeal, auricular, communicating with the glossopharyngeal nerve, pharyngeal, superior and inferior cervical cardiac, thoracic cardiac, bronchial and renal branches; anterior (anterior gastric and hepatic branches) and posterior (posterior gastric and celiac branches) vagal trunks; superior laryngeal nerve (external and internal branches) and recurrent laryngeal nerve (tracheal, esophageal and pharyngeal branches)	Heart, wall of the aorta and of its major branches; glands and smooth muscle of the respiratory tract, of the digestive tract (except for its terminal part) and of part of the urinary system; striated muscle of the pharynx, of the larynx and of the proximal part of the esophagus; carotid sinus, carotid body; mucosa of the larynx, pharynx, trachea, esophagus and other thoracic and abdominal organs; taste buds of the mucosa of the epiglottis and oropharynx; skin of the auricle, of the external acoustic meatus and of the lateral surface of the tympanic membrane
– **meningeal branch**	Vagus nerve [X]	Filaments	Meninges
vertebral	Inferior cervical ganglion	Filaments	Vertebral artery and its extracranial and intracranial branches
vestibular [VIII]	Vestibulocochlear nerve [VIII]	Utricular, utriculoampullary, anterior ampullary, lateral ampullary, posterior ampullary and saccular nerves	Macula of the utricle and the saccule and ampulla of the semicircular ducts
vestibulocochlear, VIII cranial nerve (statoacoustic)	Emerges from the brainstem between the pons and the myelencephalon, formed by the union of the vestibular and cochlear nerves	Vestibular (medial), cochlear (lateral)	Membranous labyrinth of the internal ear
vomeronasal	Present in the nasal septum of the fetus but disappears before birth		
zygomatic	Maxillary nerve [V_2]	Zygomaticotemporal and zygomaticofacial	Skin of the temple and the zygomatic region
– **zygomaticofacial branch**	Zygomatic nerve	Filaments	Skin on the protuberant part of the cheek
– **zygomaticotemporal branch**	Zygomatic nerve	Branch to the lacrimal nerve	Anterior part of the glabrous skin of the temporal fossa

N.B.: the accessory nerve (XI cranial nerve), given that it emerges at the level of the first 4-5 cervical neuromeres and supplies the superior part of the trapezius and sternocleidomastoid, is reported in the table summarizing nerves of the neck.

Summary table of the nerves of the neck			
NERVE	***ORIGIN***	***RAMIFICATIONS***	***DISTRIBUTION***
accessory (spinal accessory), XI cranial nerve	*Cranial root*: lateral face of the myelencephalon *Spinal root*: first five cervical segments of the spinal cord	Internal and external branches	*Cranial root*: via the pharyngeal branches of the vagus nerve, to the pharyngeal muscles and muscles of the palate, with the exception of the tensor veli palatini (innervated by the nerve to medial pterygoid, a branch of the mandibular nerve, third branch of the trigeminal nerve), and, via the recurrent laryngeal nerve, to the thyroarytenoid and lateral cricoarytenoid *Spinal root*: sternocleidomastoid and trapezius
ansa cervicalis (ansa of hypoglossal nerve)	*Superior root*: anastomotic branch with the hypoglossal nerve arising from the anterior ramus of the first cervical nerve *Inferior root* (or descendens cervicalis): anastomotic branches with the hypoglossal nerve arising from anterior rami of the second and third cervical nerves that flow into a common trunk which joins the superior root	Filaments	Omohyoid, sternohyoid and sternothyroid
brachial plexus	Anterior rami from the fifth to eighth cervical nerves and of the first thoracic nerve	Trunks (primary trunks) and cords (secondary trunks)	Upper limb (sensory and motor innervation)
cervical (8 pairs of spinal nerves)	Cervical segments of the spinal cord	Anterior and posterior rami	Cervical and brachial plexuses (anterior rami), skin and superficial and deep muscles in the posterior part of the neck (posterior rami)
cervical plexus	Anterior rami from the first to fourth cervical nerves	*Cutaneous branches*: lesser occipital, great auricular, transverse cervical and supraclavicular nerves; *muscular branches*: nerves to rectus capitis anterior and rectus capitis lateralis, longus capitis and longus colli, geniohyoid, thyrohyoid, omohyoid, sternohyoid, sternocleidomastoid, trapezius, levator scapulae, scalenus medius, phrenic nerve; *anastomotic branches*: gray rami communicantes with the sympathetic trunk, anastomotic branches with the hypoglossal nerve (ansa cervicalis)	Muscles and skin of the neck and the superior part of the back; diaphragm
glossopharyngeal, IX cranial nerve	Posterior lateral sulcus of the myelencephalon (sulcus of mixed nerves)	Tympanic, carotid, pharyngeal, stylopharyngeal tonsillar, lingual branches	Tongue and pharynx, fauces, palatine tonsil, baroreceptors of the carotid sinus, stylopharyngeus
jugular	Superior cervical ganglion	Filaments	Superior ganglion of the vagus nerve and inferior ganglion of the glossopharyngeal nerve
recurrent laryngeal (inferior laryngeal)	Vagus nerve	Pharyngeal, esophageal and tracheal branches	All intrinsic muscles of the larynx, excepting the cricothyroid
suboccipital	Posterior rami of the first cervical nerve	Filaments	Suboccipital muscles
superior laryngeal	Vagus nerve, near the inferior ganglion situated in correspondence to the jugular foramen	External and internal	Mucosa of the larynx, in particular of the epiglottis; inferior constrictor of pharynx and cricothyroid
superior, middle and inferior cervical ganglion	Cervical segment of the sympathetic trunk	Gray rami communicantes with the cervical nerves and white ramus communicans with the first thoracic nerve *Perivascular branches*: external carotid and vertebral nerves *Visceral branches*: laryngopharyngeal, superior, middle and inferior cervical cardiac nerves	Vessels and organs connected to the neck, spinal and meningeal vessels of the neck, cardiac plexus

continued

Summary table of the nerves of the neck			*(continued)*
NERVE	***ORIGIN***	***RAMIFICATIONS***	***DISTRIBUTION***
to geniohyoid	First cervical nerve via fibers traveling with the hypoglossal nerve	Filaments	Geniohyoid
to mylohyoid	Inferior alveolar nerve (branch of the mandibular nerve, third branch of the trigeminal nerve) just before entering the mandibular foramen	Filaments	Mylohyoid and inferior belly of the digastric
to omohyoid	Ansa cervicalis	Filaments	Omohyoid
to sternohyoid	Ansa cervicalis	Filaments	Sternohyoid
to sternothyroid	Ansa cervicalis	Filaments	Sternothyroid
to thyrohyoid (thyrohyoid branch of C1)	First cervical nerve	Filaments branching out via the hypoglossal nerve	Thyrohyoid
transverse cervical (cutaneous cervical)	Cervical plexus (from the anterior rami of C2 and C3)	Ascending and descending branches	Skin of the suprahyoid and infrahyoid regions and of the lateral cervical region
vagus, X cranial nerve	Posterior lateral sulcus of the myelencephalon (sulcus of mixed nerves)	Cervical collateral branches: meningeal, auricular, pharyngeal, superior and inferior cervical cardiac, superior laryngeal and recurrent laryngeal	In the neck: all muscles of the larynx, trachea, pharynx, esophagus
vertebral	Inferior cervical ganglion	Filaments	Spinal and meningeal vessels of the neck

N.B.: The posterior ramus of the fourth cervical nerve [C4], via its medial and lateral branches, innervates the skin of the posterior cervical region. The vagus, glossopharyngeal and recurrent laryngeal (a branch of the vagus) nerves ramify in the neck forming a network of pharyngeal branches, the pharyngeal plexus, which supplies the pharynx. The pharynx also receives laryngopharyngeal branches from the superior cervical ganglion of the sympathetic trunk.

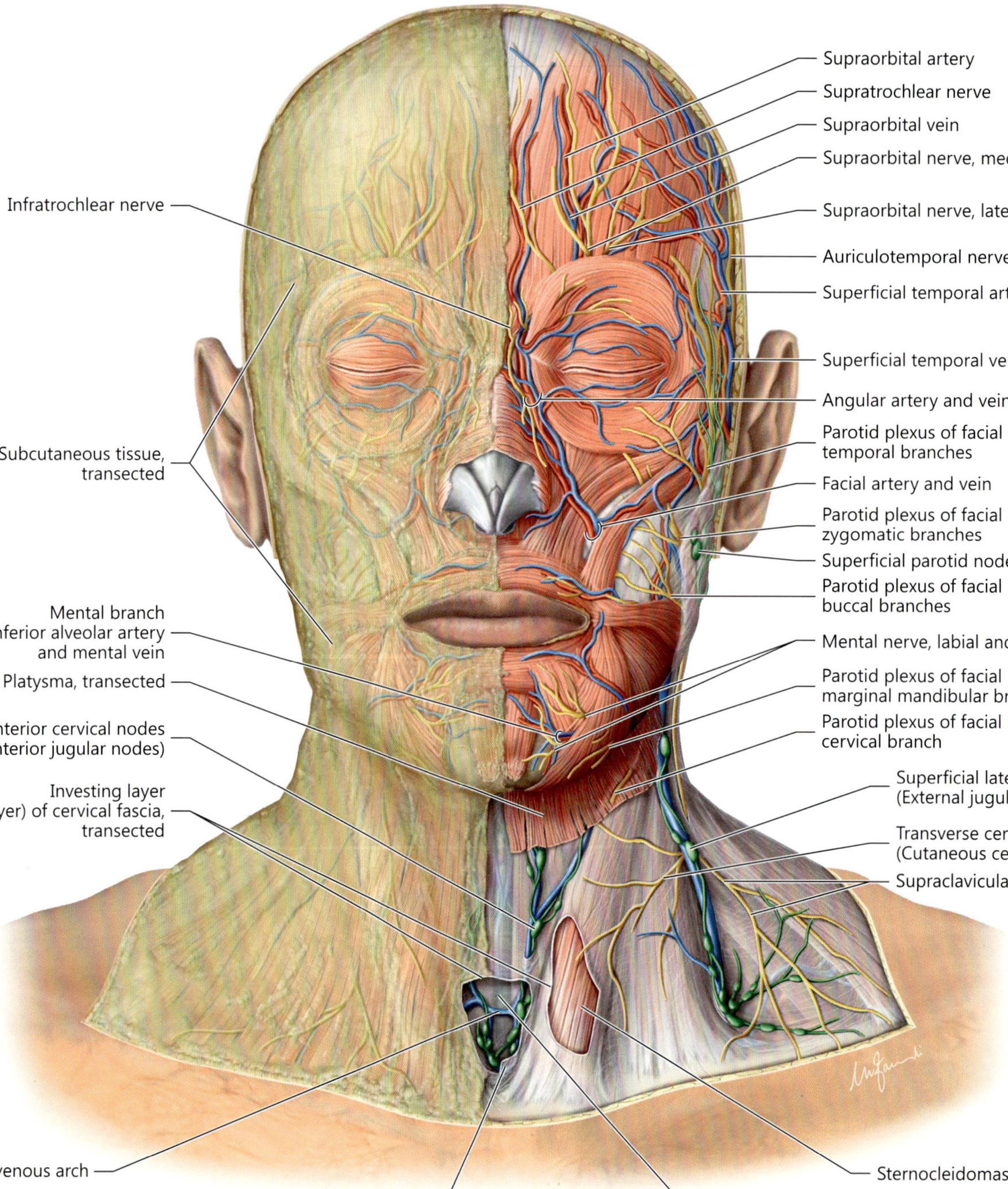

Head and **neck**, anterior view. On the left side of the head and neck, the skin and subcutaneous tissue have been removed and the platysma transected. One can see the vessels and nerves that supply the skin and muscles of the face, in particular the parotid plexus, which gives rise to the temporal, zygomatic, buccal, marginal mandibular and cervical branches of the facial nerve.

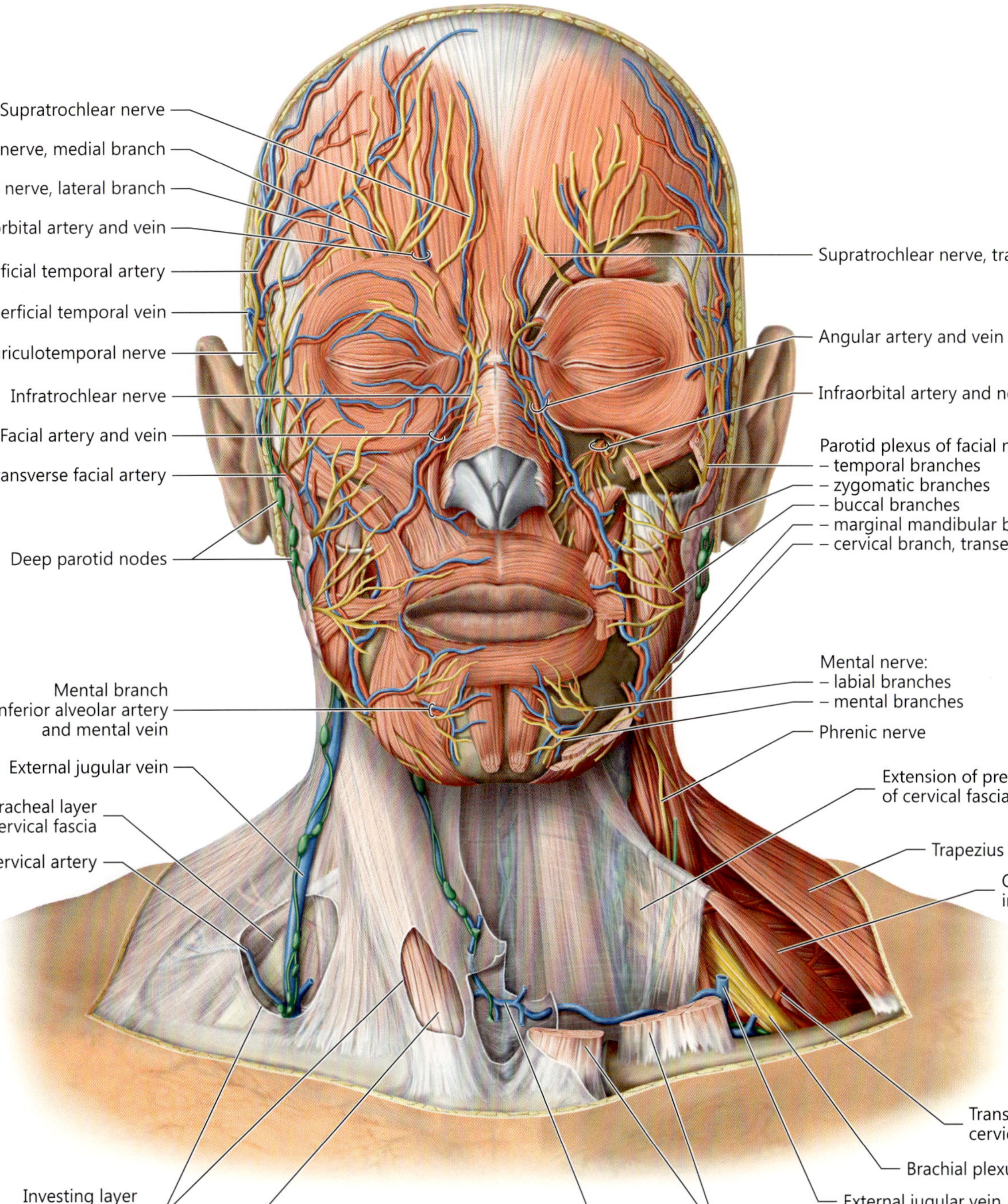

Head and **neck**, anterior view. On the right side of the head and neck, after the skin, subcutaneous tissue and platysma have been removed and the parotid fascia transected, one can see the parotid plexus of the facial nerve, the supratrochlear and supraorbital nerves, branches of the frontal nerve, and the auriculotemporal nerve, branch of the mandibular nerve. On the left side of the head, the orbicularis oculi, zygomaticus major and minor, levator labii superioris, levator anguli oris, depressor labii inferioris and depressor anguli oris have been transected. Besides the terminal branches of the parotid plexus of the facial nerve, one can see the facial artery and vein.

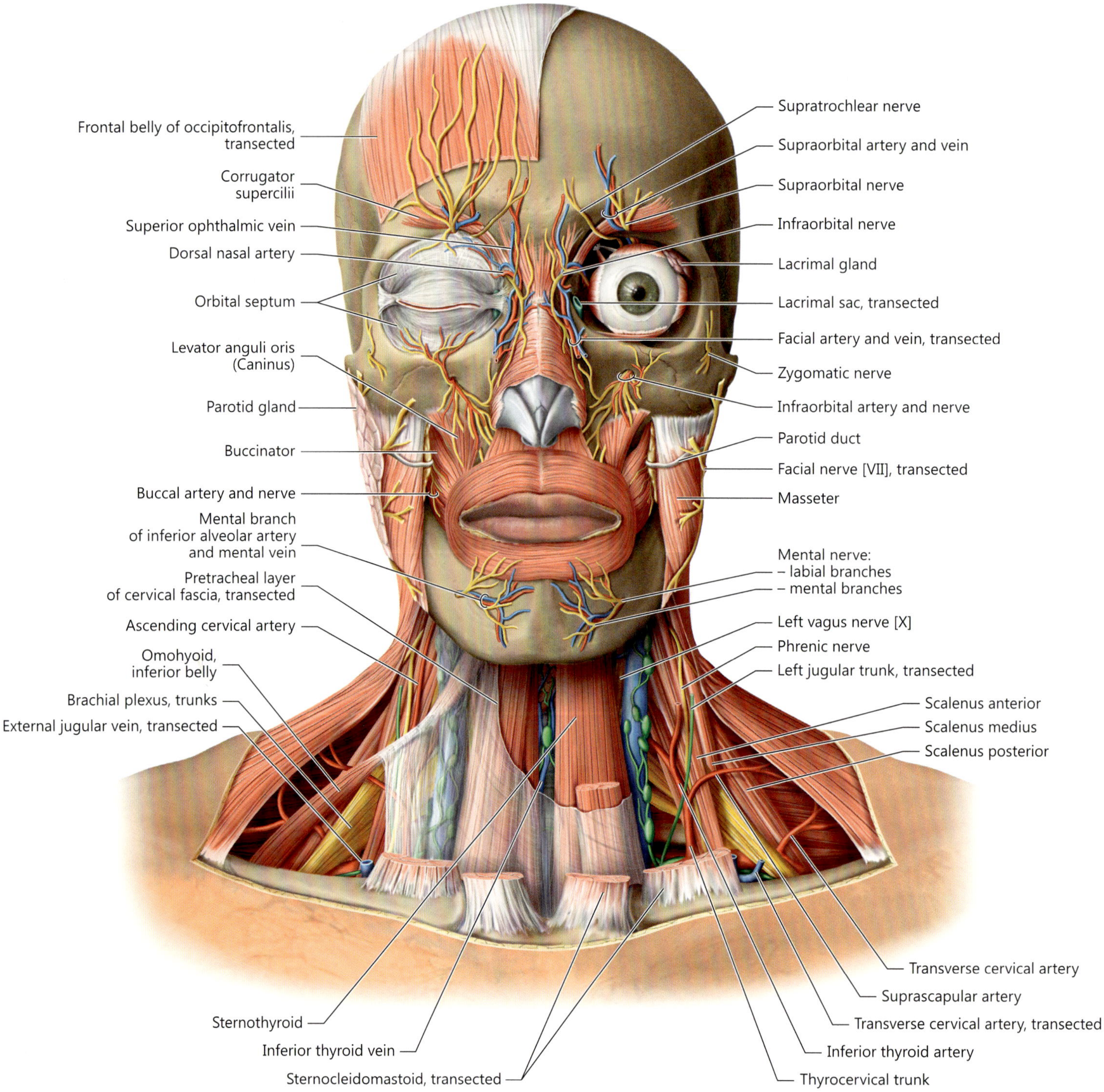

Head and **neck**, anterior view. On the right side of the cranium, the facial muscles have been transected to show the formations that emerge from the supraorbital, zygomaticofacial, infraorbital and mental foramina. On the left side, the eyeball is visible after removal of the orbital septum and tarsus of both eyelids, which together form a diaphragm separating the content of the orbit from the superficial layers of the eyelids.

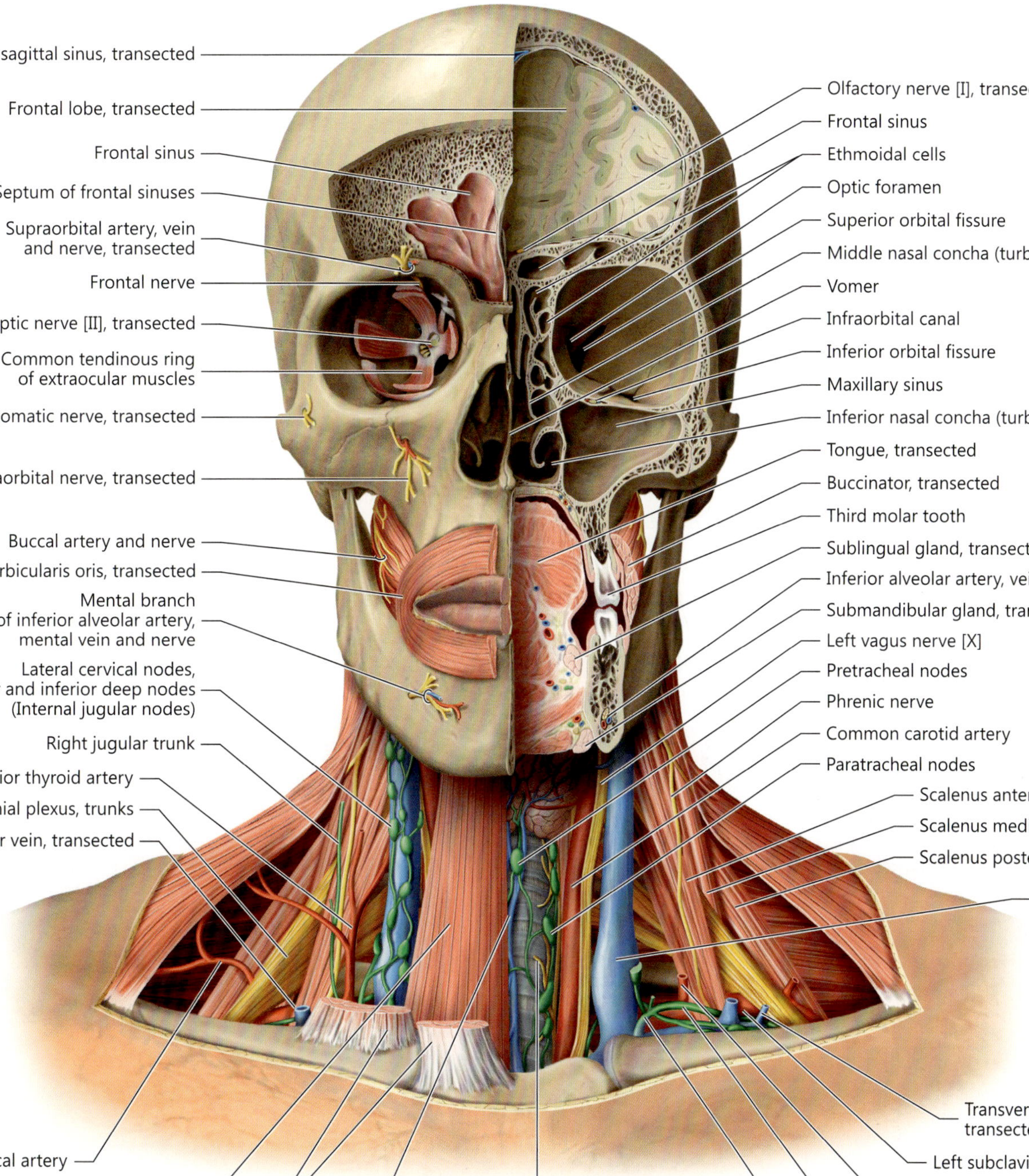

Head and **neck**, anterior view. In the right hemicranium, one can see the internal configuration of the frontal sinus after demolition of its anterior bony wall, as well as the tendinous ring of the extraocular muscles in the orbital cavity, the supraorbital, zygomaticofacial, infraorbital and mental foramina and the formations that emerge from them. In the left hemicranium, a frontal section at the level of the third molar tooth has been performed showing the ethmoidal cells, the muscles of the tongue and the floor of the mouth.

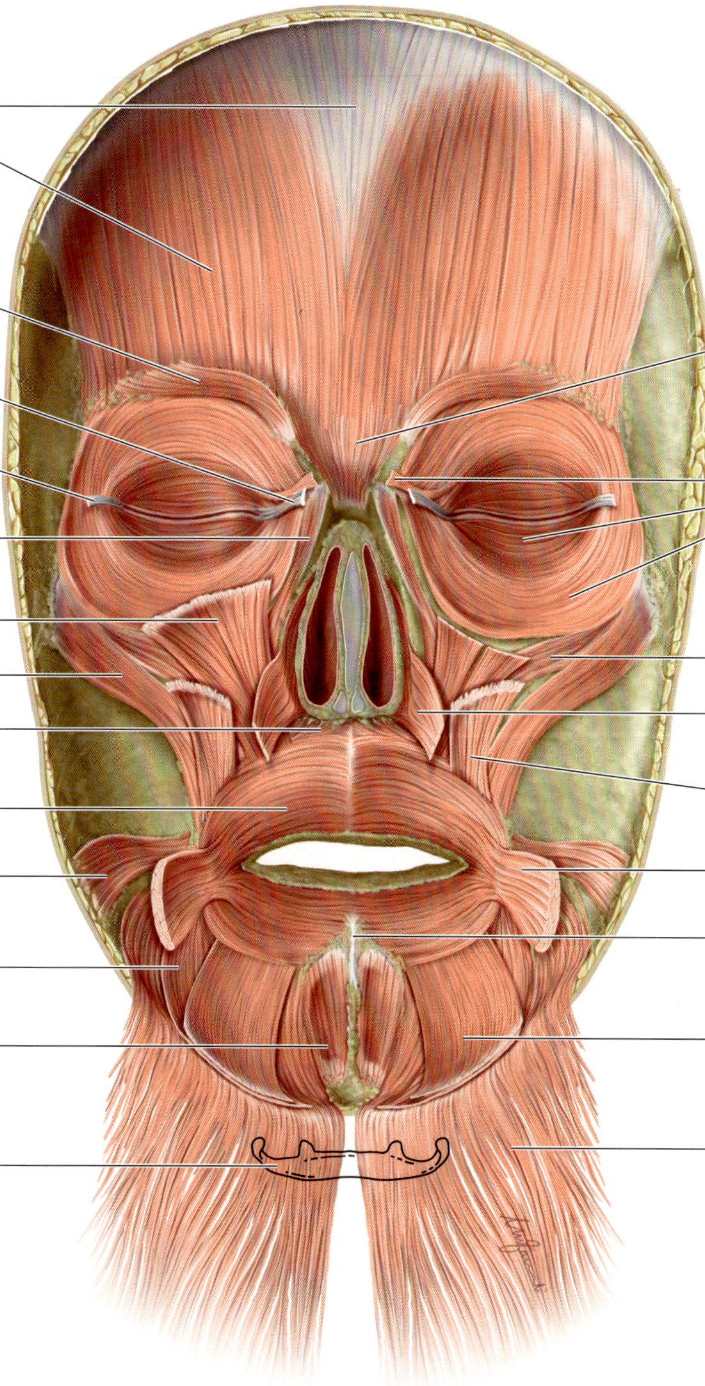

Facial muscles, view of the facial muscles and platysma, from the inside.

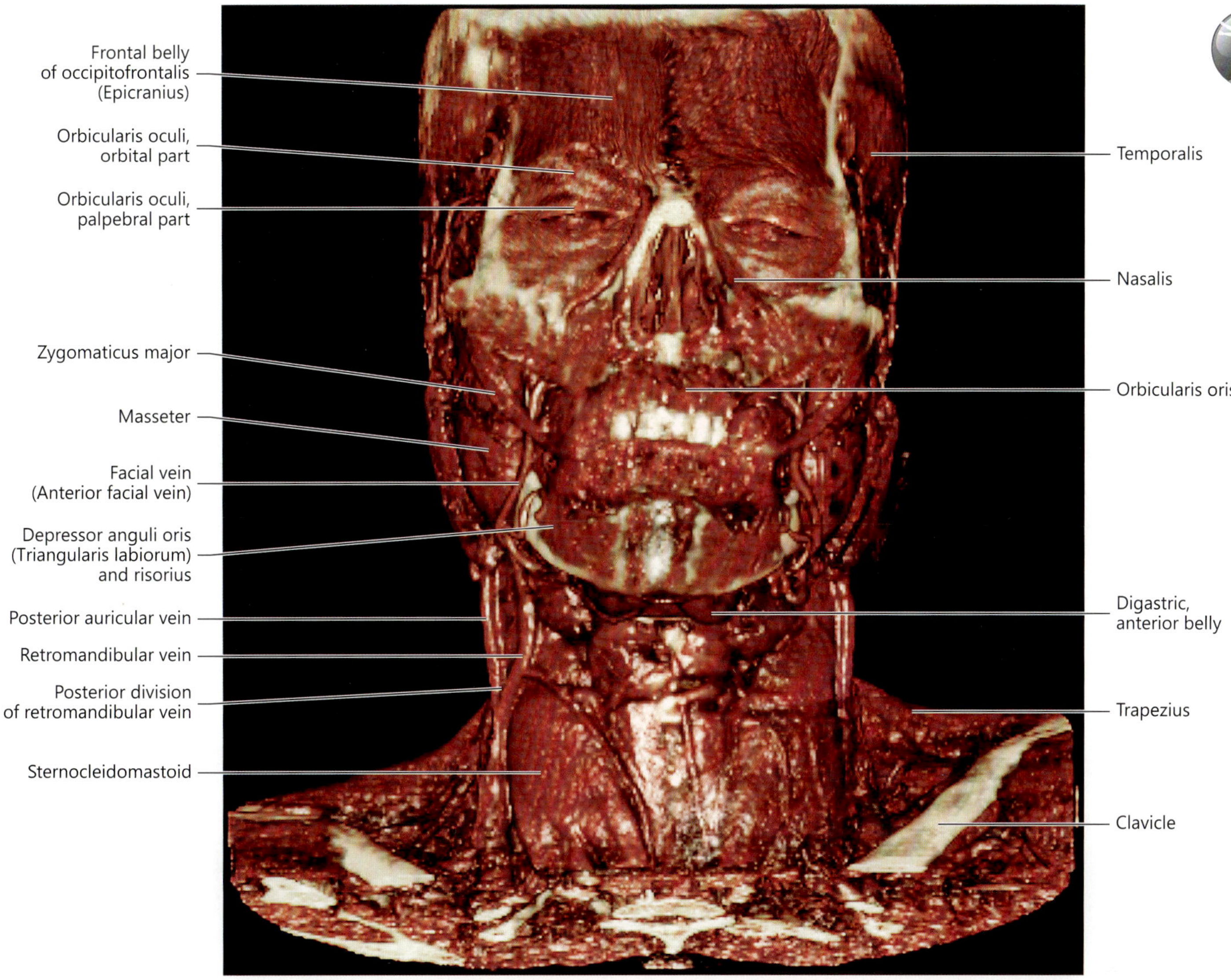

Three-dimensional image of a living human body, obtained by CT scan using a 3D volume rendering technique, showing the **cutaneous** (or **mimic**) **muscles** of the face and **masticatory muscles** of the superficial plane, anterior view. The mimic muscles constitute the superficial or subcutaneous muscle layer of the face, and their contraction causes the skin to stretch and folds to form, modifying the facial expression. The temporalis and masseter form the superficial layer of the masticatory muscles.

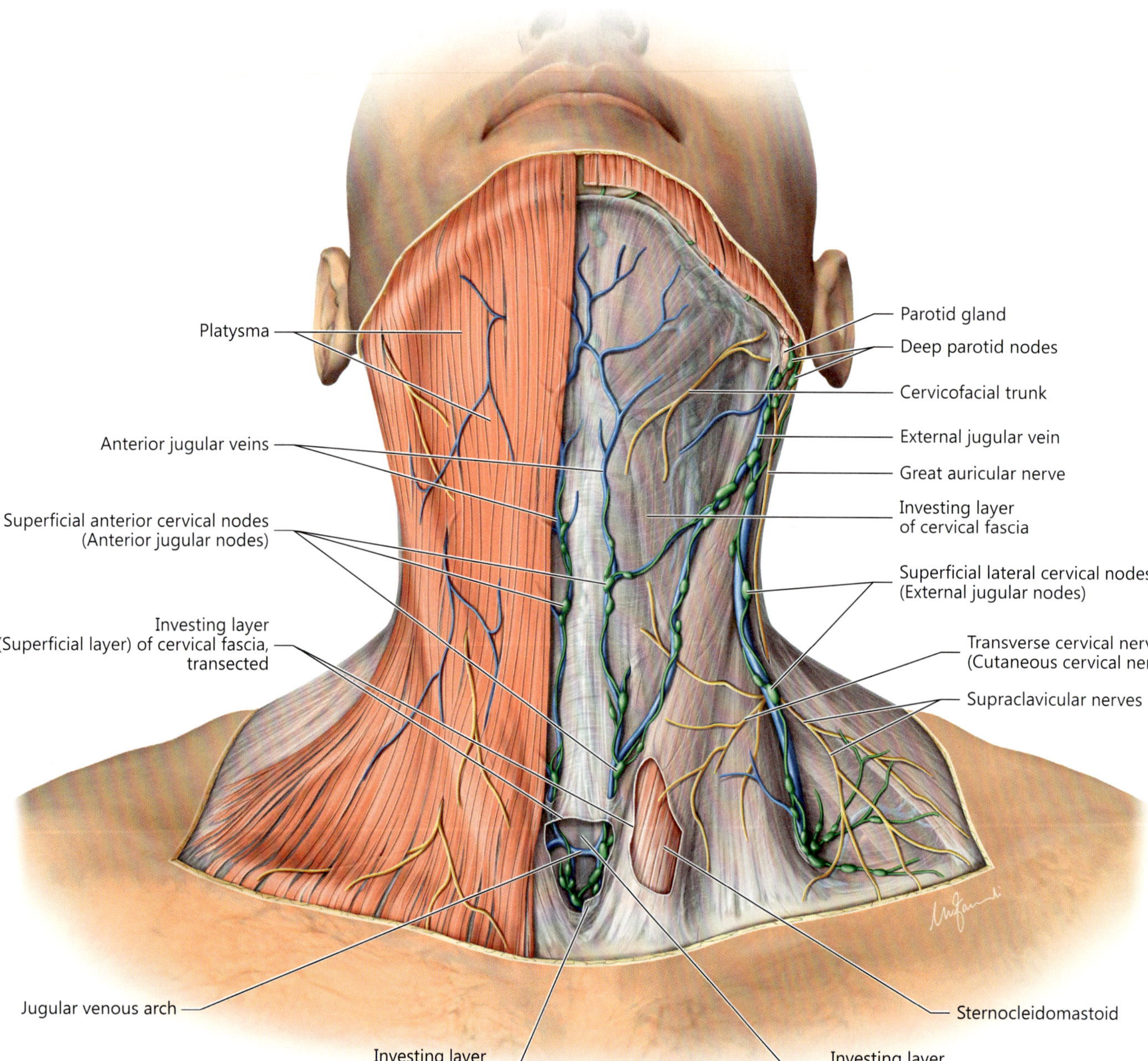

Anterior cervical region. In the right half of the neck, one can see, on a more superficial plane, the platysma, contained within the layer of subcutaneous tissue superficially to the investing layer (or superficial layer) of cervical fascia. On the left side, after removal of the platysma, one can see, superficially to the investing layer, the anterior jugular vein and the external jugular vein, with the chains of lymph nodes linked to the path they follow: the superficial anterior and superficial lateral cervical nodes (or anterior jugular nodes and external jugular nodes). In correspondence to the median line, the investing layer thickens and forms the linea alba of the neck, adhering to the underlying pretracheal layer of cervical fascia, or visceral fascia. Moving in a lateral direction, the investing layer splits to enclose the sternocleidomastoid. Posteriorly to the muscle, the fascia unites to form a single layer, only to split once again to enclose the trapezius. The fascia attaches to the sternum by splitting into two layers that go to the anterior and posterior borders of the manubrium, so delimiting the suprasternal space in which the jugular venous arch is enclosed.

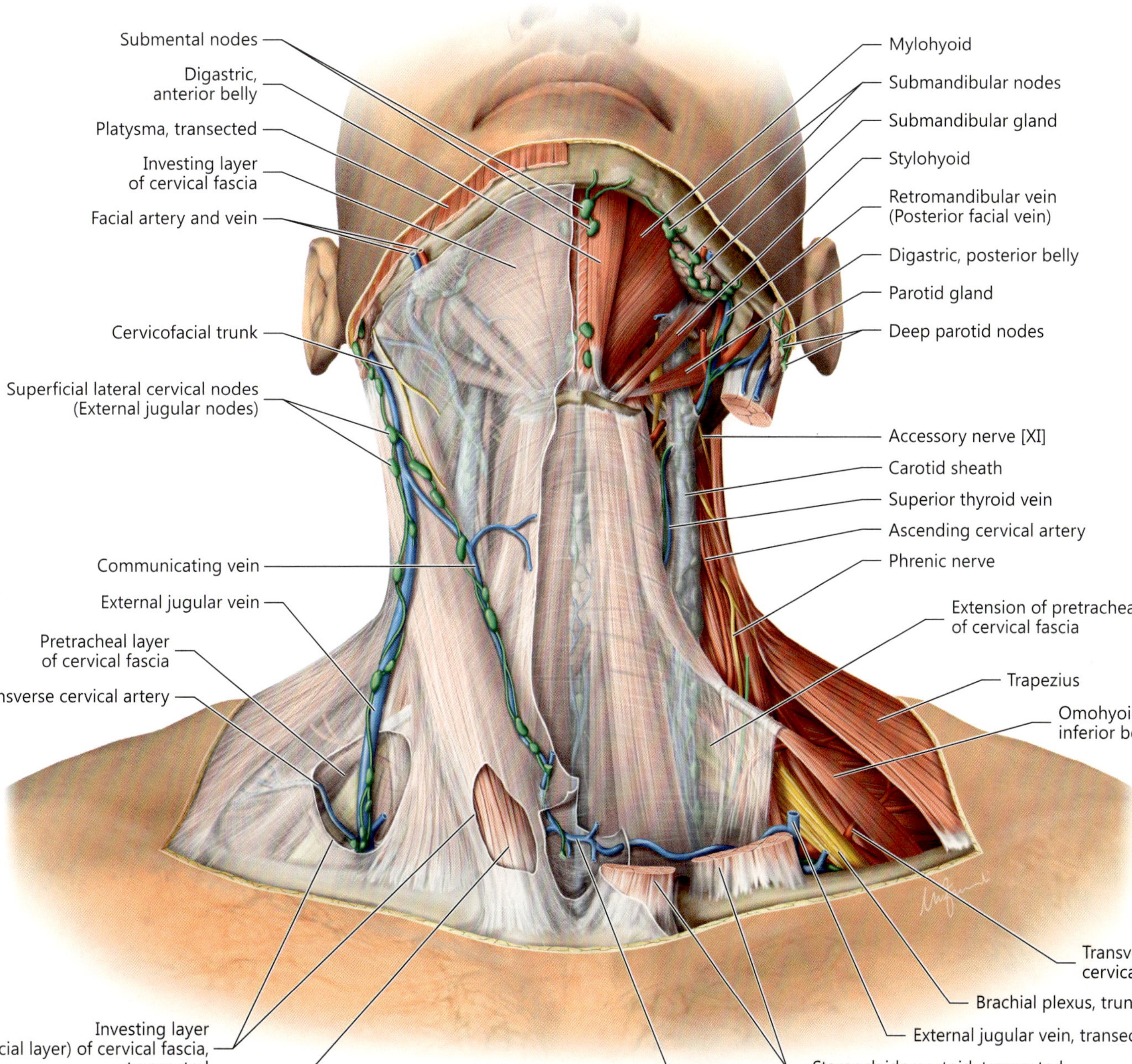

Veins of the neck, anterior view. In the right half of the neck, one can see the external jugular vein that runs down the lateral part of the neck to the middle of the clavicle where it goes deep, piercing the investing and pretracheal layers of cervical fascia, to empty into the subclavian vein at a short distance from its confluence with the internal jugular vein. On the left side, removal of the external jugular vein and investing layer reveals the pretracheal layer (visceral fascia or visceral middle layer of deep cervical fascia) between the hyoid bone and superior thoracic aperture. The pretracheal layer splits to enclose the infrahyoid muscles and, deeply, borders with the carotid sheath that encloses the neurovascular bundle of the neck. Laterally, the pretracheal layer terminates by splitting around the omohyoid. In correspondence to the superior thoracic aperture, it attaches to the posterior surface of the sternum, to the posterior border of the clavicle and adheres to the subclavian and internal jugular veins maintaining them open.

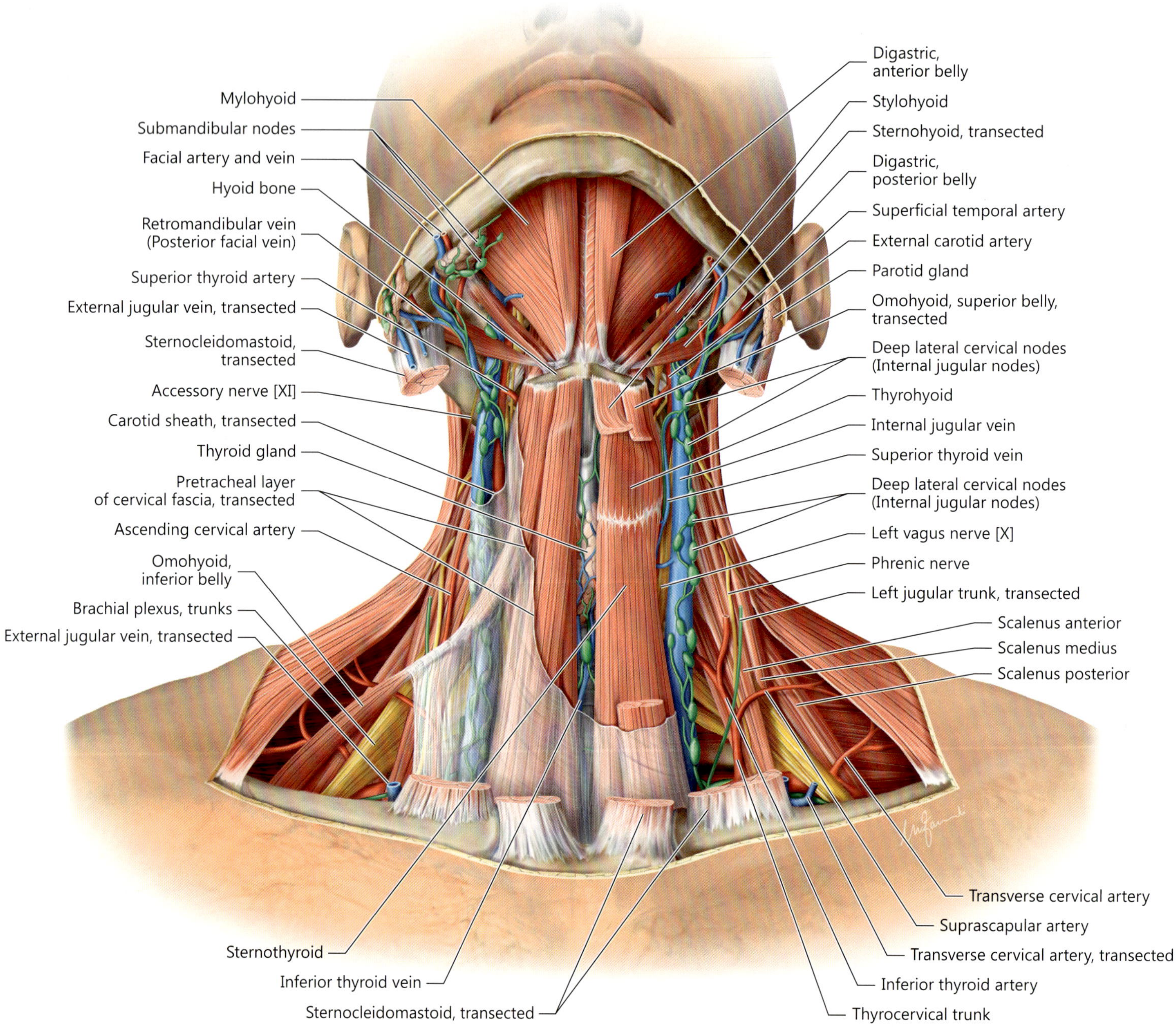

Neck, anterior view. Transection of the sternocleidomastoid, external jugular vein, investing layer and, in part, also pretracheal layer of cervical fascia enables one to observe, in the right half of the neck, the suprahyoid and infrahyoid muscles and the internal jugular vein inside the carotid sheath, which has been in part transected. On the left side, the sternohyoid and omohyoid, located on a superficial plane, have been transected and the carotid sheath removed, rendering visible the sternothyroid and thyrohyoid, located on a deeper plane, and the internal jugular vein with deep lateral cervical nodes located along the length of its course. One can also see the trunks of the brachial plexus above the clavicle, between the scalenus anterior and the scalenus medius and scalenus posterior, and the thyrocervical trunk which, arising from the subclavian artery near the medial border of the scalenus anterior, branches into the inferior thyroid and suprascapular arteries.

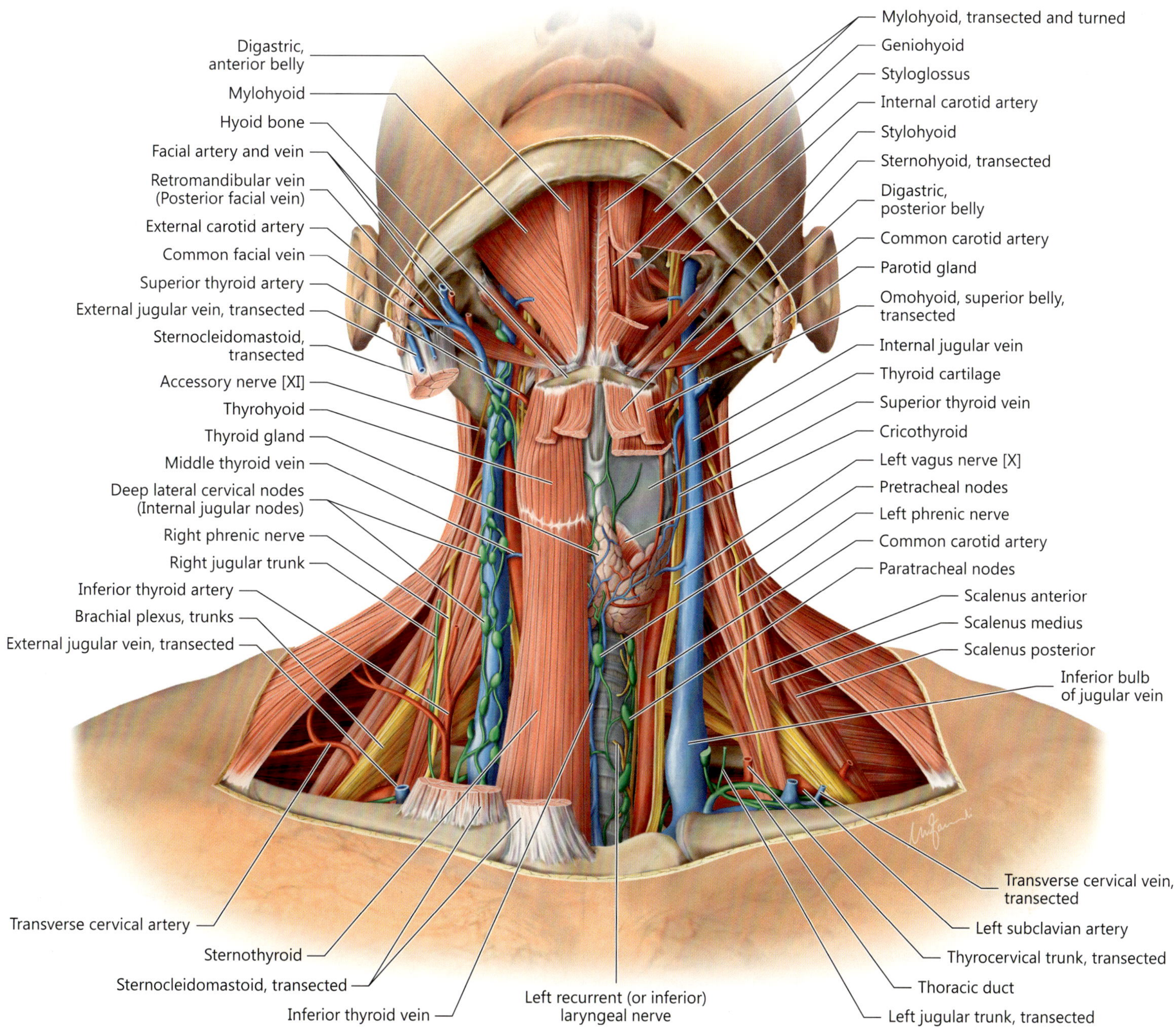

Neck, anterior view. In the right half of the neck, with the sternocleidomastoid, external jugular vein, carotid sheath and sternohyoid and omohyoid transected, it is possible to see the phrenic nerve lying on the anterior surface of the scalenus anterior, the internal jugular vein with lymph nodes present along the length of its course, the sternothyroid and thyrohyoid and the brachial plexus, between the scalenus anterior and the scalenus medius and scalenus posterior. On the left side, with the sternothyroid and thyrohyoid transected, one can see the thyroid cartilage of the larynx, the thyroid gland, the trachea with its pretracheal and paratracheal nodes, the common carotid artery and the vagus nerve. The neurovascular bundle of the neck is also visible, at the top, after transecting the anterior belly of the digastric and the mylohyoid.

Shown in detail, to the right, is the **jugular foramen** through which the glossopharyngeal [IX], vagus [X] and accessory [XI] nerves and the internal jugular vein pass.

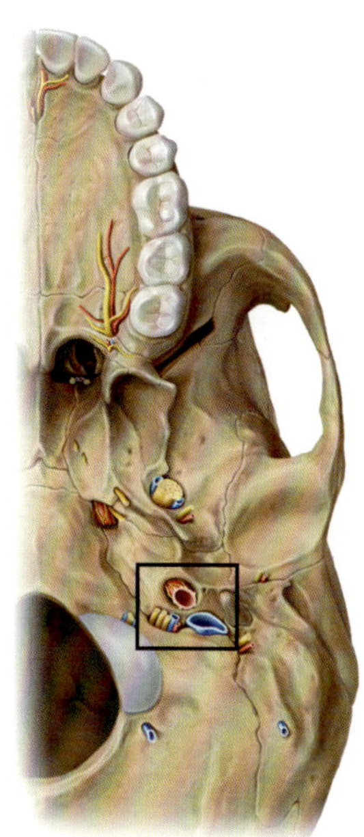

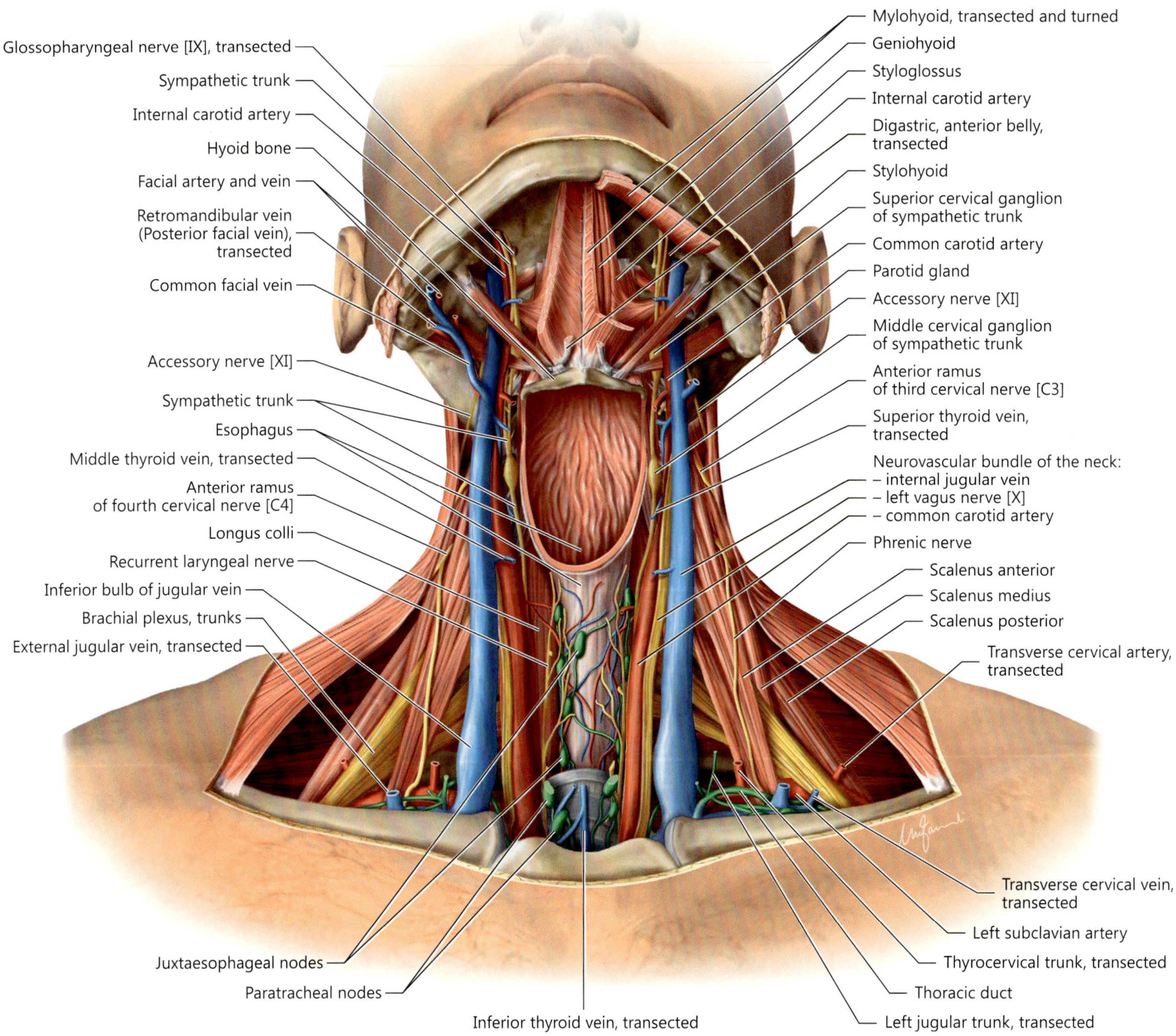

Neck, anterior view. The infrahyoid muscles, thyroid gland, larynx and lymph nodes of the internal jugular vein have been removed as well as the cervical part of the trachea, leaving exposed the posterior wall of the oropharynx and laryngopharynx. The neurovascular bundle of the neck is clearly visible, on the right and left, running anteriorly to the sympathetic trunk, which is attached to the prevertebral layer of cervical fascia (deep cervical fascia) that separates it from the longus capitis and longus colli. The vagus nerve lies in the dihedral angle, which is open posteriorly, formed by the internal carotid artery and internal jugular vein flanking each other. On the upper right side, removal of the suprahyoid muscles (with exception of the stylohyoid) makes it possible to see the common facial vein leading into the internal jugular vein. On the upper left side, the anterior belly of the digastric and the mylohyoid have been transected (the latter has also been turned), and the common facial vein has been transected.

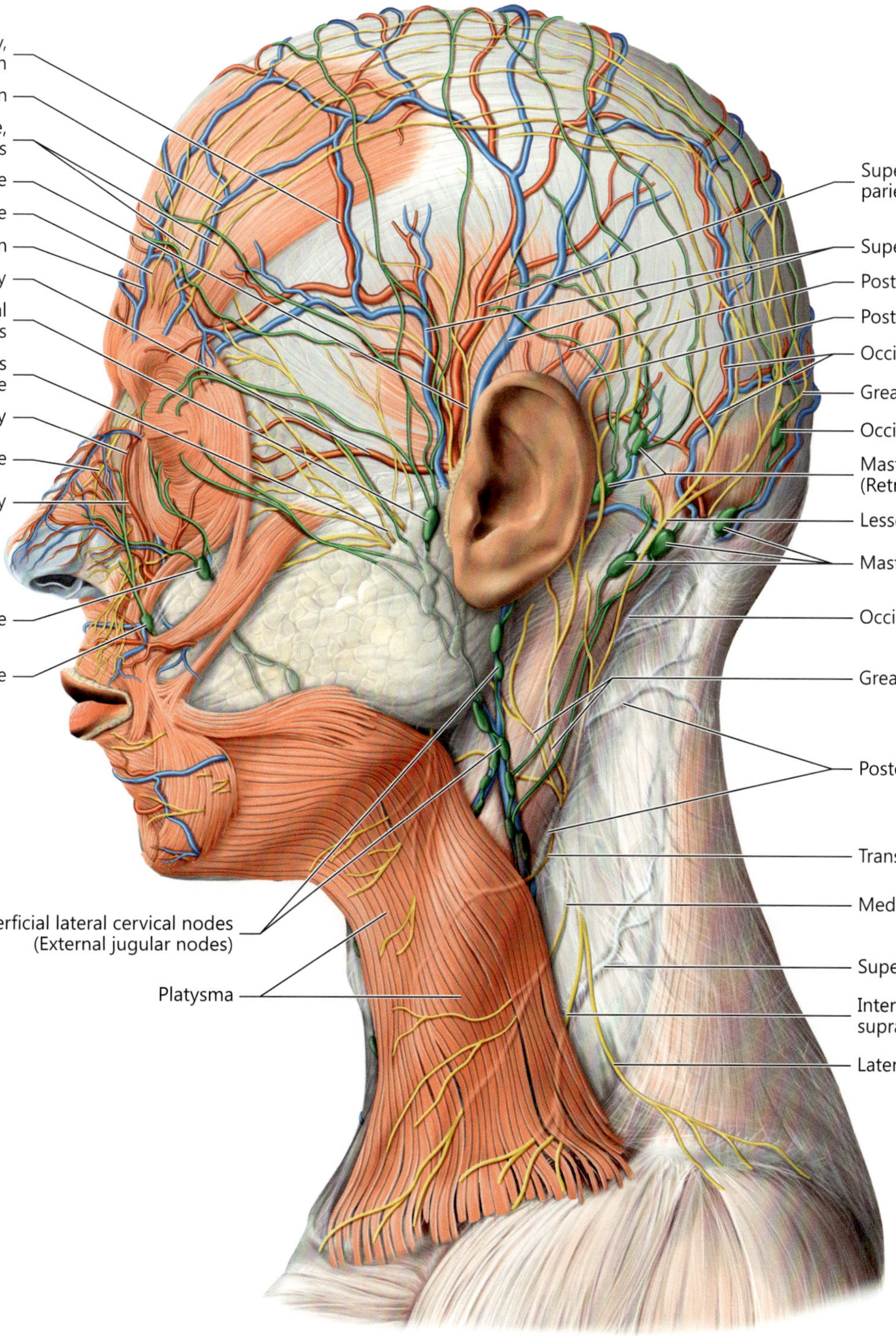

Head and **neck**, left lateral view. Superficial plane after removal of the skin and subcutaneous tissue. One can see the superficial temporal artery, terminal branch of the external carotid artery that emerges from the surface of the parotid gland and divides, in the temporal region, into a frontal and a parietal branch. The zygomatico-orbital artery, collateral branch of the superficial temporal artery, runs along the superior edge of the zygomatic arch to the lateral angle of the orbit. The occipital artery passes through the cranial insertions of the sternocleidomastoid and trapezius and climbs up on the epicranial aponeurosis. The angular artery, continuation of the facial artery, anastomoses with the dorsal nasal artery, branch of the ophthalmic artery. The superficial temporal vein originates from a subcutaneous venous plexus extending over a wide area of the scalp, and anastomoses with the contralateral vein and with the supratrochlear, supraorbital, posterior auricular and occipital veins.

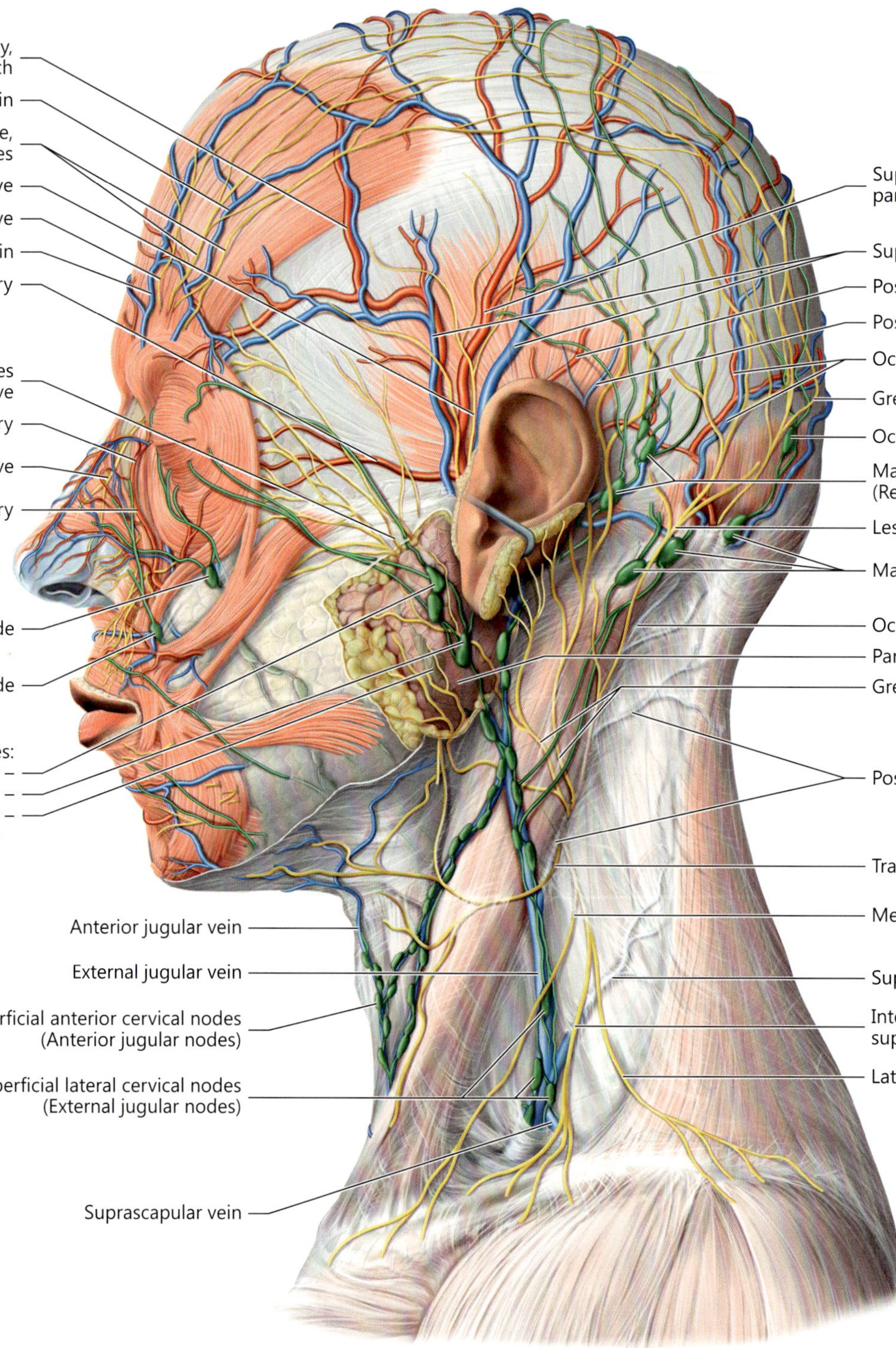

Head and **neck**, left lateral view. Superficial plane after removal of the skin, subcutaneous tissue and the platysma. The parotid fascia has also been partially transected. One can see, in particular, the external jugular and anterior jugular veins. Along the course of the two veins are the superficial anterior and superficial lateral cervical nodes (anterior jugular and external jugular nodes). One can also see the group of deep parotid nodes, the mastoid nodes and occipital nodes, the malar node and the nasolabial node. The great auricular nerve is the largest of the superficial branches of the cervical plexus. It winds around the posterior border of the sternocleidomastoid, then climbs back up its lateral surface and proceeds to the auricle, whose skin it innervates. The transverse cervical nerve, it too a cutaneous branch of the cervical plexus, turns around the posterior border of the sternocleidomastoid, then proceeds in a forward direction crossing the external jugular vein. At the level of the anterior border of the sternocleidomastoid, it innervates the suprahyoid and infrahyoid regions with superior and inferior branches. Other cutaneous branches of the cervical plexus are the supraclavicular nerves, which innervate the superior part of the thorax and the shoulder. The greater occipital nerve, a posterior ramus of C2, becomes subcutaneous in the occipital region where it divides into its terminal branches that constitute a dense plexus on the occipital belly of the occipitofrontalis and on the epicranial aponeurosis.

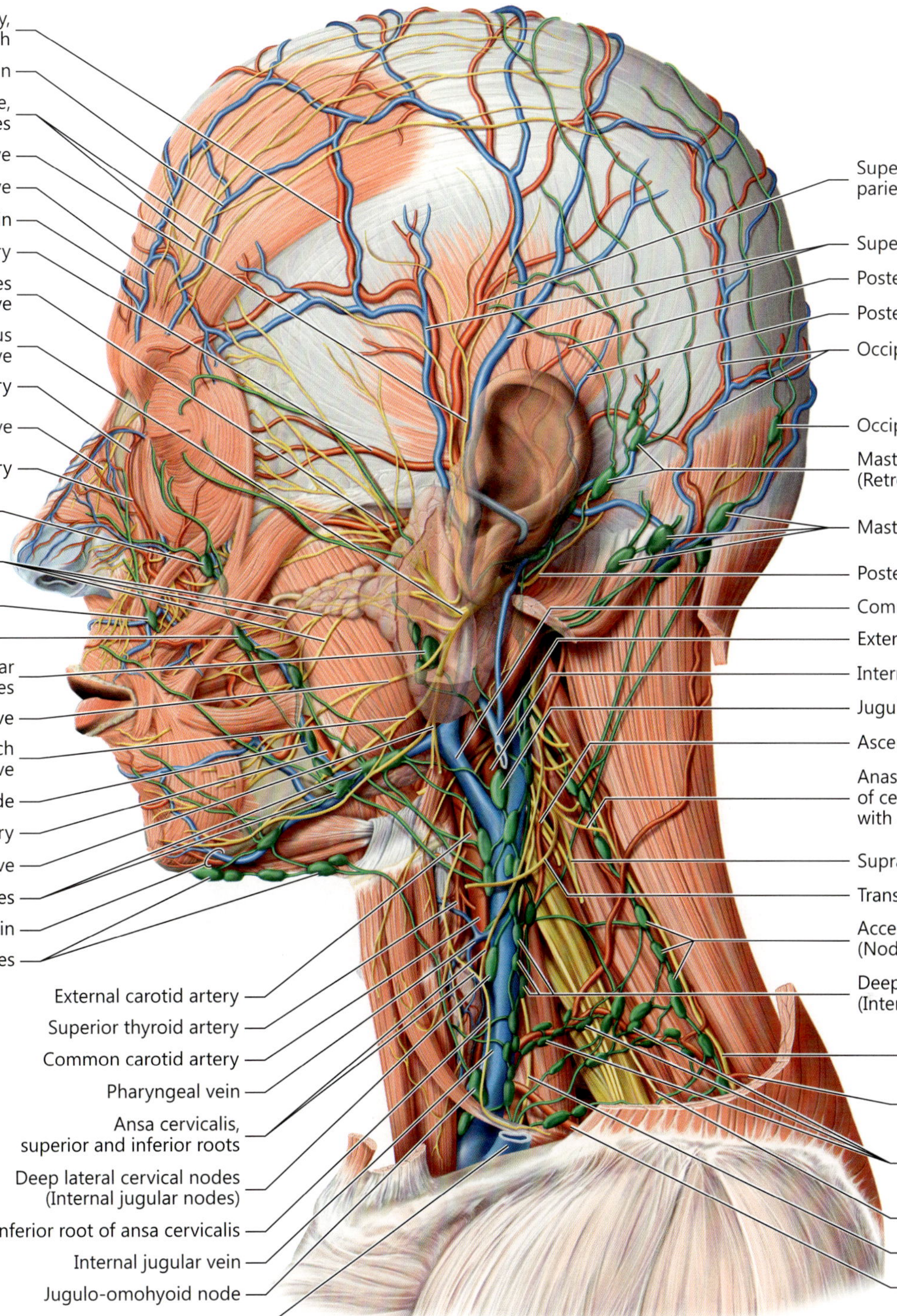

Head and **neck**, left lateral view. Deep plane. The sternocleidomastoid and trapezius and the parotid fascia have been transected. One can see, in particular, the internal jugular vein. The external jugular vein has been transected at its beginning and end. An opening has been made in the parotid gland to show the parotid plexus of the facial nerve and the auriculotemporal nerve that passes right through the gland. From the parotid plexus emerge the temporal, zygomatic, buccal, marginal mandibular and cervical branches of the facial nerve. The posterior auricular nerve originates from the facial nerve after it exits from the stylomastoid foramen. The auriculotemporal nerve, a branch of the mandibular nerve, anastomoses during its passage through the parotid gland with the parotid plexus of the facial nerve, then heads towards the exterior, between the external acoustic meatus and superficial temporal vessels, and proceeds vertically upwards in the temporal region. The chain of deep lateral cervical nodes along the internal jugular vein, that of the accessory nodes along the path of the accessory nerve, and that of the supraclavicular nodes along the transverse cervical artery constitute the posterior triangle. Clearly visible also are the facial, malar, nasolabial, buccinator and mandibular nodes, and the submandibular and submental nodes.

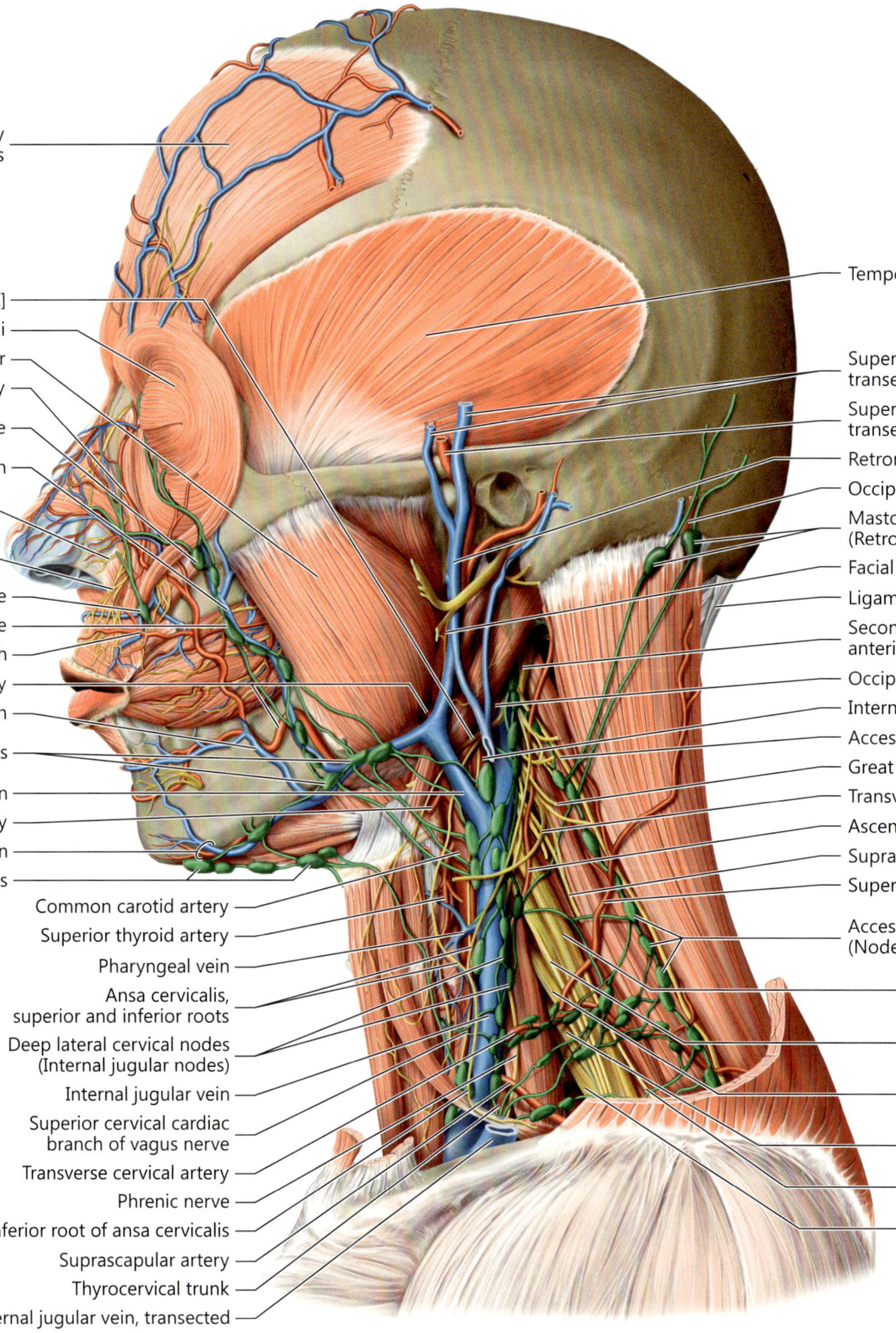

Head and **neck**, left lateral view. Deep plane. The sternocleidomastoid and trapezius, parotid gland, some facial muscles, epicranial aponeurosis and the occipital belly of the occipitofrontalis have been transected. One can see, in addition to the internal jugular vein, the facial vein and trunks of the brachial plexus, formed by the anterior rami of the fifth, sixth, seventh and eighth cervical and first thoracic nerves. The superior root of the ansa cervicalis, containing fibers from the first cervical nerve, proceeds downwards after leaving the hypoglossal nerve, in front of, or inside, the carotid sheath (which here has been removed), and unites with the inferior root of the ansa cervicalis, coming from the second and third cervical nerves. The ansa cervicalis, also known as ansa of hypoglossal nerve, innervates the omohyoid, sternohyoid and sternothyroid.

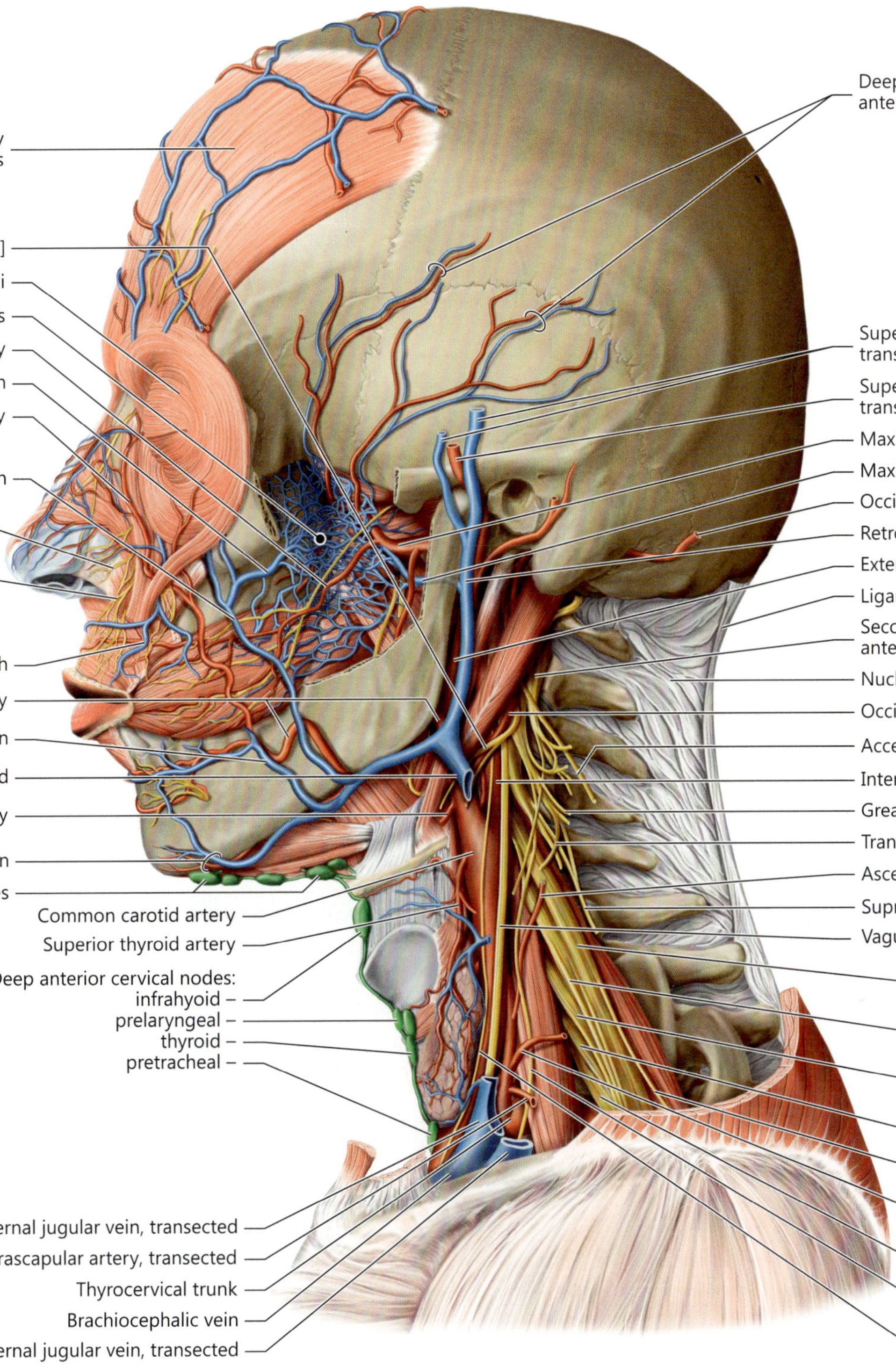

Head and **neck**, left lateral view. Deep plane. The sternocleidomastoid and trapezius, parotid gland, some facial muscles, epicranial aponeurosis, occipital belly of the occipitofrontalis, and the infrahyoid muscles, masseter, temporalis and splenius capitis have been transected. The removal of the internal jugular vein reveals the common carotid artery and the vagus nerve. Also visible are the thyroid cartilage and thyroid gland. The vagus nerve is located in the dihedral angle, which is open posteriorly, formed by the common carotid artery and internal jugular vein. One can see the group of deep anterior cervical nodes, or anterior visceral nodes, that drain the larynx, trachea and thyroid gland. In the infratemporal fossa the pterygoid plexus can be seen, situated in part between the temporalis and lateral pterygoid and partly between the lateral and medial pterygoid. From the confluence of the veins of the plexus originates the maxillary vein, which joins the superficial temporal veins forming the retromandibular vein. The pterygoid plexus communicates with the facial vein via the deep facial vein.

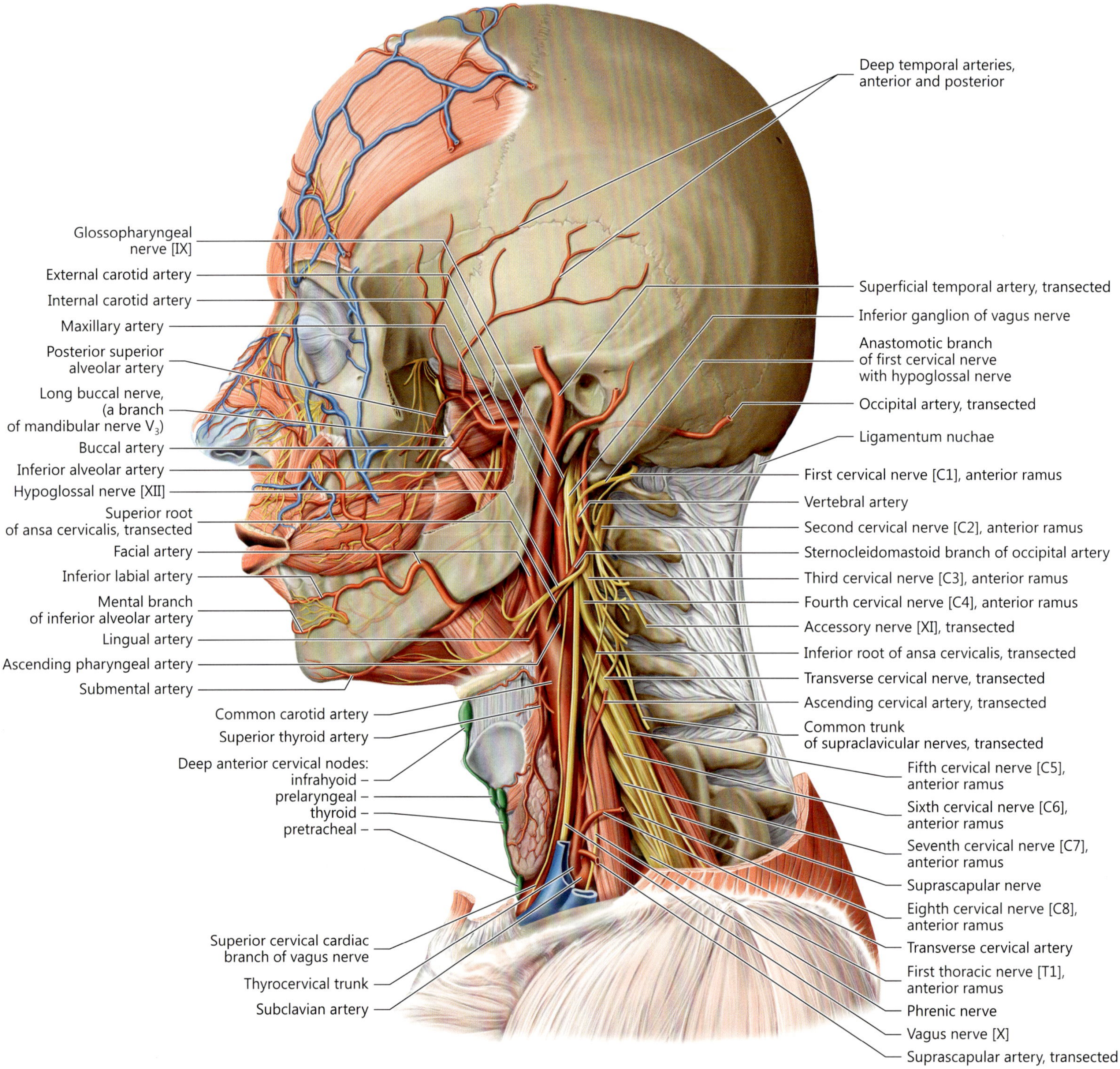

Head and **neck**, left lateral view. Deep plane. Almost the entire venous system has been removed. One can see, in addition to the brachial plexus, the cervical plexus, formed by the anterior rami of the first, second, third and fourth cervical nerves. The phrenic nerve, the largest and longest branch arising from the cervical plexus, runs obliquely downwards and medially, on the anterior surface of the scalenus anterior. In the parapharyngeal space, note the hypoglossal nerve, which crosses the internal carotid artery and vagus nerve forming a loop around the sternocleidomastoid branch of the occipital artery. The maxillary artery, the largest terminal branch of the external carotid artery, proceeds medially to the mandibular condyle, passes through the infratemporal fossa and, heading superficially (as shown here) or deeply to the lower head of the lateral pterygoid, terminates in the pterygopalatine fossa.

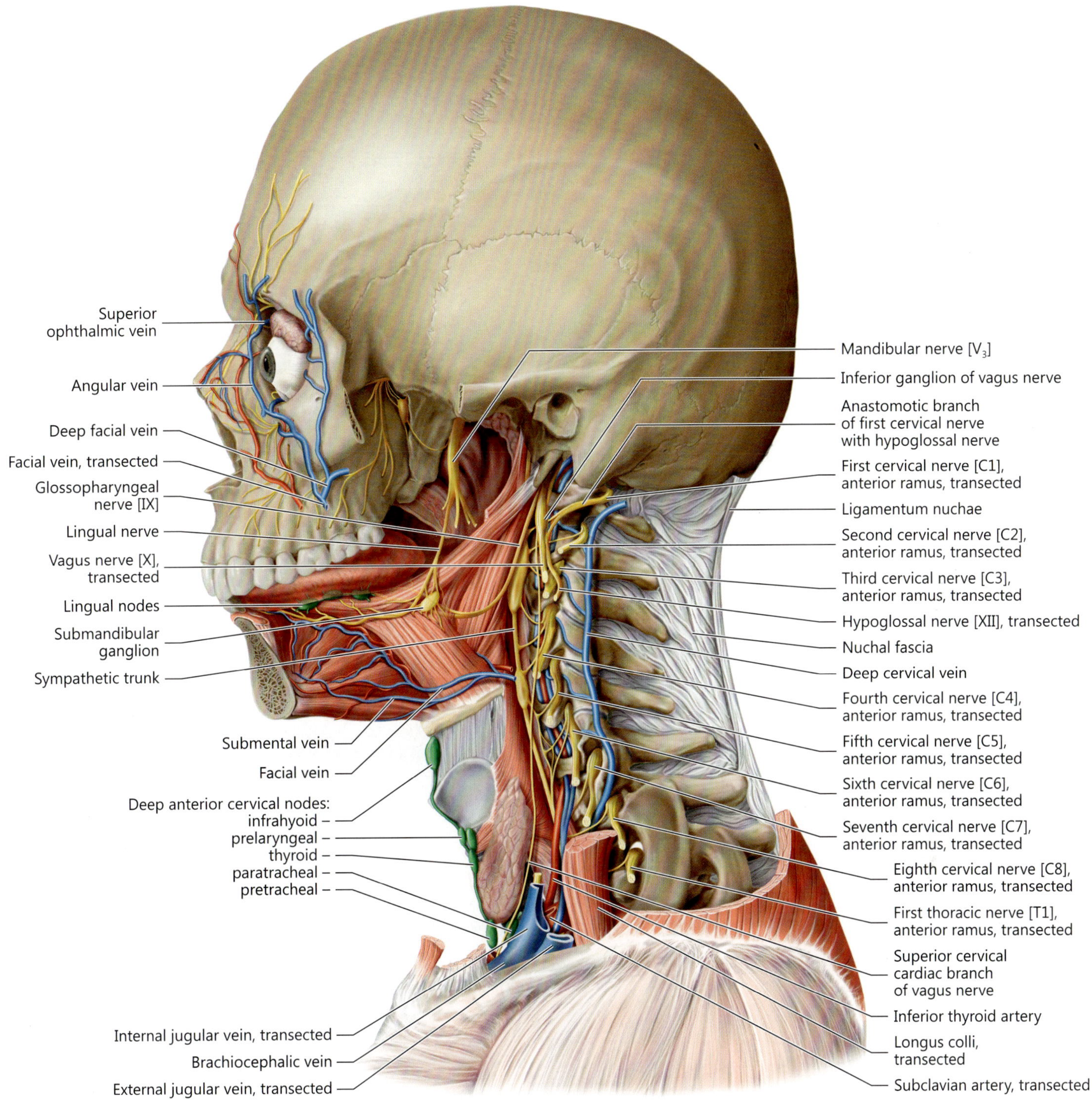

Head and **neck**, left lateral view. Deep plane. The neurovascular bundle of the neck and anterior rami of the cervical nerves have been transected, showing the sympathetic trunk. Removal of the left hemi-mandible reveals the lingual nerve and submandibular ganglion. The cervical segment of the sympathetic trunk extends from the cranial base to the superior thoracic aperture, attached to the prevertebral layer of cervical fascia, which separates it from the transverse processes of the cervical vertebrae and from the longus capitis and longus colli. Note the lingual nerve, a branch of the mandibular nerve, which makes an anterosuperiorly concave curve in a downward and forward direction. Also the glossopharyngeal nerve [IX] proceeds obliquely downwards and forwards making an anterosuperiorly concave curve. The vertebral vein originates between the occipital bone and atlas, and after descending through the foramina transversaria of the first six cervical vertebrae it heads anteriorly to empty into the brachiocephalic vein.

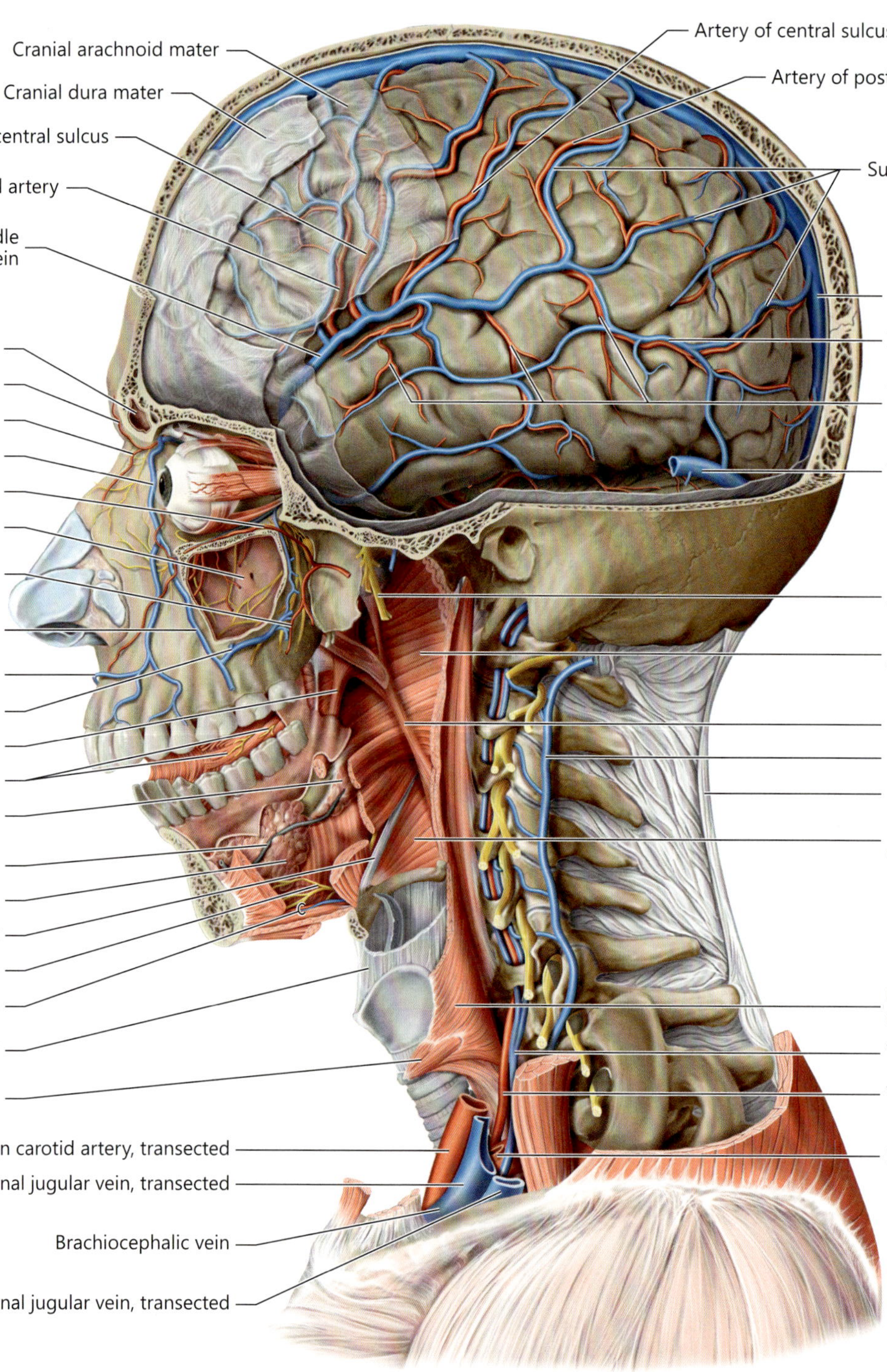

Head and **neck**, left lateral view. With most of the left hemicranium removed, one can see the superficial cerebral veins and branches of the middle cerebral artery on the surface of the left cerebral hemisphere. In the face, a parasagittal transection has been carried out making it possible to see both the orbital cavity and the interior of the maxillary sinus; one can also see the angular vein, which originates superficially from the medial angle of the eye and, running obliquely downward laterally to the root of the nose, as a facial vein, receives the deep facial vein from the pterygoid plexus. In the inferior part of the mouth, instead, the left hemi-mandible and respective soft tissues, including the entire tongue, have been removed, so as to render clearly visible the sublingual gland with its neurovascular relations. In the neck, a paramedian sagittal section reveals the deep cervical vein that originates inferiorly to the mastoid process and descends posteriorly to the transverse processes of the cervical vertebrae. It is possible, moreover, to see the vertebral vein, which originates between the occipital bone and atlas, and descends through the foramina transversaria of the first six cervical vertebrae, in a lateral position with respect to the vertebral artery. In the anterior part of the neck, a more external paramedian section allows one to see the laryngotracheal canal and its relationship to the left common carotid artery and left internal jugular vein.

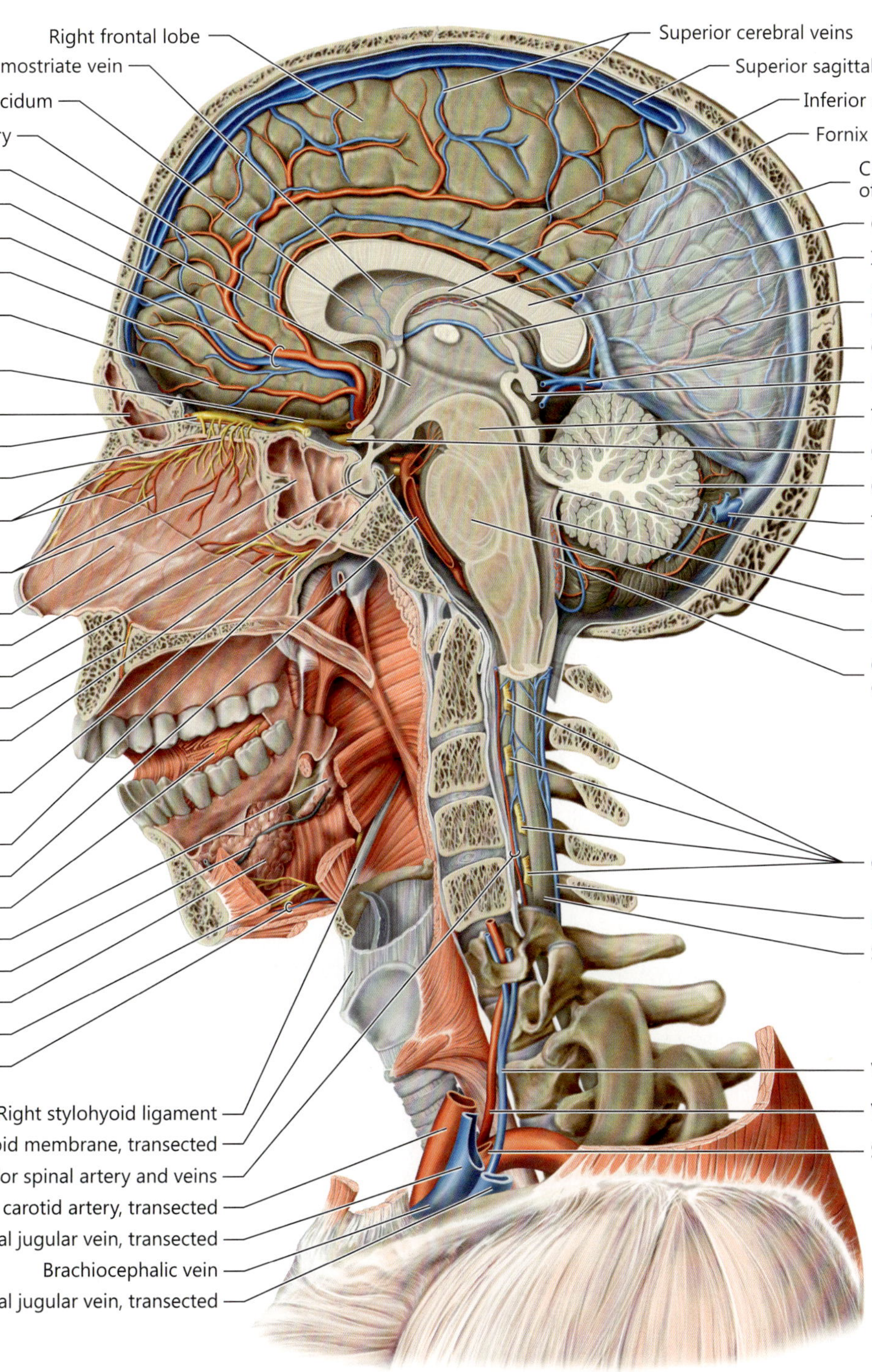

Sagittal section of head and **neck**, left lateral view, showing the contents of the cranial cavity and vertebral canal, the right nasal cavity, oral cavity, and large vessels transected at the base of the neck. The cerebral veins have an independent course with respect to the arteries and are more numerous. They can be classified into: superficial cerebral veins (of which the superior cerebral veins are visible), numbering 8-10 per hemisphere, that drain the medial and superolateral surfaces of the hemispheres and empty mostly into the superior sagittal sinus, and deep cerebral veins (of which here can be seen the internal cerebral vein and the great cerebral vein, or vein of Galen). The two internal cerebral veins, right and left, run anteroposteriorly between the two layers of the choroid membrane and terminate by uniting to form the great cerebral vein, a median unpaired venous trunk, approximately 1 cm long, situated in the transverse fissure of the brain, that runs between the cerebellum and splenium of corpus callosum terminating in the straight sinus. Below the hyoid bone, the transection plane becomes parasagittal allowing one to see, from the left, the larynx and trachea, and, lower down, the origin and partial course of the vertebral artery and vein.

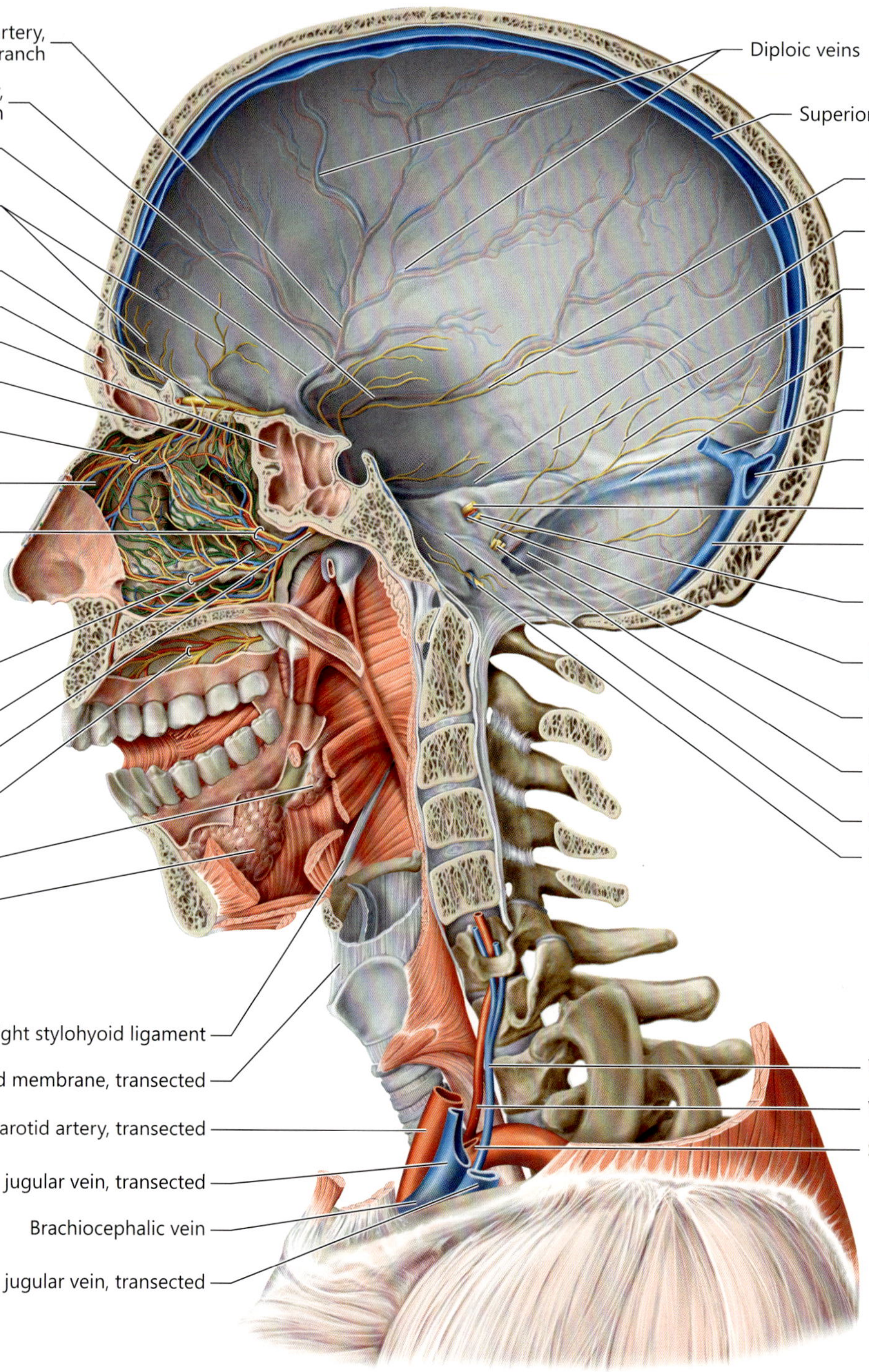

Head and **neck**, left lateral view. With the left hemicranium and brain removed, one can see the lateral wall of the cranium from the inside. The middle meningeal artery, which originates from the maxillary artery, penetrates into the middle cranial fossa through the foramen spinosum. The middle meningeal vein, a satellite of the middle meningeal artery, runs between the two layers of cranial dura mater and can be considered homologous to the dural venous sinuses. After removal of a large part of the nasal septum, it is also possible to see the lateral wall of the right nasal cavity. The posterior lateral nasal arteries originate from the sphenopalatine artery, which penetrates into the nasal cavity through the sphenopalatine foramen together with the nasopalatine nerve. The greater palatine artery emerges through the greater palatine foramen on the vault of the palate, heads forward, enters the incisive canal and anastomoses with a branch of the sphenopalatine artery. The anterior ethmoidal artery, a branch of the ophthalmic artery, passes through the anterior ethmoidal foramen together with the anterior ethmoidal nerve. Below the hyoid bone, the transection plane becomes parasagittal allowing one to see, from the left, the larynx and trachea, and, further down, the origin and partial course of the vertebral artery and vein.

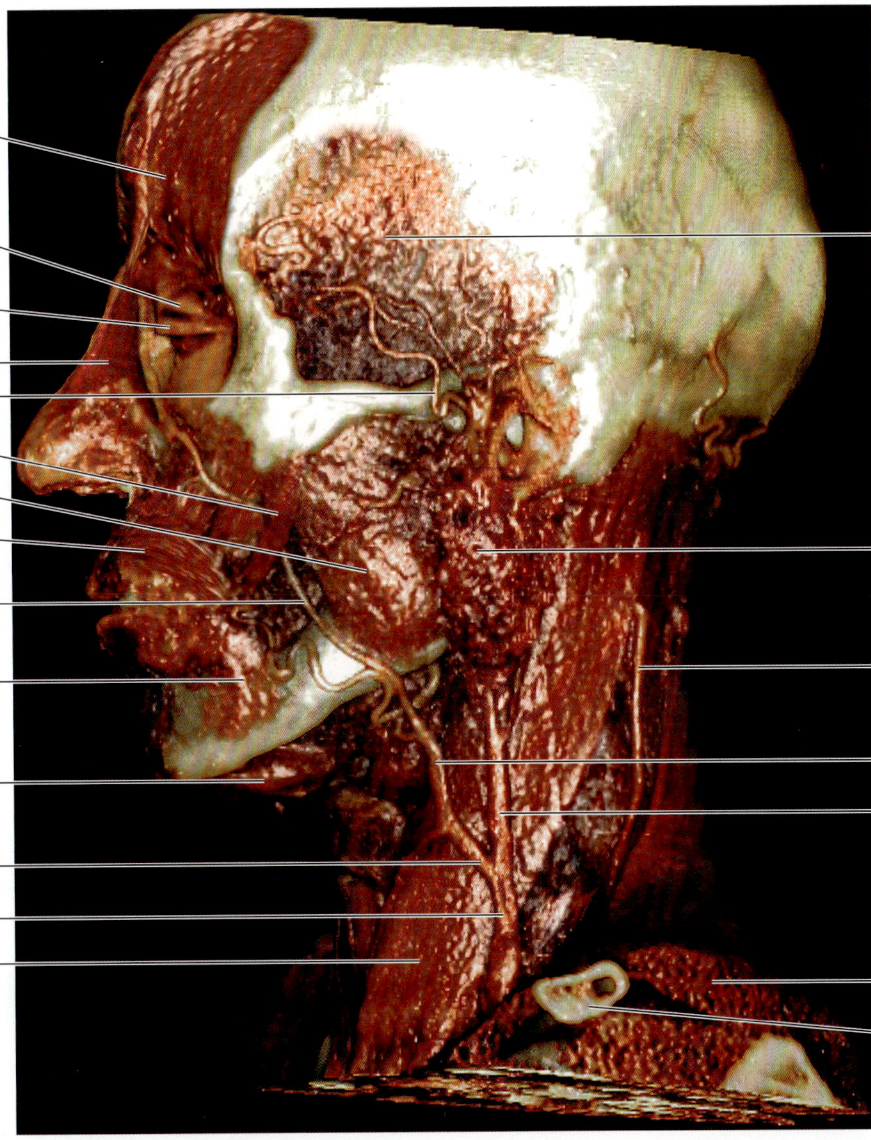

Three-dimensional image of a living human body, obtained using a 3D volume rendering technique, of the head and neck in left lateral view, showing the **cutaneous** (or **mimic**) **muscles**, the **temporalis** and **masseter** (**masticatory muscles**), the **sternocleidomastoid** and the **parotid gland**, whose superficial part or external surface, triangular in form, is visible. The anterior margin of the superficial part of the gland borders with the masseter, and is superimposed on it to some extent; the posterior margin borders with the sternocleidomastoid; the base, superior, corresponds to the cartilaginous part of the external acoustic meatus and to the zygomatic arch; the apex, inferior, is near the submandibular gland.

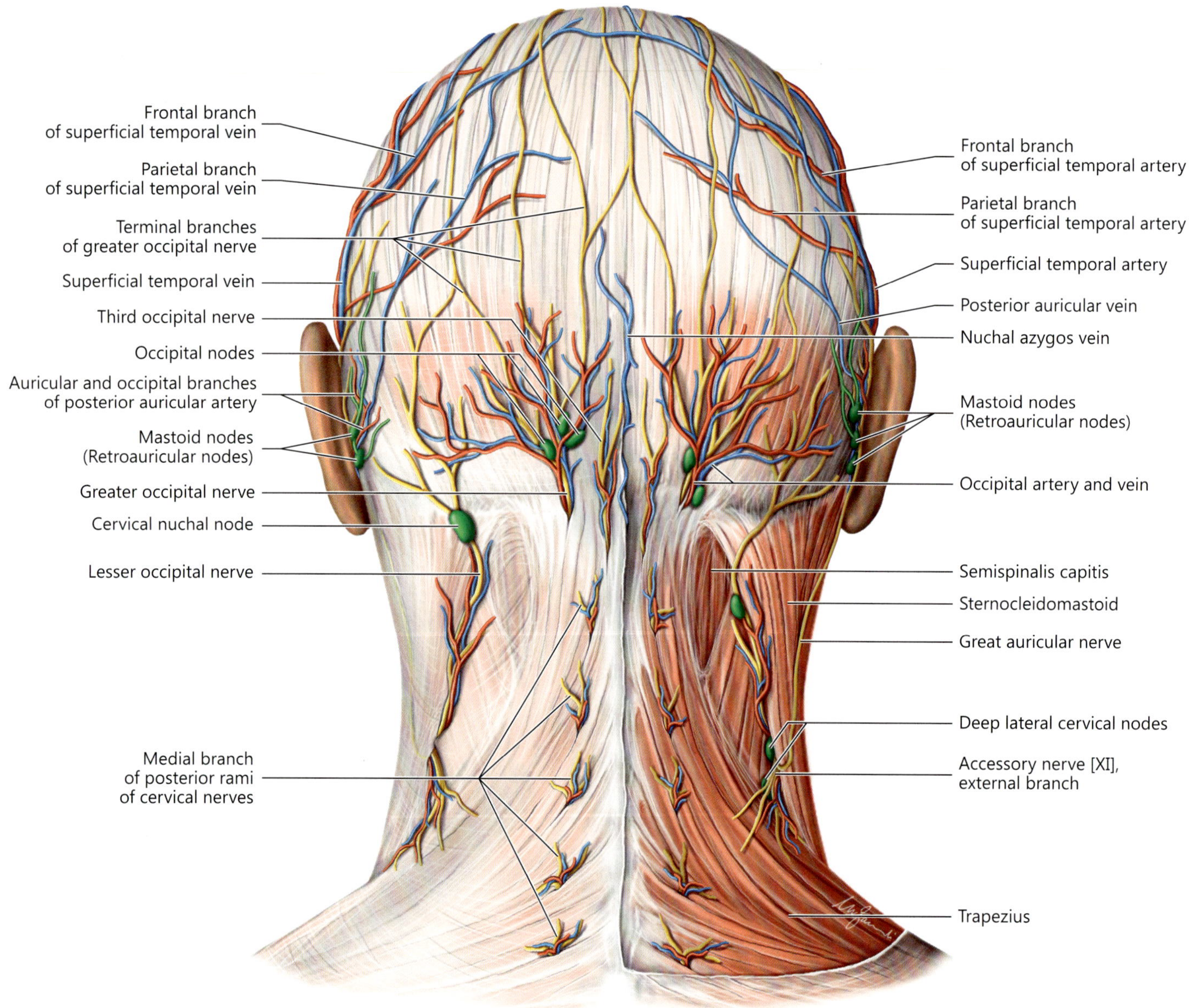

Head and **neck**, posterior view. In the left half, with the skin and subcutaneous tissue removed, one can observe in particular the occipital nodes and the mastoid or retroauricular nodes. In the right half, in addition to the skin and subcutaneous tissue, the investing layer of cervical fascia has been transected. One can see in particular the great auricular nerve, the largest of the superficial branches of the cervical plexus, which proceeds upwards on the lateral surface of the sternocleidomastoid.

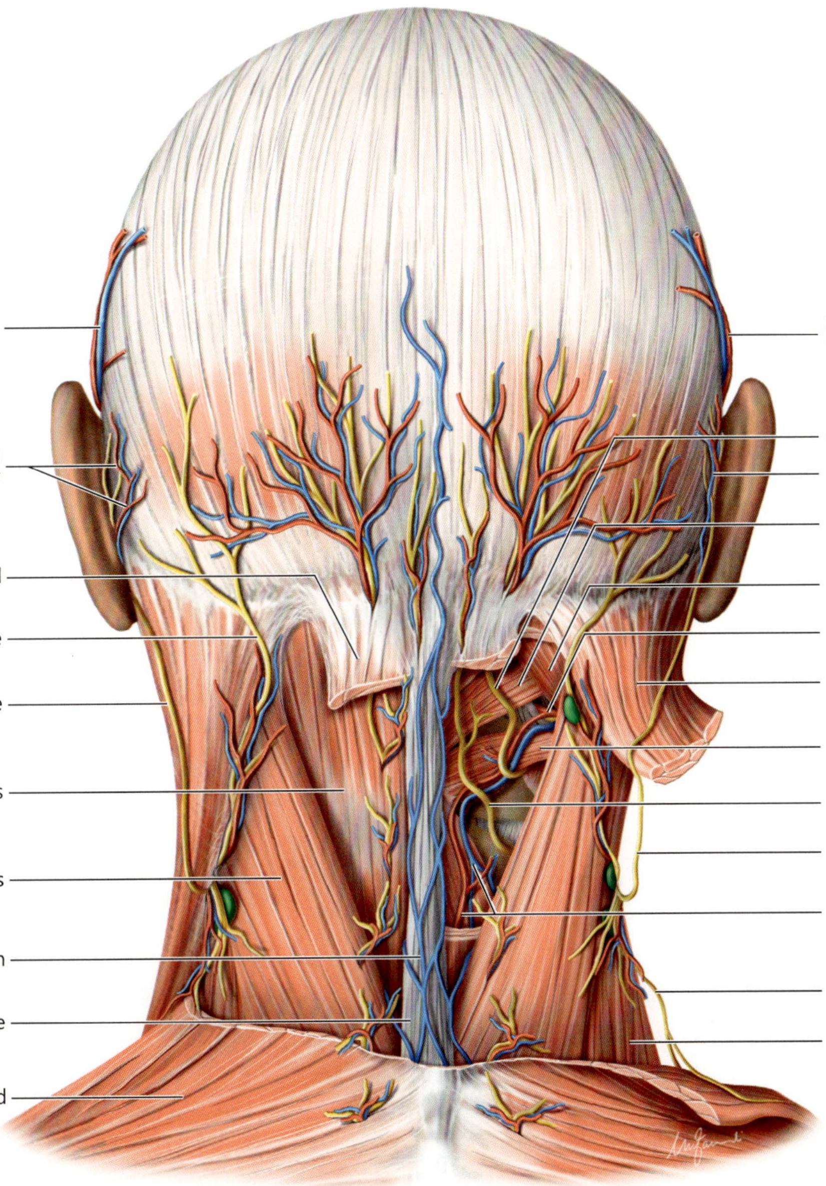

Head and **neck**, posterior view. In the left half, after removal of the skin, subcutaneous tissue and investing layer of cervical fascia, the trapezius and the nuchal fascia that separates it from the splenius capitis have been transected, revealing the semispinalis capitis. The lesser occipital nerve, a cutaneous branch of the cervical plexus, climbs up into the head along the posterior border of the sternocleidomastoid. In the right half, also the semispinalis capitis has been removed to expose the suboccipital muscles, and the sternocleidomastoid has been transected. One can see the vertebral artery and the greater occipital and third occipital nerves, posterior rami of C2 and C3, the second and third cervical nerves.

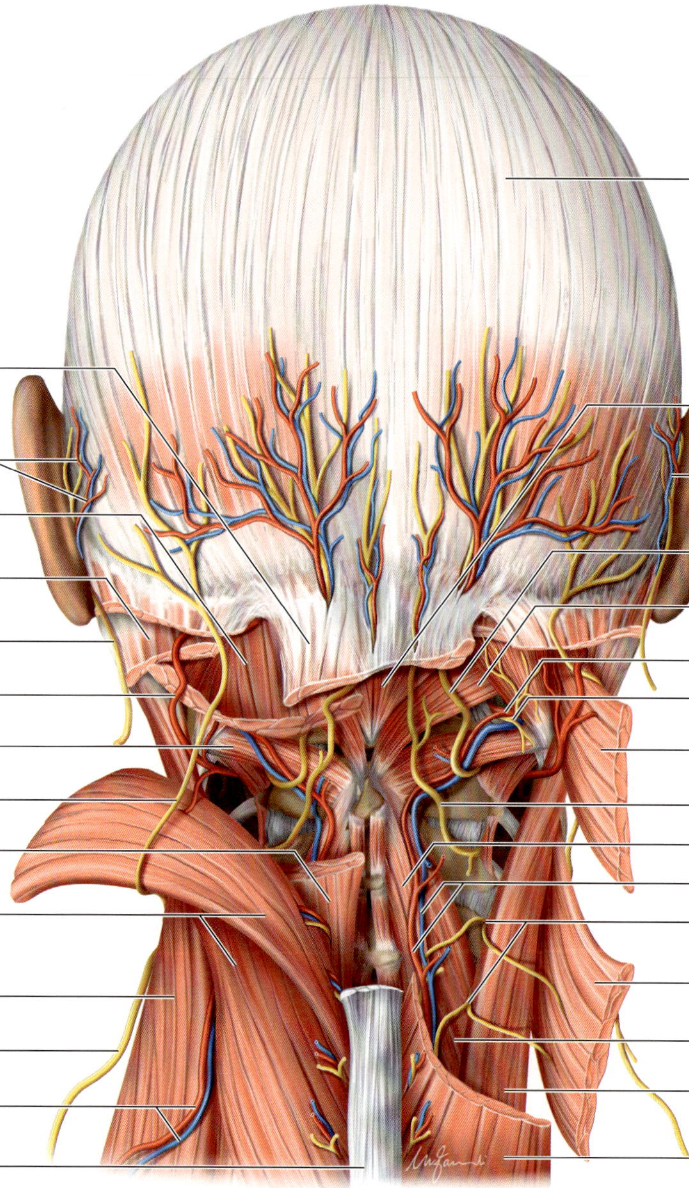

Head and **neck**, posterior view. In the left half, in addition to the trapezius, sternocleidomastoid and semispinalis capitis, the splenius capitis has been transected and turned, showing the occipital artery. On the median plane, the ligamentum nuchae has been transected. In the right half, also the levator scapulae has been transected, exposing the longissimus capitis and semispinalis cervicis. In the interstitium delimited medially by the rectus capitis posterior major and laterally by the obliquus capitis superior and obliquus capitis inferior, one can see the suboccipital nerve, a posterior ramus of C1, the first cervical nerve.

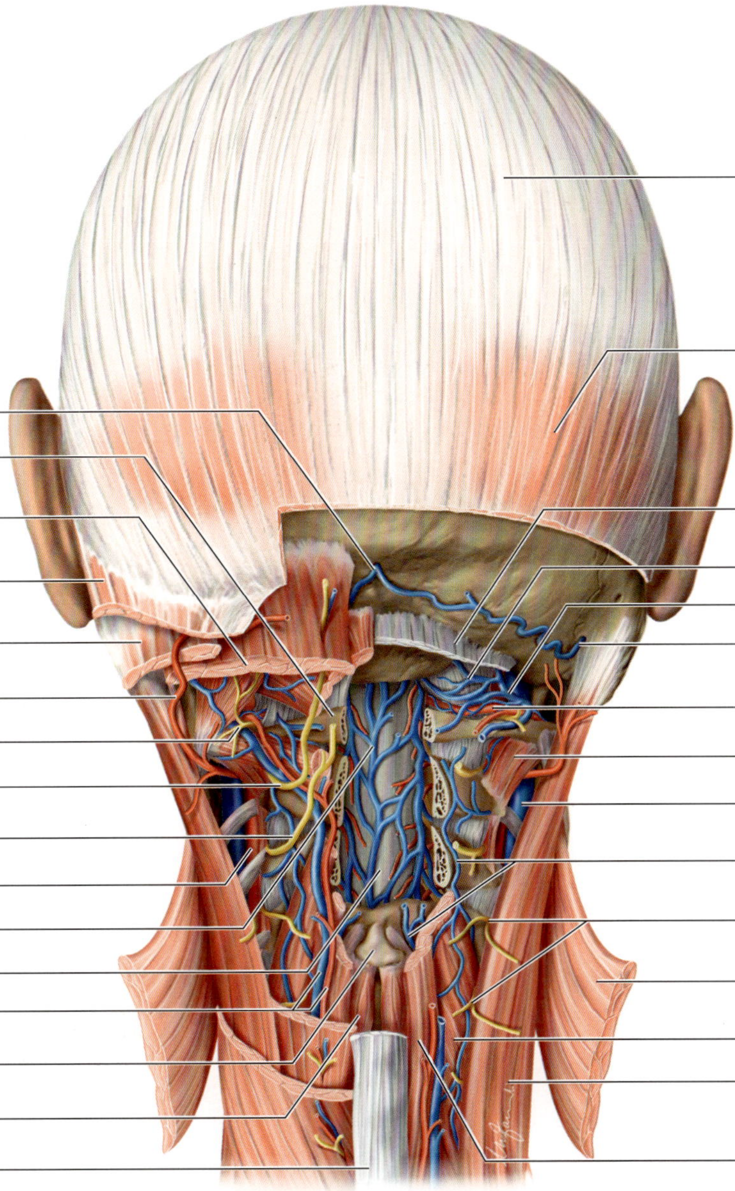

Head and **neck**, posterior view. In the left half, the trapezius, sternocleidomastoid, semispinalis capitis, semispinalis cervicis, splenius capitis and levator scapulae have been removed. On the median plane, the ligamentum nuchae has been transected and, to the right and left, the arches of the first three cervical vertebrae have been transected, revealing the posterior external vertebral venous plexus. In the right half, the insertion of the occipital belly of the occipitofrontalis and the atlanto-occipital membrane have also been transected, showing the suboccipital venous plexus, the occipital, condylar and mastoid emissary veins, and the atlantic part of the vertebral artery.

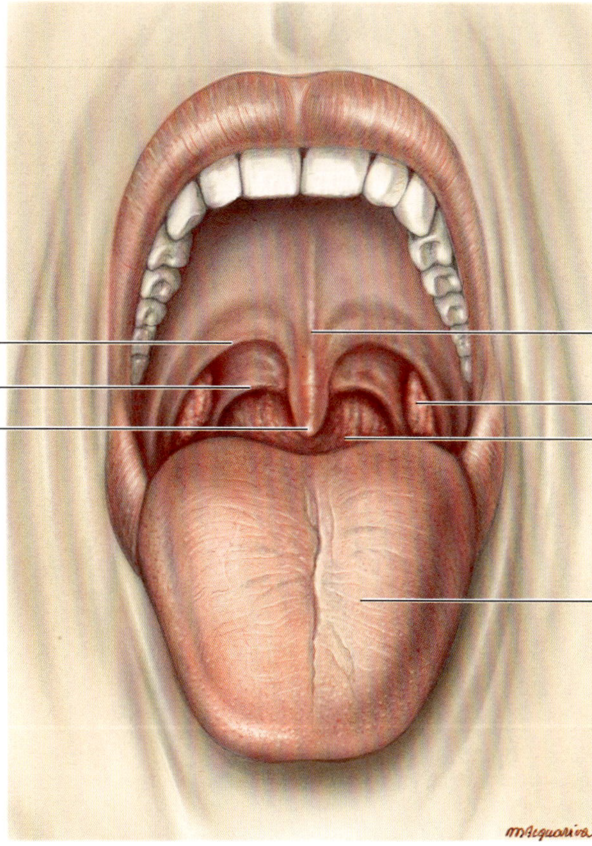

Oral cavity and isthmus of the fauces viewed from the front.

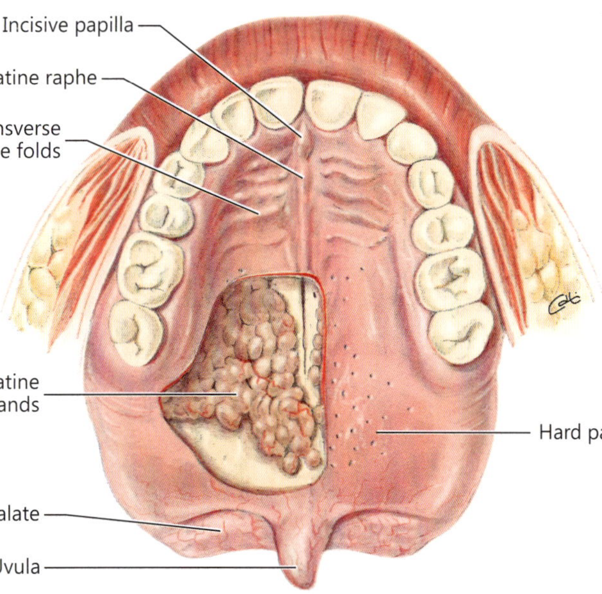

Palate. In the anterior third of the hard palate, the mucous membrane displays the transverse palatine folds and, in median position, the palatine raphe. Posteriorly, with the mucous membrane removed, one can see the lobules of the palatine glands, which extend also to the soft palate.

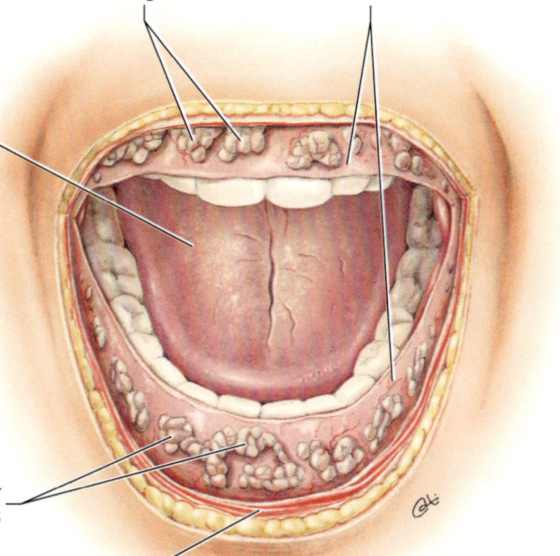

After the skin and muscle layer have been removed, the lower labial mucosa turned and the upper labial mucosa pulled downwards, one can see the distribution of lobules of the **labial glands** that form a glandular layer deep to the lamina propria of labial mucosa. The glandular lobules appear less densely concentrated near the commissures.

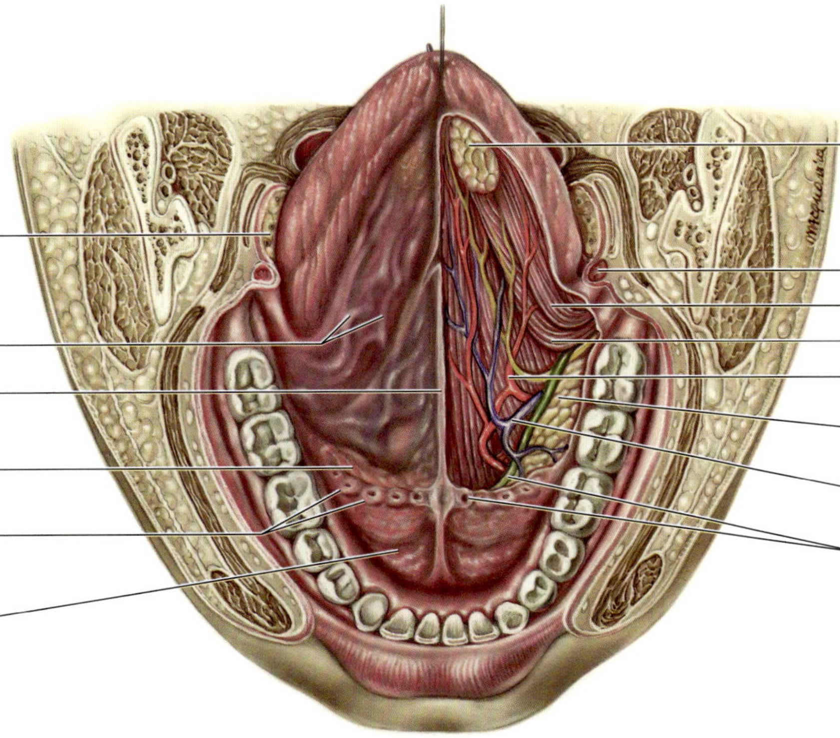

Sublingual fold. Transverse section of the head passing through the oral fissure. The tongue raised backwards shows the sublingual fold. On the right side, where the mucosa is intact, the veins of the submucosa can be seen showing through. On the left, the mucosa has been removed, and one can see affluents of the lingual vein and branches of the deep lingual artery. In addition, in the sublingual fold, numerous orifices where the submandibular and sublingual glands open into the sulcus are visible.

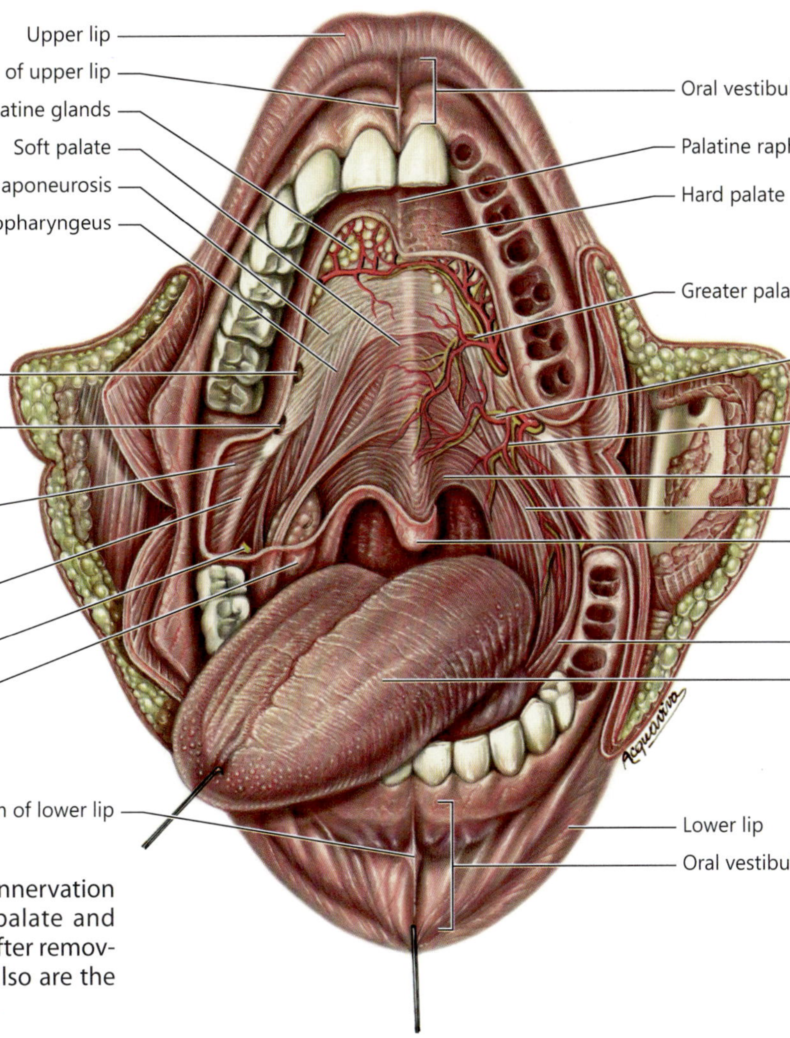

Arterial blood supply and innervation of the **hard palate**, soft palate and palatoglossal arch, visible after removal of the mucosa. Evident also are the muscles of the **soft palate**.

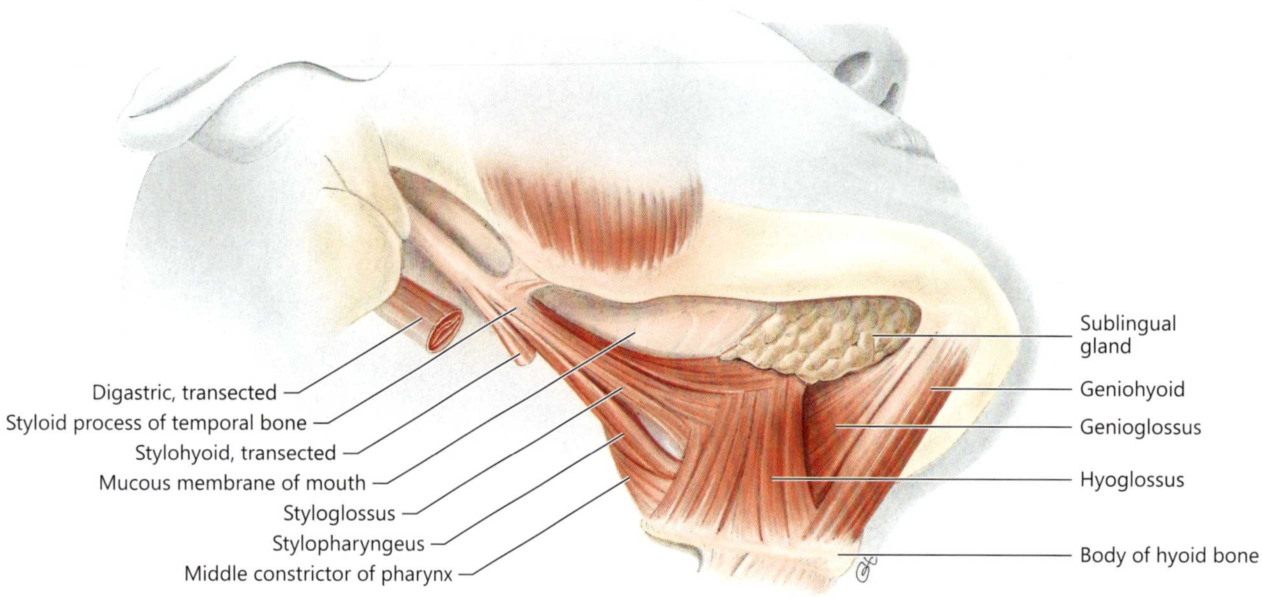

Diagram showing the **extrinsic muscles of the tongue**. This view of the deep layer of the suprahyoid region shows, alongside the extrinsic muscles that originate from the hyoid bone, also the muscles that originate from the styloid process and mandible.

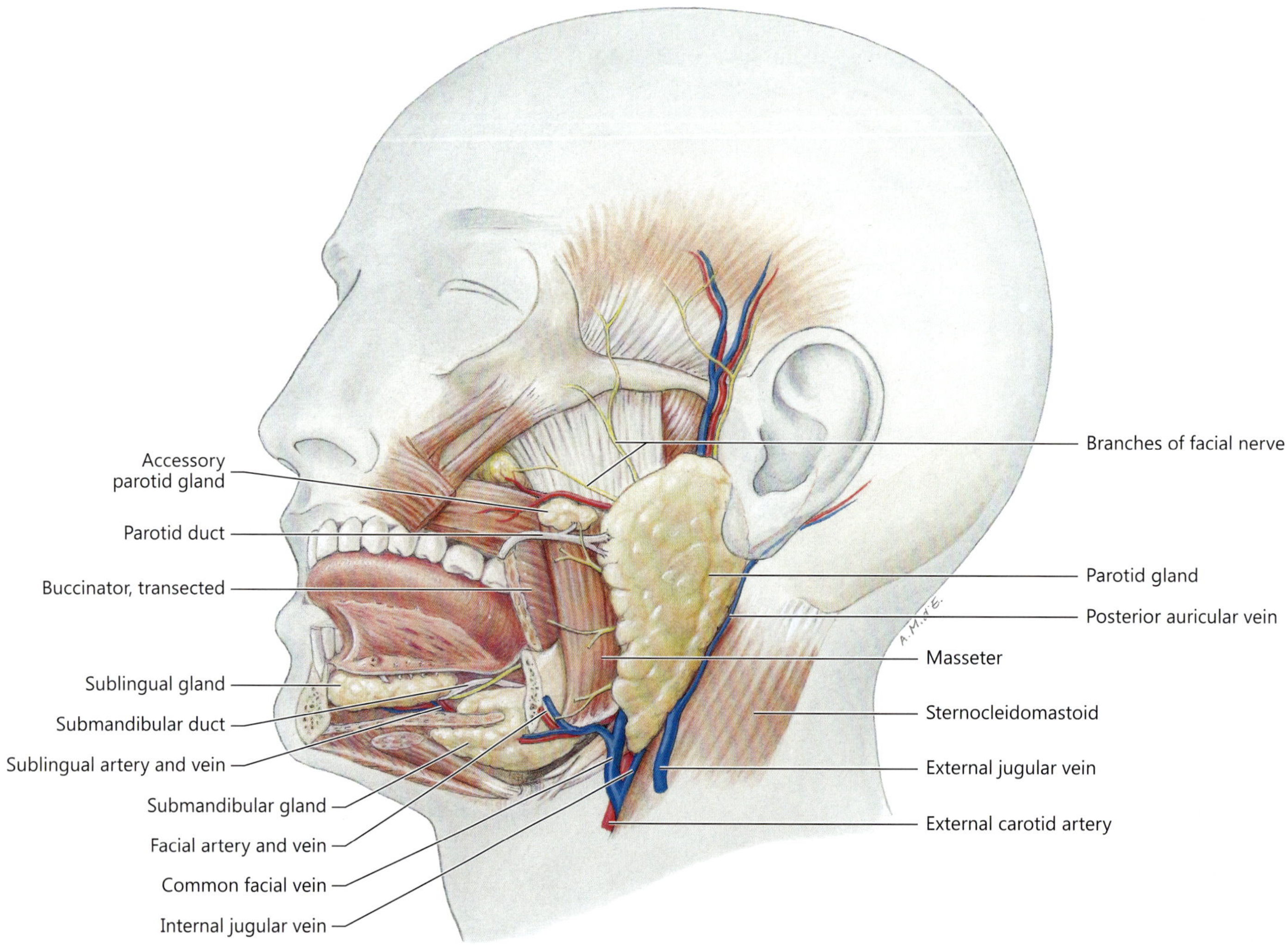

Diagram showing the location of the left **submandibular** and **sublingual glands** in relation to the floor of the mouth. The submandibular duct is flanked by the anterior prolongation of the homonymous gland, which, running above the mylohyoid, borders directly with the sublingual gland.

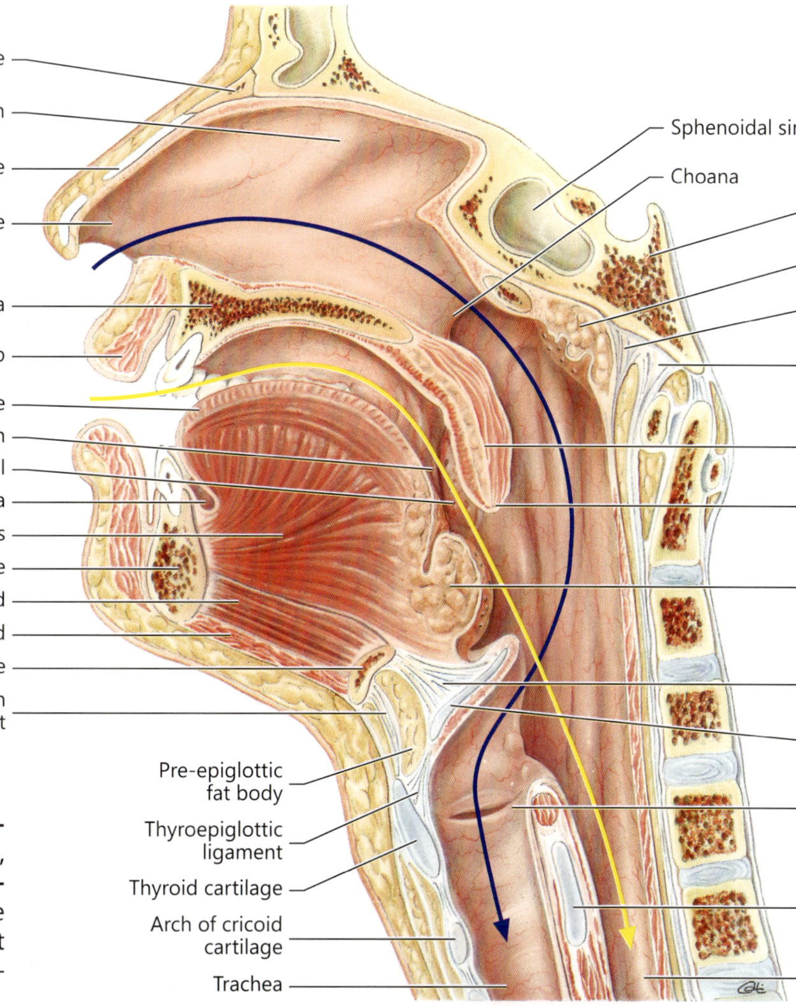

Diagram illustrating the **crossing**, at the level of the pharynx, **of the airways** (in *blue*) and **digestive tract** (in *yellow*). The place of crossing is at the point of the laryngeal inlet, in correspondence to the epiglottis.

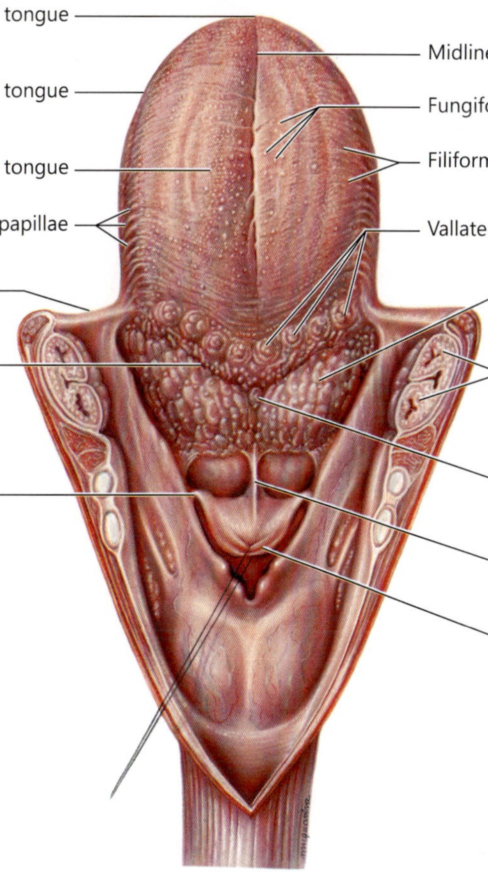

Dorsal surface of the tongue. Note the different external configuration of the body of the tongue with respect to the root. The *terminal sulcus* represents the boundary between the two regions. The tongue here is viewed from behind, after ample demolition of the posterior wall of the pharynx.

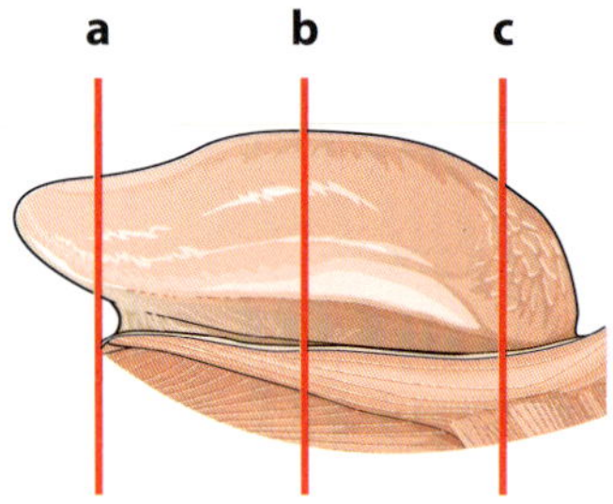

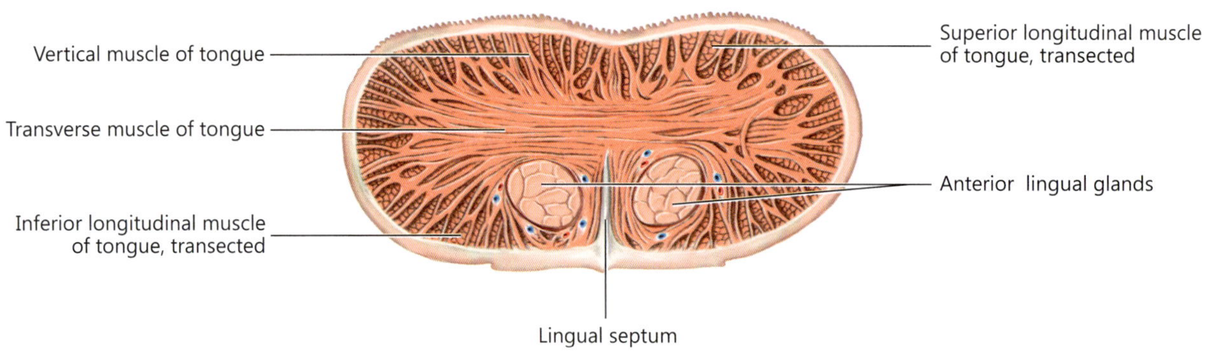

a

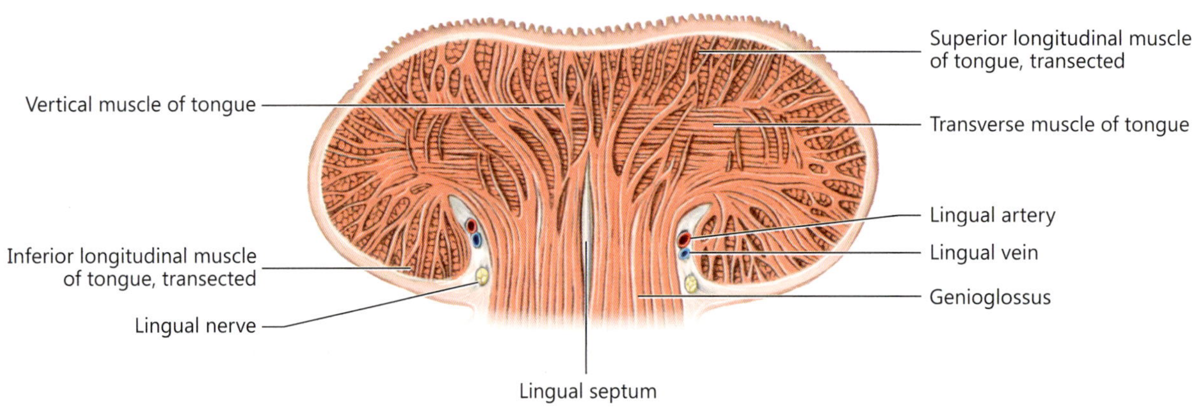

b

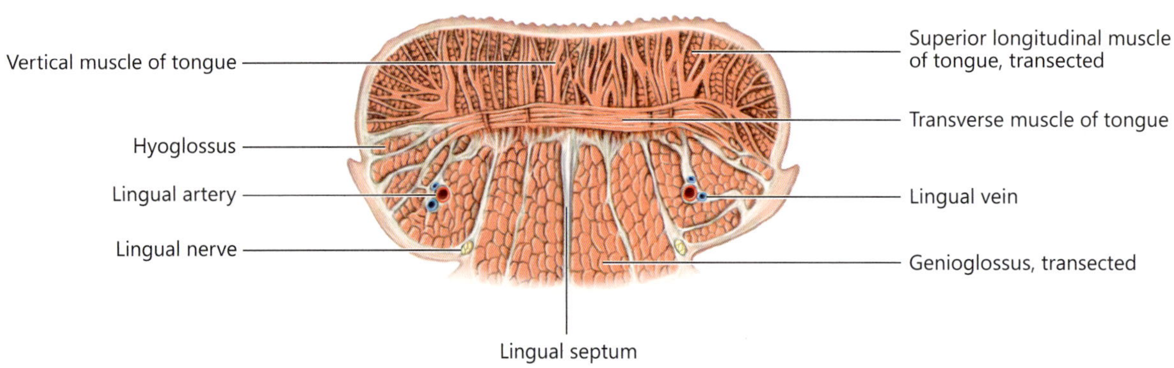

c

Structure of the tongue in frontal sections conducted at the level of: the body (**a**) and root of the tongue (**b** and **c**; see scheme above). The organ has a prevalently fibromuscular constitution and is covered, on the surface, by the mucous membrane. The tongue, as a whole entity, contains glands (here the anterior lingual glands are represented).

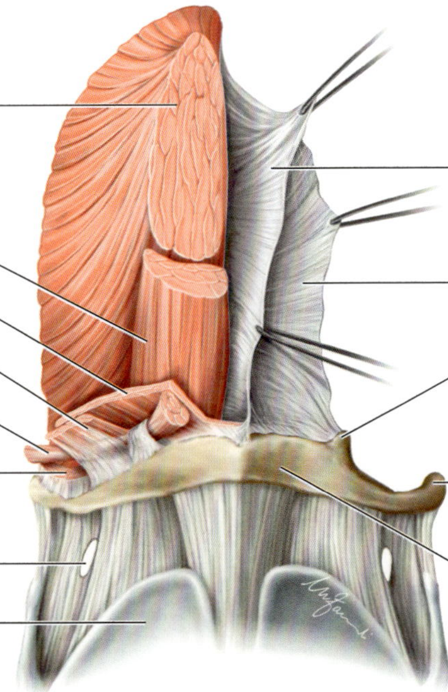

Inferior surface and **root of the tongue**. This view highlights the **fibrous skeleton of the tongue**, on the left side, formed by the lingual septum and hyoglossal membrane. The *hyoglossal membrane* is a broad thin lamina, located on an almost frontal plane, that inserts on the body of the hyoid bone, between the lesser horns, and extends into the root of the tongue. The *lingual septum* has a crescent-shaped form and extends, starting from the inferior surface of the hyoglossal membrane and hyoid bone, on a median sagittal plane between the two genioglossus muscles.

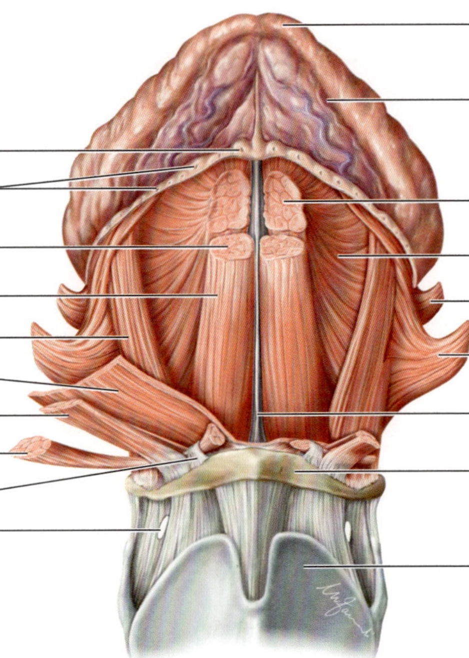

Inferior surface and **root of the tongue**. One can see the extrinsic muscles of the tongue. These include the genioglossus and hyoglossus, and the palatoglossus and styloglossus, which here have been transected. The floor of the mouth is formed by the mylohyoid and geniohyoid, in part transected, classified as part of the suprahyoid muscles. The fimbriated folds run from front to back and from the interior to exterior in the lateral parts of the inferior surface of the tongue.

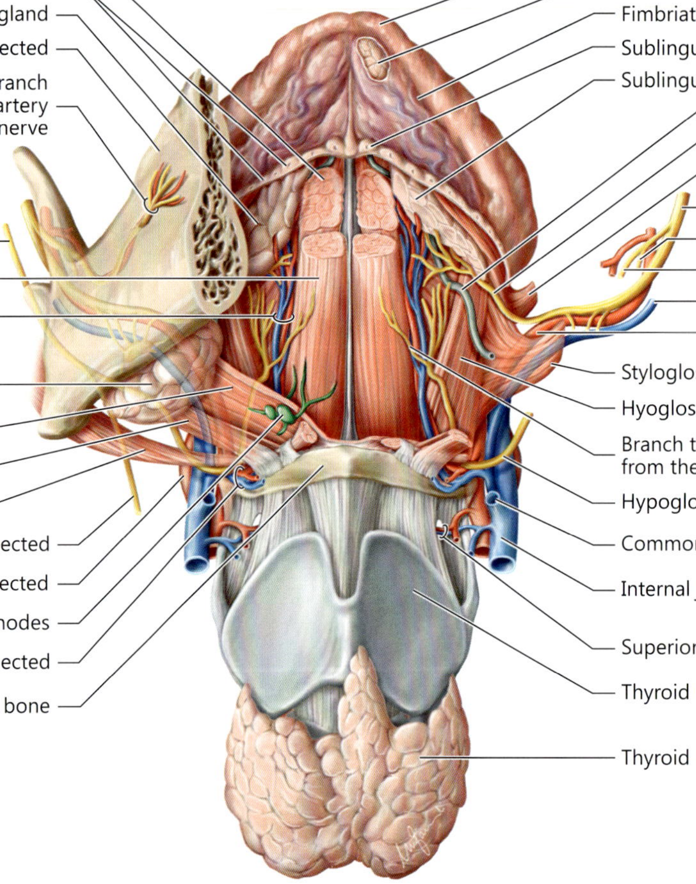

Floor of the mouth, anterior view. The tongue has been raised displaying its inferior surface. On the right, the body of the mandible has been transected in part and one can see the genioglossus and geniohyoid, transected at the point of their insertions into the superior and inferior mental, or genial, spines. One can see the sublingual and submandibular glands, the lingual artery and vein and, visible through the body of the mandible, the hypoglossal nerve. In the left half, with the mandible removed and the mylohyoid, stylohyoid and posterior belly of the digastric transected, one can see the lingual nerve, a branch of the mandibular nerve, the sublingual duct, and the retromandibular, common facial and internal jugular veins, transected. At the bottom, beneath the right and left laminae of the thyroid cartilage, one can see the thyroid gland.

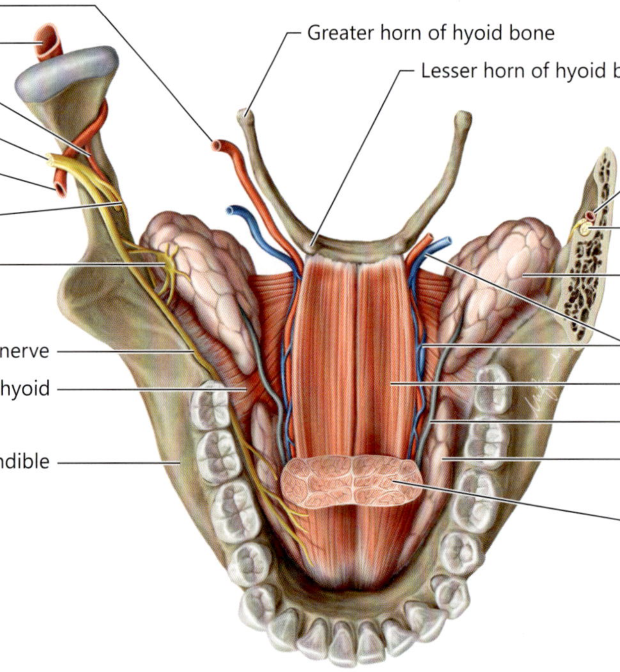

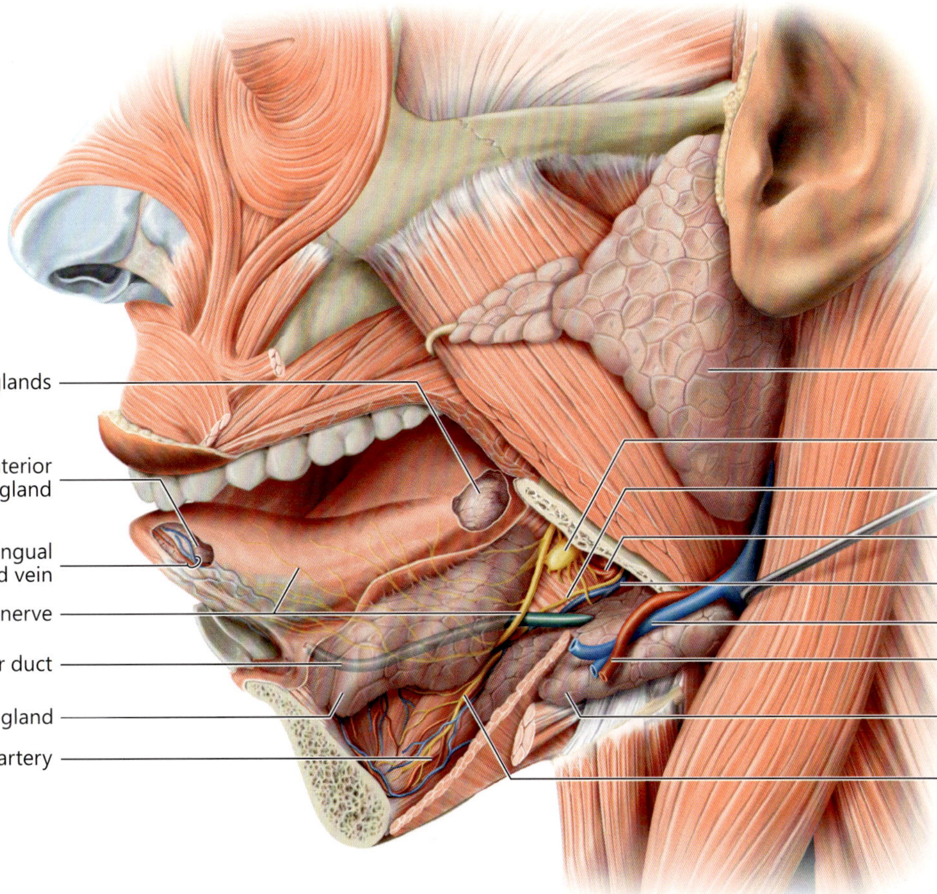

Left lateral view of the **oral cavity** after removal of part of the left body of the mandible and of the mylohyoid, stylohyoid, hyoglossus, genioglossus, digastric, buccinator, and masseter. One can see the major salivary glands (submandibular and sublingual glands) and some lingual glands. Also the parotid gland is visible in the parotid space. The lingual nerve, a branch of the mandibular nerve [V_3], enters the tongue on the lateral surface of the hyoglossus, in correspondence to the upper part of the submandibular space. Passing between the hyoglossus and the posterior border of the mylohyoid, it reaches the sublingual space, crossing below and in a lateromedial direction the submandibular duct. It then runs between the hyoglossus and genioglossus, located medially, and the sublingual gland, situated laterally. The hypoglossal nerve [XII], after reaching the submandibular space, passes into the interstitium between the hyoglossus and mylohyoid, deep to the submandibular gland and its excretory duct, anastomosing with the lingual nerve situated superiorly.

➤

Submandibular and **sublingual glands**, superior view after removal of the tongue. The submandibular ganglion receives afferent branches from the lingual nerve, a branch of the mandibular nerve. These are preganglionic fibers that arise from the superior salivatory nucleus, emerge from the brainstem with the intermediate nerve of the facial nerve, pass into the chorda tympani and unite with the lingual nerve along its course in the infratemporal fossa. Some postganglionic fibers travel directly to the submandibular gland, others return to the lingual nerve, which distributes them to the sublingual gland and to the minor salivary glands.

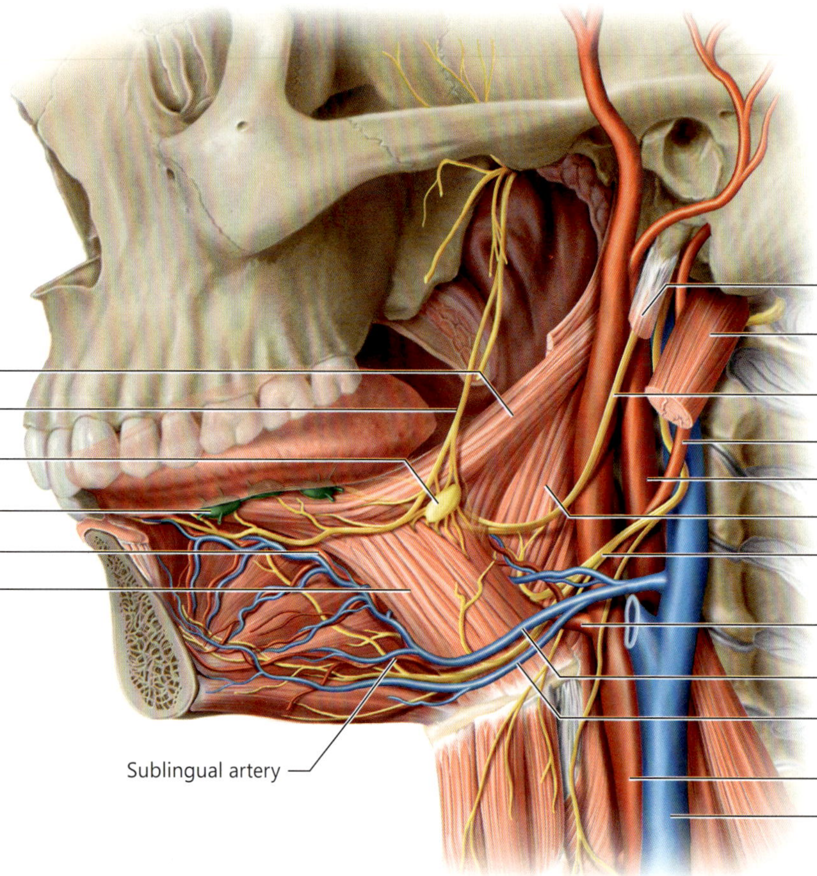

Vessels and nerves of the tongue. Left lateral view after removal of the left hemi-mandible, mylohyoid, stylohyoid, genioglossus, digastric, buccinator and masseter, and of the salivary glands. The submandibular ganglion receives afferent branches from the lingual nerve, a branch of the mandibular nerve [V_3]. Some efferent branches of the ganglion travel back to the lingual nerve, through which they are distributed. The glossopharyngeal nerve [IX], after emerging from the jugular foramen, follows an oblique path downwards and forwards, passing between the internal carotid artery and the internal jugular vein, then between the stylopharyngeus and styloglossus and, finally, attached to the stylopharyngeus. The hypoglossal nerve [XII], after its initial course behind the styloid muscles and neurovascular bundle of the neck, passes between the internal carotid artery and internal jugular vein, deep to the stylohyoid and posterior belly of the digastric, then winds around the occipital artery and, further down, superficially, crosses the lingual artery.

➤

a, Distribution of **papillae on the surface of the tongue**. **b**, Three-dimensional graphic reconstruction of the filiform, vallate, foliate (situated at the edges of the body of the tongue and vestigial in man), and fungiform papillae. The filiform papillae contain only mechanoreceptors and respond to stimuli of a mechanical nature; the others contain also taste buds and, hence, respond also to chemical stimuli. **c**, Each taste bud is made up of a variety of taste sensory cells (organ of taste), each of which is specialized in mediating a certain type of flavor (in the image shown, the color of the cells corresponds to a specific flavor) in such a way that each taste bud perceives all the flavors. The apical surface of the taste cells forms microvilli, also termed taste hairs, which enter into contact, through the taste pore, with the chemical stimuli. At the basal extremity, the taste sensory cells in the posterior third of the tongue receive peripheral projections of protoneurons of the inferior or petrosal ganglion of the glossopharyngeal nerve [IX], whose central projections reach the nucleus of the solitary tract. The taste sensory cells of the anterior two-thirds of the tongue receive instead peripheral projections of the protoneurons of the geniculate ganglion of the intermediate nerve of the facial nerve [VII], whose central projections also reach the nucleus of the solitary tract. **d**, Recent functional and molecular studies have demonstrated that, in contrast to what is commonly held, the sensitivity to different modes of taste is not spatially distributed on the tongue, i.e. there is not a specific map of flavors. Each part of the tongue, in particular the zones marked by different colors, is sensitive to all flavors, as described above in **c** in regard to taste buds.

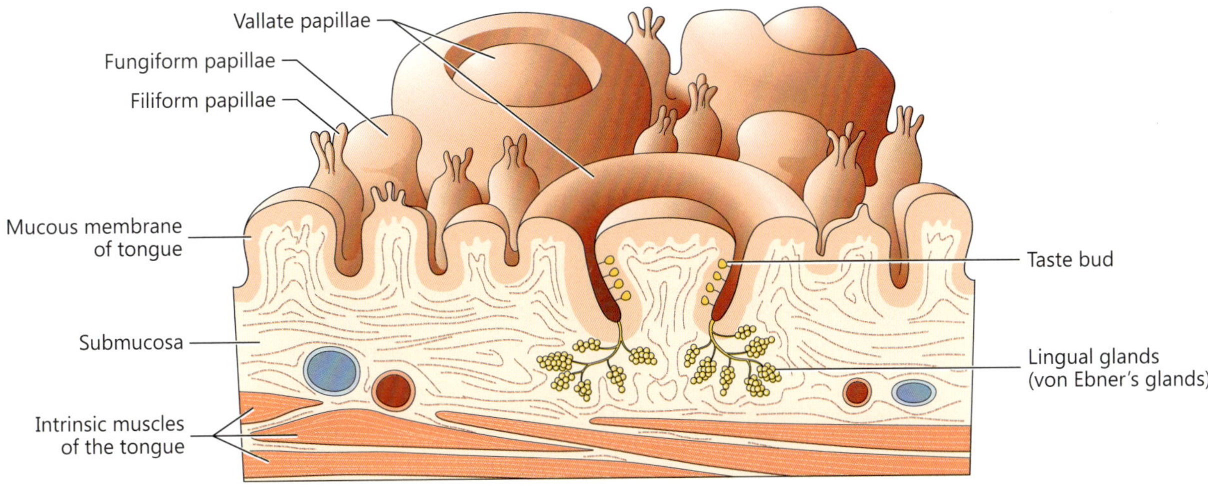

The **mucous membrane of the tongue** has a velvet-like texture owing to the presence of diverse types of papillae. The filiform papillae are features of the lamina propria of the mucosa which present at their apex fine secondary evaginations of a filamentous aspect. The fungiform papillae, also offshoots of the lamina propria, are mushroom-shaped with a narrow base and swollen apex. The vallate papillae, also termed circumvallate papillae, do not protrude from the lamina propria but are cylindrical features of connective tissue that have a circular sulcus or dip. The taste buds are contained in the epithelium covering the sides of the sulcus.

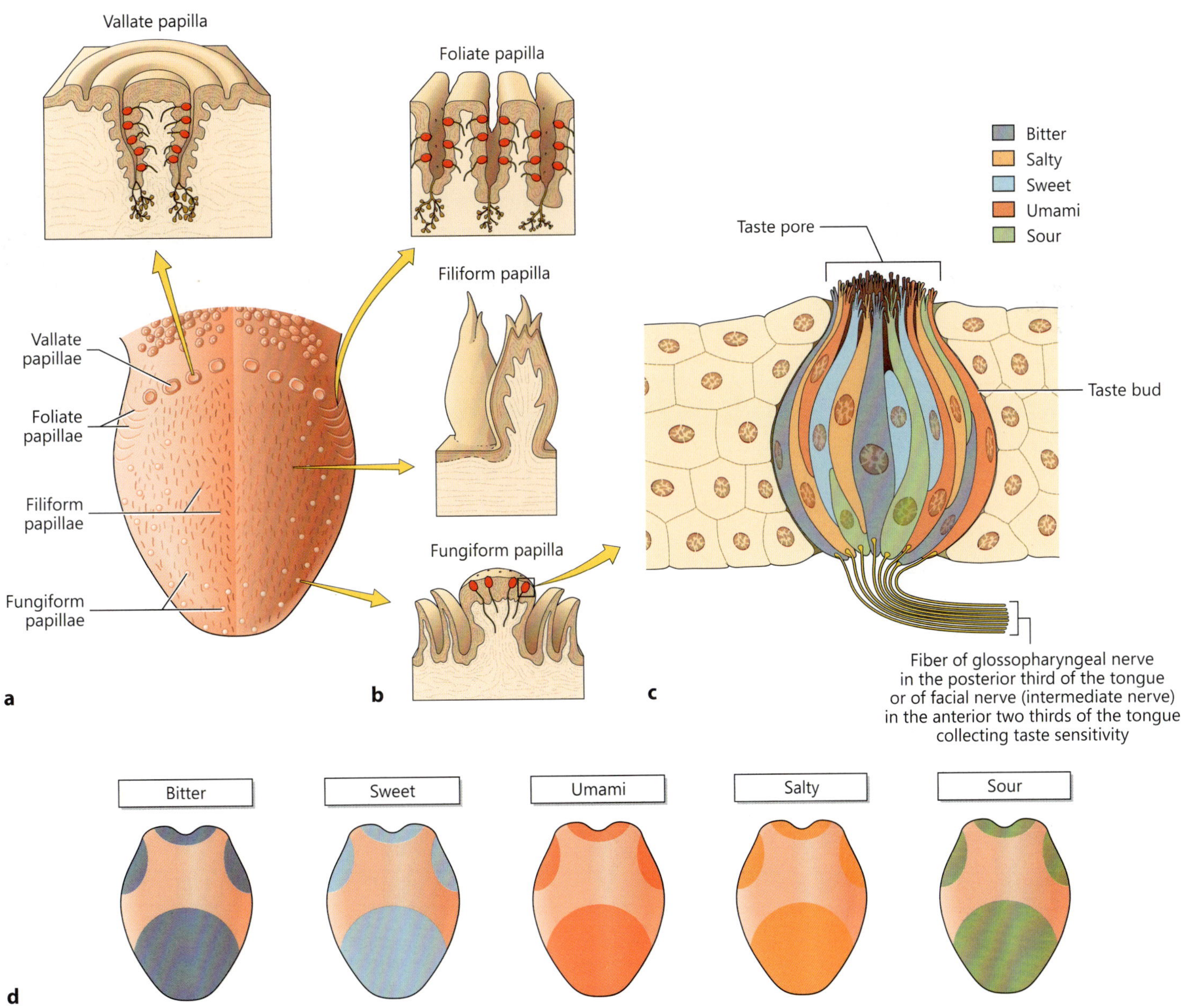

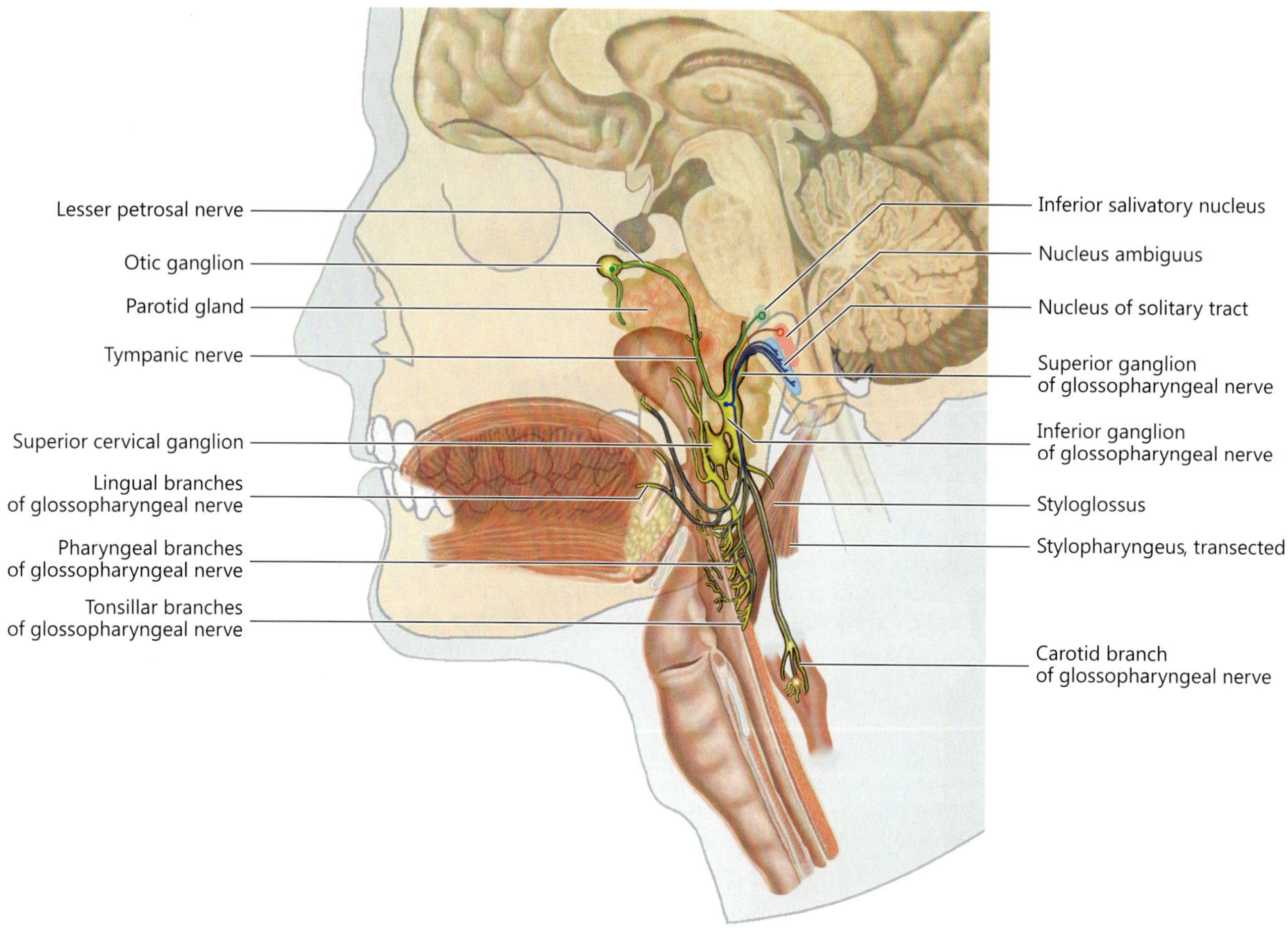
Lesser petrosal nerve
Otic ganglion
Parotid gland
Tympanic nerve
Superior cervical ganglion
Lingual branches of glossopharyngeal nerve
Pharyngeal branches of glossopharyngeal nerve
Tonsillar branches of glossopharyngeal nerve
Inferior salivatory nucleus
Nucleus ambiguus
Nucleus of solitary tract
Superior ganglion of glossopharyngeal nerve
Inferior ganglion of glossopharyngeal nerve
Styloglossus
Stylopharyngeus, transected
Carotid branch of glossopharyngeal nerve

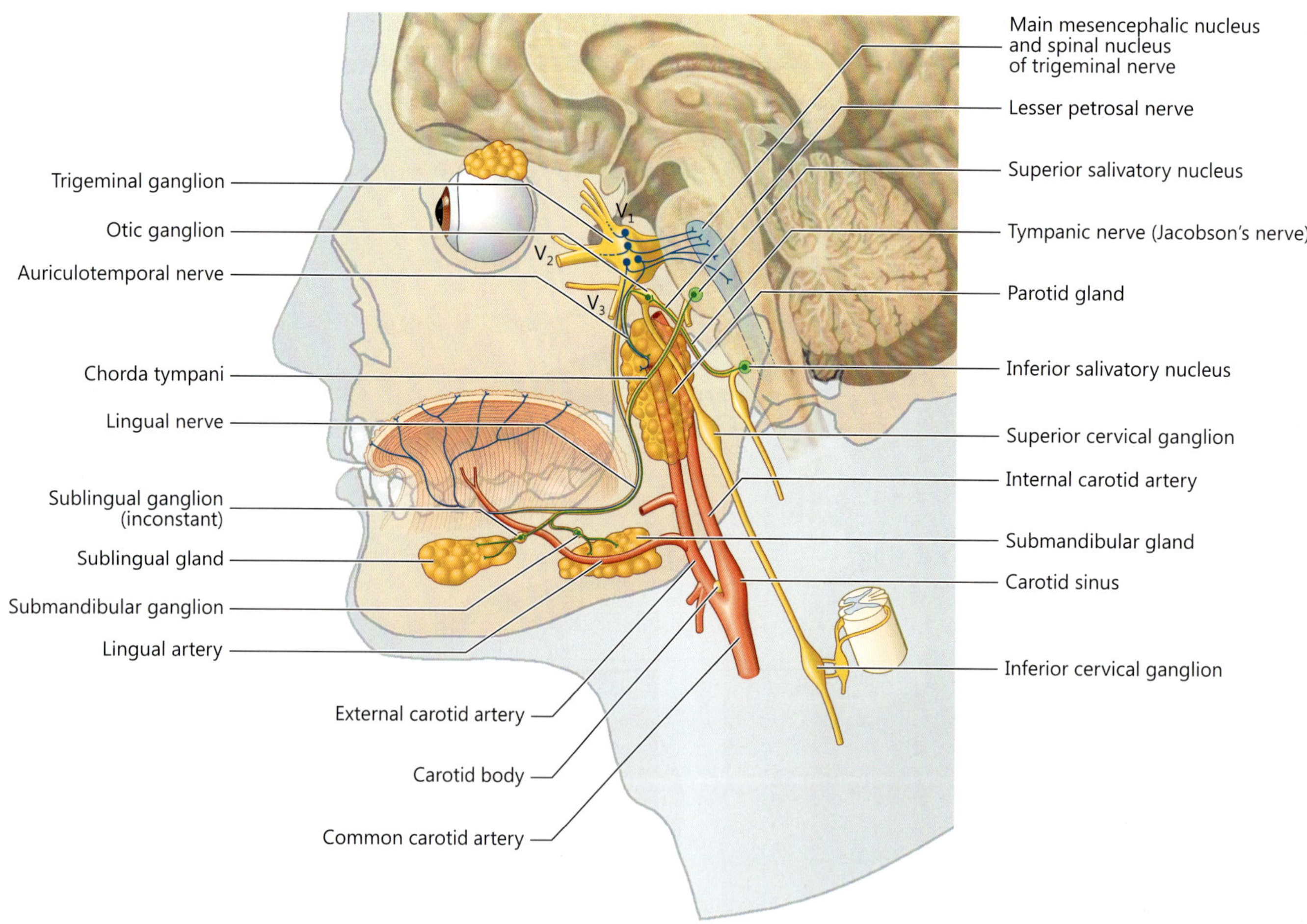
Trigeminal ganglion
Otic ganglion
Auriculotemporal nerve
Chorda tympani
Lingual nerve
Sublingual ganglion (inconstant)
Sublingual gland
Submandibular ganglion
Lingual artery
External carotid artery
Carotid body
Common carotid artery
V1
V2
V3
Main mesencephalic nucleus and spinal nucleus of trigeminal nerve
Lesser petrosal nerve
Superior salivatory nucleus
Tympanic nerve (Jacobson's nerve)
Parotid gland
Inferior salivatory nucleus
Superior cervical ganglion
Internal carotid artery
Submandibular gland
Carotid sinus
Inferior cervical ganglion

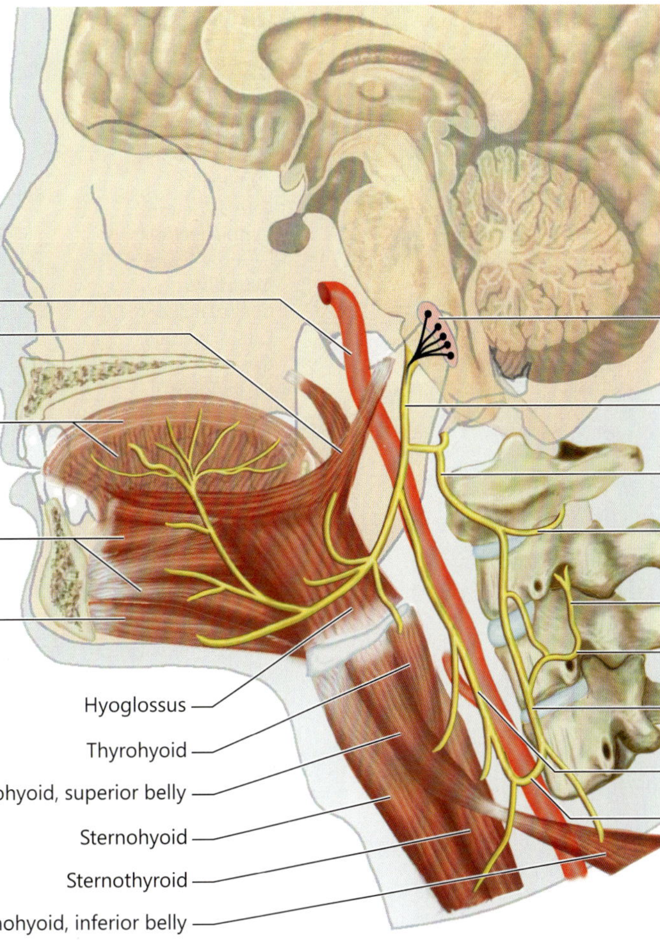

Course and distribution of the **hypoglossal nerve** [XII]. The nerve, which is exclusively somatic motor, supplies the muscles of the tongue and also the supra- and infrahyoid muscles. These latter are actually innervated by the anterior rami of the first cervical nerves, through the ansa cervicalis. The superior root of the ansa cervicalis, also known as the descending branch of the hypoglossal nerve, contains only fibers coming from the first cervical nerve [C1]. The inferior root of the ansa cervicalis, also known as the descending cervical nerve, is formed of fibers coming from the second [C2] and third [C3] cervical nerves. The two roots unite to form the ansa cervicalis, known also as ansa of the hypoglossal nerve, whose branches innervate the sternohyoid, sternothyroid and inferior belly of the omohyoid. The superior belly of the omohyoid is innervated by a branch of the superior root of the ansa cervicalis. The thyrohyoid is innervated by a branch containing fibers coming from the first cervical nerve [C1] that separates from the hypoglossal nerve after the latter has given rise to the superior root of the ansa cervicalis.

➤

At the top of the previous page, course and branches of the **glossopharyngeal nerve** [IX]. Its somatic motor component supplies the stylopharyngeus. The somatic sensory fibers (general somatic sense) receive sensory input from a limited zone of the auricle. The motor or visceral effector component reaches the parotid and minor salivary glands. Visceral sensory fibers conduct special visceral stimuli (specific taste sense) from the taste buds of the posterior third of the tongue and visceral stimuli (visceral general sense) from the chemoreceptors of the carotid body, from the baroreceptors of the carotid sinus, and from the mucosa of the tympanic cavity, pharyngotympanic tube, nasopharynx, isthmus of fauces, palatine tonsil and the posterior third of the tongue.

At the bottom of the previous page, diagram showing the connections of the **otic**, **submandibular** and **sublingual ganglia**. The three ganglia receive parasympathetic fibers (*green*) from the superior salivatory nucleus (of the facial nerve) and inferior salivatory nucleus (of the glossopharyngeal nerve). The otic ganglion receives preganglionic fibers coming from the inferior salivatory nucleus that exit from the brainstem with the glossopharyngeal nerve [IX] and pass into the tympanic nerve and then into the lesser petrosal nerve. Most of the postganglionic fibers enter into the auriculotemporal nerve and reach the parotid gland; others go to the minor salivary glands by means of peripheral branches of the mandibular nerve [V_3]. Some postganglionic vasodilator fibers go to peripheral innervation zones of the mandibular nerve [V_3]. The submandibular and sublingual (inconstant) ganglia receive preganglionic fibers coming from the superior salivatory nucleus, which emerge from the brainstem with the intermediate nerve, a component of the facial nerve [VII], pass into the chorda tympani and then unite with the lingual nerve, a branch of the mandibular nerve [V_3]. Some postganglionic fibers supply the submandibular gland, others reach the lingual nerve and from there supply the sublingual and minor salivary glands.

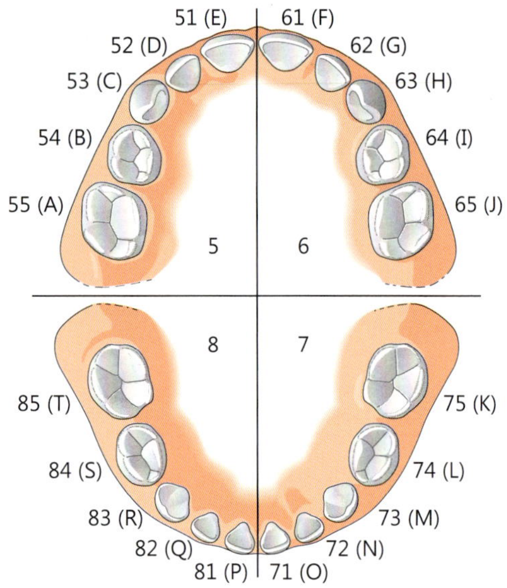

a

Deciduous teeth		
	ERUPTION	EXFOLIATION
Maxilla		
Second molars	23-31 months	10-12 years
First molars	14-18 months	9-11 years
Canines	17-23 months	9-12 years
Lateral incisors	10-16 months	7-8 years
Central incisors	6-10 months	6-7 years
Mandible		
Central incisors	8-12 months	6-7 years
Lateral incisors	9-13 months	7-8 years
Canines	16-22 months	10-12 years
First molars	13-19 months	9-11 years
Second molars	25-33 months	10-12 years

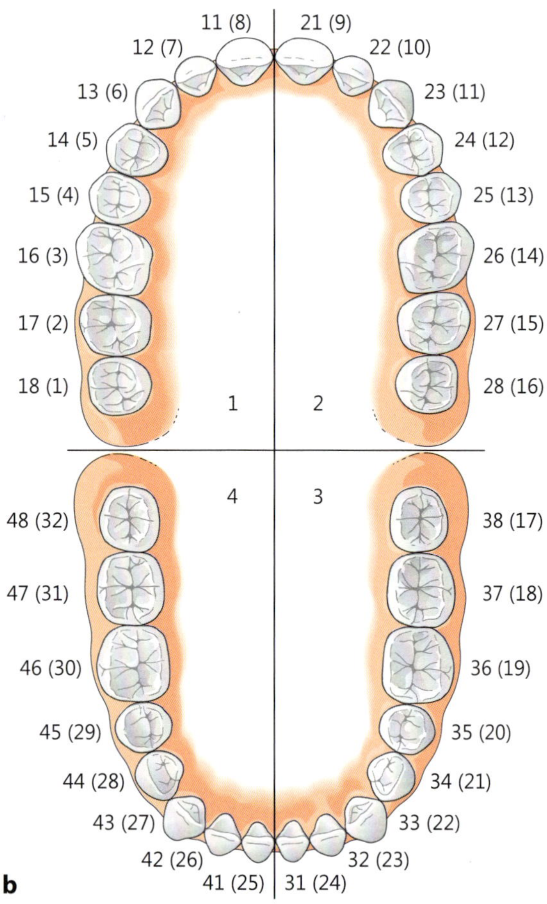

b

Permanent teeth		
	ERUPTION	ROOT COMPLETION
Maxilla		
First molars	6-7 years	9-10 years
Central incisors	7-8 years	10 years
Lateral incisors	8-9 years	11 years
First premolars	10-11 years	12-13 years
Second premolars	10-12 years	12-14 years
Canines	11-12 years	13-15 years
Second molars	12-13 years	14-16 years
Third molars	17-21 years	18-25 years
Mandible		
First molars	6-7 years	9-10 years
Central incisors	6-7 years	9-11 years
Lateral incisors	7-8 years	10 years
Canines	9-10 years	12-14 years
First premolars	10-12 years	12-13 years
Second premolars	11-12 years	13-14 years
Second molars	11-13 years	14-15 years
Third molars	17-21 years	18-25 years

Dentition. a, numbering and representation of **deciduous teeth** according to the Fédération Dentaire International (FDI) and American Dental Association (ADA; indicated in brackets). In the FDI numbering, each tooth is classified by two digits: the first indicates the hemiarcade, the second, the type of tooth. The hemiarcade is indicated by the number 5, 6, 7, or 8 (in order, right and left maxillary hemiarcades and left and right mandibular hemiarcades), while the tooth (central incisor, lateral incisor, canine, 1st molar, 2nd molar) is indicated by a number from 1 to 5. In the ADA system of numbering, deciduous teeth are represented by the letters of the English alphabet from A to T starting from the upper right 2nd molar and proceeding left to the upper left 2nd molar, then continuing inferiorly from the lower left 2nd molar to the lower right 2nd molar; **b**, numbering of **permanent teeth** according to the Fédération Dentaire International (FDI) and American Dental Association (ADA; indicated in brackets). In the FDI numbering, each tooth is classified by two digits: the first indicates the hemiarcade, the second, the type of tooth. The hemiarcade is indicated by the number 1, 2, 3, or 4 (in order, right and left maxillary hemiarcades, and left and right mandibular hemiarcades), while the tooth (central incisor, lateral incisor, canine, 1st premolar, 2nd premolar, 1st molar, 2nd molar, 3rd molar) is indicated by a number from 1 to 8. In the ADA system of numbering, permanent teeth are numbered from 1 to 32 starting from the upper right 3rd molar and proceeding left to the upper left 3rd molar, then continuing inferiorly from the lower left 3rd molar to the lower right 3rd molar.

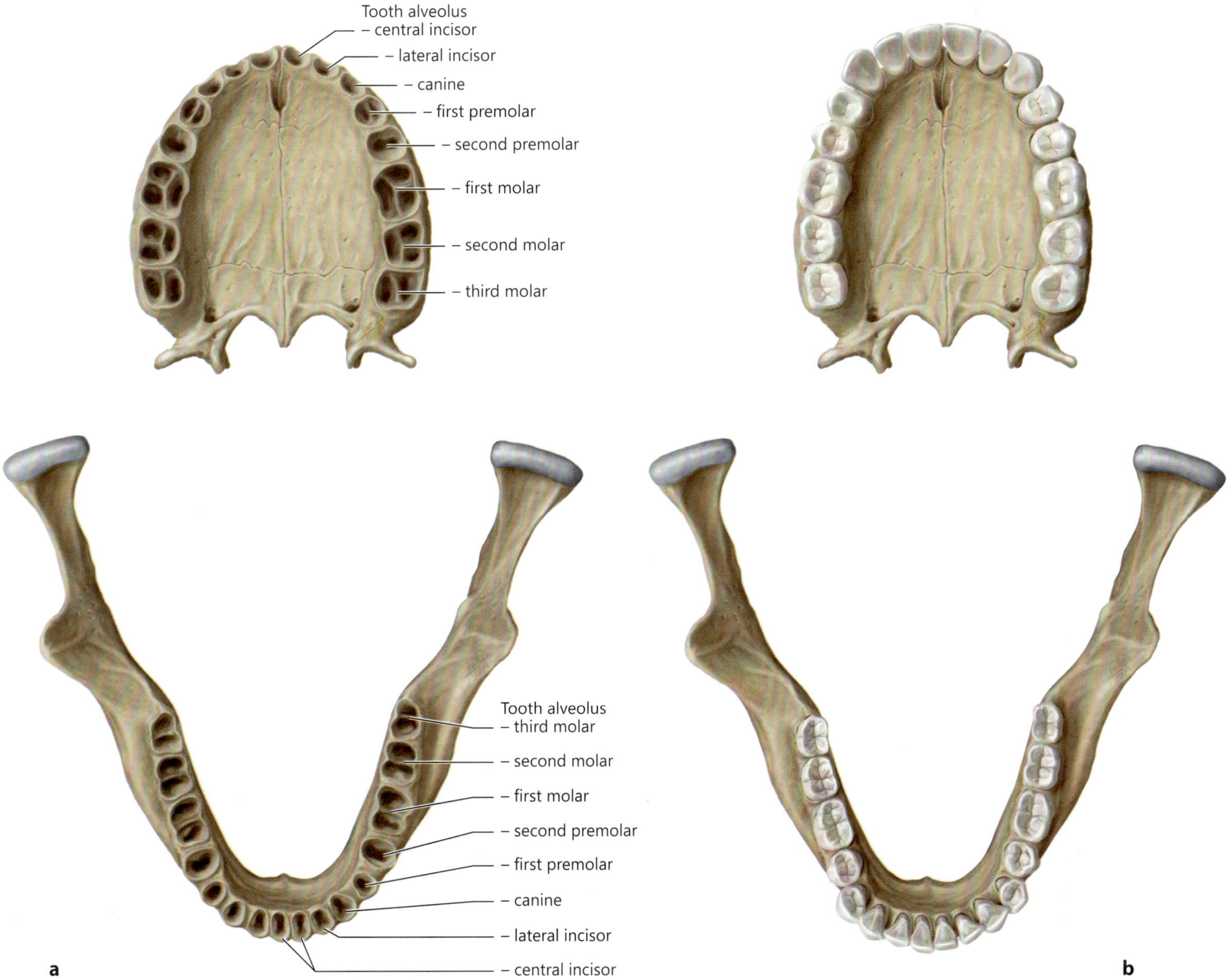

Maxillary, or upper (above), **and mandibular**, or lower (below), **alveolar arches** (**a**) **and dental arcades** (**b**), without and with dentition, viewed respectively from below and from above. Monoradicular teeth are held in dental alveoli with a single cavity, pluriradicular teeth in alveoli with a cavity subdivided by septa.

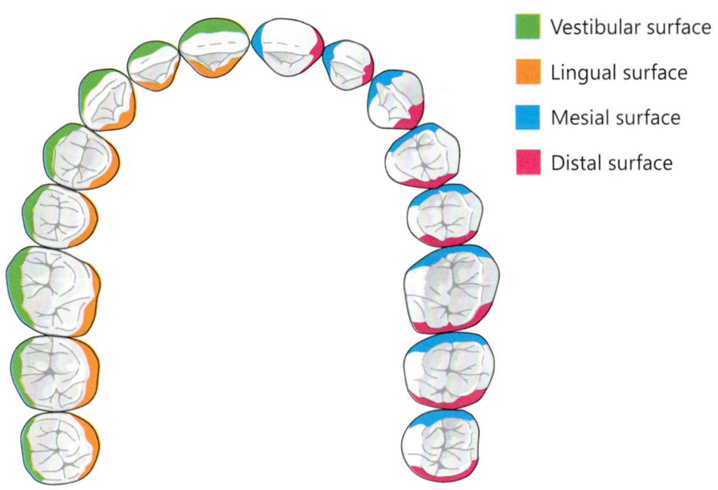

Terminology of position and surfaces of the teeth	
Vestibular	Facing towards the oral vestibule *Vestibular surface*: the external surface of the teeth
Lingual	Facing towards the tongue *Lingual surface*: internal surface of the teeth (many use the term "palatine" for the corresponding surfaces of the superior teeth)
Mesial	Facing the median line *Mesial surface*: surface of the tooth turned towards the median line; faces the tooth that precedes it
Distal	Facing in the opposite direction with respect to the median line *Distal surface*: surface of the tooth furthest from the median line; faces the tooth that follows it

The mesial and distal surfaces are indicated as *proximal surfaces*.

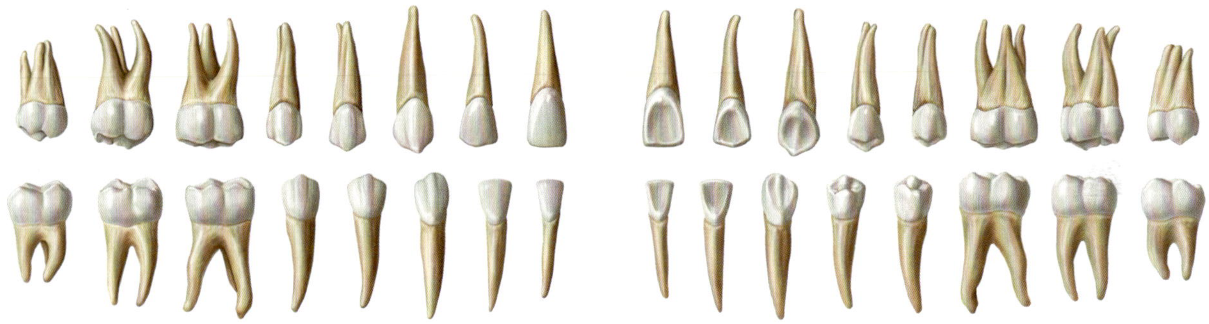

Dentition. **a**, **Permanent teeth** of the right **upper hemiarcade**, viewed from the vestibular surface and from the lingual surface. The premolars present a slight bifidity of the roots; the molars are triradicular; **b**, **permanent teeth** of the right **lower hemiarcade** viewed from the vestibular surface and from the lingual surface. The premolars are monoradicular, while the molars present two roots.

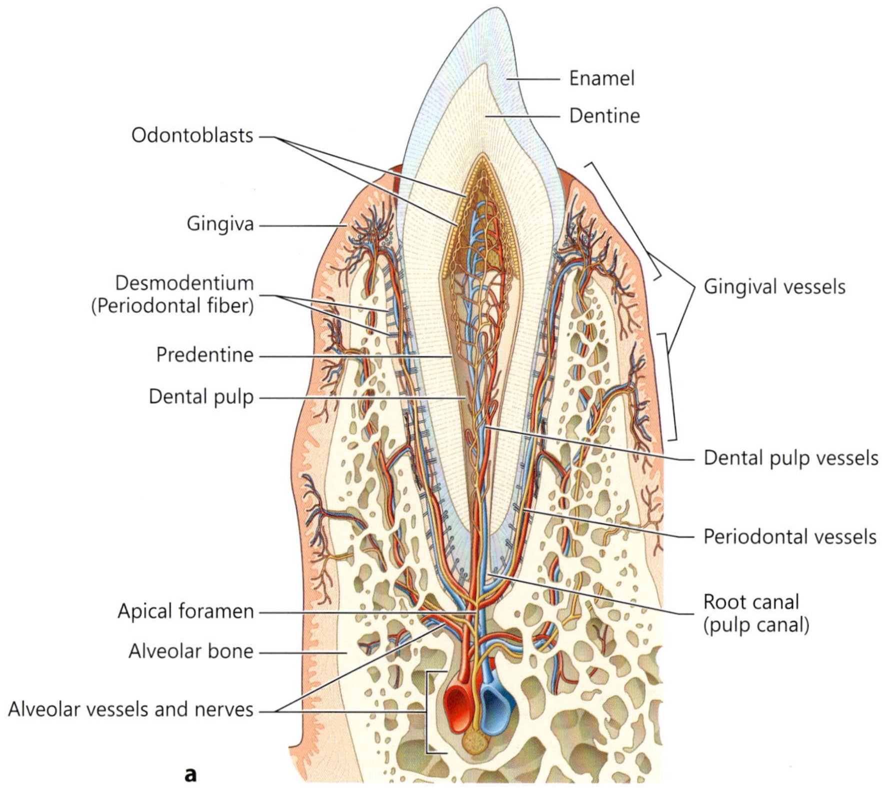

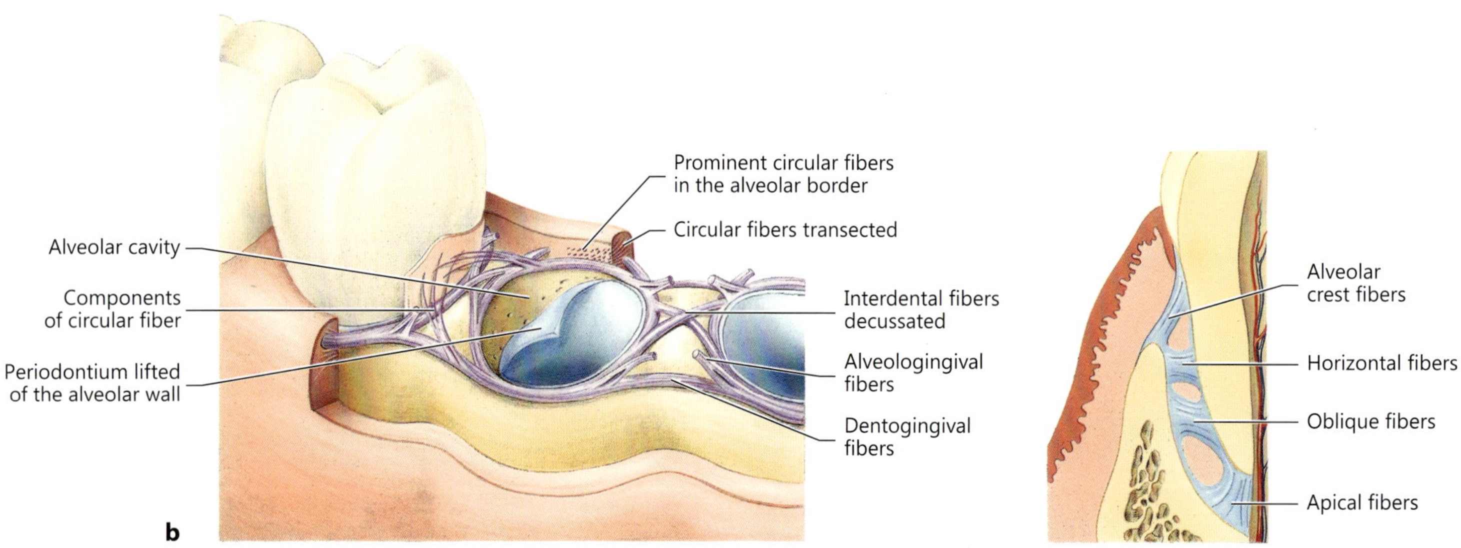

Dentition. **a**, Irroration of the oral tissues. The blood vessel supply and innervation of the desmodentium and dental pulp are shown; **b**, general structure of the periodontium (system of fixation of the tooth).

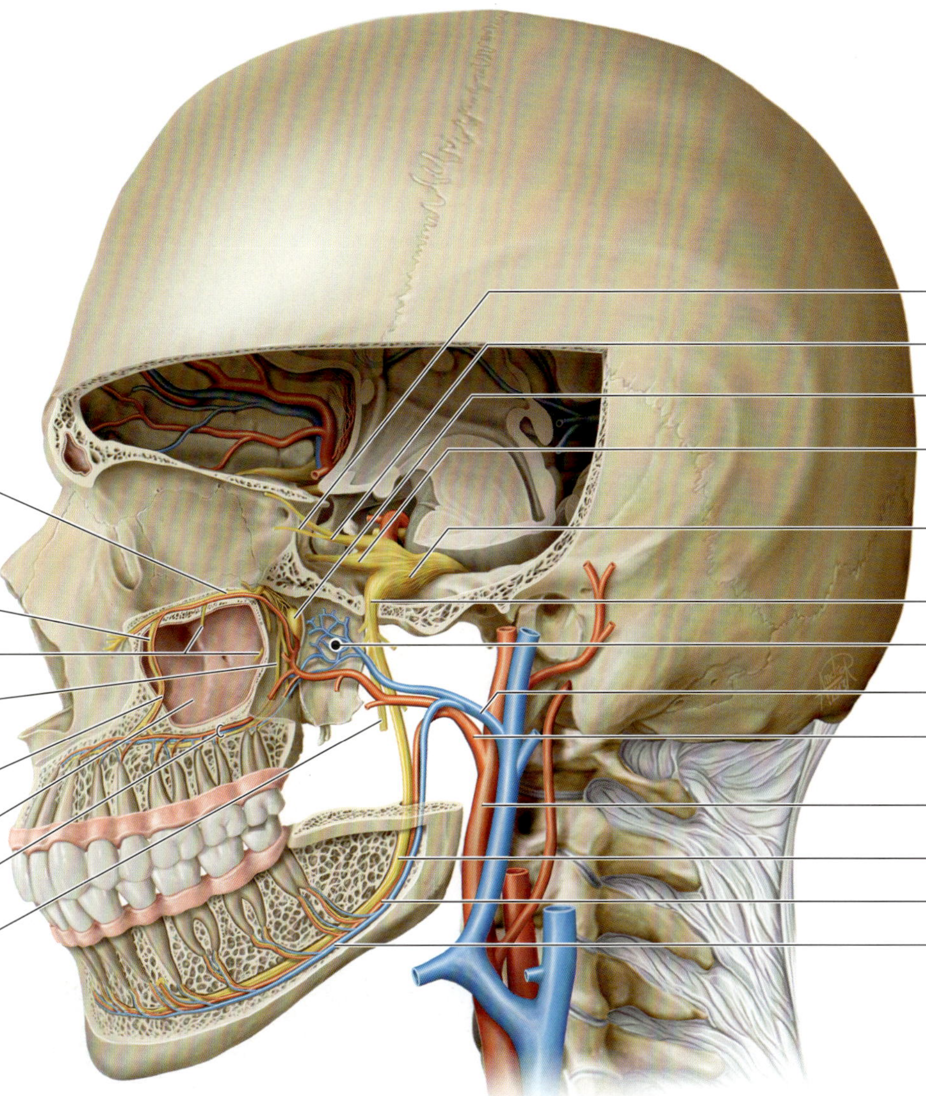

Viscerocranium transected at different levels, left lateral view. The left lateral wall of the neurocranium has also been partially removed to show the trigeminal or semilunar ganglion in the middle cranial fossa, near the apex of the petrous part of the temporal bone. The **mandibular nerve** [V_3] exits from the middle cranial fossa through the foramen ovale to reach the upper part of the infratemporal fossa where it divides into two large trunks, anterolateral and posteromedial. The **inferior alveolar nerve** arises from the posteromedial trunk and heads downwards, forwards and laterally describing an anterosuperiorly concave arch. After reaching the mandibular foramen on the medial surface of the mandible, it enters the mandibular canal together with the inferior alveolar artery, a branch of the **maxillary artery**. The posterior superior alveolar branch of the superior alveolar nerves arises from the **maxillary nerve** [V_2], whereas the anterior and middle superior alveolar branches originate from the infraorbital nerve, a terminal branch of the maxillary nerve [V_2], while it travels through the infraorbital canal. These branches pass in canaliculi excavated in the wall of the maxillary sinus, through which they reach the alveolar process of the maxilla. The posterior superior alveolar artery, a branch of the maxillary artery, descends forwards down on the maxillary tuberosity, dividing into small branches that penetrate into the alveolar canals of the maxilla. The anterior superior alveolar arteries, of which one single branch is represented here, arise from the infraorbital artery, a branch of the maxillary artery, within the orbital cavity, and penetrate into the incisive canals of the maxilla.

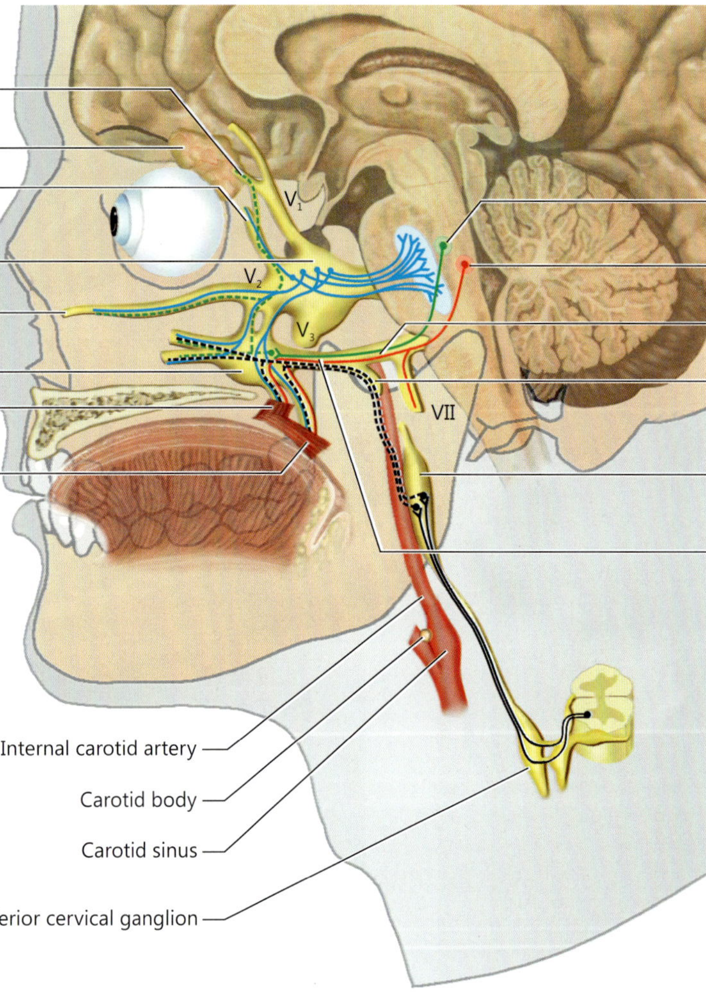

Connections of the **pterygopalatine ganglion** (or sphenopalatine ganglion). Motor and somatosensory fibers (*red* and *blue*) and sympathetic fibers (*black*) pass through the pterygopalatine ganglion, but only the parasympathetic fibers (*green*) originating from the superior salivatory nucleus sinapse there.

Diagram showing the course and distribution of the **trigeminal nerve** ☞ pag. 86.

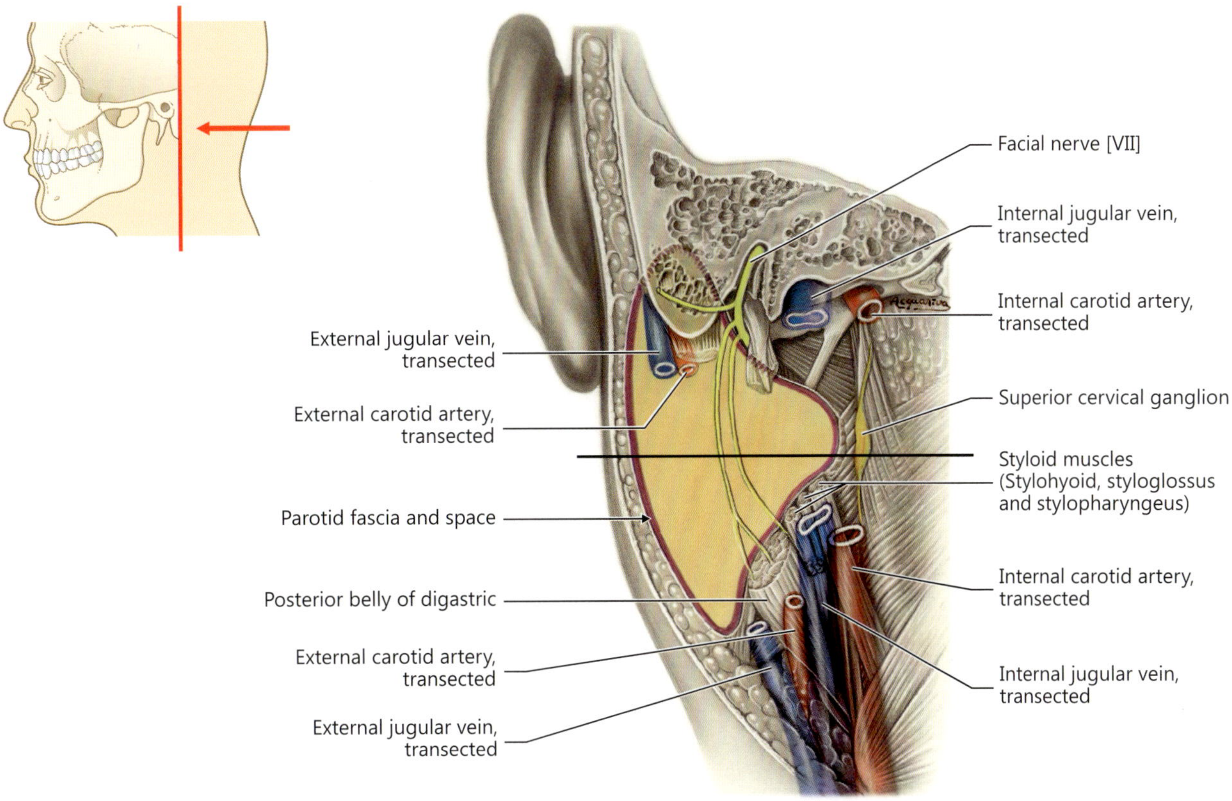

Superior and inferior, superficial and deep boundaries of the **parotid space** (area in *yellow*) in frontal section. The principal muscles, blood vessels and nerve formations related to the parotid space and the gland contained within it are represented. The horizontal line indicates the plane of transection that is illustrated in the following figure.

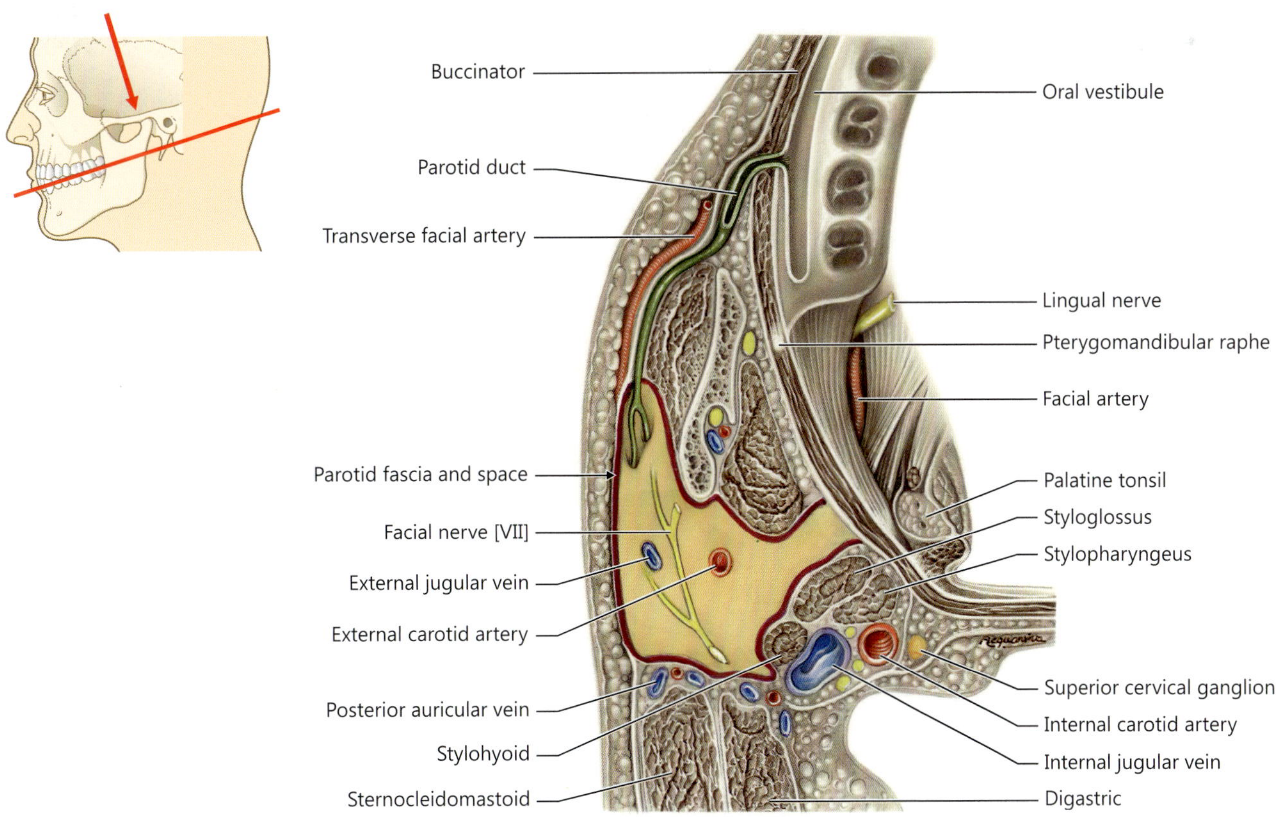

Transverse section of the **parotid space** (area in *yellow*) passing through the plane indicated in the preceding figure. Besides the superficial and deep relations of the parotid gland, also its anterior and posterior relations are illustrated.

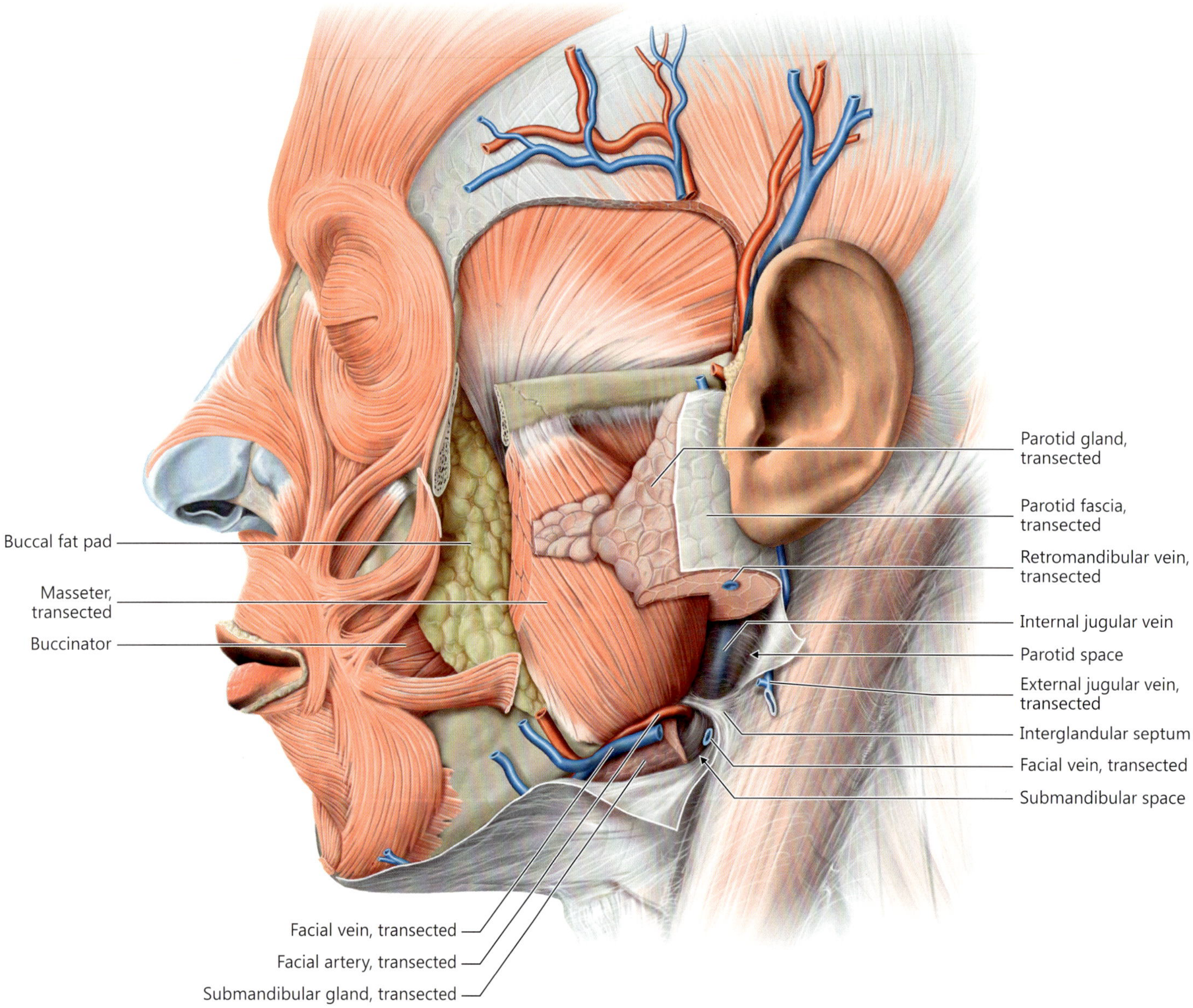

Head, left lateral view. After removing the skin and subcutaneous tissue, the zygomatic arch, masseter, parotid fascia and parotid gland have been transected. In the thickness of the posterior part of the cheek is the buccal fat pad, which occupies a space delimited laterally by the medial surface of the masseter and medially by the lateral surface of the buccinator. The parotid and submandibular glands are divided by a fibrous lamina formed by the fusion of the superficial and deep layers of the parotid fascia: the interglandular septum.

➤

Schematic representation showing the path of the **maxillary artery** in the **infratemporal fossa**. The maxillary artery is the largest terminal branch of the external carotid artery. After its origin behind the neck of the mandible within the parotid gland, it passes medially to the neck of the mandible and crosses the infratemporal fossa. This part of the artery, known as the pterygoid portion, can run either along the lateral surface of the lateral pterygoid, between the lower head of the lateral pterygoid and inferior part of the temporalis (in approximately 60% of cases), or along its medial surface, between the lower head of the lateral pterygoid and the medial pterygoid (in approximately 40% of cases), and it terminates in the pterygopalatine fossa.

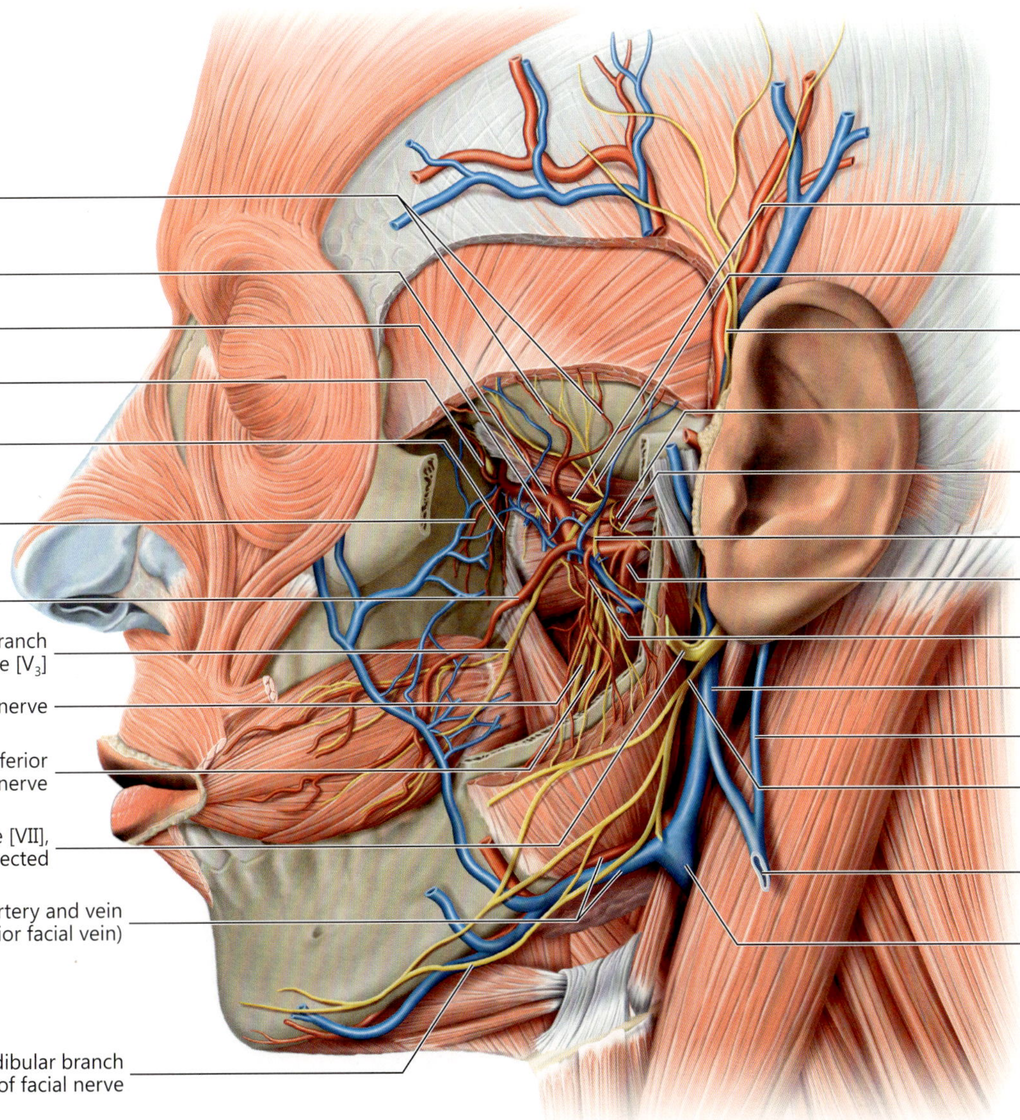

Infratemporal fossa, deep plane. Left lateral view after removal of the zygomatic arch and part of the temporalis. The maxillary artery, largest terminal branch of the external carotid artery, originates behind the neck of the mandible inside the parotid gland, passes medially to the neck of the mandible and crosses the infratemporal fossa heading laterally (as shown in the image and in the diagram below on the right), or medially (diagram below on the left) to the lower head of the lateral pterygoid, and terminates in the pterygopalatine fossa. In the infratemporal fossa one can see the inferior alveolar, masseteric, buccal, and anterior and posterior deep temporal arteries and the pterygoid branches of the maxillary artery, while in the pterygopalatine fossa one can see the posterior superior alveolar artery and infraorbital artery and the terminal branch of the maxillary artery, represented by the sphenopalatine artery.

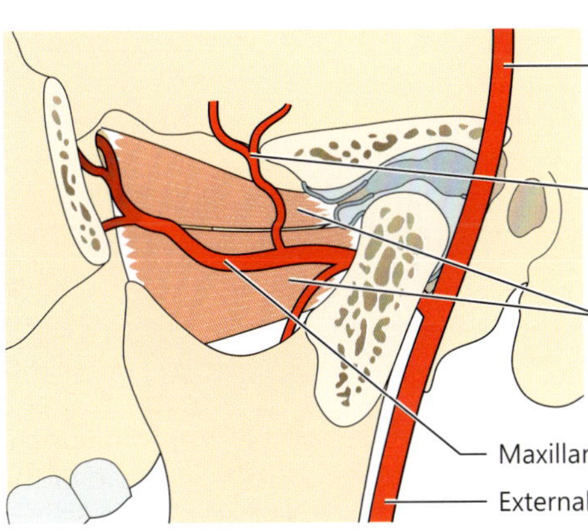

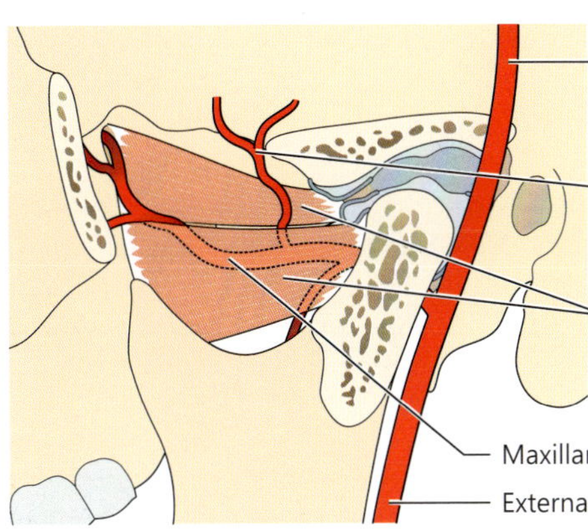

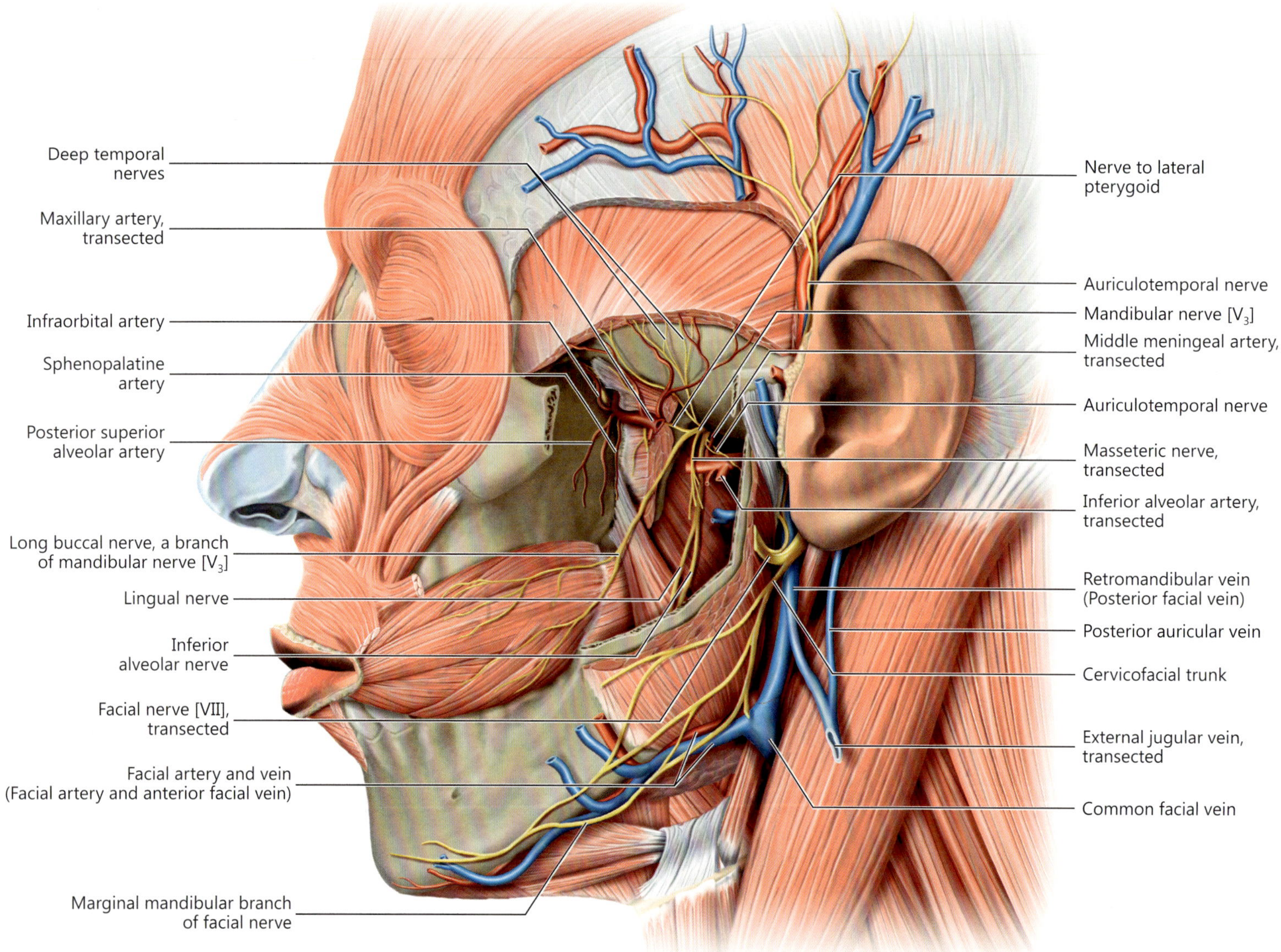

Infratemporal fossa, deep plane. Left lateral view after removal of the zygomatic arch, part of the temporalis and upper and lower heads of the lateral pterygoid. The mandibular nerve [V_3] arrives in the upper part of the infratemporal fossa after passing through the foramen ovale and here divides into two trunks, anterolateral and posteromedial. From the former arise the deep temporal, buccal, masseteric and lateral pterygoid nerves, from the latter the lingual, inferior alveolar, auriculotemporal and medial pterygoid nerves. The auriculotemporal nerve separates from the posterior trunk of the mandibular nerve with two roots that encircle the middle meningeal artery.

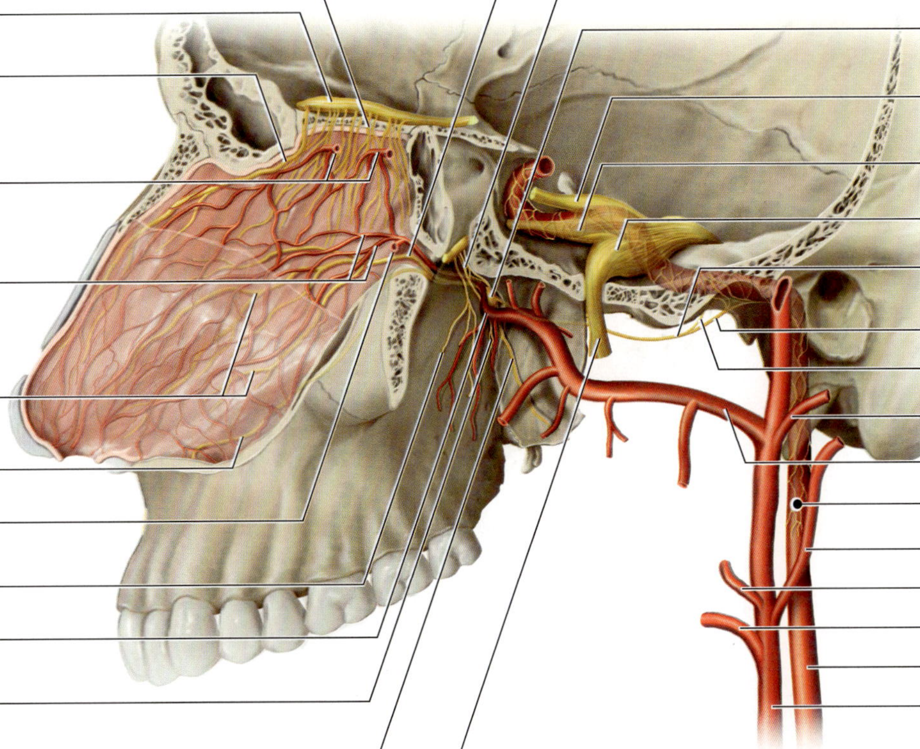

Left lateral view of the medial wall of the left **nasal cavity** after removal of its lateral wall. One can see the nasal and palatine branches of the maxillary nerve [V_2]. Also the medial wall of the pterygopalatine fossa has been removed in order to show the pterygopalatine (or sphenopalatine) ganglion, which receives the nerve of the pterygoid canal (or Vidian nerve), into which the greater petrosal nerve, a branch of the facial nerve [VII], flows as well as the deep petrosal nerve, coming from the internal carotid plexus. To it travel also the ganglionic branches to the pterygopalatine ganglion of the maxillary nerve (or the nasopalatine or pterygopalatine nerves). Efferent branches of the pterygopalatine ganglion are the pharyngeal, greater palatine and lesser palatine nerves and the posterior superior nasal branches of the maxillary nerve, of which the largest is the nasopalatine nerve. One can also see the trigeminal or semilunar ganglion, located in the middle cranial fossa near the apex of the petrous part of the temporal bone.

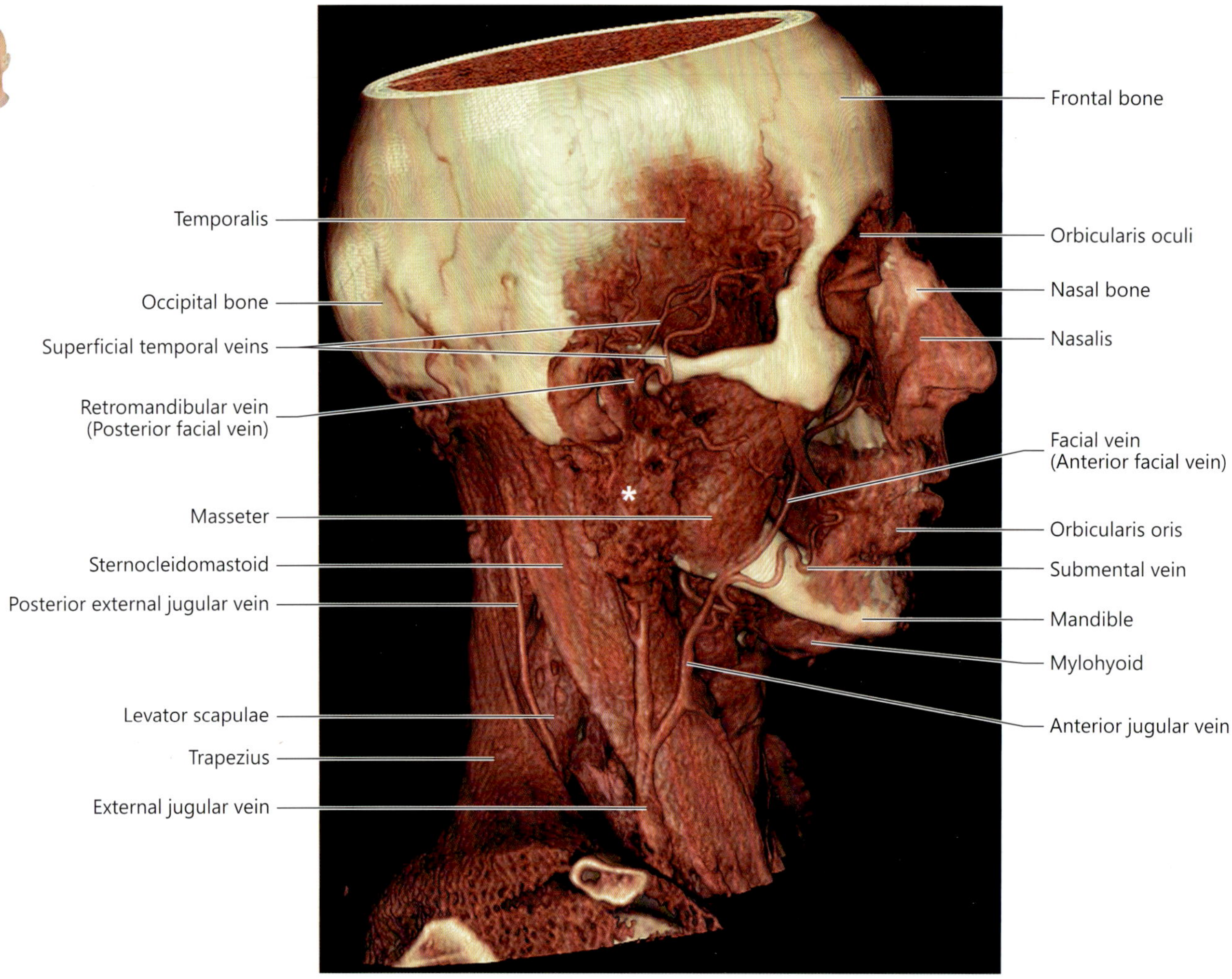

Three-dimensional image of a living human body, obtained using a 3D volume rendering technique, showing some of the **bony structures of the cranium** and muscle structures of the neck. The parotid space is indicated with an asterisk and reported in the figure below.

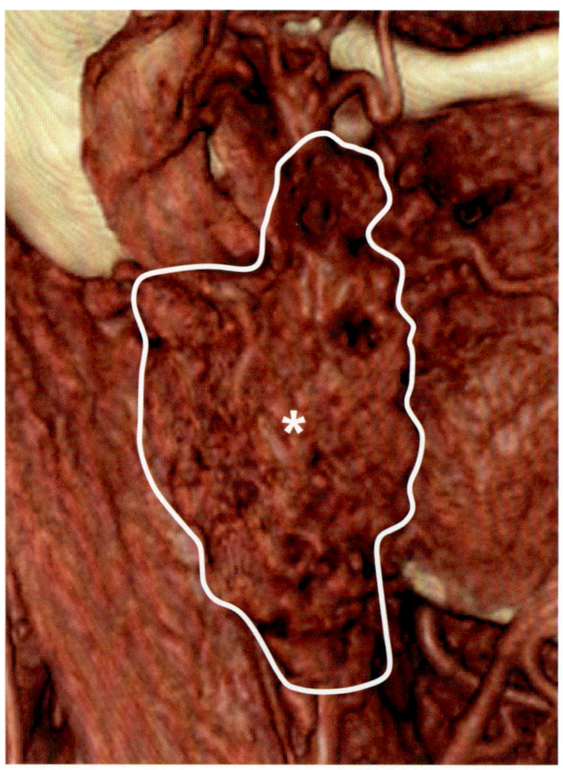

Close-up detail of the **parotid space**, showing its boundaries on the skin plane, i.e. below the auricle and external acoustic meatus, behind the ramus of the mandible and in front of the sternocleidomastoid.

Isthmus of Fauces

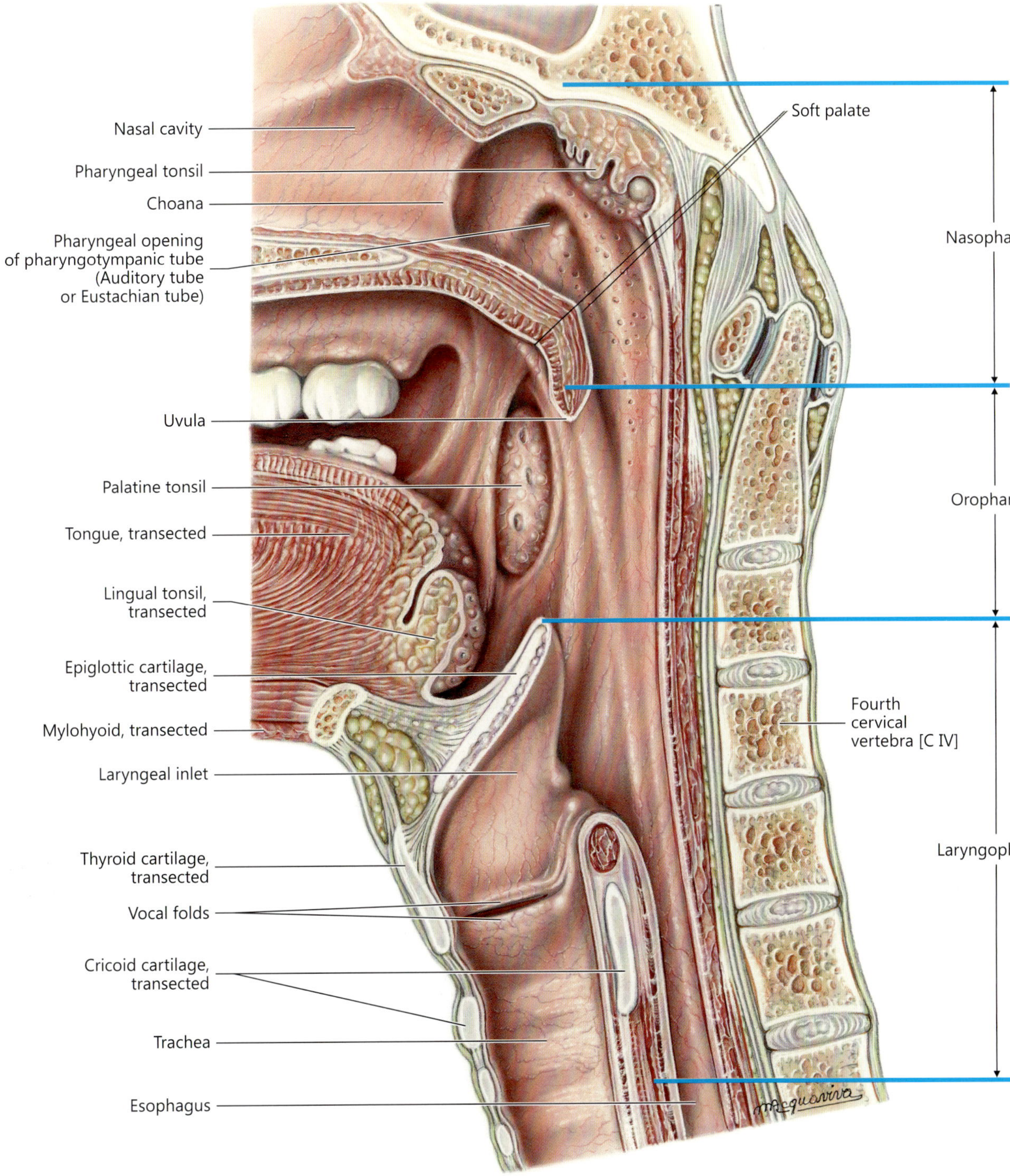

Sagittal section of the head and neck showing the lateral wall of the **isthmus of the fauces**. The palatine tonsil is enclosed in the space between the palatoglossal arch (anteriorly) and the palatopharyngeal arch (posteriorly). Also visible are the lateral wall of the pharynx, with the pharyngeal opening of the pharyngotympanic tube (auditory tube), the initial part of the esophagus and, in front of it, the larynx and initial part of the trachea.

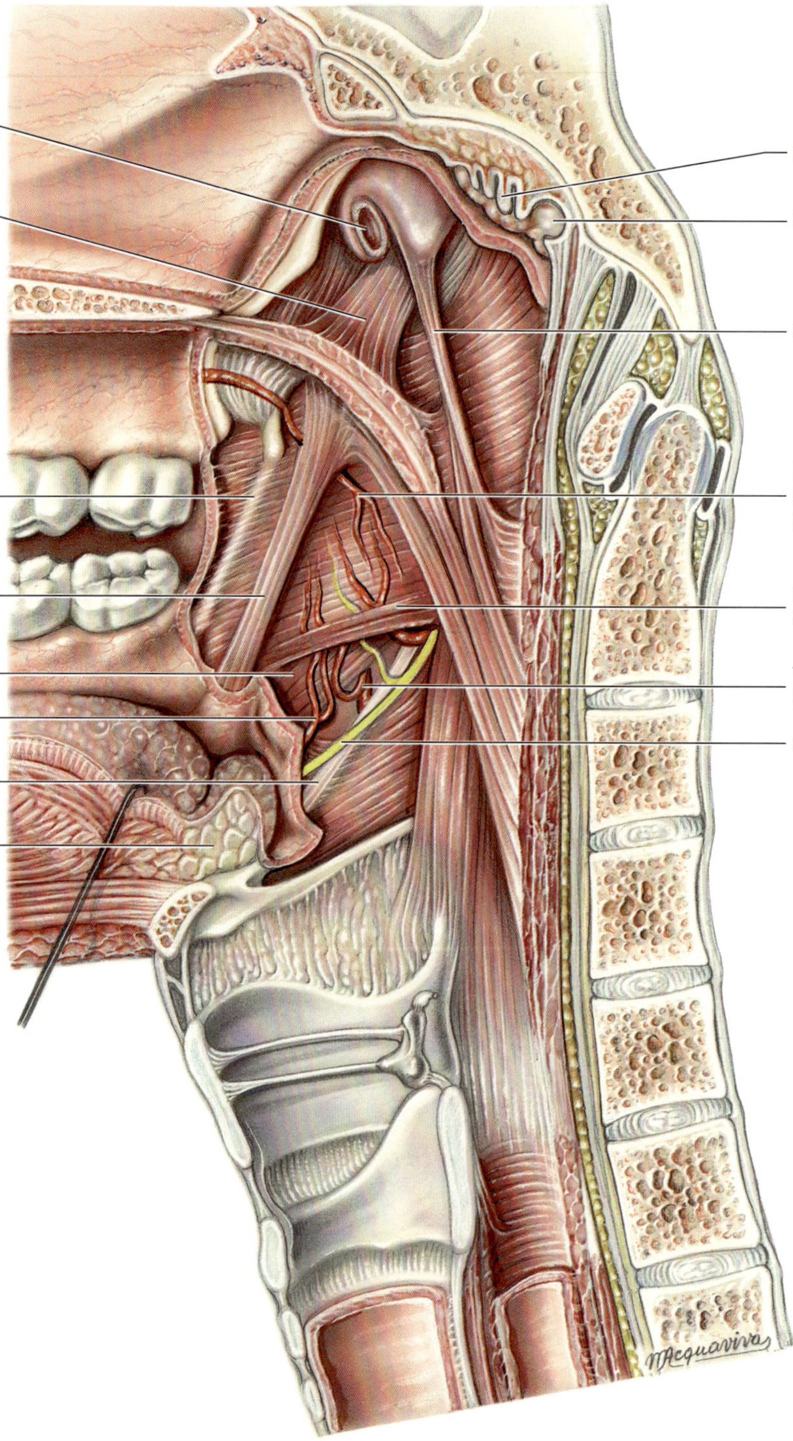

Lateral wall of the **isthmus of the fauces**, after removing the mucosa of the palate and palatine tonsil. Some of the muscles and deep nerves related to the palatine tonsil can be seen, as well as the muscular plane that supports the organ. Also highlighted is the musculature of the lateral wall of the pharynx.

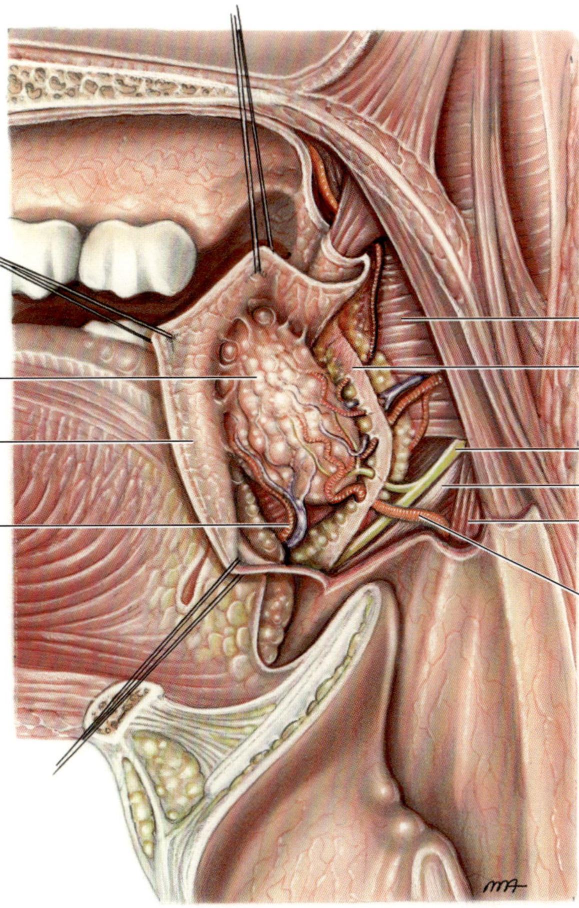

After section of the peritonsillar mucosa and its detachment with respect to the deep planes, one has a view of the neurovascular peduncles of the **palatine tonsil**.

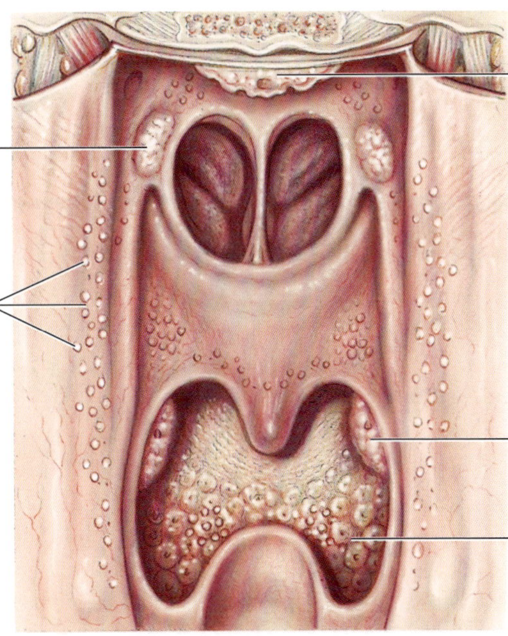

Pharyngeal lymphoid ring (Waldeyer's ring). Ring-like arrangement of lymphoid tissue in the pharynx. The ring is formed by the pharyngeal tonsil, tubal tonsils, palatine tonsils and lingual tonsil.

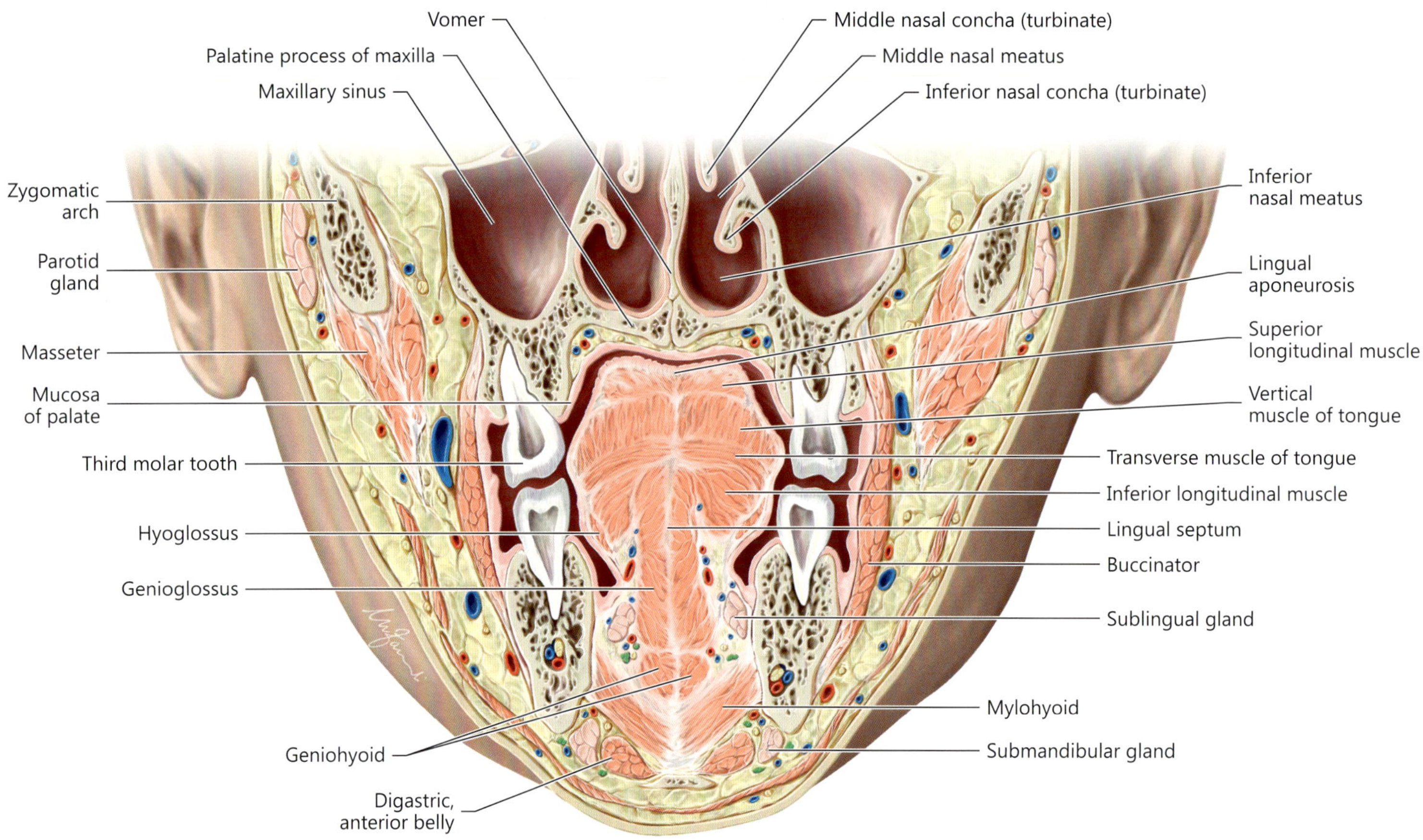

Muscles of the tongue and floor of the mouth, frontal section at the level of the third molar.

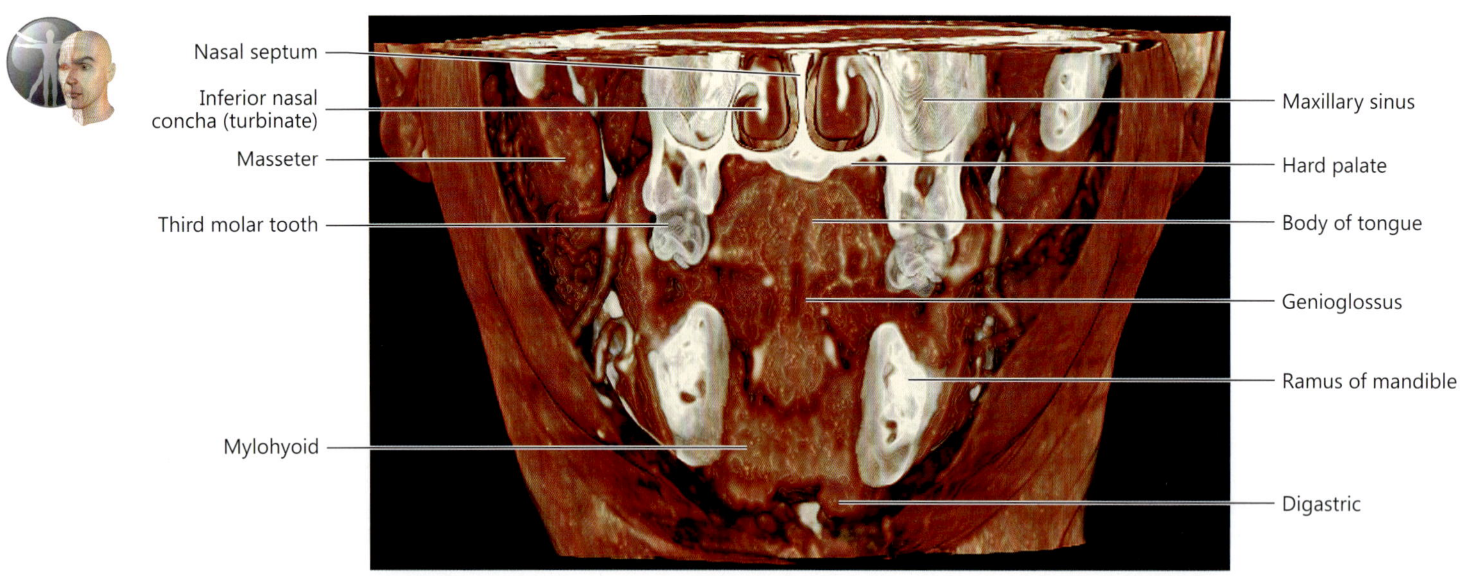

Three-dimensional image of a living human body, obtained using a 3D volume rendering technique, showing the **tongue** and **muscles of the floor of the mouth**, frontal section at the level of the third molar.

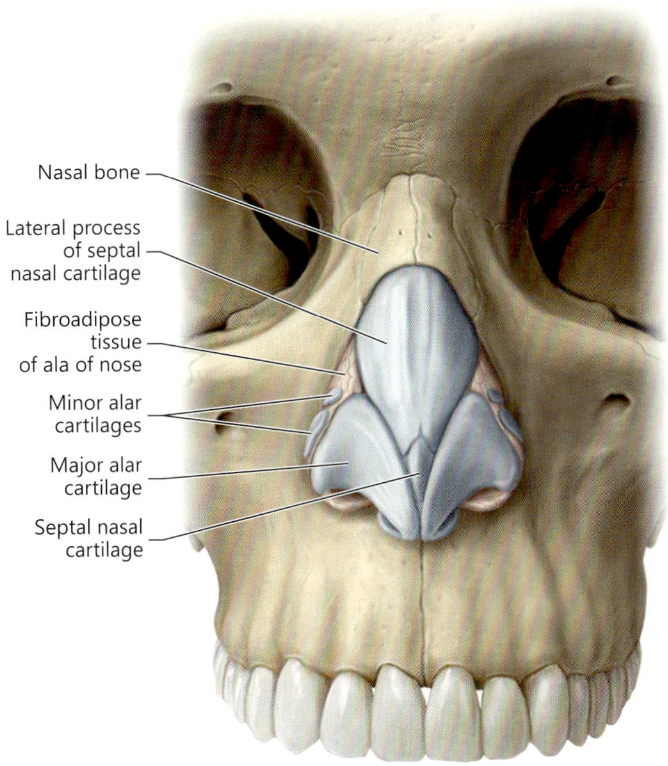

Constitution of the **external nose**, viewed in anterior projection. The major and minor alar cartilages and septal nasal cartilage form the skeleton of the mobile part of the nasal pyramid.

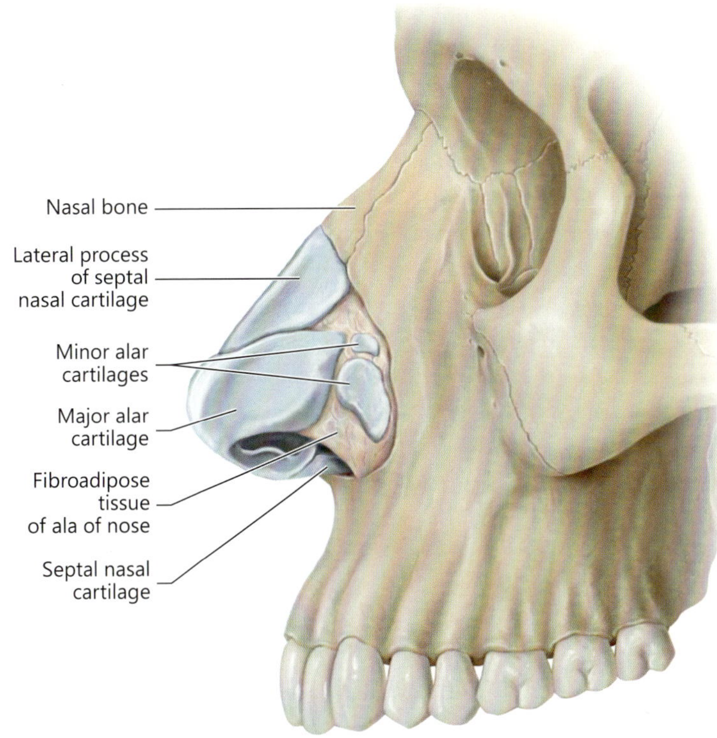

Constitution of the **external nose**, viewed in left lateral projection. The nasal pyramid is formed of bone at the apex, while the intermediate and basal parts have a cartilaginous constitution.

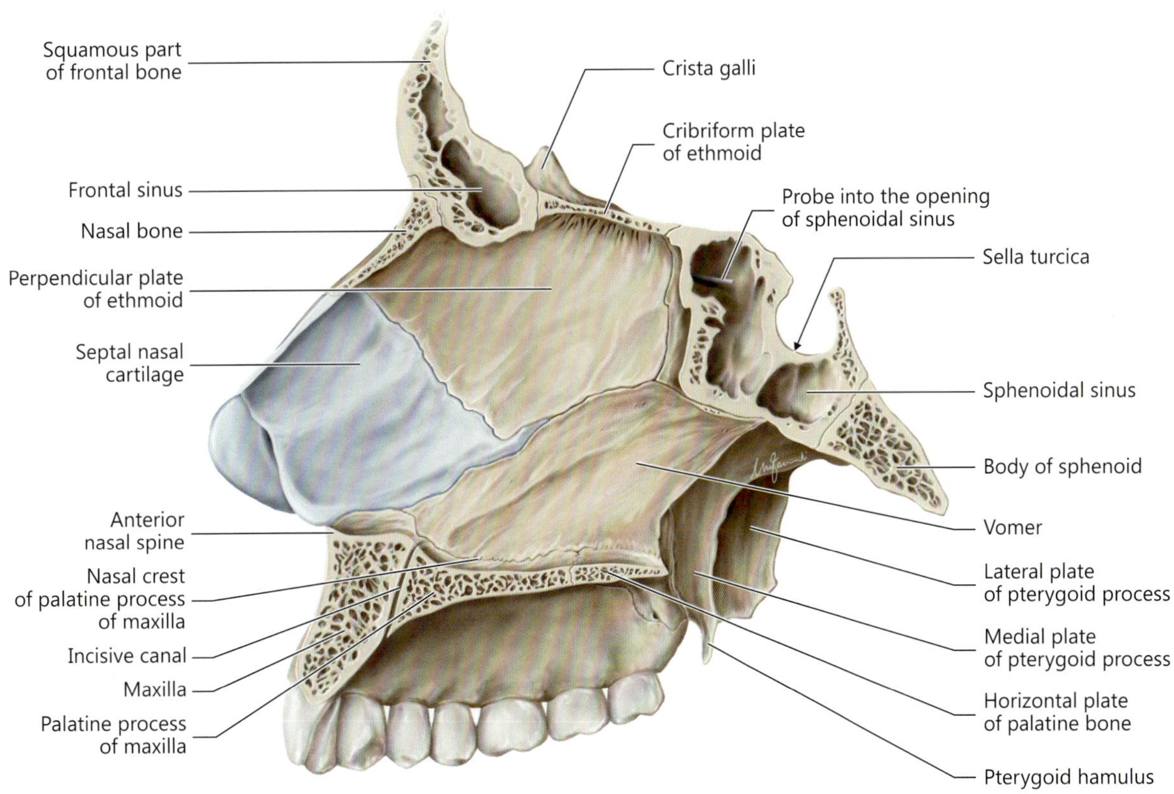

Constitution of the **nasal septum**, viewed in left lateral projection. One can see the two bony components of the septum, the vomer and perpendicular plate of the ethmoid, which unite forming an angle open to the front into which the septal nasal cartilage fits.

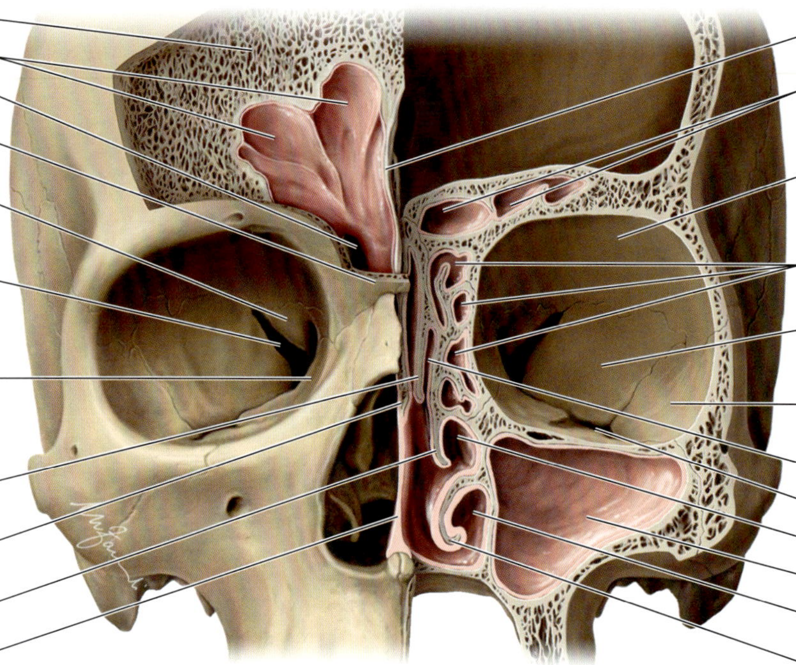

Nasal cavity, **orbital cavity**, and **paranasal sinuses** (anterior view). On the right, the squamous part of the frontal bone has been transected, displaying the frontal sinus. On the left, a frontal section has been performed passing through the orbital surface of the frontal bone to display the ethmoidal cells, nasal meatuses and maxillary sinus. The three nasal conchae protrude from the lateral wall of the nasal cavity: from top to bottom, the superior, middle and inferior nasal conchae, which constitute the roof of the respective meatuses. Respiratory mucosa lines both sides of the conchae and, through the communicating orifices, also the paranasal sinuses. The ethmoidal cells, contained prevalently in the ethmoid, open for the most part into the middle nasal meatus, some into the superior nasal meatus.

For further detail ☞ pages 170-171 of volume 1.

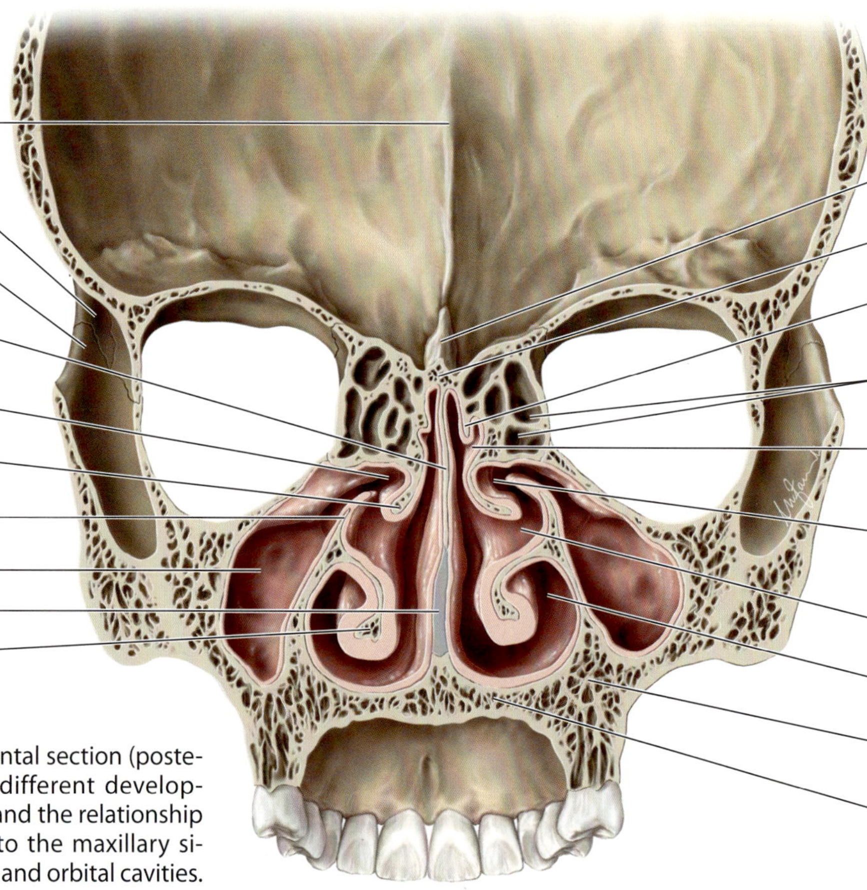

Nasal cavities in a frontal section (posterior view). Note the different development of the conchae and the relationship of the nasal cavities to the maxillary sinuses, ethmoidal cells and orbital cavities.

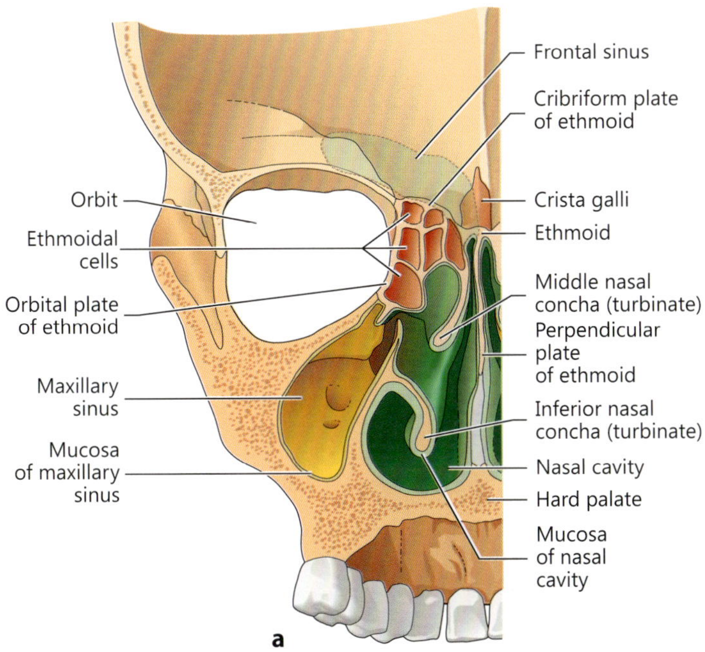

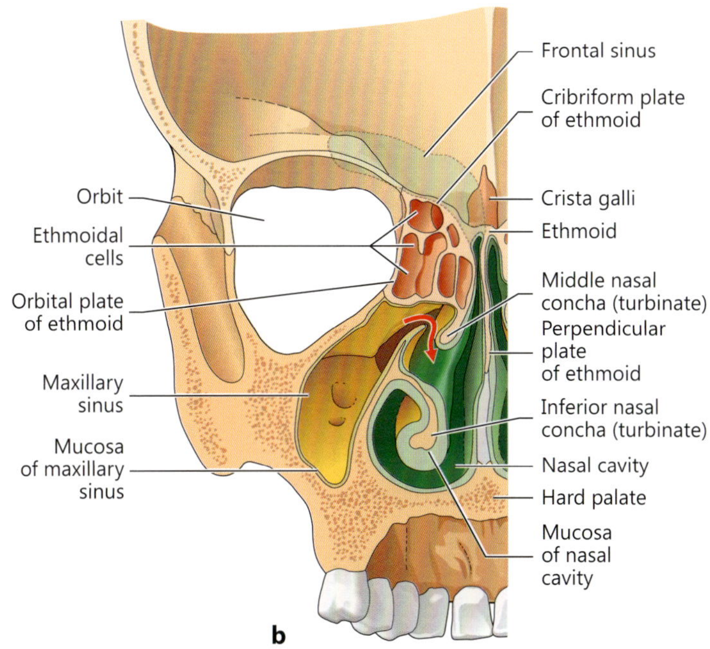

Schematic representation showing frontal sections of the **nasal cavity**. In **a**, the nasal cavity has been transected passing through the ethmoidal infundibulum. The transection in **b** highlights the entry of the maxillary sinus into the nasal cavity (arrow).

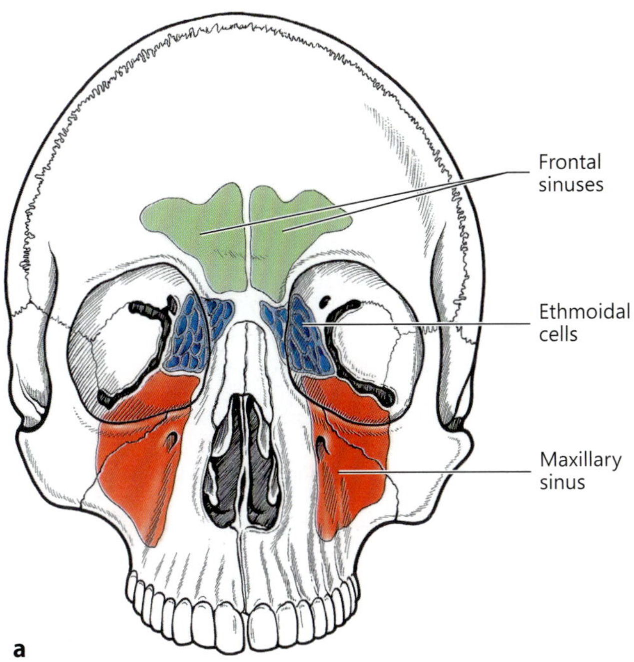

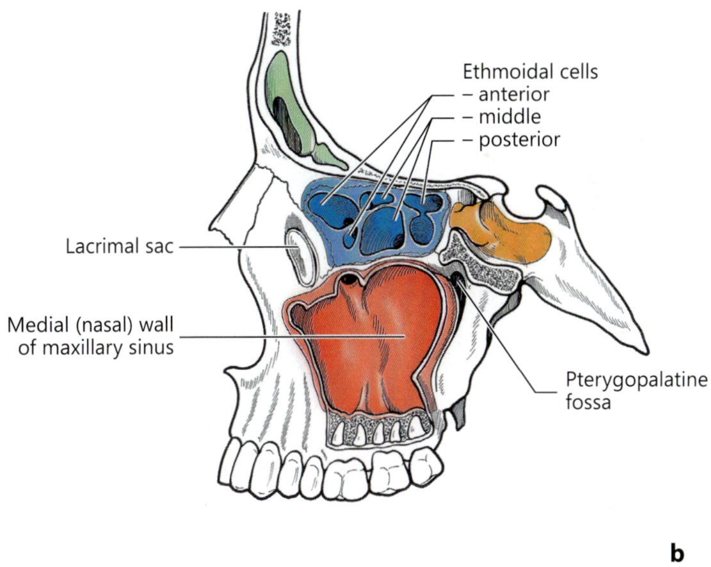

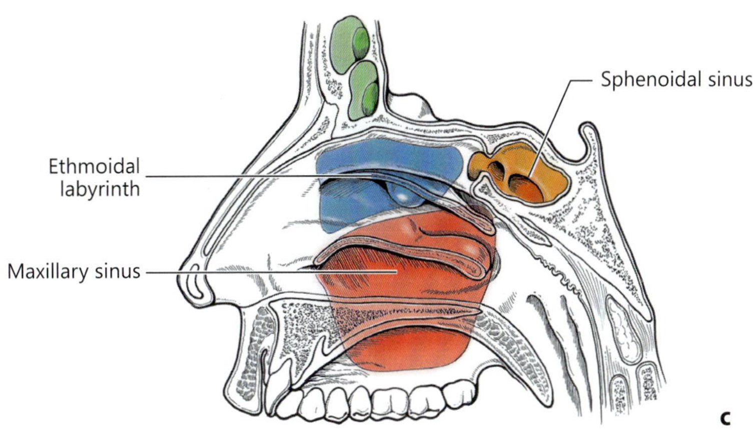

General conformation of the **paranasal sinuses**, in transparent view, in relation to the craniofacial skeleton. In **a**, anterior projection, in **b** and **c**, respectively, lateral and medial projections. The **maxillary sinuses** are visible in the three-dimensional image of a living human body on page 381 of volume 1.

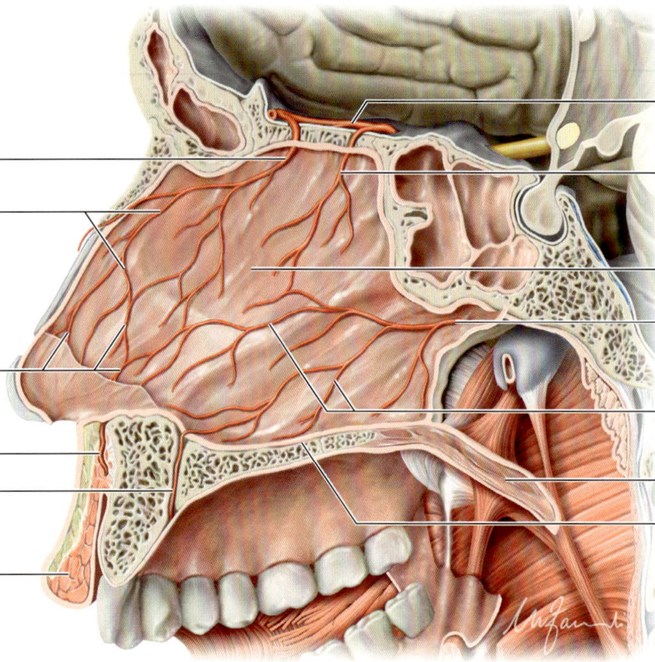

Paramedian sagittal section of the left **nasal cavity**. One can see the arterial branches that supply the nasal septum. The anterior and posterior ethmoidal arteries, branches of the ophthalmic artery, supply nasal branches that cross the cribriform plate. Anterior septal branches of the anterior ethmoidal artery anastomose with posterior septal branches of the sphenopalatine artery, a branch of the maxillary artery, which penetrates into the nasal cavity through the sphenopalatine foramen. Also the superior labial branch of the facial artery supplies a branch to the nasal septum. The greater palatine artery, a branch of the descending palatine artery, itself a branch of the maxillary artery, after emerging on the palatal vault, heads forward and enters the incisive canal and anastomoses with a branch of the sphenopalatine artery. The Kiesselbach's area, in the anteroinferior part of the nasal septum, corresponds to the vascular plexus formed by anastomoses of the anterior ethmoidal, sphenopalatine, greater palatine and superior labial arteries.

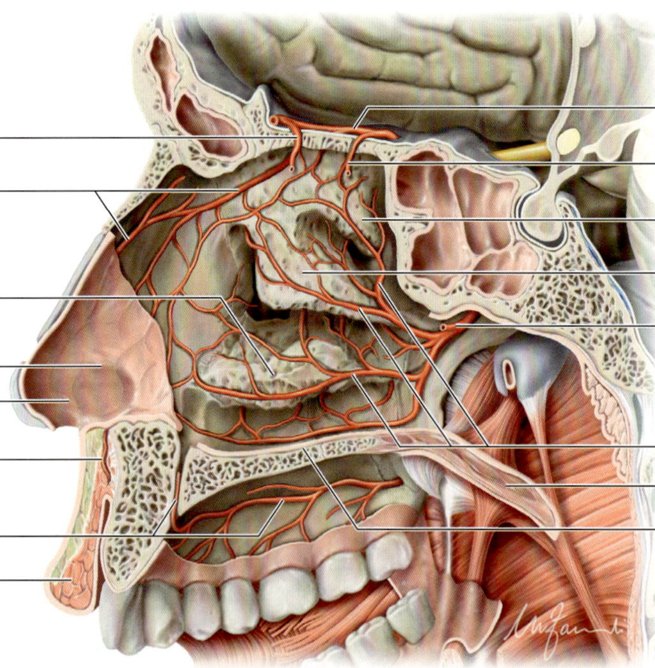

Sagittal section of the right **nasal cavity**, left lateral view. One can see the arterial branches that supply the lateral wall of the nasal cavity: the anterior lateral nasal branches, which stem from the anterior ethmoidal artery, a branch of the ophthalmic artery, and the posterior lateral nasal arteries, branches of the sphenopalatine artery, which anastomose with the ethmoidal arteries and with nasal branches of the greater palatine artery.

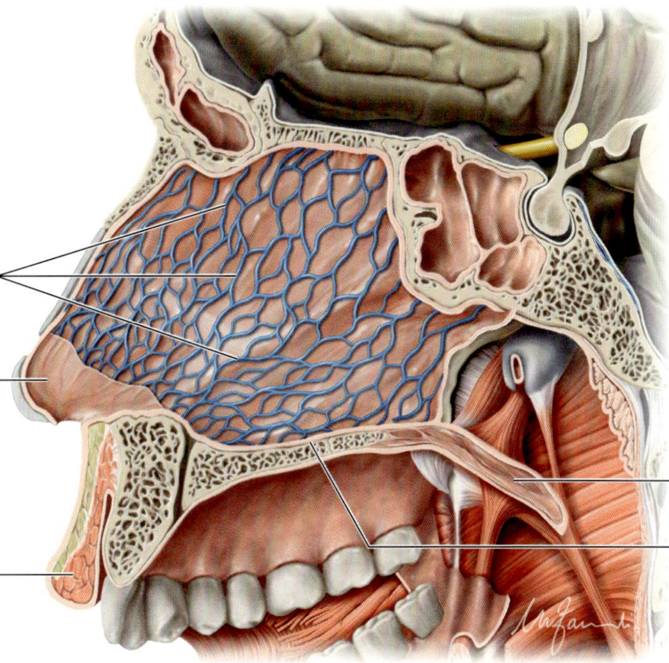

Paramedian sagittal section of the left **nasal cavity**, showing the superficial venous plexus in the lamina propria of the respiratory region at the level of the nasal septum.

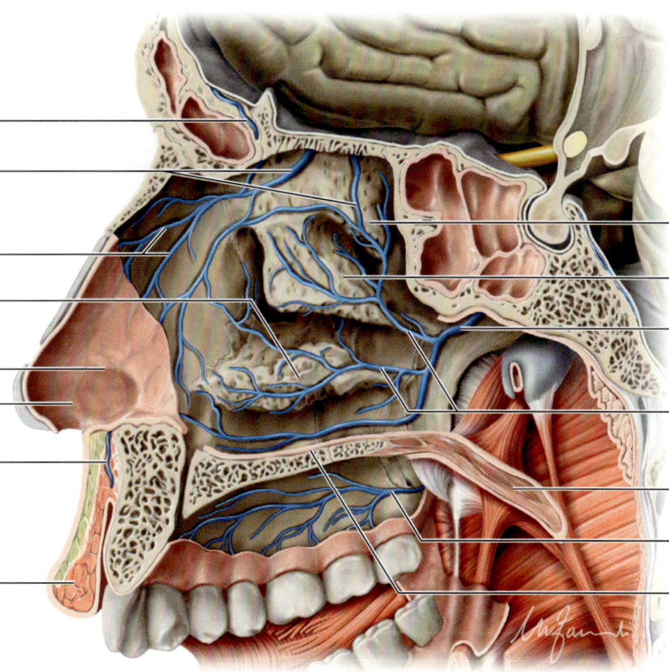

Sagittal section of the right **nasal cavity**, left lateral view. The veins of the nasal cavity terminate: posteriorly, in the sphenopalatine vein, which drains into the pterygoid plexus; superiorly, in the ethmoidal veins, which drain into the superior ophthalmic vein; and anteriorly, in the superior labial vein, an affluent branch of the facial vein. The presence in man of the vein of the foramen cecum remains a controversial issue. The vein should provide intracranial drainage of the nasal mucosa into the superior sagittal sinus through one of the frontal veins.

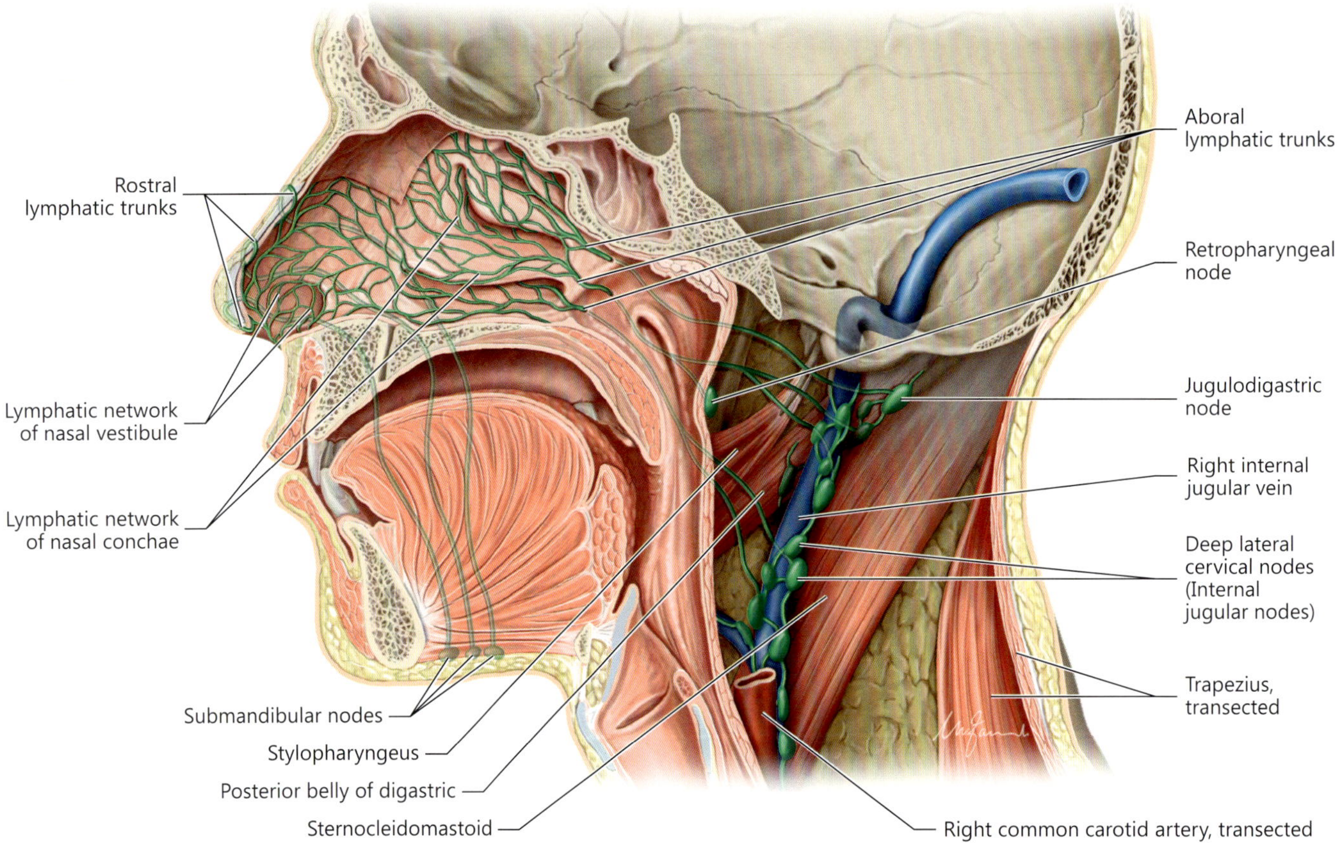

Sagittal section of the right **nasal cavity** (anteriorly) and oblique section on a plane passing through the mastoid process of the temporal bone and basilar part of the occipital bone (posteriorly). One can see the lymphatic network of the mucosa of the nasal cavity, the efferent trunks of which drain into the submandibular, retropharyngeal, deep lateral cervical (internal jugular) and jugulodigastric nodes.

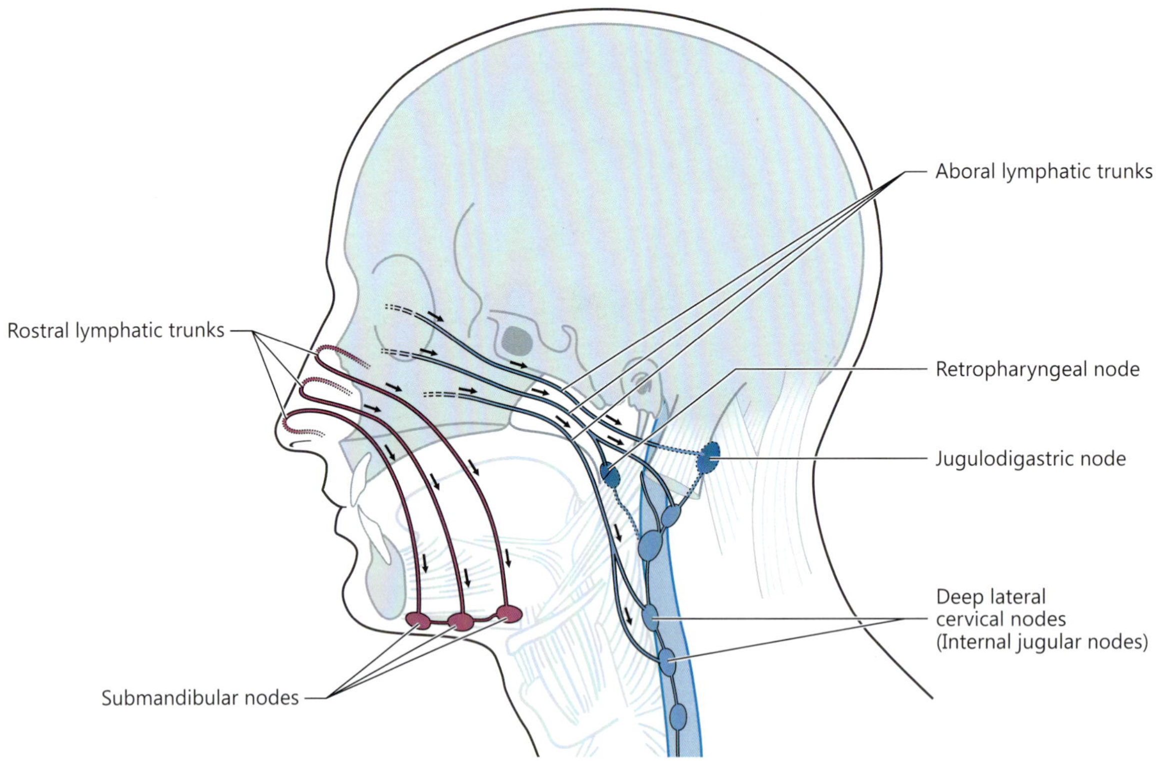

Schematic representation showing the **pathways of lymphatic drainage** of the mucosa of the nasal cavity to the submandibular, retropharyngeal, deep lateral cervical (internal jugular) and jugulodigastric nodes.

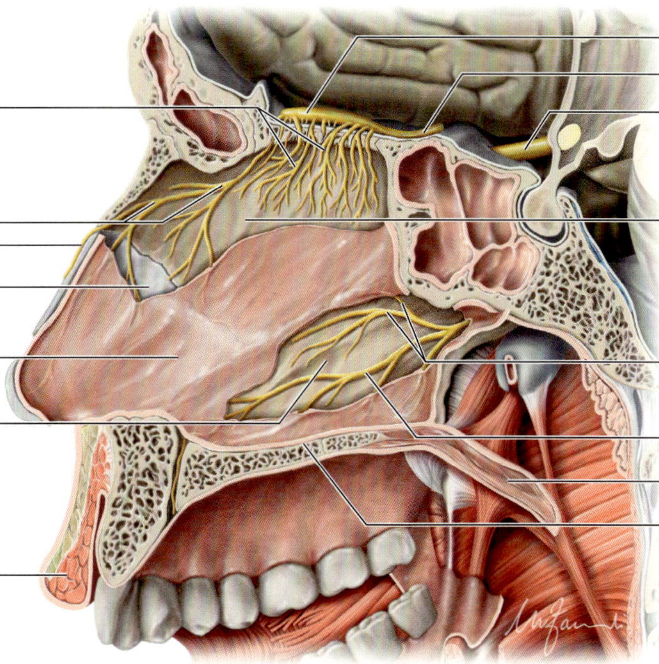

Paramedian sagittal section of the left **nasal cavity**, left lateral view. The anterior ethmoidal nerve, a branch of the nasociliary nerve, itself a branch of the ophthalmic nerve [V_1], supplies internal medial nasal branches, while posterior superior medial nasal branches are supplied by the maxillary nerve [V_2]. The nasopalatine nerve, a branch of the maxillary nerve [V_2], following the sulcus of the vomer running obliquely forwards and downwards, descends down the wall of the nasal septum reaching the incisive canal, through which it enters the oral cavity. The olfactory nerve [I] is composed of filaments which, crossing the cribriform foramina of the ethmoid, penetrate into the inferior surface of the olfactory bulb, situated in the anterior cranial fossa, above the cribriform plate of the ethmoid.

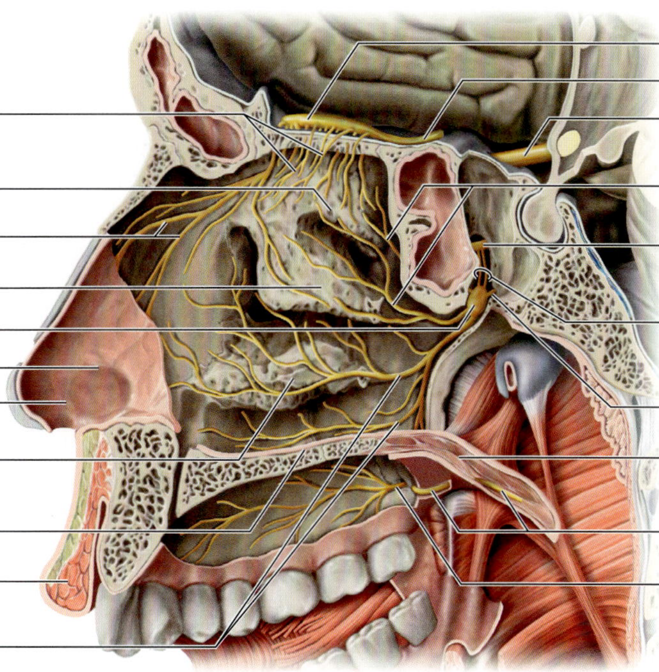

Sagittal section of the right **nasal cavity**, left lateral view. From the anterior ethmoidal nerve, a branch of the ophthalmic nerve [V_1], lateral nasal branches head to the vault and lateral wall of the nasal cavity. The medial surface of the pterygopalatine ganglion gives off numerous fibers that pass into the nasal cavity through the sphenopalatine foramen. The lateral group consists of posterior superior lateral nasal branches of the maxillary nerve [V_2] that go to the lateral wall of the nasal cavity, which is reached also by the posterior inferior nasal branches of the greater palatine nerve, which originates from the inferior part of the pterygopalatine ganglion and descends through the greater palatine canal to the palate. Also the lesser palatine nerves originate from the inferior part of the pterygopalatine ganglion, and pass through the lesser palatine canals from which they emerge to head behind, through the lesser palatine foramina, to the soft palate.

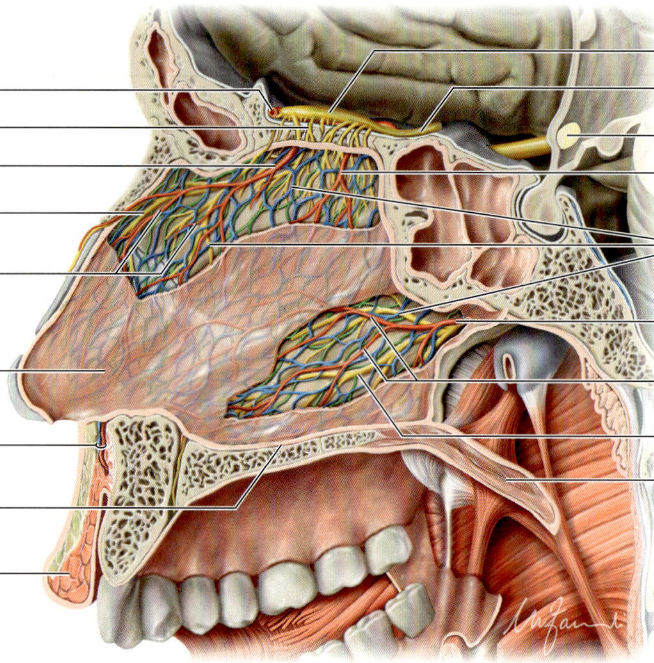

Paramedian sagittal section of the left **nasal cavity**. The olfactory region and part of the respiratory region of the mucosa of the nasal cavity have been transected to display the particularly rich **vascular network** of the **nasal mucosa**, which in some zones such as the middle part of the nasal septum is highly developed.

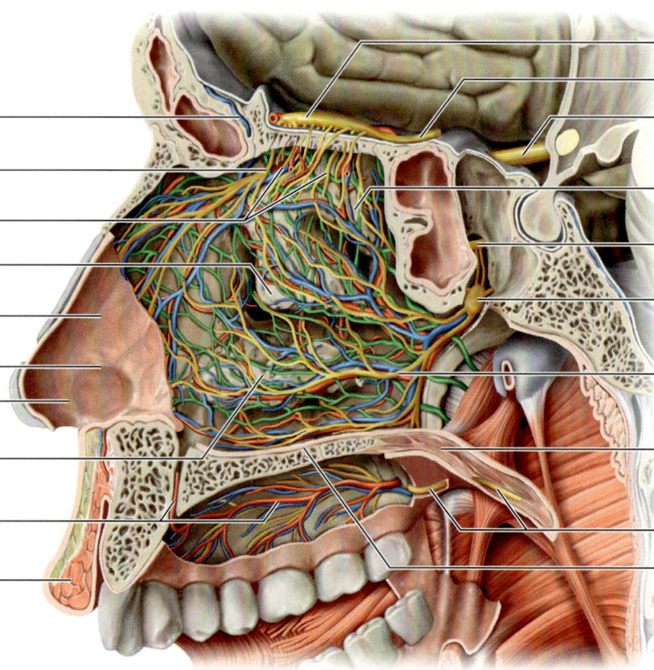

Sagittal section of the right **nasal cavity**, left lateral view. The vascular system is particularly well developed, especially in certain zones such as the inferior nasal meatus. The arteries, starting from deep branches situated near the periosteum, run perpendicularly to the surface of the respiratory region forming an intermediate plexus in the lamina propria and ramifying into a dense subepithelial capillary network. In correspondence to the middle and inferior nasal conchae, there is a **superficial venous plexus** that gives the lamina propria a cavernous tissue-like appearance due to the presence of large venous caverns partitioned by fine fibrous septa.

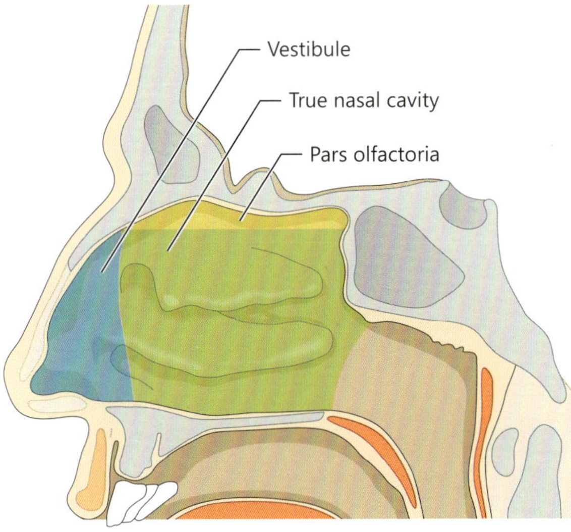

Subdivision of the **nasal cavity**.

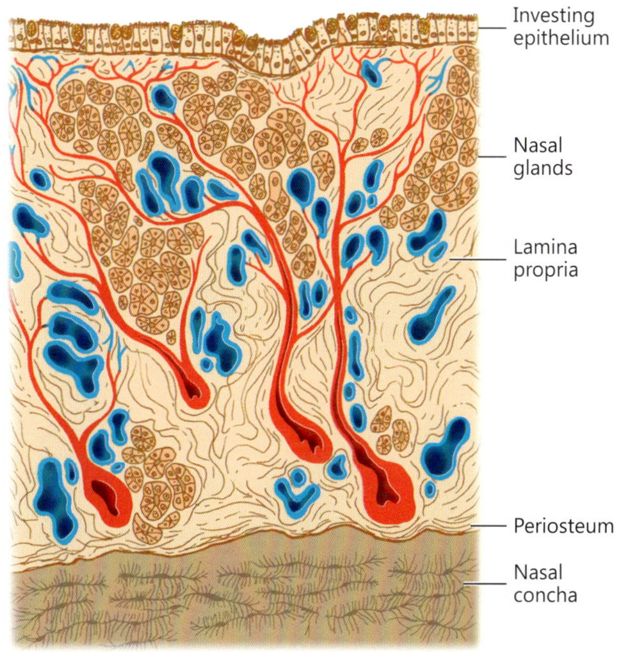

Schematic representation showing the structure of the **respiratory region**. The rich vascular supply is indicated in *red* (arterial part) and *blue* (venous part). There is direct continuity between the two systems through arteriovenous anastomoses.

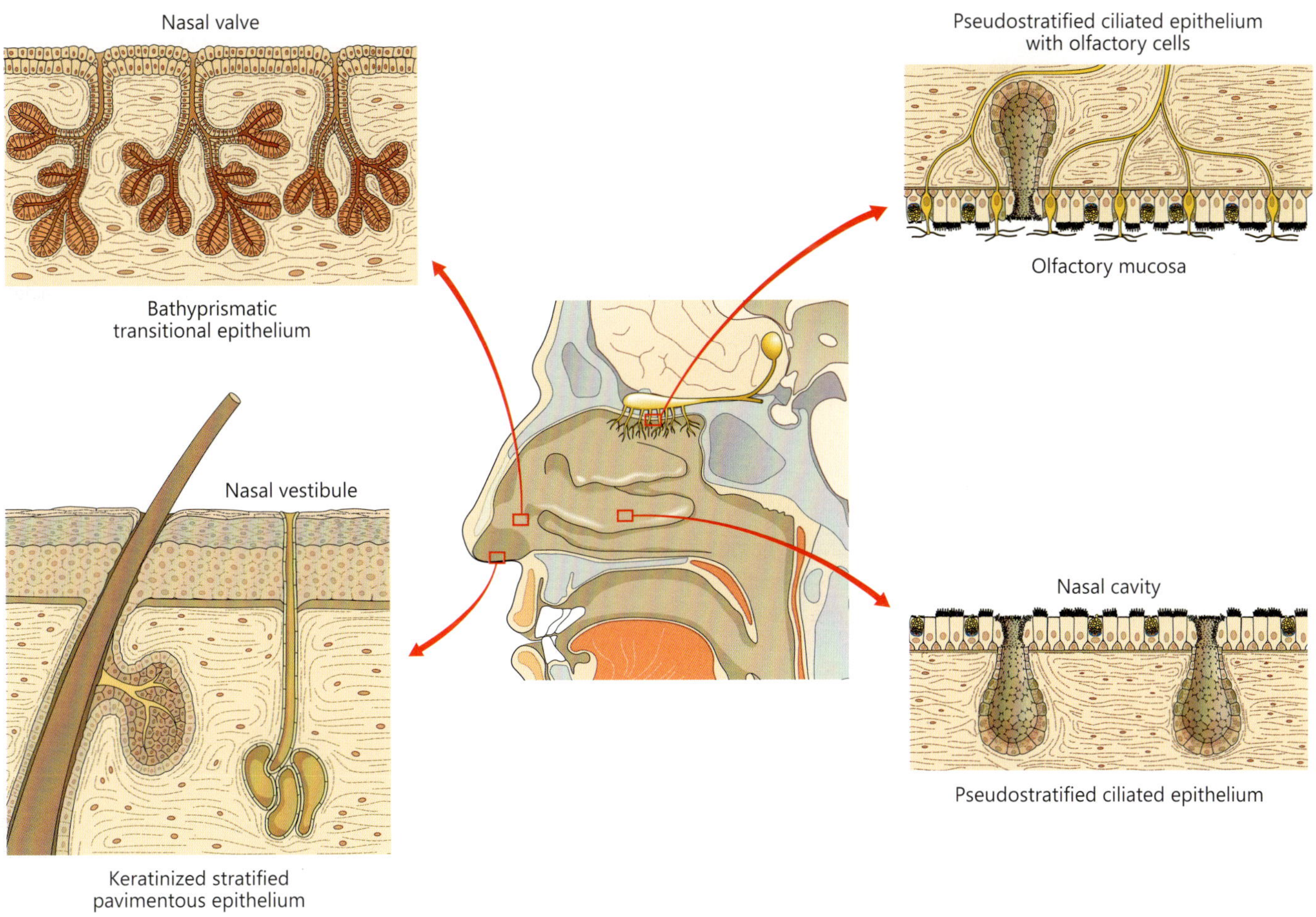

Nasal mucosa: histological variations according to the nasal cavity zone.

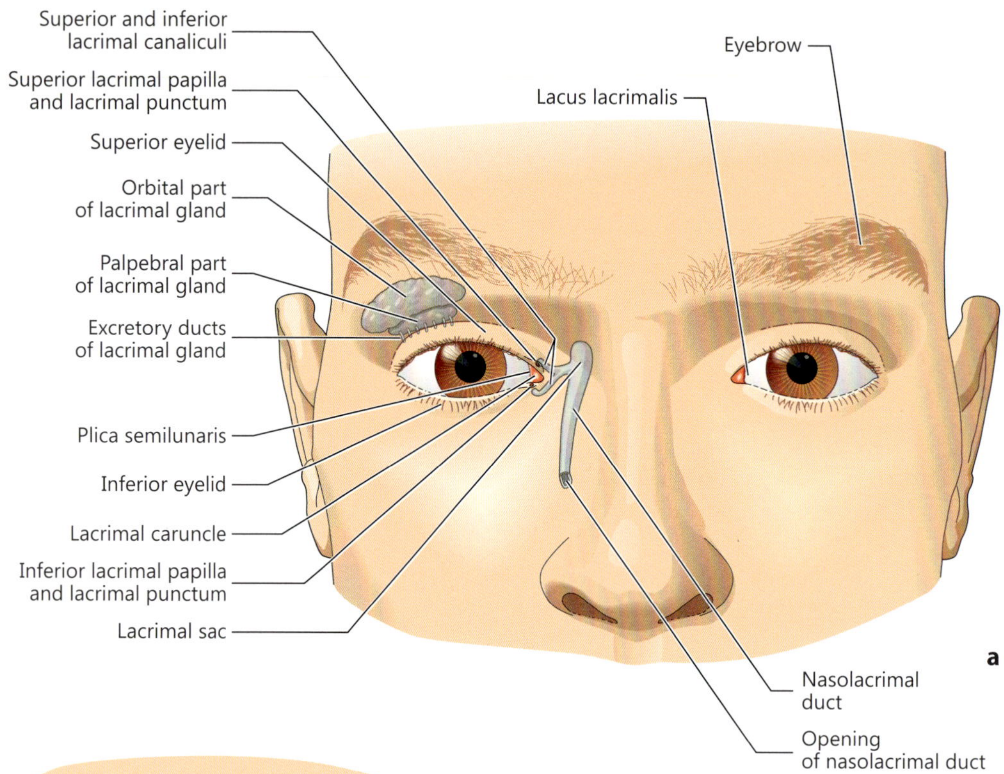

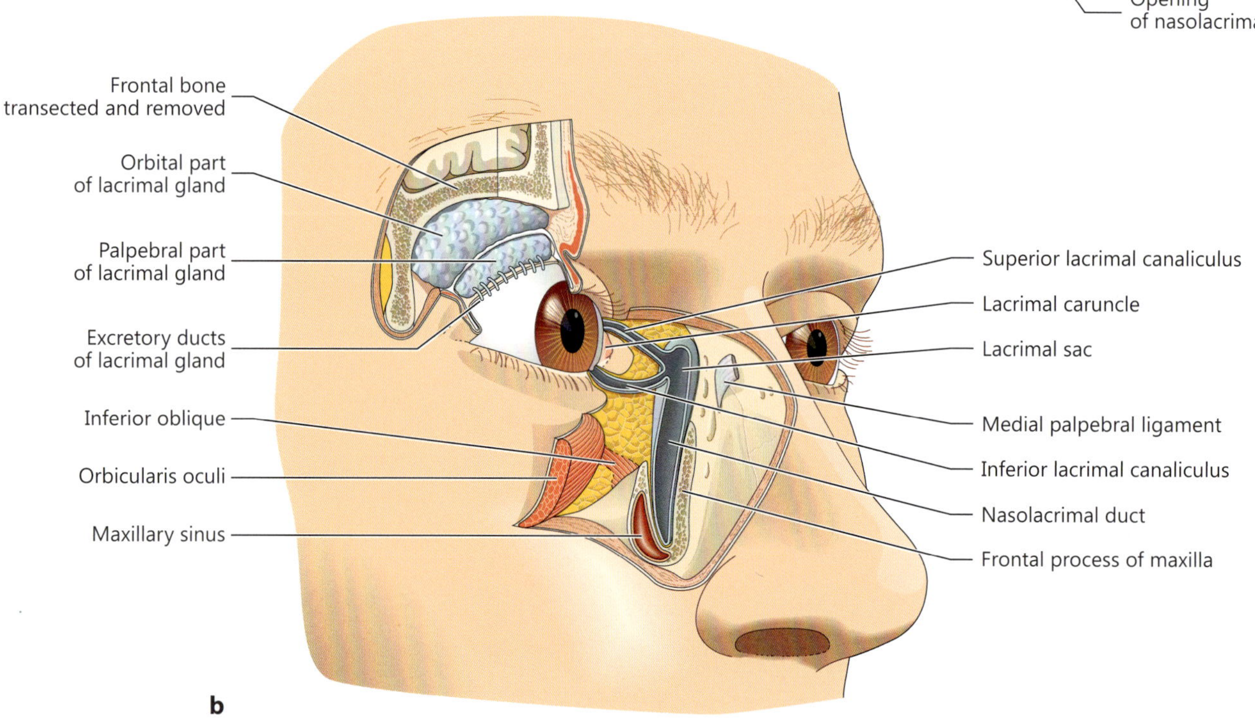

a, Eye and accessory structures as seen through the palpebral fissure. In transparent view, the formations of the protective apparatus of the eyeball. **b**, Organs of the lacrimal apparatus.

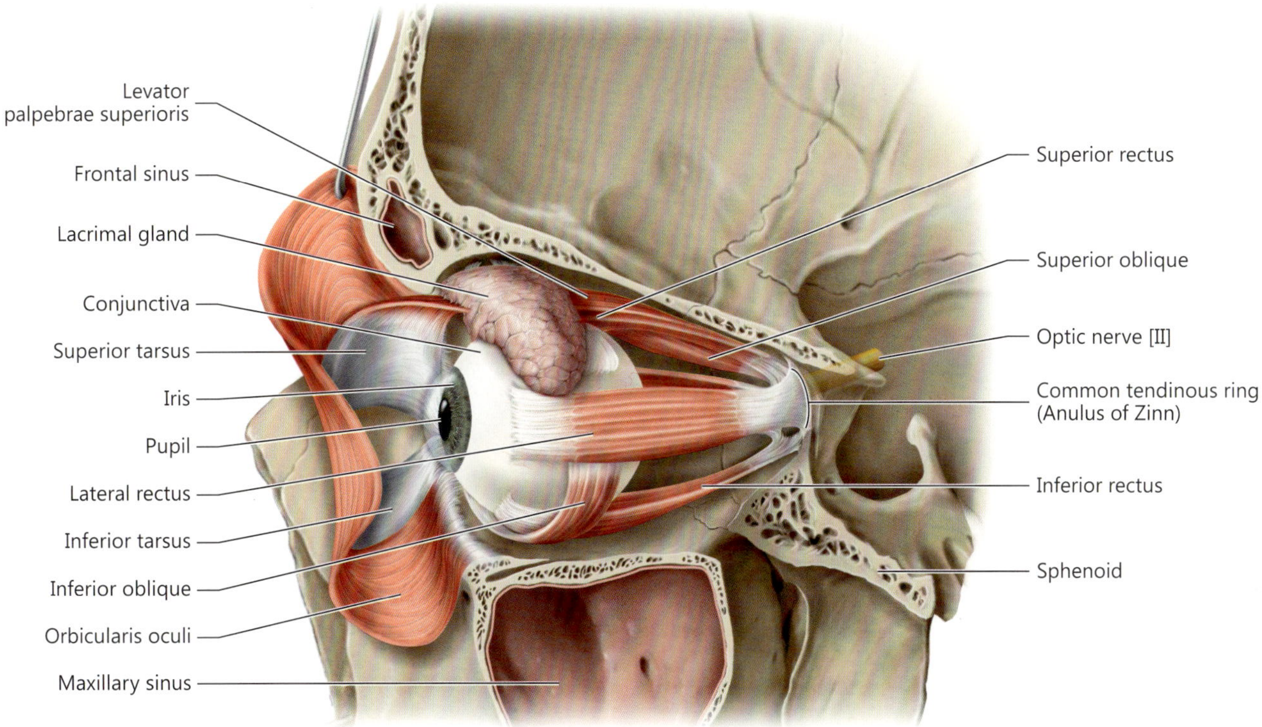

Extraocular muscles. Left eye, lateral view after removal of the lateral wall of the orbit.

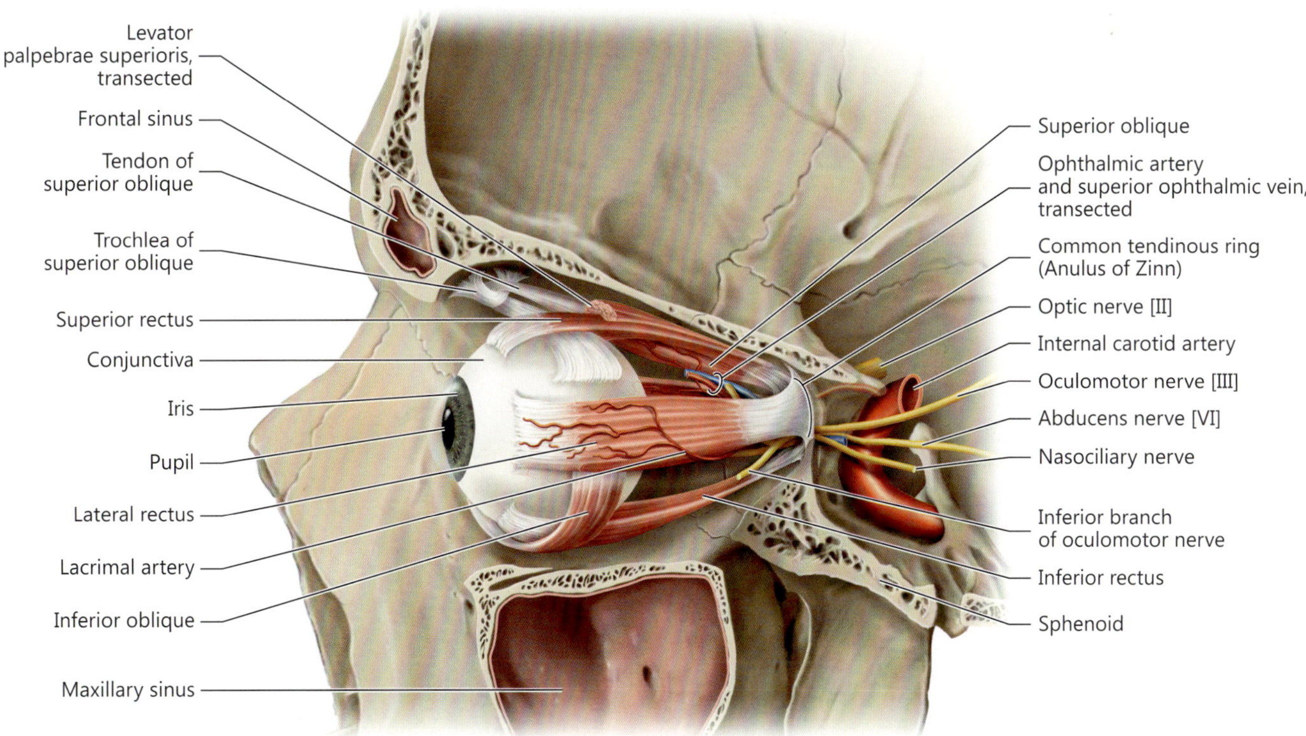

Common tendinous ring (**anulus of Zinn**). The tendinous ring is the origin of the rectus muscles and, partially, of the levator palpebrae superioris and superior oblique. Through its superior compartment run the optic nerve [II] and ophthalmic artery, while through its inferior compartment run the oculomotor nerve [III], superior ophthalmic vein, abducens nerve [VI] and the nasociliary nerve, a branch of the ophthalmic nerve [V_1].

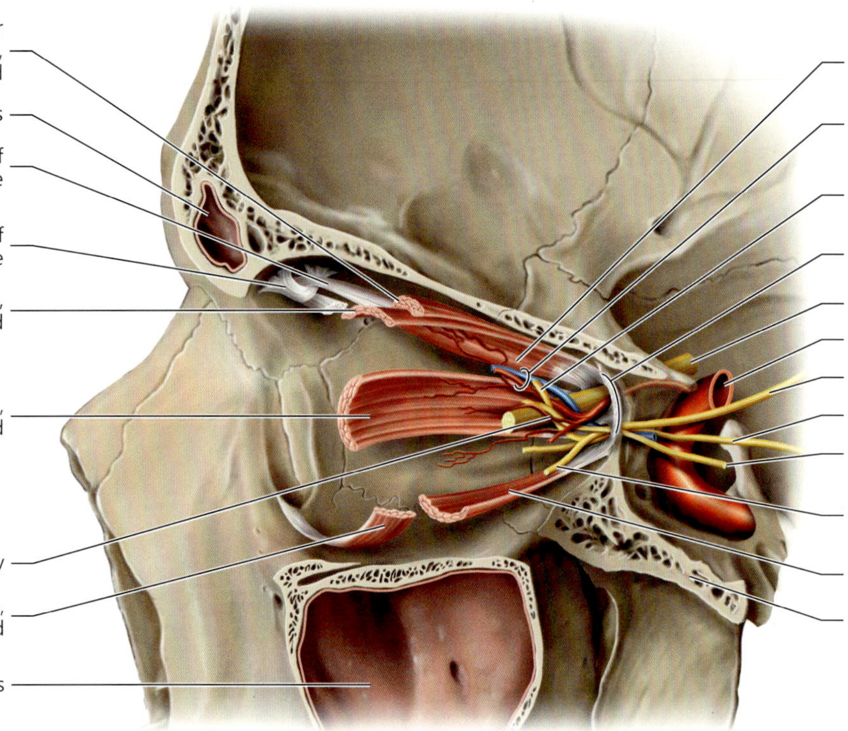

Extraocular muscles of the left eye, lateral view after removal of the lateral wall of the orbit, lateral rectus and eyeball.

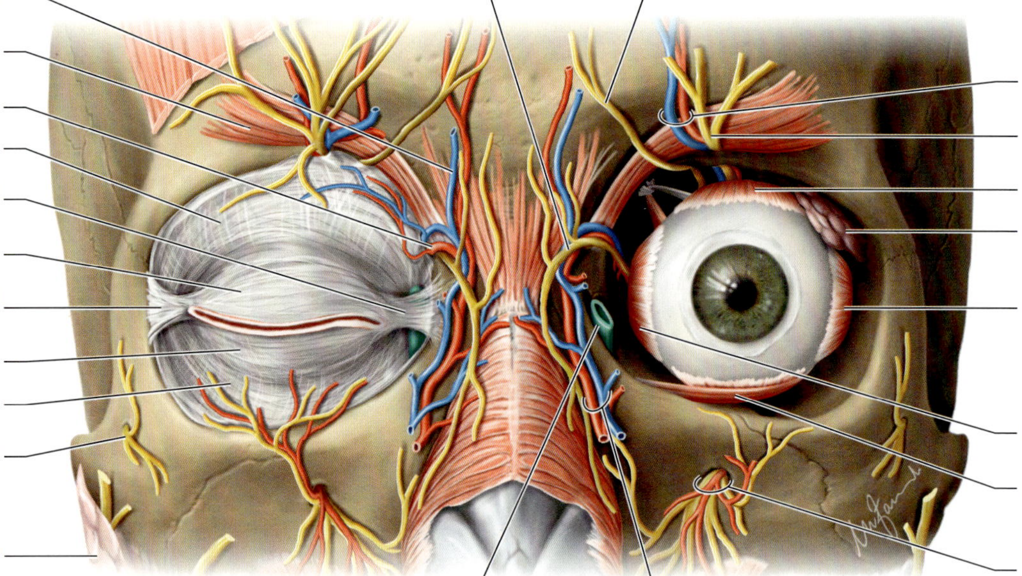

In the right eye, the orbicularis oculi has been transected, showing the orbitopalpebral part of the orbital contents, in front of the **orbital septum**. In the left eye, also the orbital septum has been transected, revealing the orbitobulbar part behind the septum. The **supratrochlear nerve**, a branch of the frontal nerve, itself a branch of the ophthalmic nerve [V_1], exits from the orbital cavity above the trochlea of the **superior oblique**. The **supraorbital nerve**, which is the other branch of the frontal nerve, exits from the orbital cavity together with the **supraorbital artery**, a branch of the ophthalmic artery, and the **supraorbital vein**, which gives rise to the angular vein, passing through the supraorbital notch or foramen of the frontal bone. The **infraorbital nerve**, which represents the last tract of the maxillary nerve [V_2], exits from the infraorbital canal through the infraorbital foramen, together with the **infraorbital artery**, a branch of the maxillary artery.

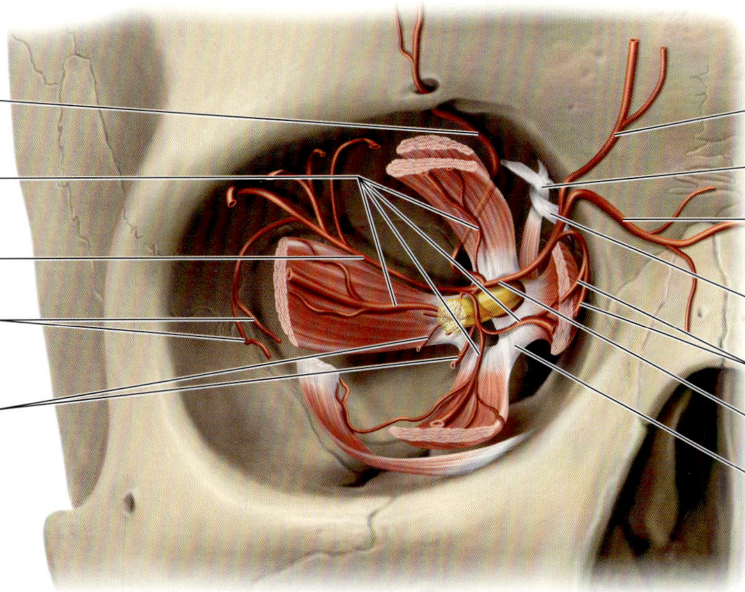

Arteries of the orbit, anterior view after removal of the eyeball. At the level of the medial angle of the eye, the **ophthalmic artery** divides into its terminal branches, i.e. the **medial palpebral arteries**, **dorsal nasal artery** and **supratrochlear** (or frontal) **artery**. The **lateral palpebral arteries** are terminal branches of the lacrimal artery, which is a branch of the ophthalmic artery that arises just after its entrance in the orbital cavity and runs along the superior border of the lateral rectus to supply the lacrimal gland. The **supraorbital artery** originates from the tract of the ophthalmic artery where it crosses the optic nerve, and passes between the superior rectus and levator palpebrae superioris, in the vault of the orbital cavity, exiting through the supraorbital notch or foramen. The **muscular arteries** are branches of the ophthalmic artery that supply the extraocular muscles, accompanying the branches of the oculomotor nerve [III]. The **long posterior ciliary arteries** originate from the tract of the ophthalmic artery that runs under the optic nerve.

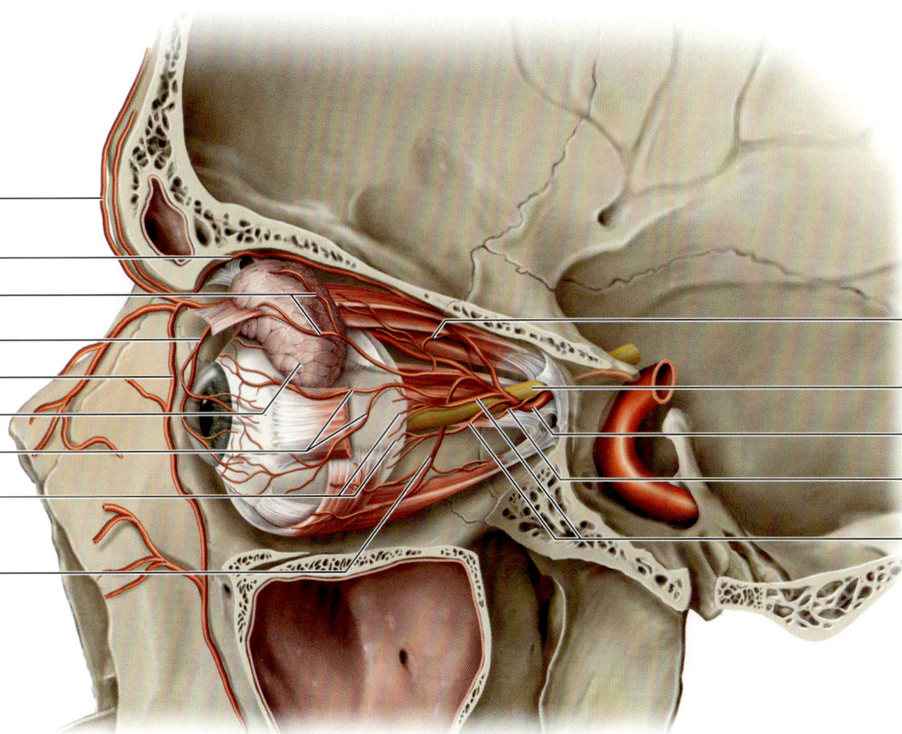

Lateral view of the left **orbital cavity** after removal of the lateral wall. The **central retinal artery**, first and smallest collateral branch of the ophthalmic artery, runs in a lateral position with respect to the optic nerve, and then penetrates its inferomedial surface. The **lacrimal artery** runs along the superior border of the lateral rectus. The **long posterior ciliary arteries** originate from the tract of the ophthalmic artery laterally to the optic nerve and branch into the **short posterior ciliary arteries**. The **muscular arteries** travel to the orbital muscles accompanying the branches of the oculomotor nerve [III] and give rise to the **anterior ciliary arteries**. The **supraorbital artery** passes between the superior rectus and levator palpebrae superioris and exits from the orbit through the supraorbital foramen. Terminal branches of the ophthalmic artery are the **medial palpebral**, **dorsal nasal** and **supratrochlear** (or frontal) **arteries**.

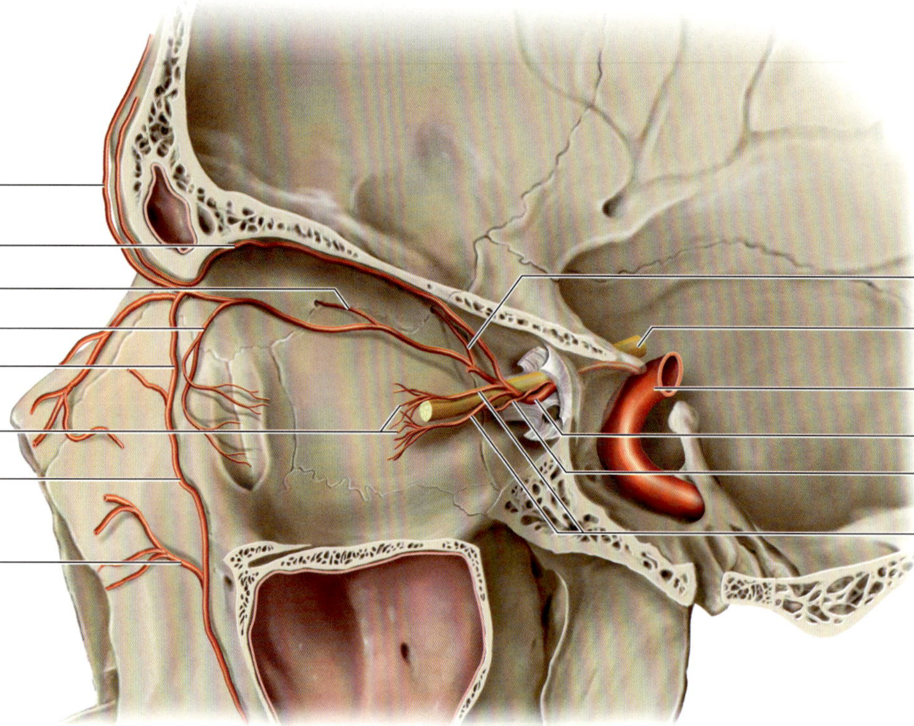

Medial wall of the **orbit**. Paramedian sagittal section, left lateral view, after removal of the eyeball and accessory visual structures. The **internal carotid artery** enters the cranial cavity through the internal opening of the carotid canal of the temporal bone and, turning upwards, makes an S-shaped curve to enter the cavernous sinus, here removed. At a point corresponding to the anterior clinoid process of the lesser wing of the sphenoid, it gives off the **ophthalmic artery** which passes through the optic canal and enters the orbital cavity running laterally beneath the optic nerve [II]. The **central retinal**, **long** and **short posterior ciliary**, **supraorbital**, and the **posterior** and **anterior ethmoidal arteries** enter, respectively, the posterior and anterior ethmoidal foramina; the medial palpebral, supratrochlear (or frontal) and dorsal nasal arteries are terminal branches of the ophthalmic artery.

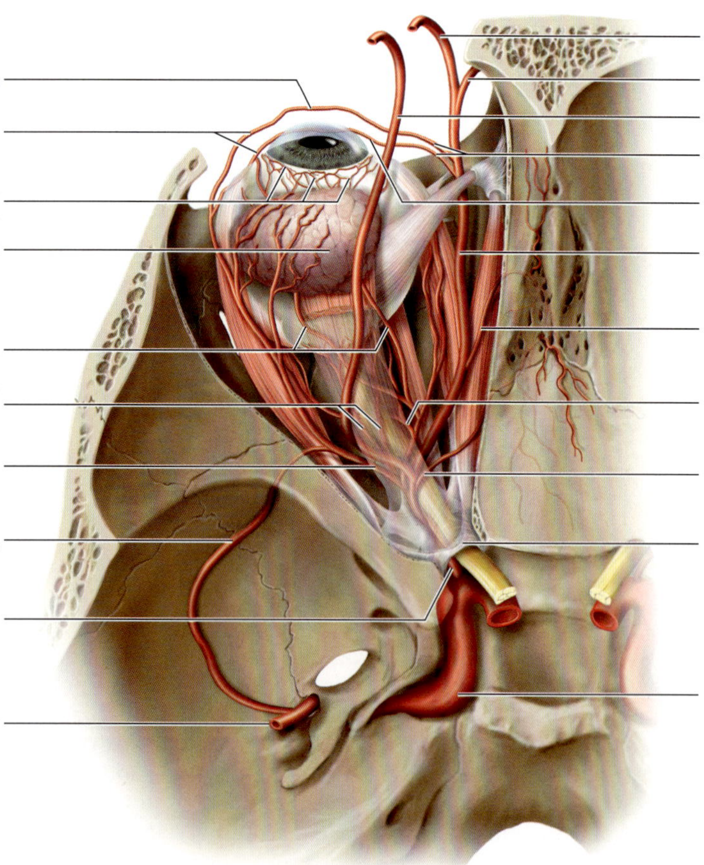

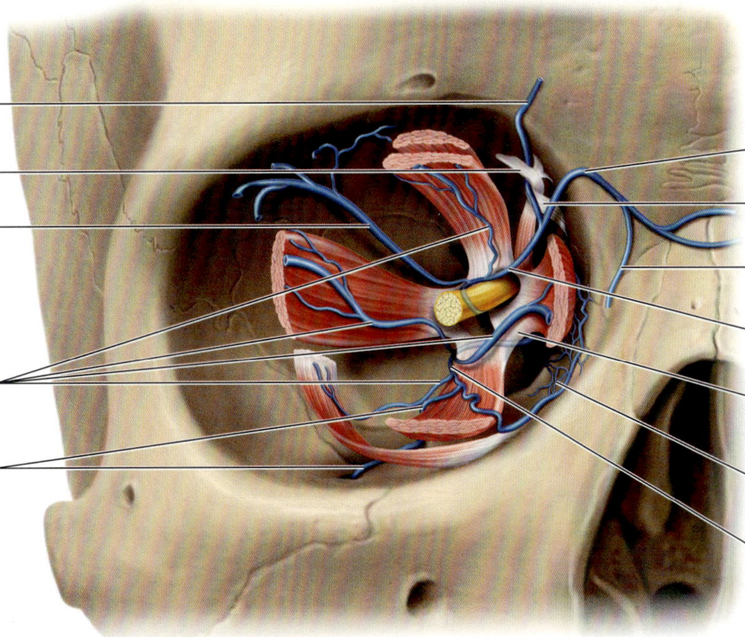

Veins of the orbit, anterior view. The **superior ophthalmic vein**, originating from the confluence of the **nasofrontal vein** and a venous root connected to the supraorbital vein, runs in the superior part of the orbital cavity. Its course corresponds more or less to that of the ophthalmic artery. The **inferior ophthalmic vein**, originating from a venous network connected to the venules of the lacrimal sac, runs in the inferior part of the orbit, above the inferior rectus. Among the affluent branches of the ophthalmic veins are the **muscular veins**, satellites of the muscular arteries or muscular branches of the ophthalmic artery. The **lacrimal vein**, a satellite of the lacrimal artery, empties into the superior ophthalmic vein.

➤ Transverse section of the cranium passing just below the roof of the **orbital cavity**, superior view. The **ophthalmic artery**, an offshoot of the internal carotid artery after leaving the cavernous sinus, supplies the orbital cavity and its contents, the eyelids, the dura mater of the anterior cranial fossa, and the vault and lateral walls of the nasal cavities. The **lacrimal artery** runs along the superior border of the lateral rectus and gives rise to the recurrent meningeal branch, which passes through the lateral part of the superior orbital fissure and anastomoses with the middle meningeal artery. The **lateral palpebral arteries**, terminal branches of the lacrimal artery, anastomose with the **medial palpebral arteries**, terminal branches of the ophthalmic artery, forming the superior and inferior **palpebral arches**. The **long posterior ciliary arteries** branch into **short posterior ciliary arteries**, while the **anterior ciliary arteries** originate from the muscular arteries, supplying the muscles of the orbit. The **major circulus arteriosus of the iris** is formed by anastomoses of division branches of the long posterior ciliary arteries with branches of the anterior ciliary arteries and between the branches of the long posterior ciliary arteries themselves.

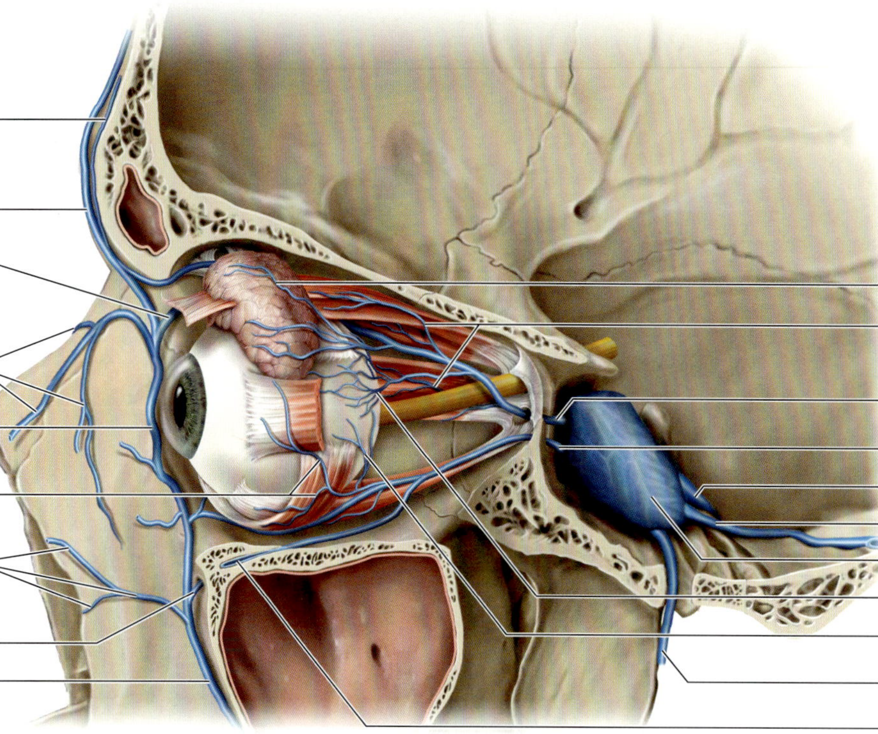

Lateral view of the left **orbital cavity** after removal of the lateral wall. The **superior ophthalmic vein** arises from the confluence of the nasofrontal vein with a venous root connected to the supraorbital vein and, after passing through the superior orbital fissure, empties into the cavernous sinus. Among its affluent branches are the lacrimal vein, muscular veins and superior vorticose veins. The **inferior ophthalmic vein** originates in correspondence to the medial inferior angle of the orbit, runs along the floor of the orbit above the inferior rectus and, after crossing the superior orbital fissure, terminates in the cavernous sinus. Tributaries of it are the muscular veins and inferior vorticose veins. The **angular vein** originates superficially at the medial angle of the eye from the confluence of the frontal, supraorbital and nasofrontal veins, runs obliquely downwards and finally heads in a posterolateral direction constituting the **facial vein**.

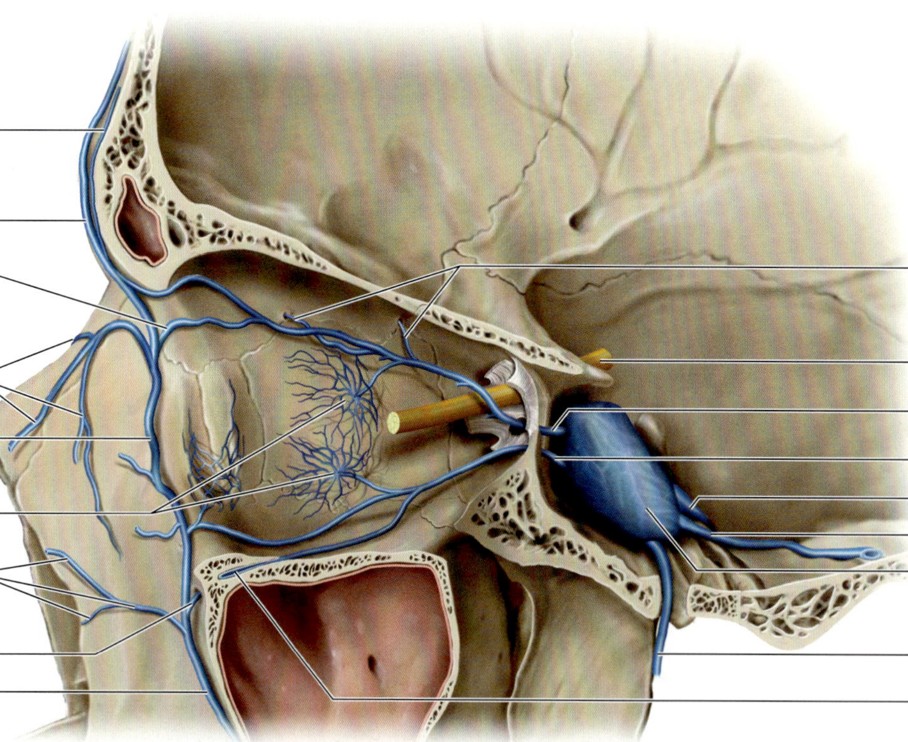

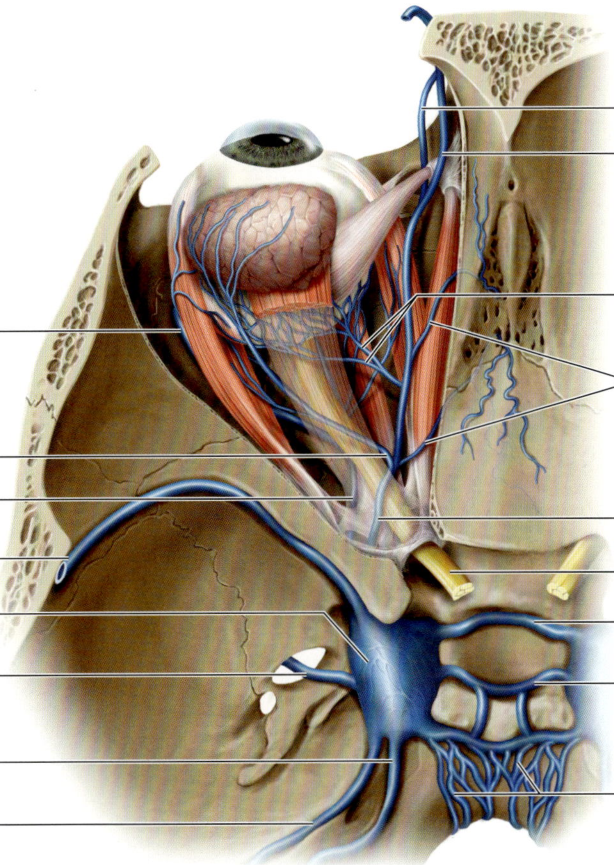

Transverse section of the cranium passing just under the roof of the **orbital cavity**, superior view. The **veins of the orbit** are shown. The **superior ophthalmic vein**, the largest vein of the organ of sight, originates from the confluence of the nasofrontal and supraorbital veins and empties into the anterior extremity of the cavernous sinus. Its affluents are the **ethmoidal veins**, **lacrimal vein** and **superior vorticose veins**. The **cavernous sinus**, extending from the medial extremity of the superior orbital fissure to the apex of the petrous part of the temporal bone, receives also the **inferior ophthalmic vein**. The cavernous sinuses of the two sides are in communication with each other by means of the **intercavernous sinuses** and drain into the **superior** and **inferior petrosal sinuses**, into the basilar plexus and the pterygoid plexus via the **emissary vein of the foramen ovale** or a venous network of the foramen ovale. The **infraorbital vein**, satellite of the infraorbital artery, runs through the infraorbital canal and groove, exits from the orbital cavity through the inferior orbital fissure and drains into the pterygoid plexus.

➤

Medial wall of the **orbit**. Paramedian sagittal section, left lateral view, after removal of the eyeball and accessory visual structures. The **cavernous sinus** is situated laterally to the sella turcica of the sphenoid, between the medial extremity of the superior orbital fissure and the apex of the petrous part of the temporal bone. Running through its cavity are numerous trabeculae and blood and nerve vessels. The internal carotid artery, here not shown, passes through the cavernous sinus in a posteroanterior direction. The **superior ophthalmic vein**, whose course in the superior part of the orbital cavity corresponds more or less to that of the ophthalmic artery, originates from the confluence of the nasofrontal vein and a venous root connected to the supraorbital vein. After passing through the superior orbital fissure, it empties into the anterior extremity of the cavernous sinus, which receives also the **inferior ophthalmic vein**, which arises in correspondence to the inferior and medial angle of the orbit from a venous network connected to the venules of the lacrimal sac and lower eyelid.

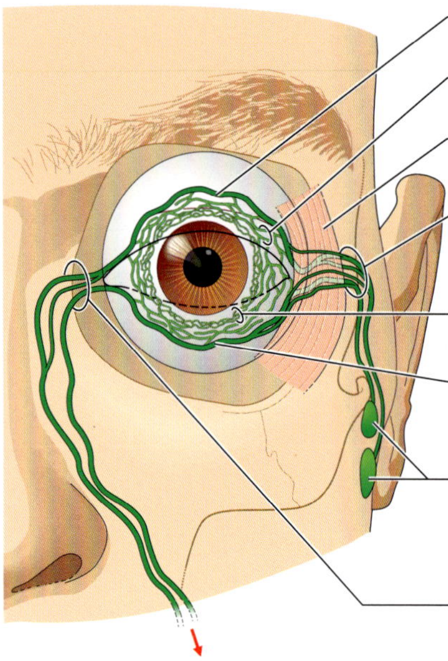

The **lymphatic capillaries of the bulbar conjunctiva** constitute a pericorneal lymphatic ring around the corneoscleral junction, approximately 1 mm wide, in continuity with a radial lymphatic network disposed around the cornea. This network flows into two collectors, a superior and an inferior one, which proceed into the medial and lateral lymphatic collectors, at the angles of the eye. The medial group converges towards the root of the nose, follows the facial vein and reaches the submandibular nodes. The lateral group drains into the preauricular and infra-auricular deep parotid nodes.

The **superficial lymphatic network of the eyelids**, localized in the skin, and the deep or conjunctival lymphatic network, situated in correspondence to the palpebral conjunctiva and bulbar conjunctiva, drain through medial and lateral lymphatic collectors, which constitute the paths of lymphatic drainage for the eyelids, into, respectively, the submandibular nodes and the preauricular and infra-auricular deep parotid nodes.

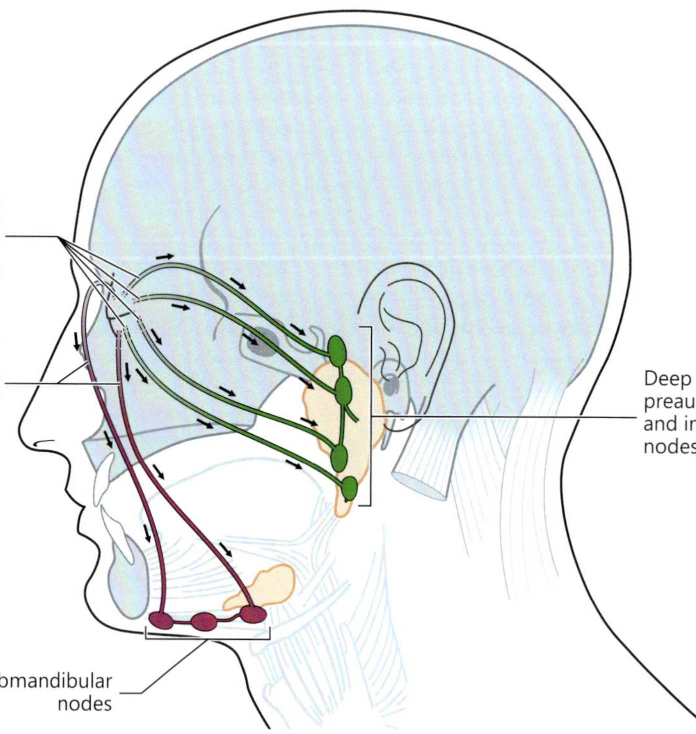

➤

Lateral view of the left **orbital cavity** after removal of the lateral wall. At the boundary with the superior orbital fissure, the **ophthalmic nerve** [V_1] divides into the **nasociliary**, **frontal** and **lacrimal nerves**. The lacrimal nerve, through a communicating branch with the zygomaticotemporal nerve, a branch of the zygomatic nerve, itself a branch of the maxillary nerve [V_2], receives postganglionic fibers to the lacrimal gland arising from the pterygopalatine ganglion. The long, or sensory, root of the **ciliary ganglion** is a collateral branch of the nasociliary nerve whose fibers, passing through the ciliary ganglion without being interrupted, follow the short ciliary nerves up to the eyeball. The ciliary ganglion has two other roots: a short, or parasympathetic, one and a sympathetic one. The short root is a collateral branch of the oculomotor nerve [III] containing preganglionic fibers from the accessory nuclei of the oculomotor nerve (nucleus of Edinger-Westphal). The postganglionic fibers supply the sphincter pupillae and ciliary muscle. The sympathetic root comes directly from the internal carotid plexus and contains postganglionic vasomotor fibers arising from the superior cervical ganglion. The long root of the ciliary ganglion also contains postganglionic fibers from the superior cervical ganglion that, through the internal carotid plexus, anastomose with the ophthalmic nerve [V_1] on their way to the dilator pupillae via the short ciliary nerves.

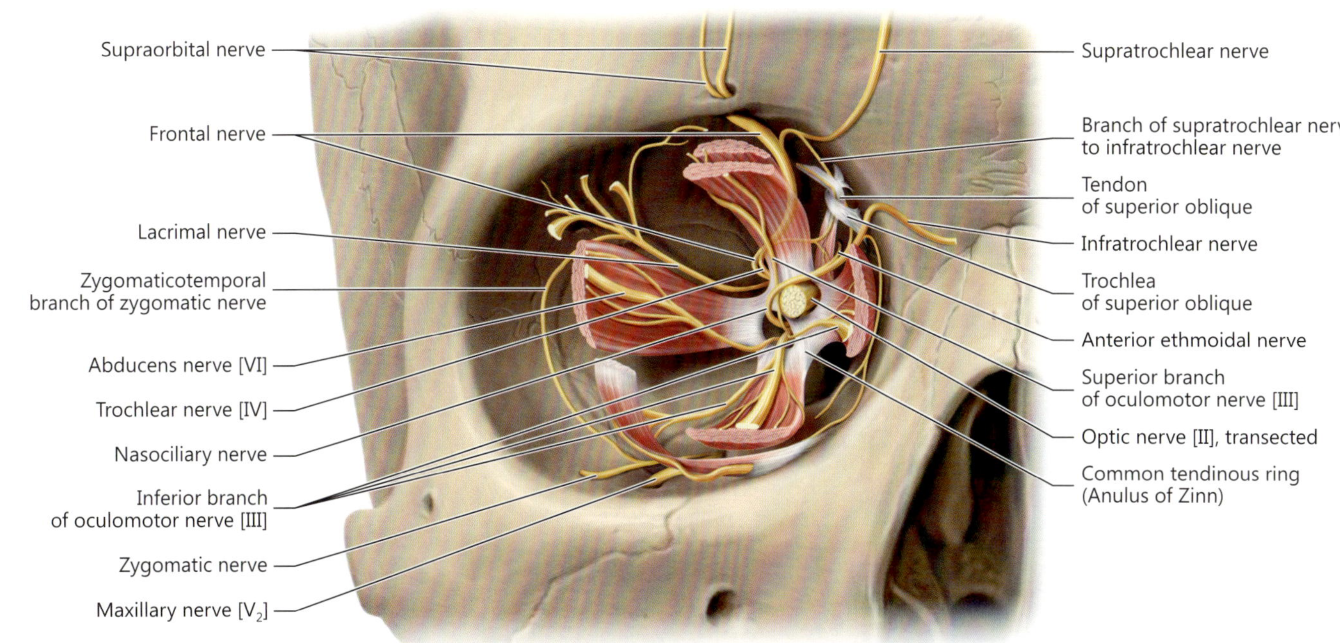

Nerves of the orbit, anterior view. The **oculomotor nerve** [III], at its arrival in correspondence to the posterior clinoid process, runs in the superior lateral wall of the cavernous sinus, and at the level of the superior orbital fissure divides into two branches, superior and inferior, that enter the orbital cavity through the common tendinous ring. The superior branch innervates the superior rectus and levator palpebrae superioris, while the inferior branch innervates the medial rectus, inferior rectus and inferior oblique. Also the **abducens nerve** [VI], which innervates the lateral rectus, and the **nasociliary nerve**, a branch of the ophthalmic nerve [V_1], pass through the ring. The abducens nerve [VI], after its course in the cavernous sinus laterally to the internal carotid artery, enters the orbital cavity through the superior orbital fissure and passes inside the tendinous ring in a position between the superior and inferior branches of the oculomotor nerve and inferolaterally to the nasociliary nerve. The nasociliary nerve, which has branched off from the ophthalmic nerve [V_1] before entering the orbital cavity, passes through the common tendinous ring and continues in a medial direction crossing over the ophthalmic artery and the optic nerve [II]. The **trochlear nerve** [IV] passes instead above the ring, together with the **lacrimal** and **frontal nerves**, branches of the ophthalmic nerve, to supply the superior oblique. The **supratrochlear** and **supraorbital nerves** are the two terminal branches of the frontal nerve, while the **infratrochlear** and **anterior ethmoidal nerves** are terminal branches of the nasociliary nerve.

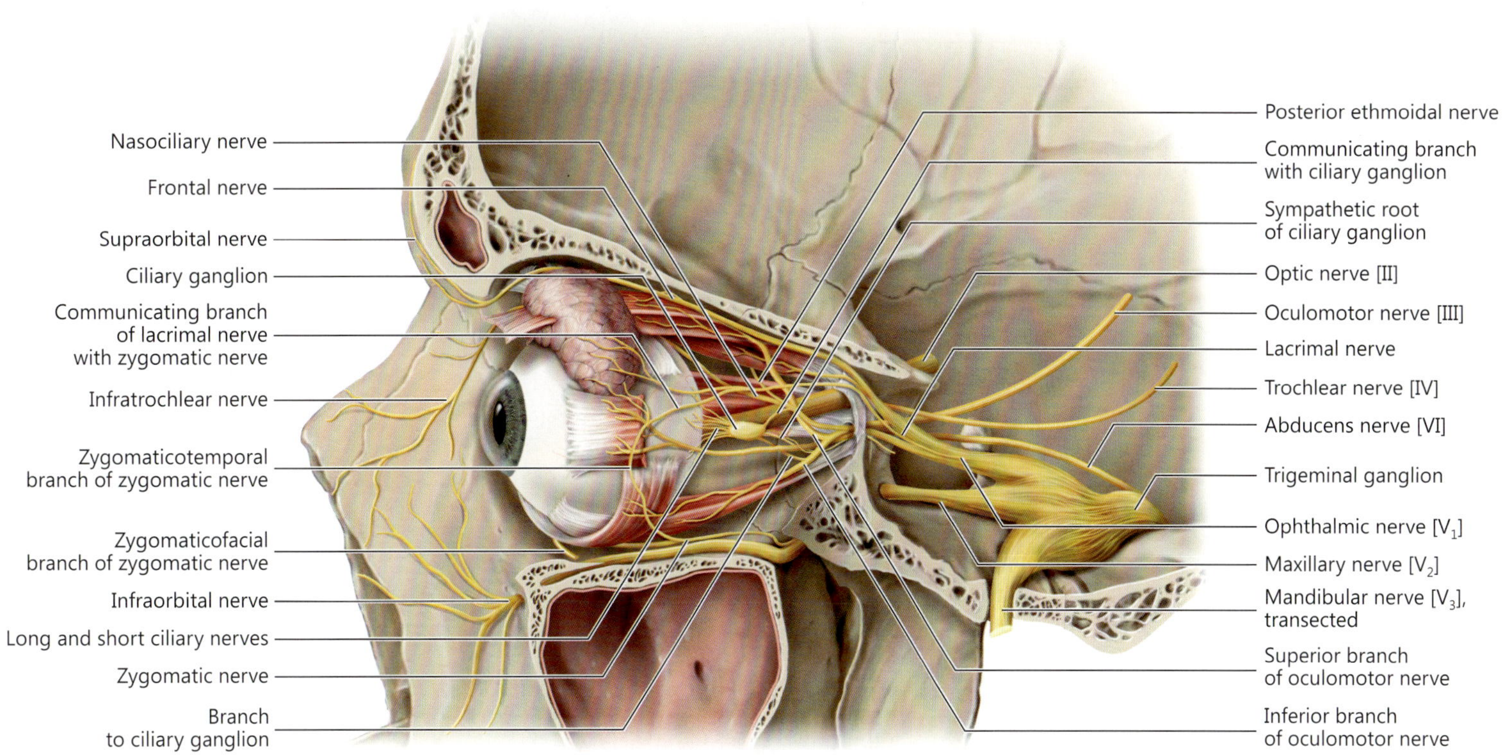

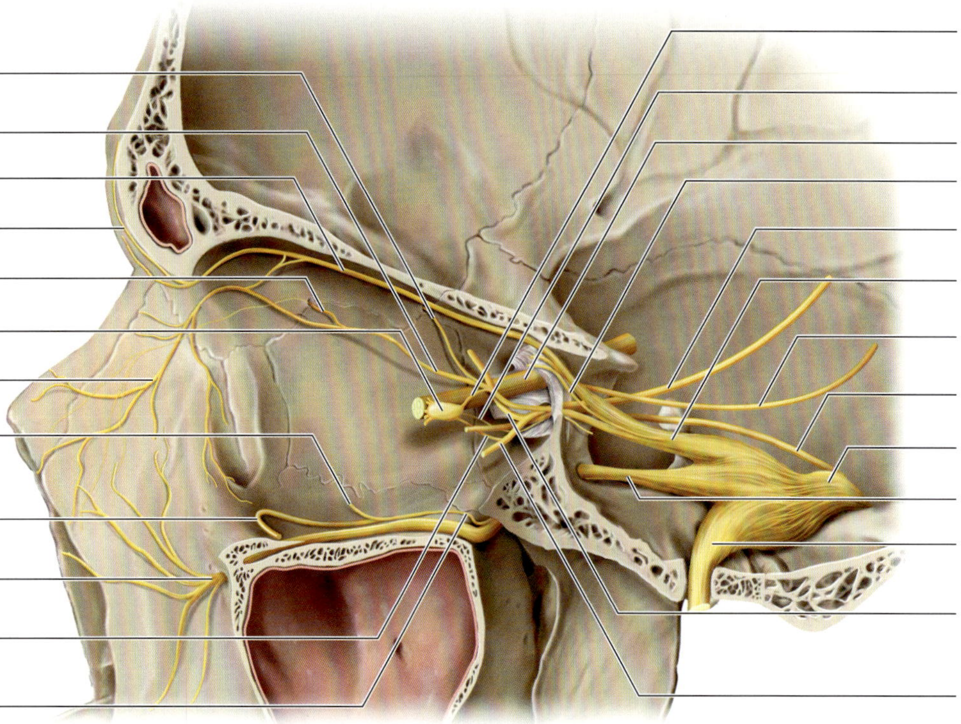

Medial wall of the **orbit**. The **nasociliary nerve**, a medial division of the ophthalmic nerve [V_1], enters the orbital cavity passing through the common tendinous ring (anulus of Zinn) and continues in a medial direction with two terminal branches, the anterior ethmoidal and infratrochlear nerves. The **oculomotor nerve** [III] divides into two branches, superior and inferior, that pass through the common tendinous ring, together with the abducens nerve [VI]. The **trochlear nerve** [IV] passes into the orbital cavity above the common tendinous ring, together with the frontal and lacrimal nerves, intermediate and lateral divisions of the ophthalmic nerve [V_1]. The **maxillary nerve** [V_2] enters the orbital cavity through the inferior orbital fissure and continues its path forward on the floor of the orbit and in the infraorbital canal, as the infraorbital nerve. The **zygomatic nerve**, a branch of the maxillary nerve, divides off from the maxillary nerve at the border with the inferior orbital fissure and heads laterally forwards dividing into two terminal branches, the zygomaticotemporal and zygomaticofacial nerves.

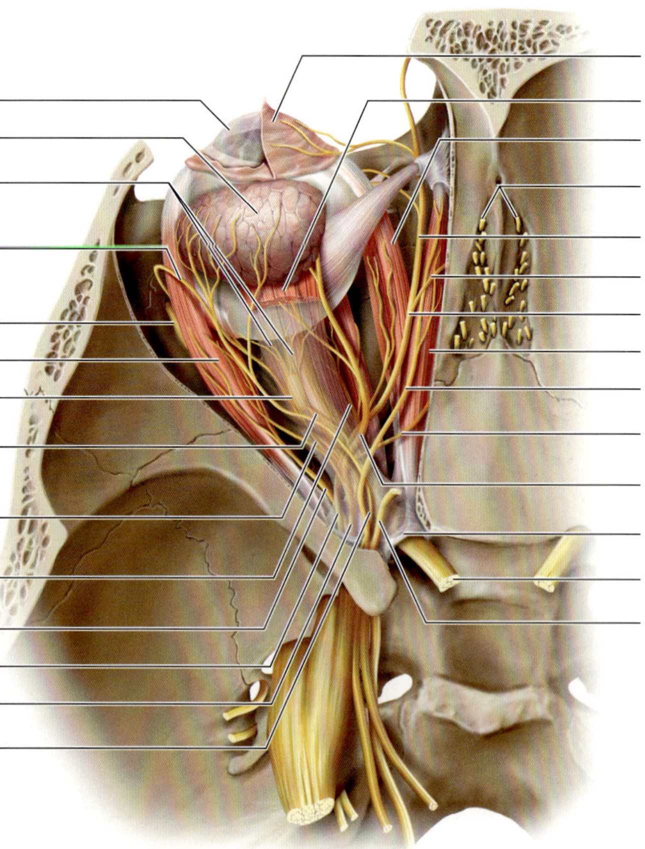

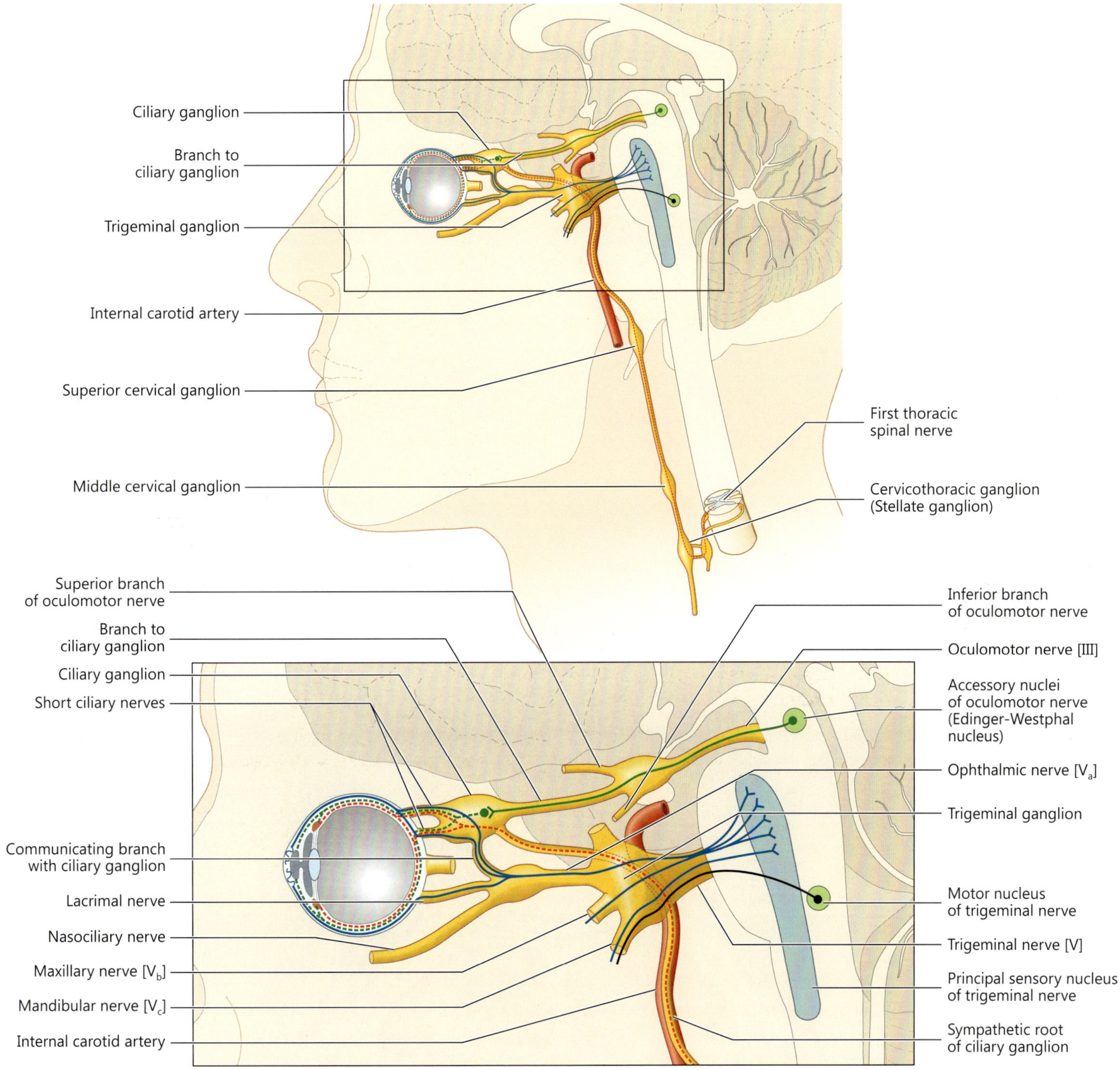

Diagram showing the connections of the **ciliary ganglion** (in the box). The only fibers that form synapses in the ganglion are the parasympathetic ones (*green*); sympathetic fibers (*red* dotted line) and sensory fibers (*blue*) pass through the ganglion without sinapsing there. The three types of fiber constitute, respectively, the parasympathetic root, sympathetic root, and sensory root of the ciliary ganglion.

◄
Transverse section of the cranium passing just below the roof of the **orbital cavity**, superior view. One can see the nerves that enter the orbital cavity, through the optic canal and superior compartment of the common tendinous ring: the **optic nerve** [II]; through the superior orbital fissure, inside the common tendinous ring in its inferior part, the superior and inferior branches of the **oculomotor nerve** [III], and the **abducens nerve** [VI] and **nasociliary nerve**, a branch of the ophthalmic nerve [V_1]; outside the common tendinous ring, the **trochlear nerve** [IV] and **frontal** and **lacrimal nerves**, branches of the ophthalmic nerve [V_1]. The common tendinous ring (anulus of Zinn), funnel-shaped with the superior part corresponding to the optic foramen, which is the opening of the optic canal, is the point of origin of the rectus muscles of the eyeball and, partially, of the levator palpebrae superioris and superior oblique.

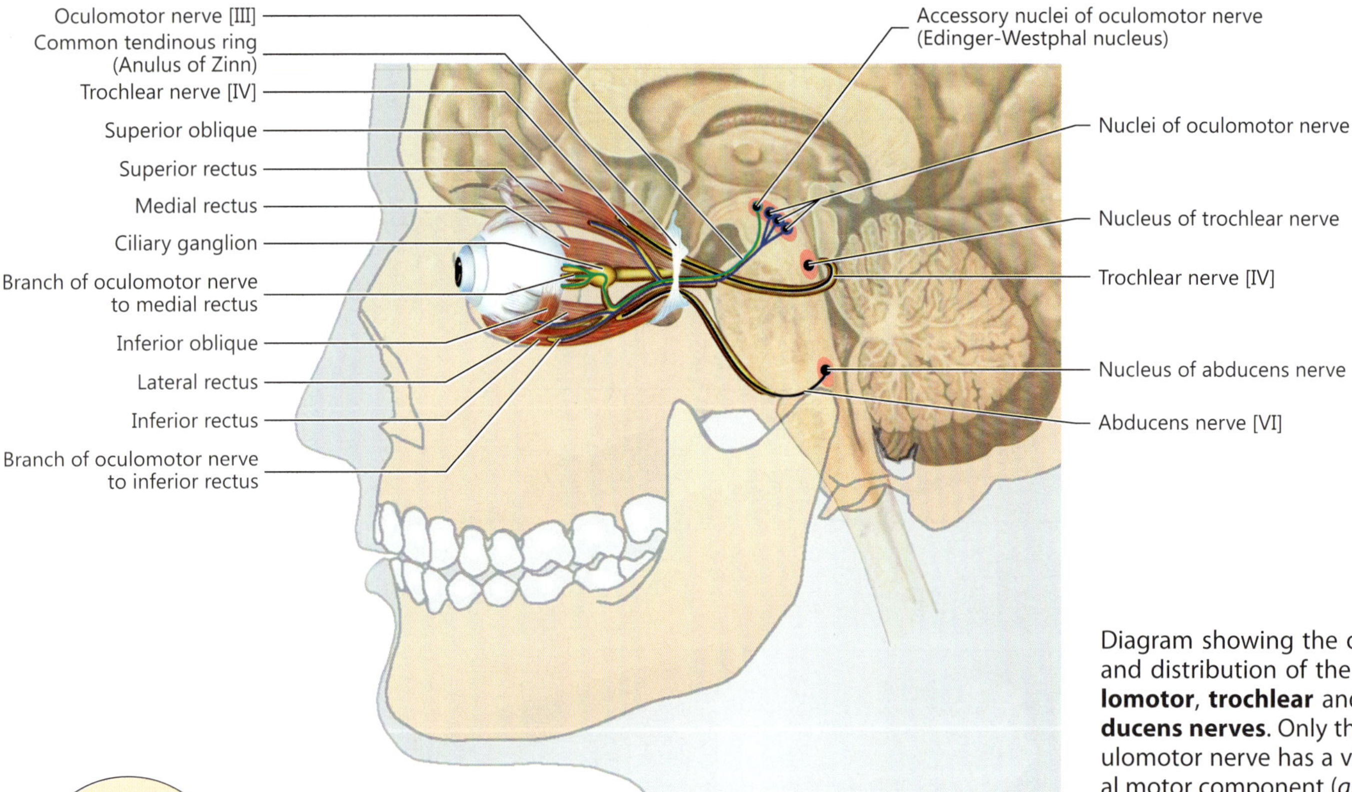

Diagram showing the origin and distribution of the **oculomotor**, **trochlear** and **abducens nerves**. Only the oculomotor nerve has a visceral motor component (*green*).

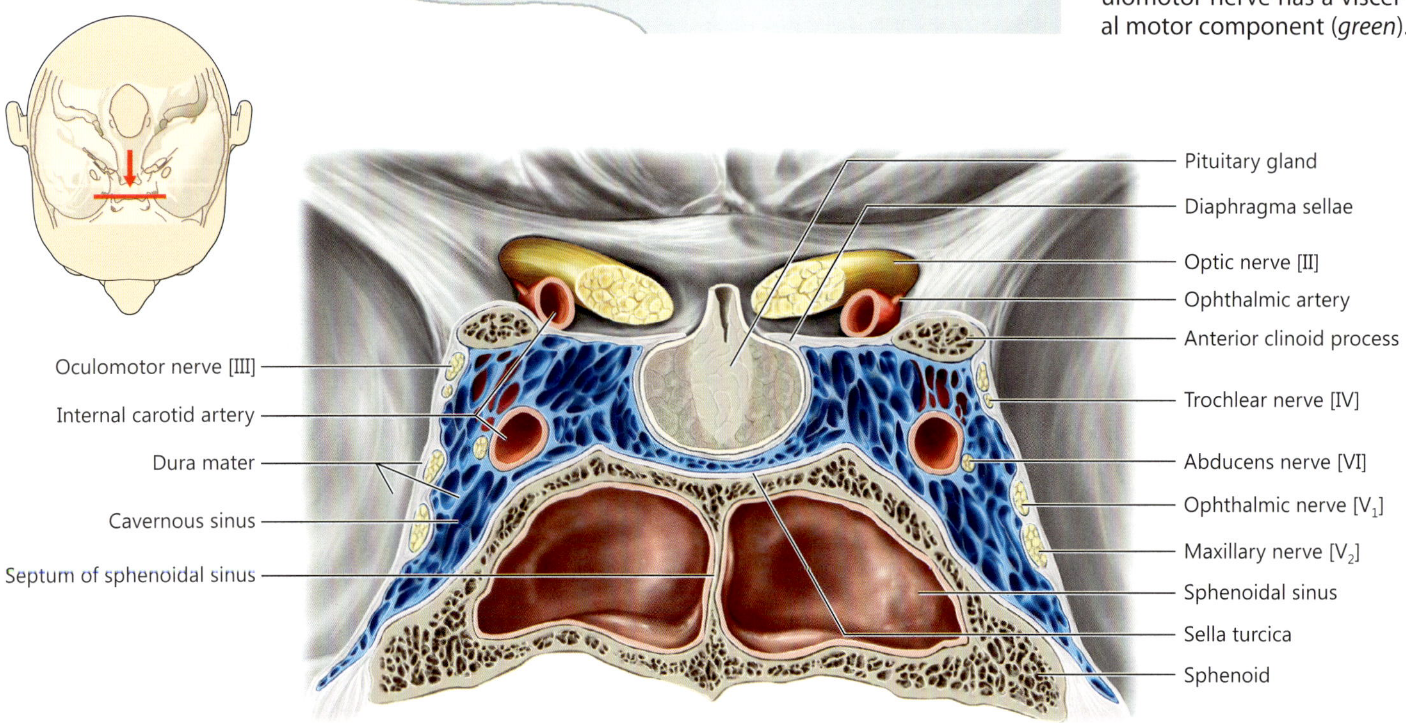

Frontal section of the head passing through the **anterior clinoid processes** of the sphenoid. The **cavernous sinus**, paired, is situated lateral to the sella turcica of the sphenoid, which contains the pituitary gland. Running through its cavity are numerous trabeculae or fibrous bands. The **internal carotid artery** passes through the cavernous sinus in a posteroanterior direction, and the **abducens nerve** [VI] runs inferolaterally to it. Within the lateral wall of the cavernous sinus run the **oculomotor** [III], **trochlear** [IV], **ophthalmic** [V_1] and **maxillary** [V_2] **nerves**.

➤

Medial wall of the **orbit**. Paramedian sagittal section, left lateral view after removal of the eyeball and accessory visual structures. The **vorticose veins**, in general four, one for each quadrant of the eyeball, subdivided into superior and inferior (here one can see the medial ones), drain blood from the choroid as well as from the ciliary body and iris, and are tributaries of the **superior** and **inferior ophthalmic veins**, which receive also the **anterior ciliary veins**, draining blood from the anterior part of the ciliary body and aqueous humor from the scleral venous sinus, and the (posterior) **ciliary veins**, that collect blood coming from the posterior part of the sclera.

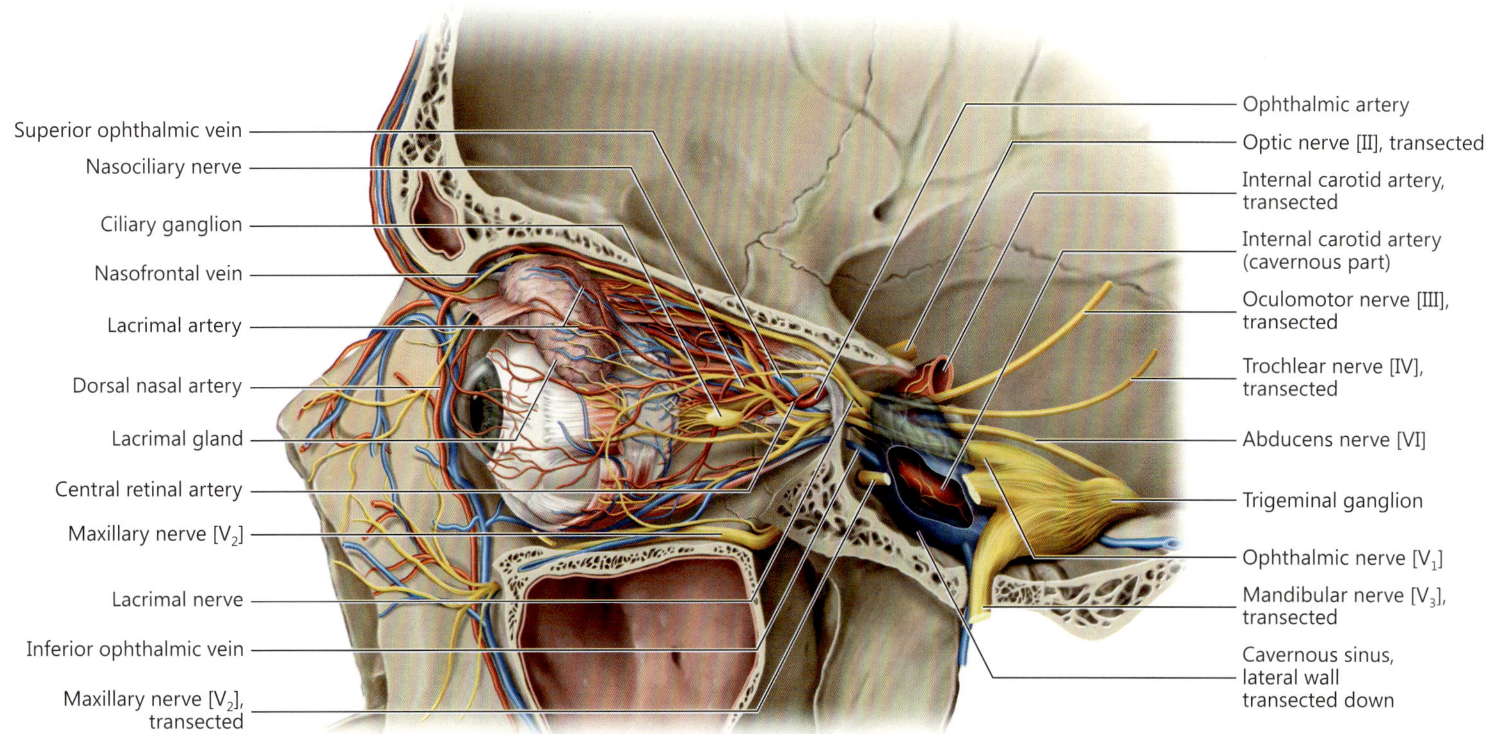

Lateral view of the left **orbital cavity** and middle cranial fossa after removal of the lateral wall. The lateral wall of the cavernous sinus has been transected in part to display its contents. The **oculomotor nerve** [III], in correspondence to the posterior clinoid process of the sphenoid, pierces the internal layer of the dura mater penetrating into the superior lateral wall of the cavernous sinus, within which run also the **trochlear nerve** [IV], beneath the oculomotor nerve [III], the **ophthalmic nerve** [V_1], which runs obliquely, from bottom to top, crossing under the trochlear [IV] and oculomotor [III] nerves, and, in the lowest region, also the **maxillary nerve** [V_2]. The **internal carotid artery** enters the cavernous sinus with an S-shaped curve and at its exit crosses laterally the **optic nerve** and passes through the arachnoid mater so coming to an end. Inside the cavernous sinus, the internal carotid artery is surrounded by sympathetic nerve fibers constituting the cavernous plexus, formed by the **internal carotid nerve**, a perivascular branch of the cervical segment of the sympathetic trunk that accompanies the internal carotid artery and its intracranial branches.

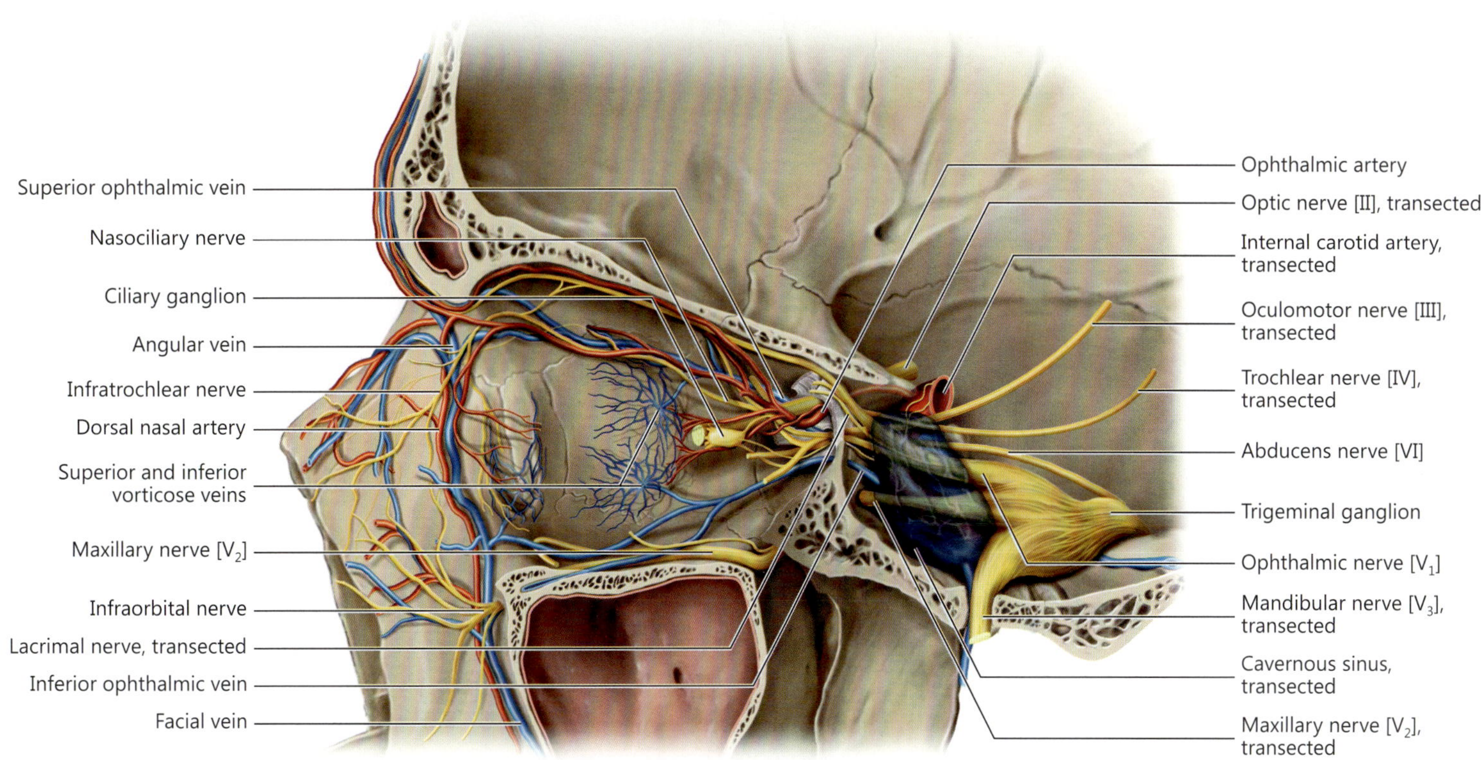

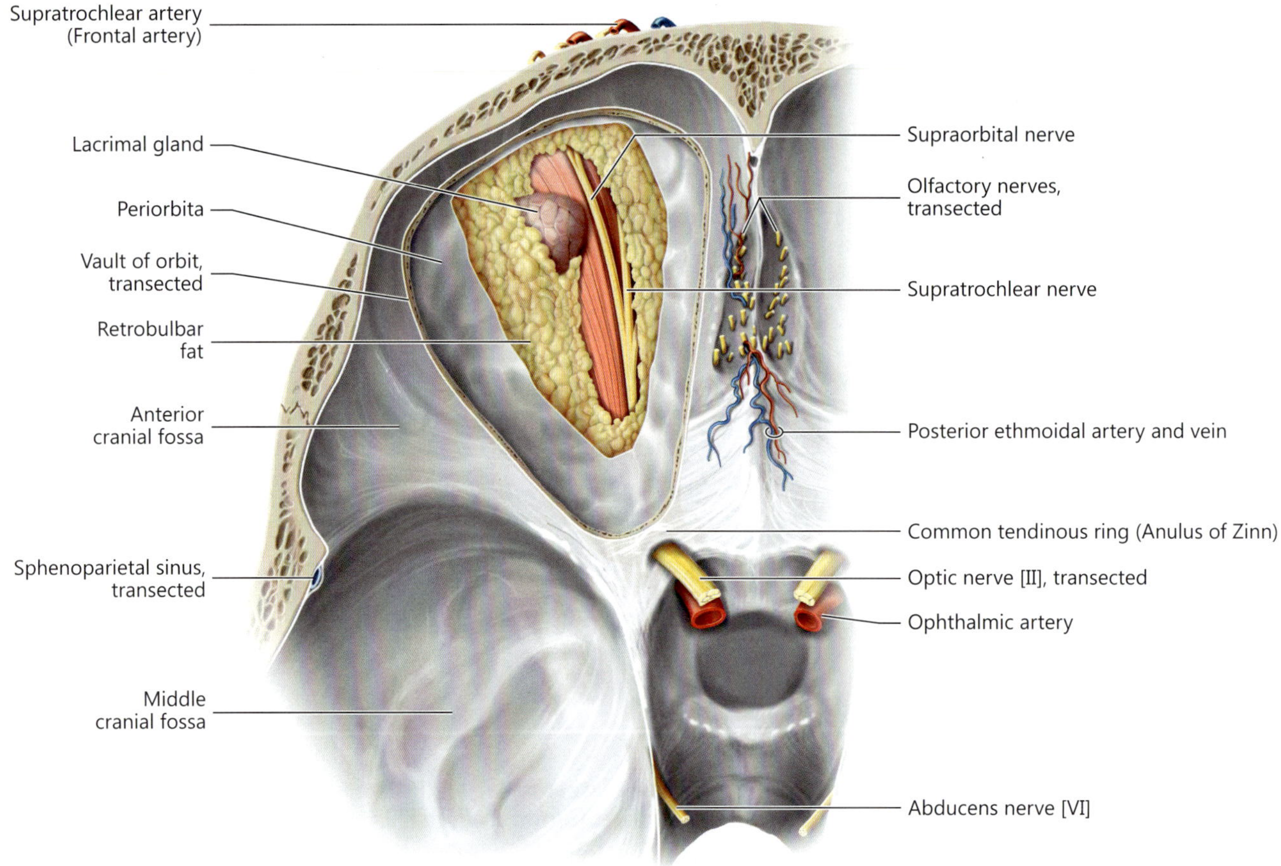

Transverse section of the cranium passing just below the roof of the **orbital cavity**, superior view. One can see the retrobulbar fat that fills the spaces of the orbital cavity located between the periosteum, which covers its internal surface, called the periorbita, and the organs contained in it.

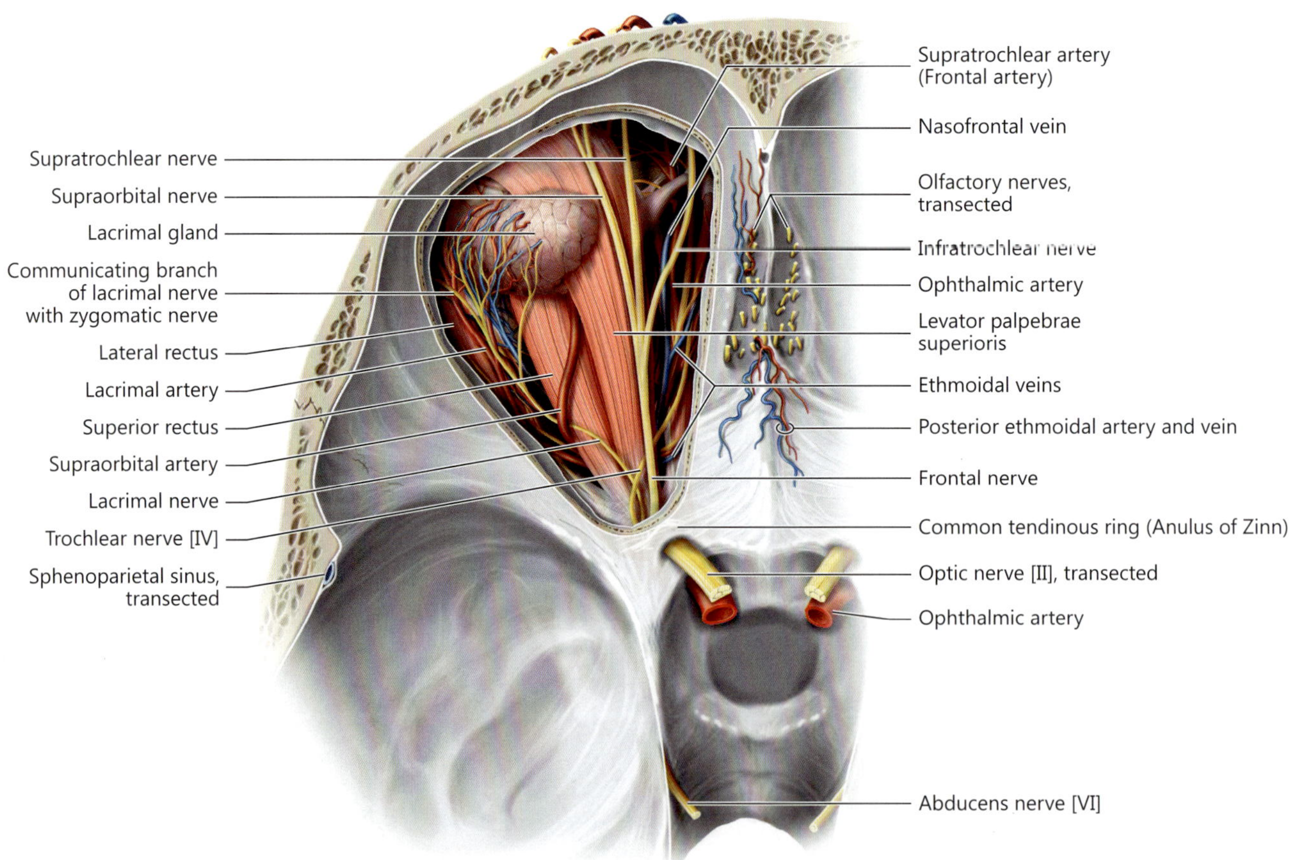

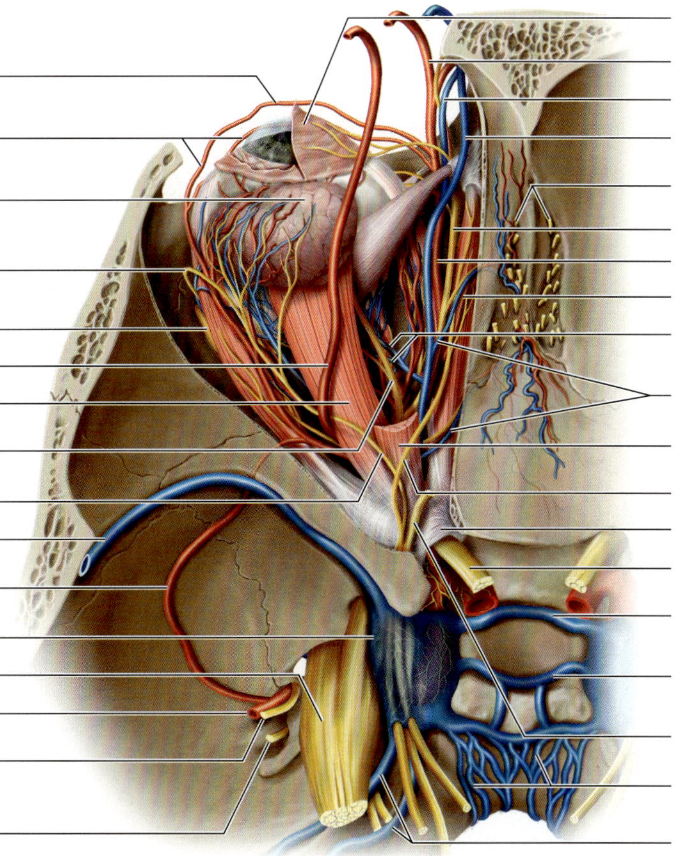

Transverse section of the cranium passing just below the roof of the **orbital cavity**, superior view. The levator palpebrae superioris has been transected to show the contents of the medial part of the orbit. One can see the three nerves that enter the orbital cavity passing above and lateral to the common tendinous ring: the **trochlear nerve** [IV], that crosses from above the tendon of the levator palpebrae superioris, the **frontal nerve**, an intermediate terminal branch of the ophthalmic nerve [V_1], and the **lacrimal nerve**, a lateral terminal branch of the ophthalmic nerve.

◄

Transverse section of the cranium passing just below the roof of the **orbital cavity**, superior view. The **frontal nerve**, an intermediate terminal branch of the ophthalmic nerve [V_1], runs on the vault of the orbital cavity in direct contact with the periosteum, above the levator palpebrae superioris, and divides into two branches whose paths diverge slightly: the **supratrochlear** and **supraorbital nerves**. The **lacrimal nerve**, a lateral terminal branch of the ophthalmic nerve, runs in the external part of the orbital vault, near the periosteum, following the superior border of the lateral rectus together with the **lacrimal artery**, and advancing forwards it reaches the lacrimal gland, in the vicinity of which it receives a **communicating branch with the zygomatic nerve**, a branch of the maxillary nerve [V_2], containing postganglionic fibers from the pterygopalatine ganglion coming to innervate the lacrimal gland.

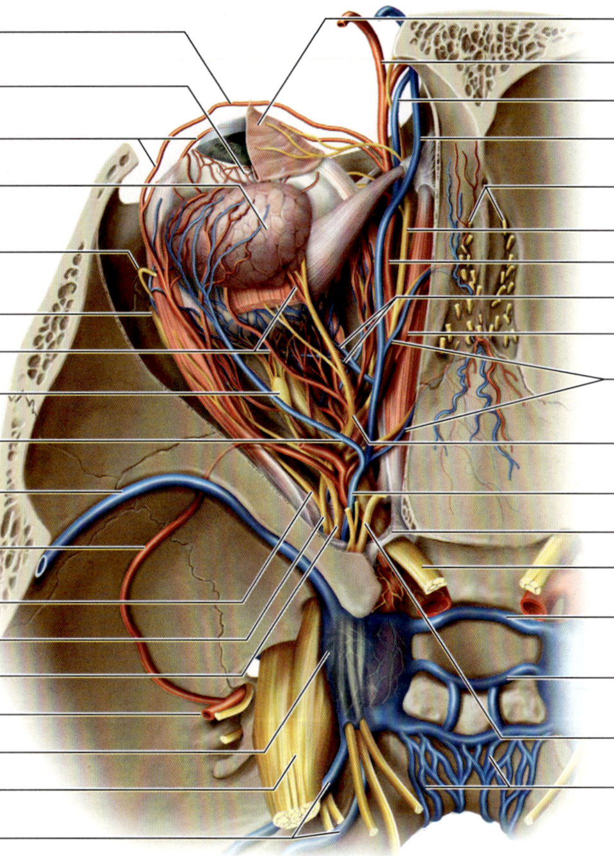

Transverse section of the cranium passing just below the roof of the **orbital cavity**, superior view. One can see the contents of the orbit, after removal of the superior rectus and levator palpebrae superioris, and the **vascular and nerve formations** that penetrate into the **orbital cavity** through the superior orbital fissure: the **trigeminal ganglion** in the middle cranial fossa, near the apex of the petrous part of the temporal bone; the **cavernous sinus**, and the formations contained within it, laterally to the sella turcica of the sphenoid; the **basilar plexus** on the clivus of the occipital bone; and the **olfactory nerves** that pass through the small holes of the cribriform plate of the ethmoid and penetrate into the anterior cranial fossa.

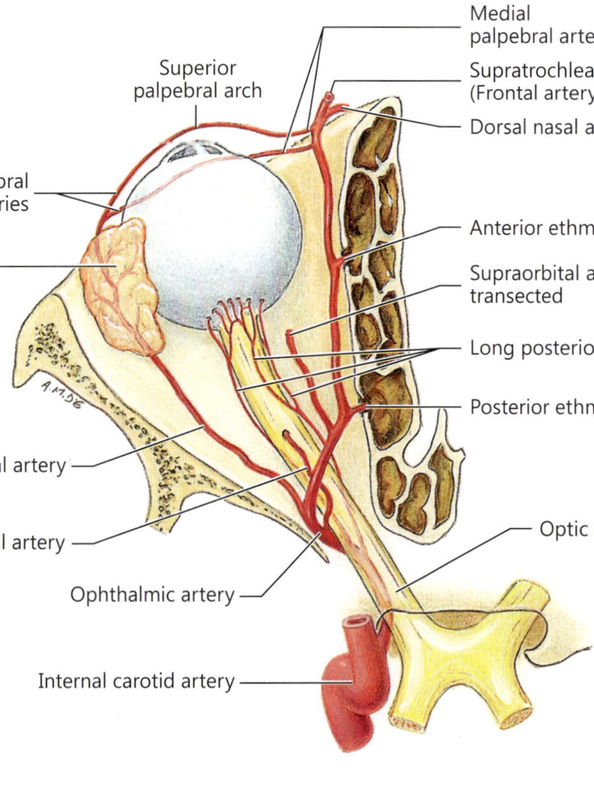

Left **ophthalmic artery** and its branches viewed from above, after demolition of the orbit and removal of part of its contents.

Three-dimensional image of a living human body, obtained by CT scan using a 3D volume rendering technique, showing the **extraocular muscles of the right eyeball** viewed laterally.

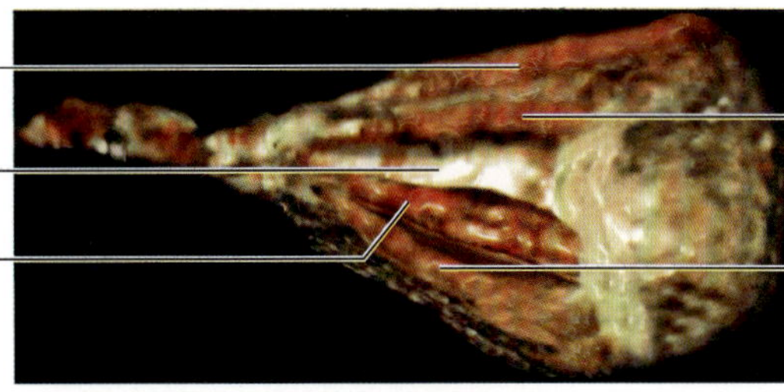

Three-dimensional image of a living human body, obtained by CT scan using a 3D volume rendering technique, showing the **extraocular muscles of the eyeballs** viewed superiorly.

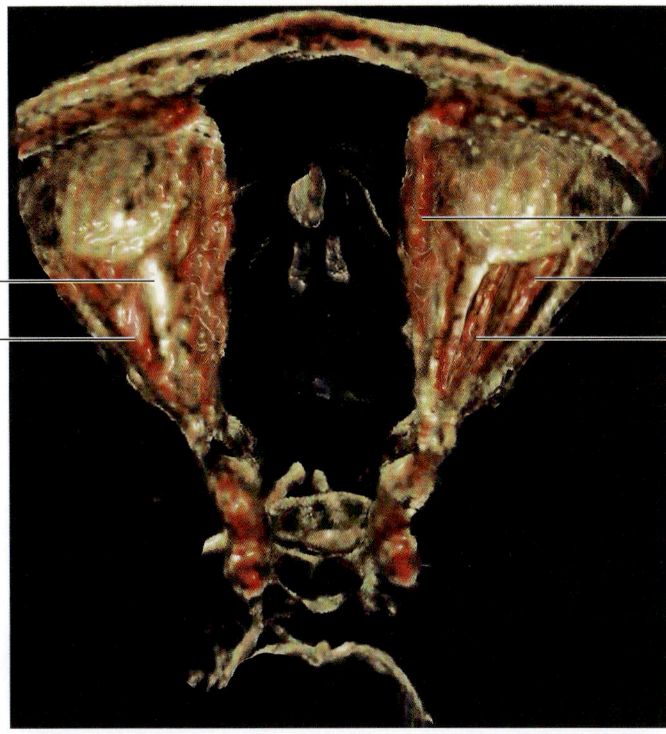

Extraocular muscles*

MUSCLE	ORIGIN	INSERTION	INNERVATION	ACTION
Inferior oblique	Floor of the orbital cavity (orbital surface of the maxilla) under the lacrimal fossa	Corneoscleral junction between the insertions of the lateral rectus and superior rectus	Oculomotor nerve [III]	Superior and lateral rotation of the eyeball
Inferior rectus	Inferior segment of the common tendinous ring (Anulus of Zinn)	Inferior part of the sclera just behind the corneoscleral junction	Oculomotor nerve [III]	Inferior and slightly medial rotation of the eyeball
Lateral rectus	Lateral border of the common tendinous ring (Anulus of Zinn)	Lateral part of the sclera just behind the corneoscleral junction	Abducens nerve [VI]	Lateral rotation of the eyeball
Levator palpebrae superioris	Roof of the orbital cavity (orbital part of the frontal bone)	Superior tarsus, skin of the superior eyelid, and superior conjunctival fornix	Oculomotor nerve [III]	Raising of the superior eyelid
Medial rectus	Medial segment of the common tendinous ring (Anulus of Zinn)	Medial part of the sclera just behind the corneoscleral junction	Oculomotor nerve [III]	Medial rotation of the eyeball
Superior oblique	Lesser wing of the sphenoid above the optic canal	After passing through the trochlea the muscle fibers change direction and insert on the superior part of the sclera, deep to the insertion of the superior rectus	Trochlear nerve [IV]	Inferior and lateral rotation of the eyeball
Superior rectus	Superior border of the common tendinous ring (Anulus of Zinn)	Superior part of the sclera just behind the corneoscleral junction	Oculomotor nerve [III]	Superior and slightly medial rotation of the eyeball

* In addition to the extraocular muscles there are three intrinsic muscles: the ciliary muscle, sphincter pupillae and dilator pupillae, not considered in this section of the Atlas dedicated to the musculoskeletal system since they are formed of smooth muscle fibers. Among the accessory visual structures are the superior tarsal and inferior tarsal muscles, also composed of smooth muscle fiber, that form the muscle layer of the eyelids.

Eye movements ☞ page 390 of volume 1.

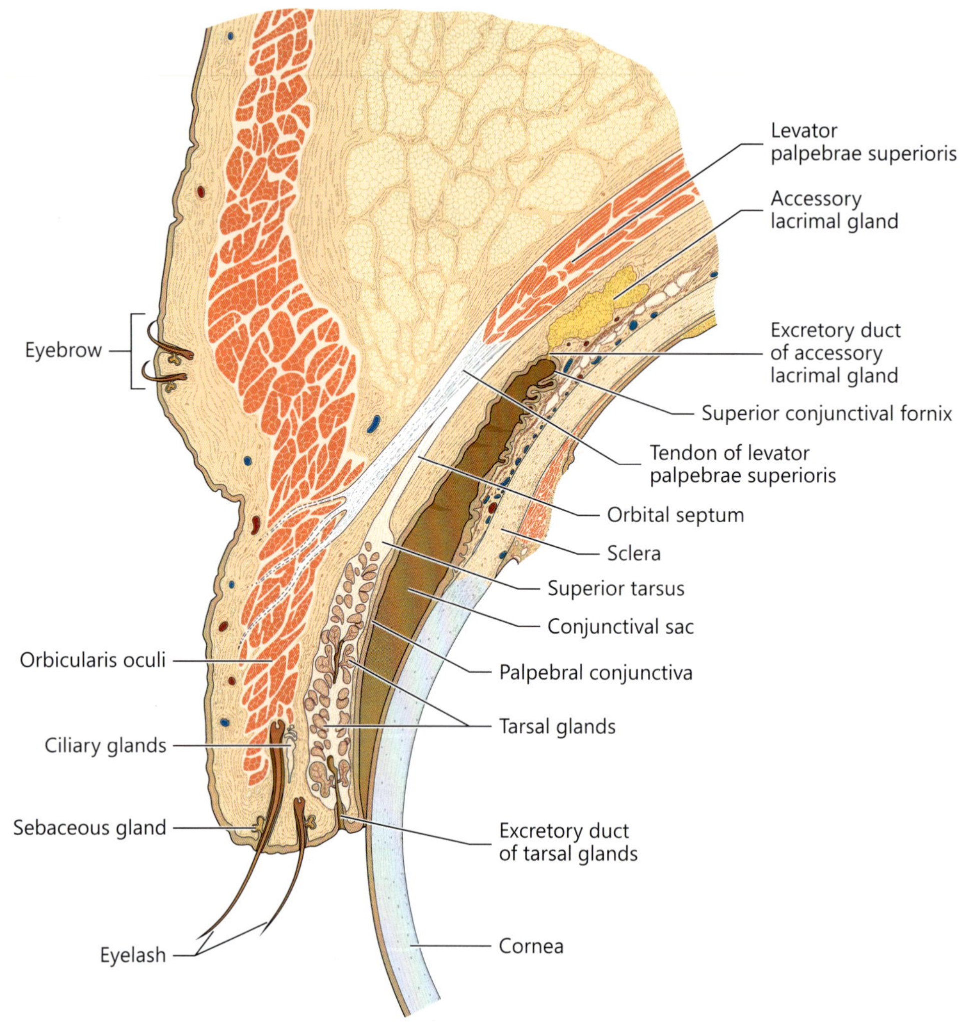

Superior eyelid, sagittal section. The diagram shows the relationship between the various formations of connective tissue, muscles and glands.

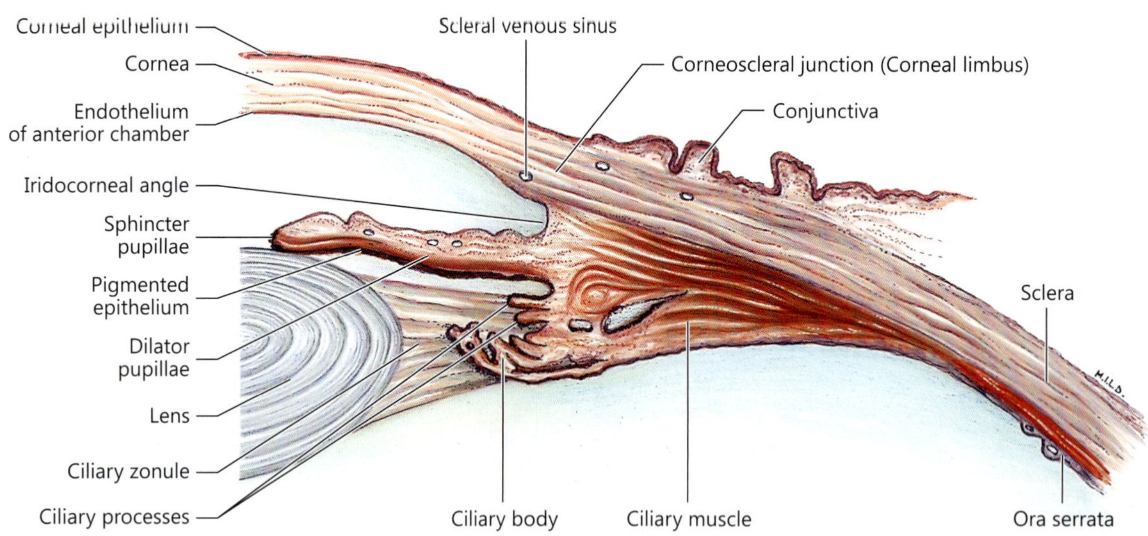

Anterior segment of the eye viewed in a **meridian section of the eyeball**. One can see the relationships of the sclera and cornea with the conjunctiva, ciliary processes and iris.

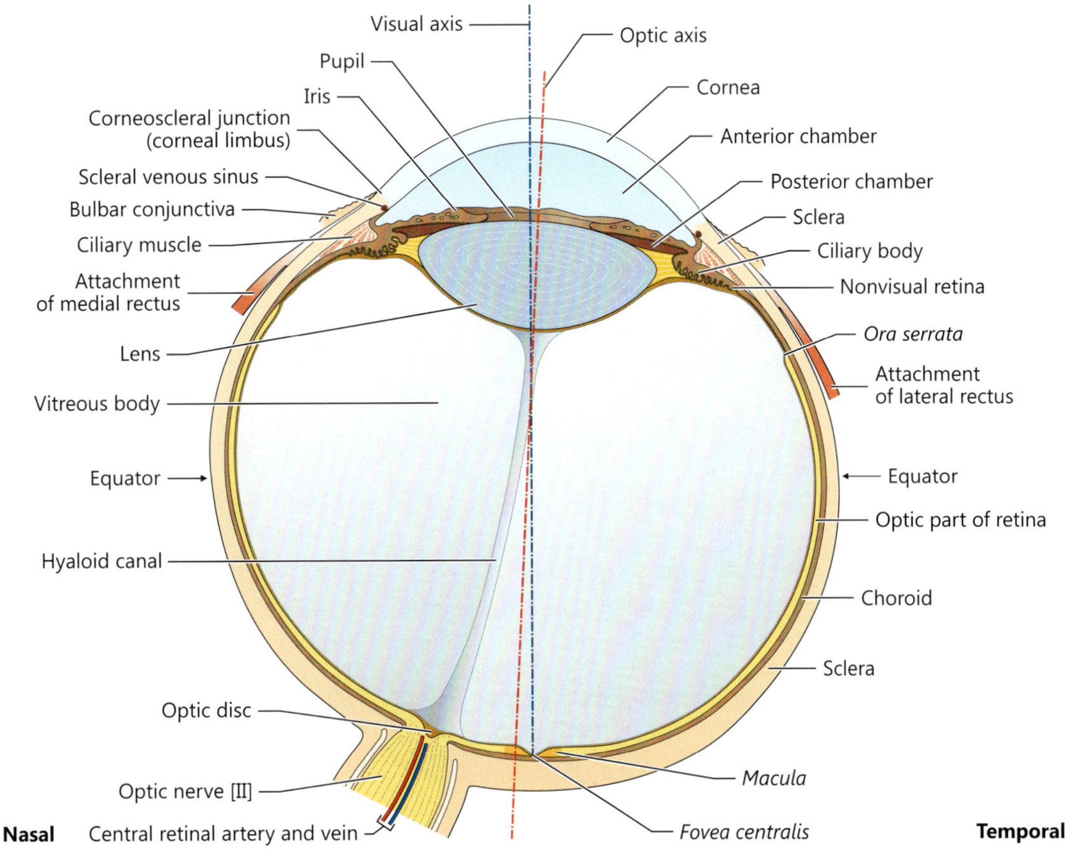

Schematic representation of the general structure of the right **eyeball** transected on the horizontal plane. The aqueous humor is shown in *blue*. The sclera is continuous with the cornea. The tendons of the extraocular muscles (such as the lateral rectus and medial rectus shown in the figure) insert into the sclera. The optic axis or external axis of the eyeball (*red*) and the visual axis (*blue*) are indicated.

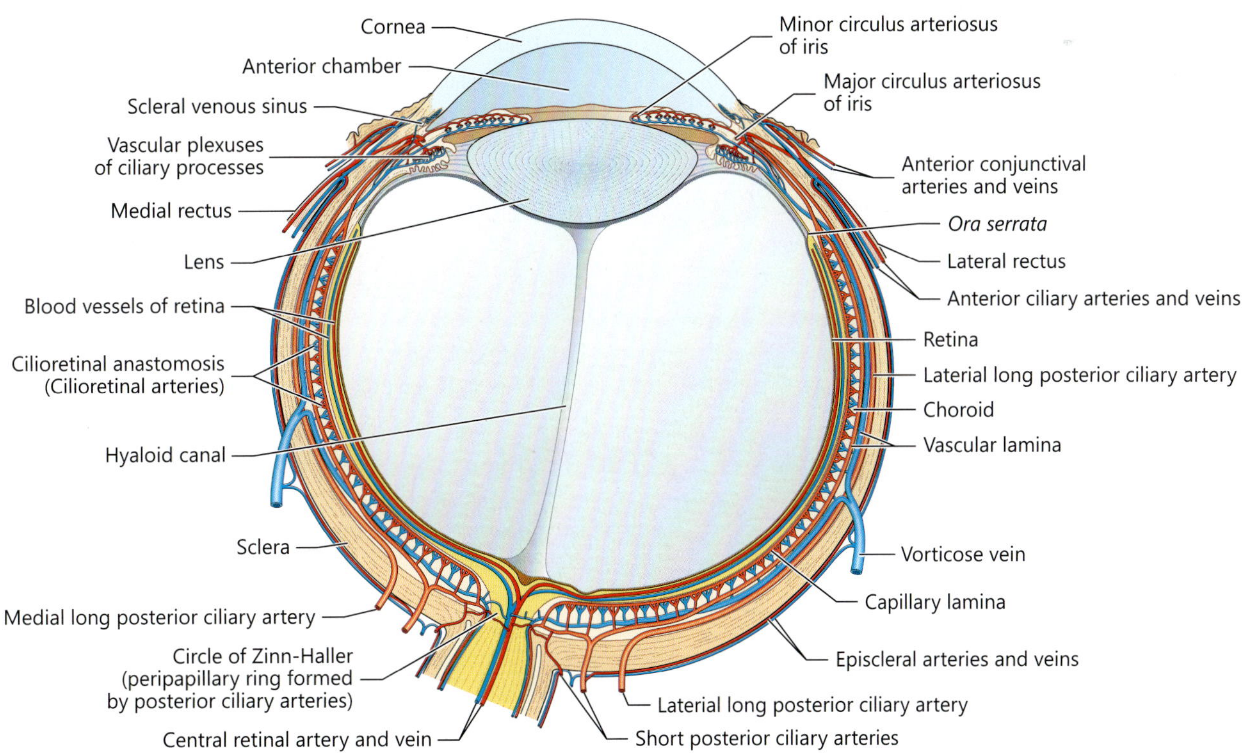

Diagram showing the **blood circulation of the eyeball**. The principal sources of arterial blood for the layers, or tunics, of the eyeball are the central retinal artery and the ciliary arteries. These vessels cross the wall of the eyeball in correspondence, respectively, to the optic nerve and the corneoscleral junction (or corneal limbus) (anterior ciliary arteries). The vorticose veins, which cross the wall of the eyeball itself, emerge in the equatorial region of the eyeball.

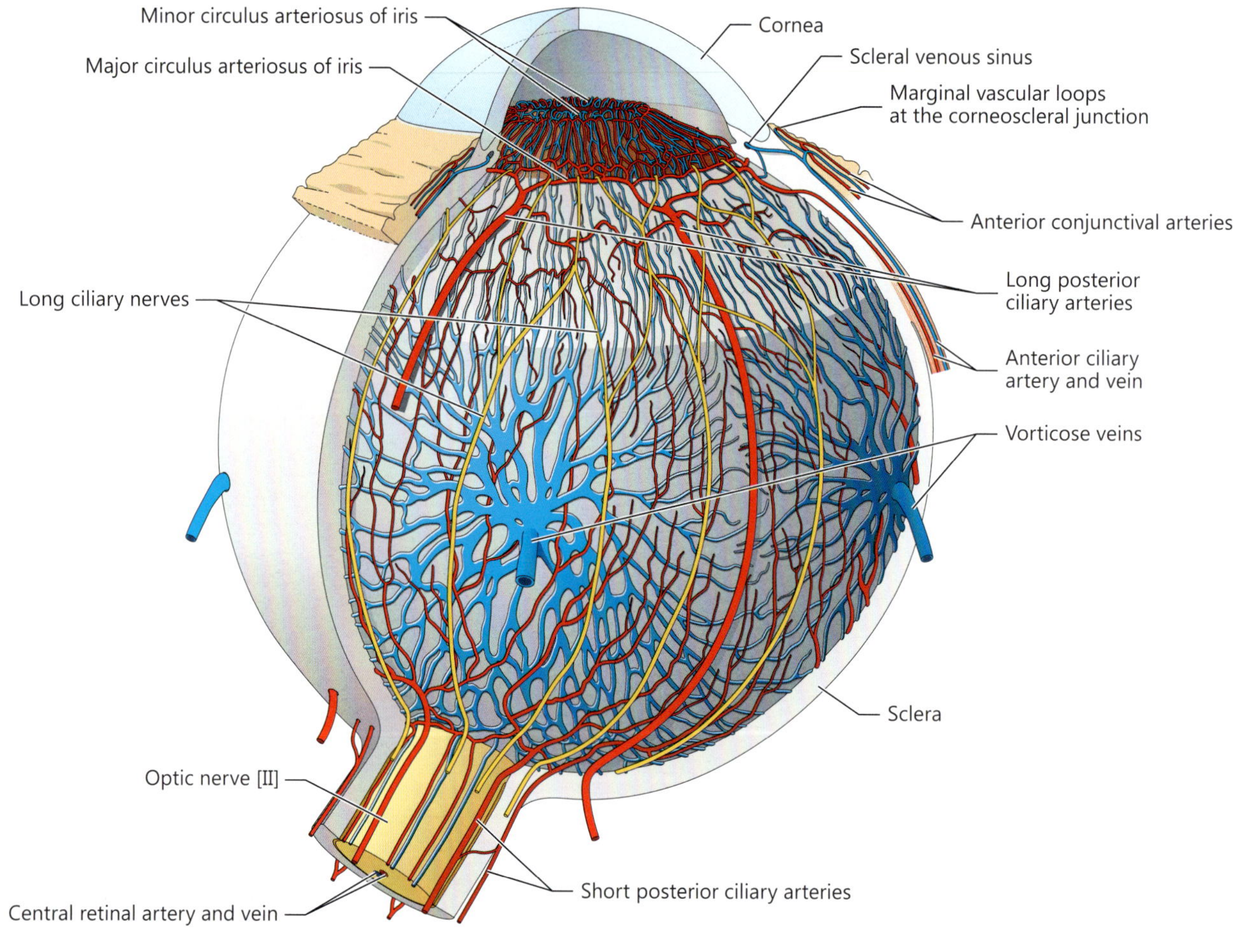

Blood vessels of the eyeball.

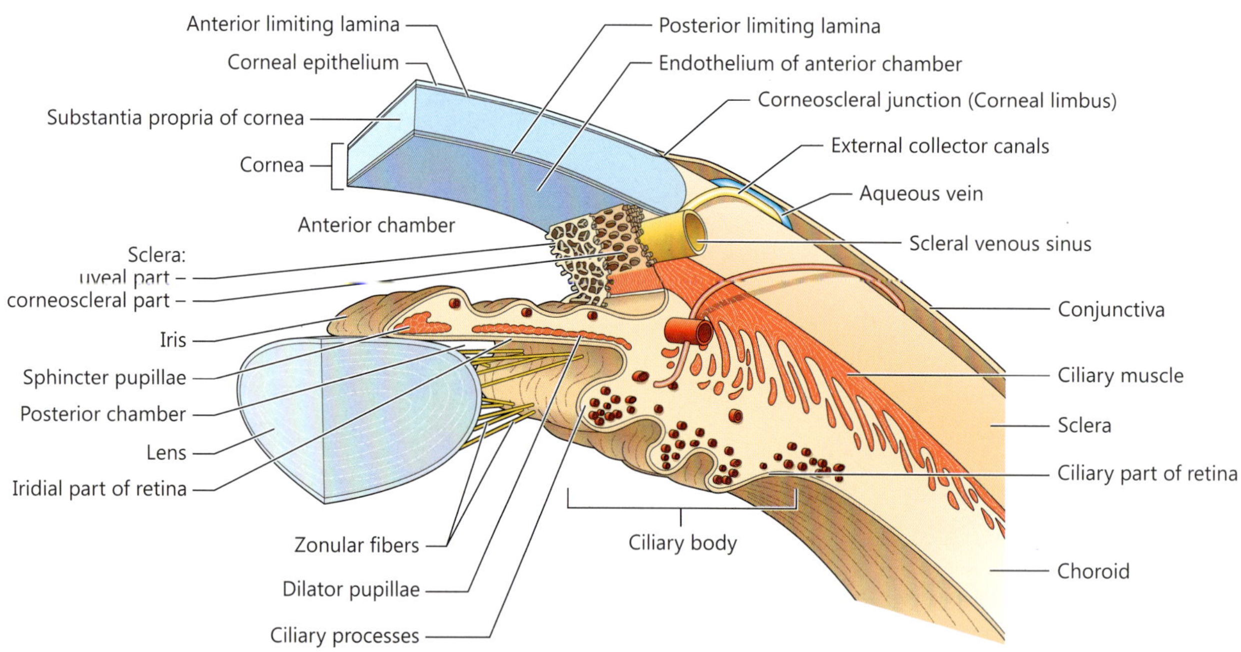

Eyeball, schematic representation of a horizontal section of the anterior part. The fibrous layer of the eyeball is visible, with the sclera, corneoscleral junction and cornea characterized by a 5-layer structure, and the vascular layer, with the iris, ciliary body and choroid, and the anterior and posterior chambers. The lens is shown suspended by fibers that constitute the zonule of Zinn (zonular fibers); these fibers, separating from the ciliary body where they originate, move to the equator of the lens where they insert.

Note: The aqueous vein, a tributary of the anterior ciliary vein, receives aqueous humor from the scleral venous sinus. The external collector canals transport aqueous humor from the scleral venous sinus to the scleral veins.

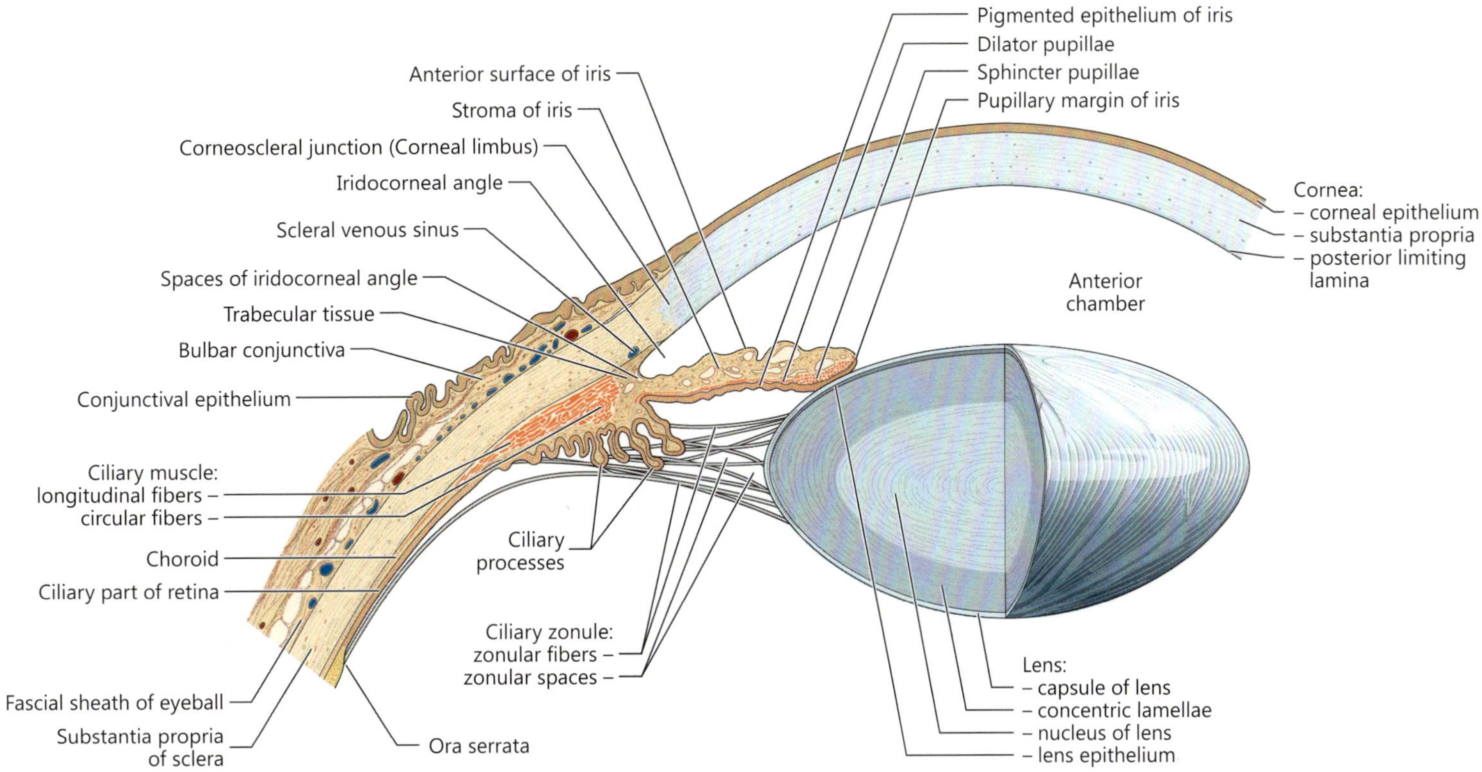

Eye, structure of the anterior (iridociliary) part of the vascular layer.

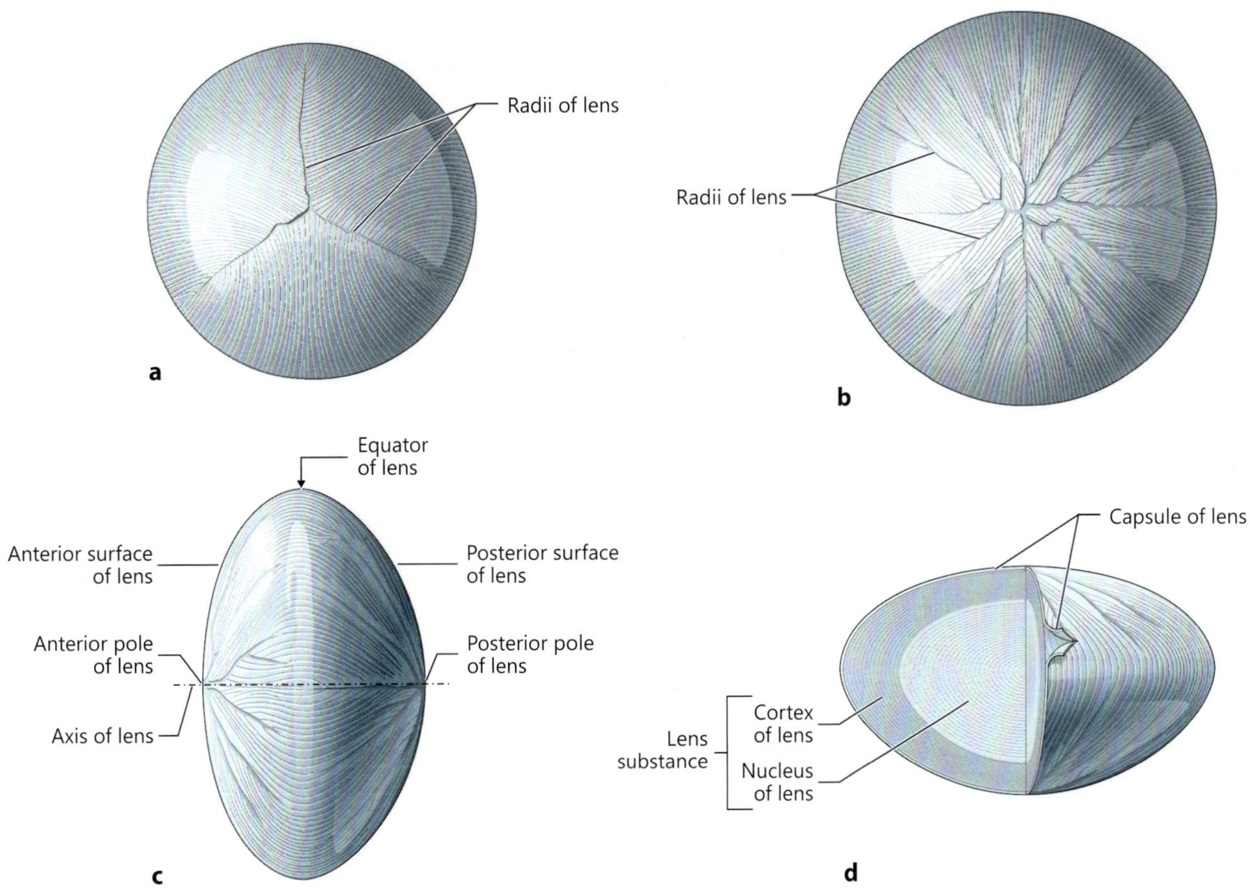

Lens, external and internal conformation. **a**, Anterior surface of the lens, in the child, with a triradiate star figure. **b**, Anterior surface of the lens, in the adult, with a multiradiate star figure. **c**, Lateral projection. **d**, Equatorial section, in which the nucleus of the lens is clearly visible.

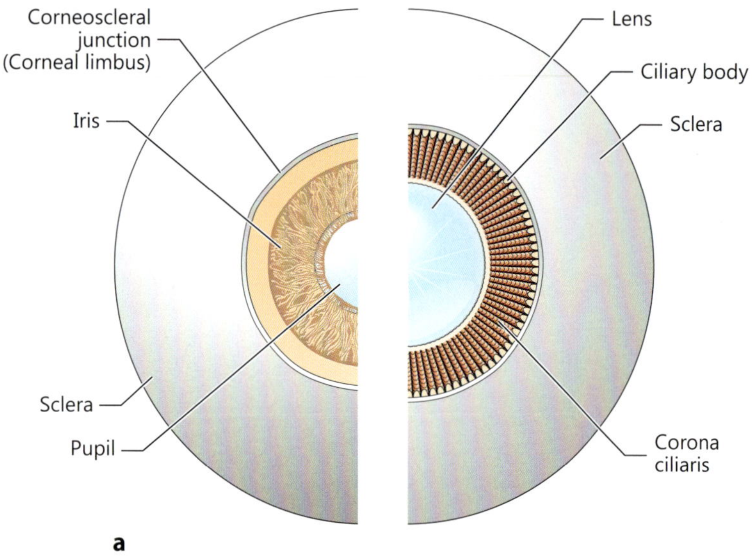

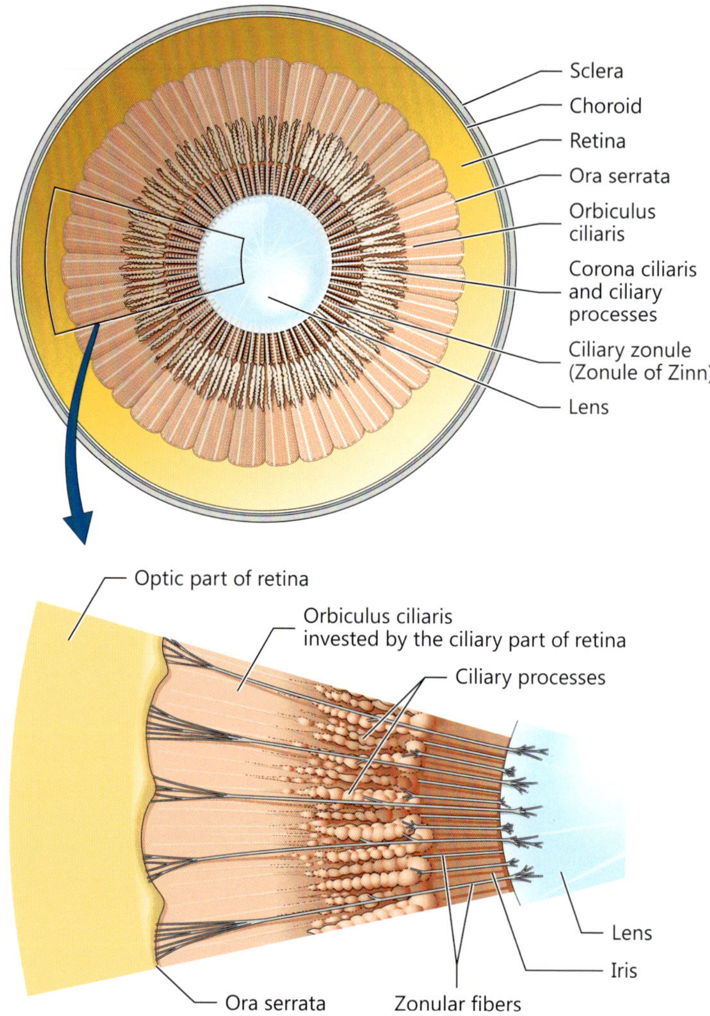

Eyeball, frontal section. **a**, The cornea (on the left) and half of the iris (on the right) have been removed in order to display the pupil, bounded by the iris (on the left), and the lens with its suspensory apparatus (on the right). **b**, Anterior segment viewed posteriorly.

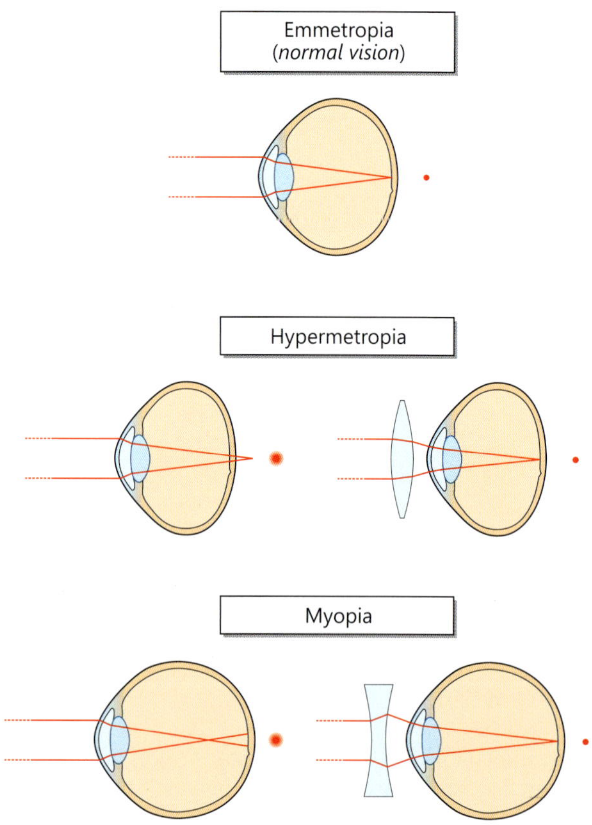

In an **emmetropic eye** accommodated for an object at infinity, the focus of the dioptric system of the eye is located on the retina, where the parallel light rays (coming from infinity) converge to form a focused image. In **hypermetropia**, the dioptric power of the eye is not sufficient to make the parallel rays converge on the retina (generally because the anteroposterior length of the eyeball is reduced with respect to the norm). On the contrary, in the **myopic eye** the excessive length of the eyeball makes the rays converge in front of the retina. In both cases, therefore, in the eye accommodated for infinity, the images that form on the retina are out of focus. Hypermetropia can be corrected with convergent lenses (and myopia with divergent lenses) whose dioptric power, added to (or subtracted from) that of the eye's dioptric system, brings the image into focus on the retina. Convergent lenses are also called positive (their dioptric power adds to that of the eye), while divergent lenses are termed negative (their dioptric power subtracts from that of the eye).

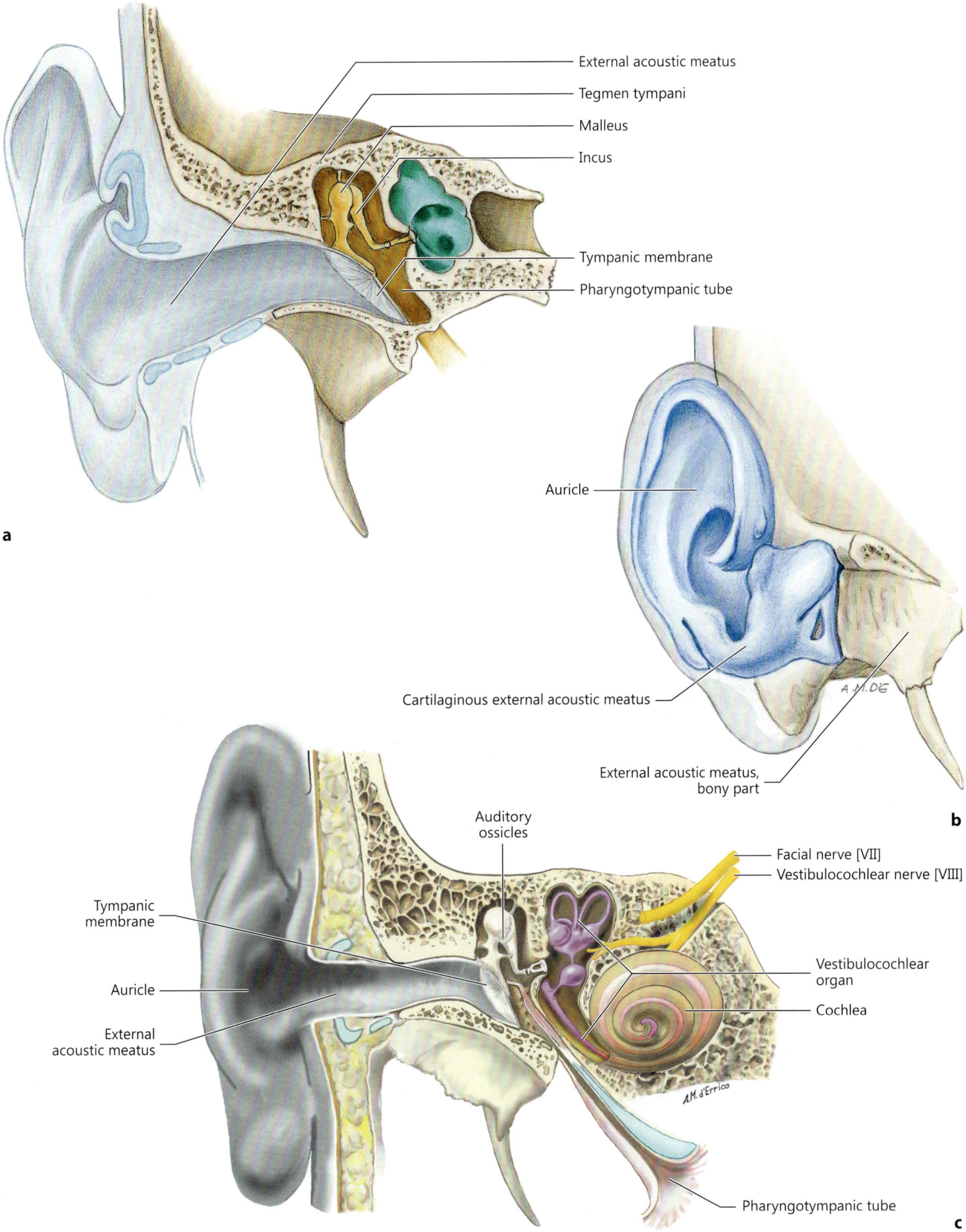

Structure of the **auditory system**. **a**, In *blue*, the **external ear**; in *yellow*, the **middle ear**; in *green*, the **internal ear**. **b**, Indicated in *blue* are the **cartilaginous parts of the external ear**: the auricle and the cartilaginous external acoustic meatus, which proceeds into a segment consisting of a bony part. **c**, **Internal ear**: vestibulocochlear organ. Indicated in *purple* are the **vestibular** and **cochlear labyrinths**.

For a three-dimensional image illustrating the membranous labyrinth, see volume 1, page 383.

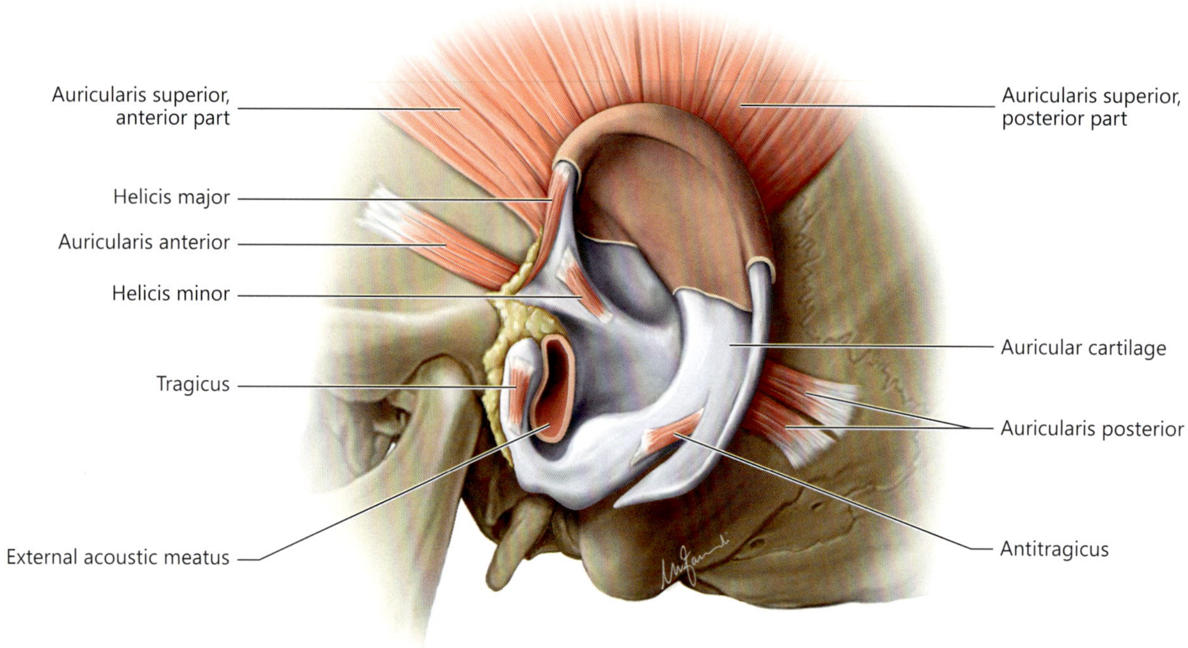

Left ear, external lateral view. Visible beneath the skin are the muscles and cartilage of the **auricle**, in particular the auricularis muscles, helicis muscles, tragicus and antitragicus.

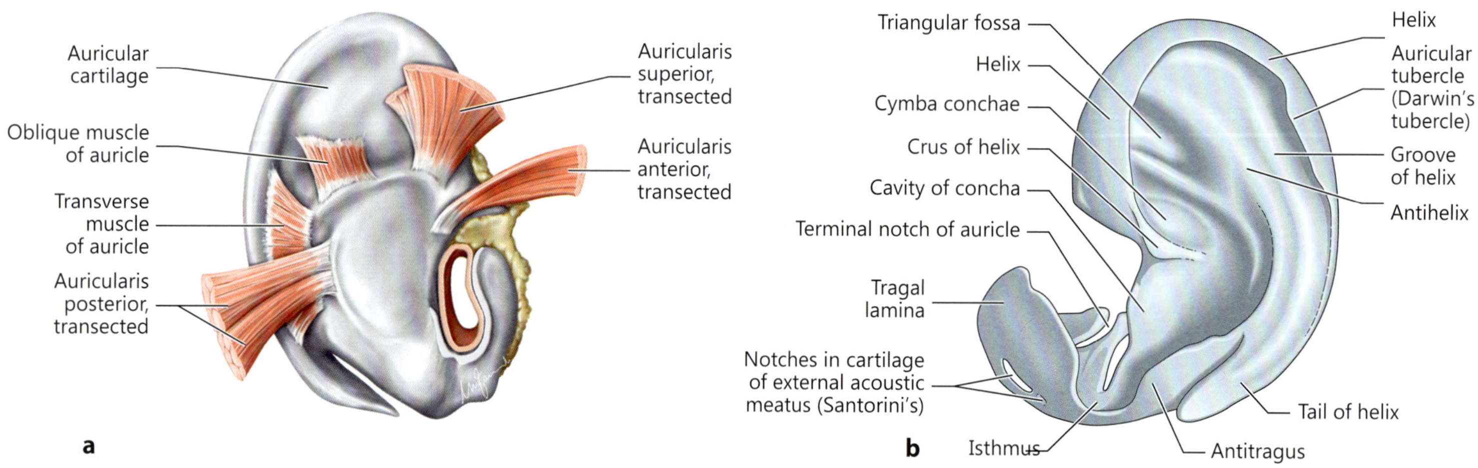

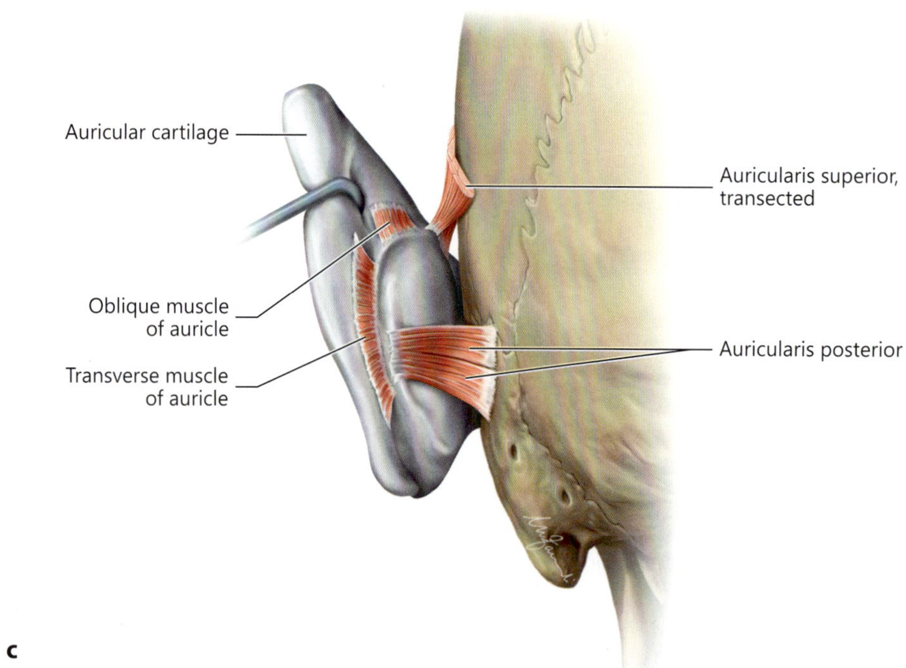

Left ear. **a**, Medial view, showing the oblique and transverse muscles of the **auricle** and auricular cartilage. **b**, Lateral view of the **cartilaginous skeleton**. **c**, Posterior view of the cartilage and muscles of the **auricle**.

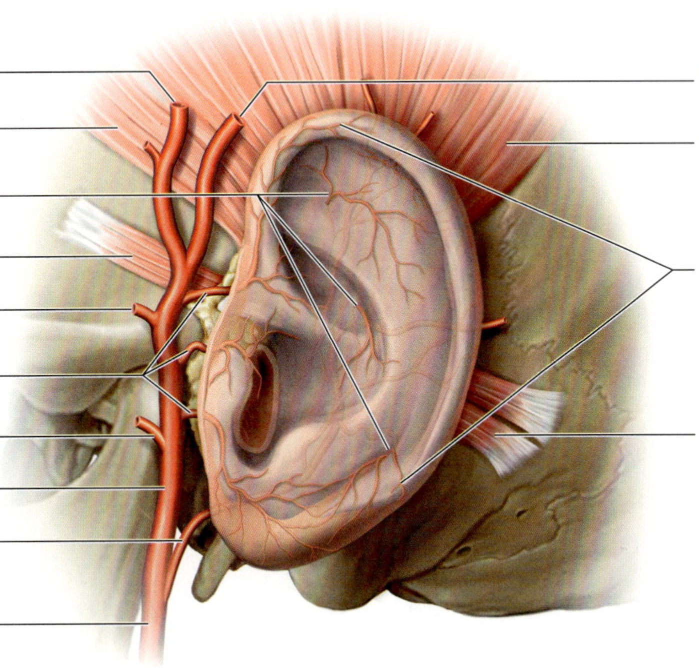

Arteries of the auricle, lateral view of the left external ear. Anterior auricular branches of the **superficial temporal artery**, a branch of the external carotid artery, supply the anterior half of the lateral surface of the auricle. The medial surface and posterior half of the lateral surface of the auricle are supplied by the **posterior auricular artery**, a branch of the external carotid artery. Anastomoses are abundant among the different arterial branches supplying the auricle.

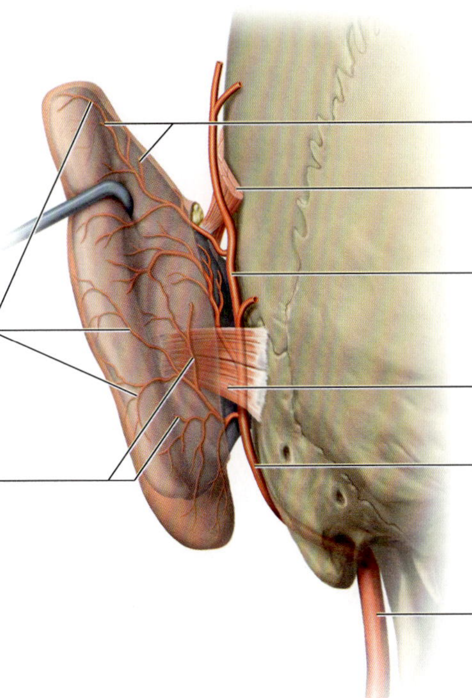

Arteries of the auricle, posterior view of the left external ear. The **posterior auricular artery**, a branch arising from the external carotid artery, ascends to the groove between the auricle and mastoid process of the temporal bone where it continues as an **auricular branch of the posterior auricular artery**, supplying the territory of the medial surface and posterior half of lateral surface of the auricle.

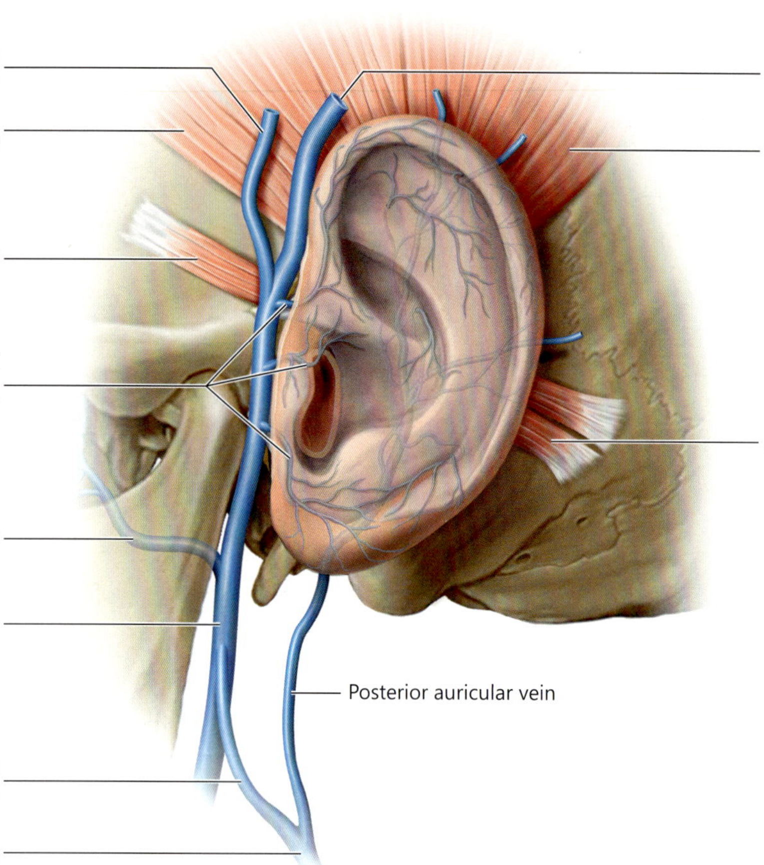

Veins of the auricle, lateral view of the left external ear. The **anterior auricular veins** drain into the **superficial temporal vein**, which unites with the **maxillary vein** forming the **retromandibular vein** or **posterior facial vein**.

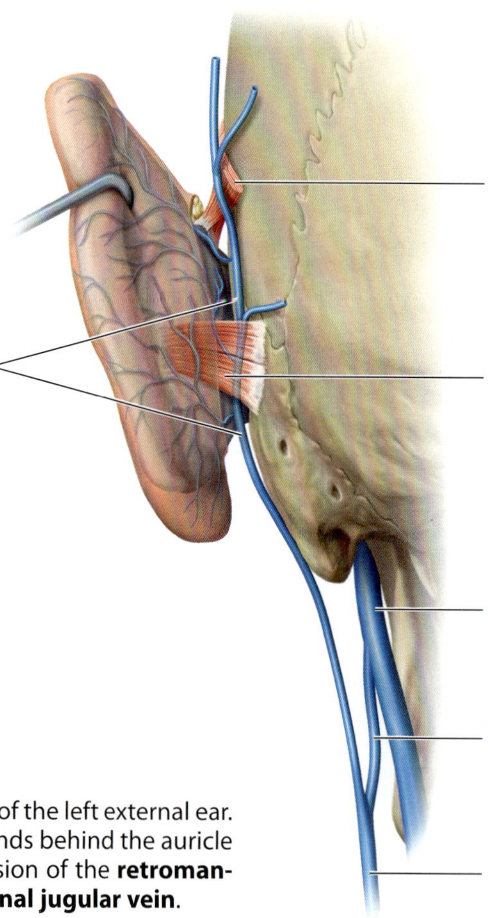

Veins of the auricle, posterior view of the left external ear. The **posterior auricular vein** descends behind the auricle and, uniting with the posterior division of the **retromandibular vein**, gives rise to the **external jugular vein**.

Lymphatic drainage of the auricle. The lymphatic network of the medial surface of the auricle drains into an **infra-auricular node**, belonging to the **group of deep parotid nodes**, situated in contact with the internal jugular vein, in front of the sternocleidomastoid. The lymphatic network of the lateral surface anterior to the concha of the auricle drains into the **preauricular superficial** and **deep parotid nodes**, above and below the concha into the **mastoid nodes**, while at the level of the ear lobe it drains into the **infra-auricular deep parotid nodes**.

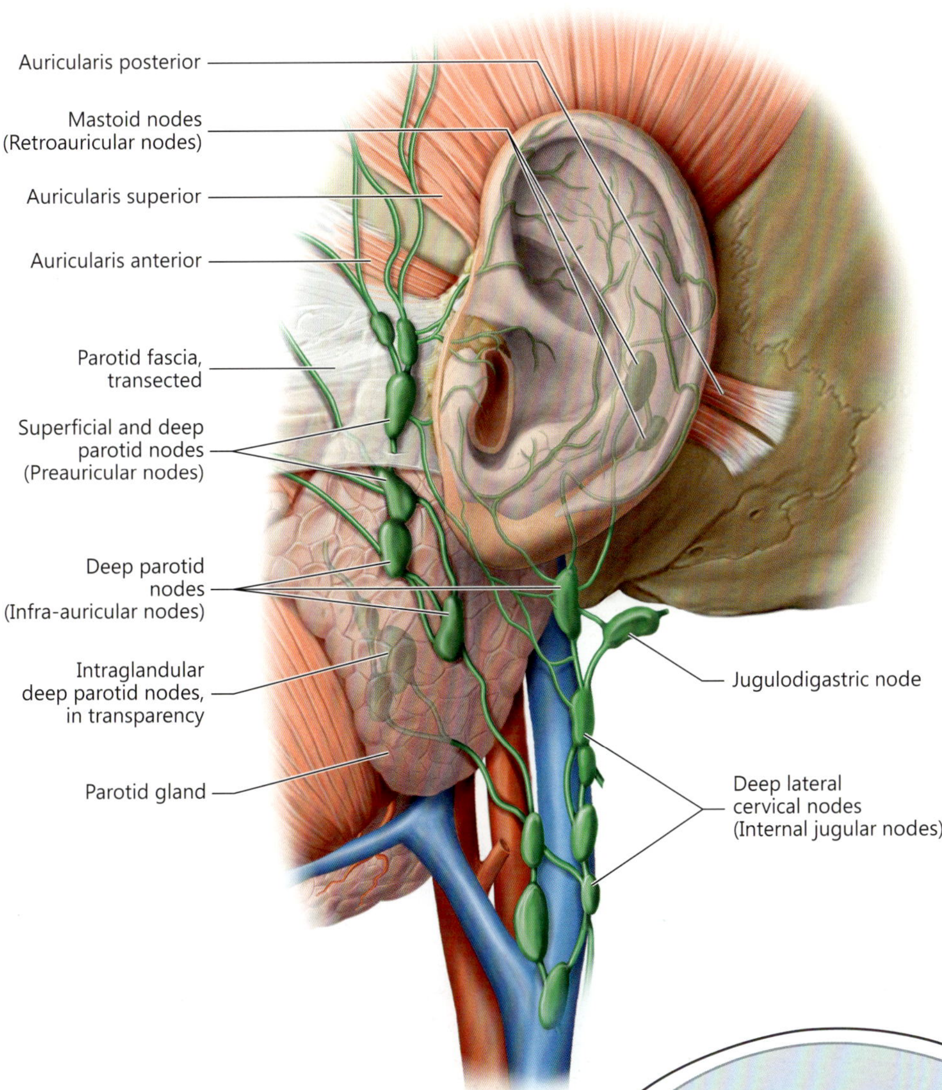

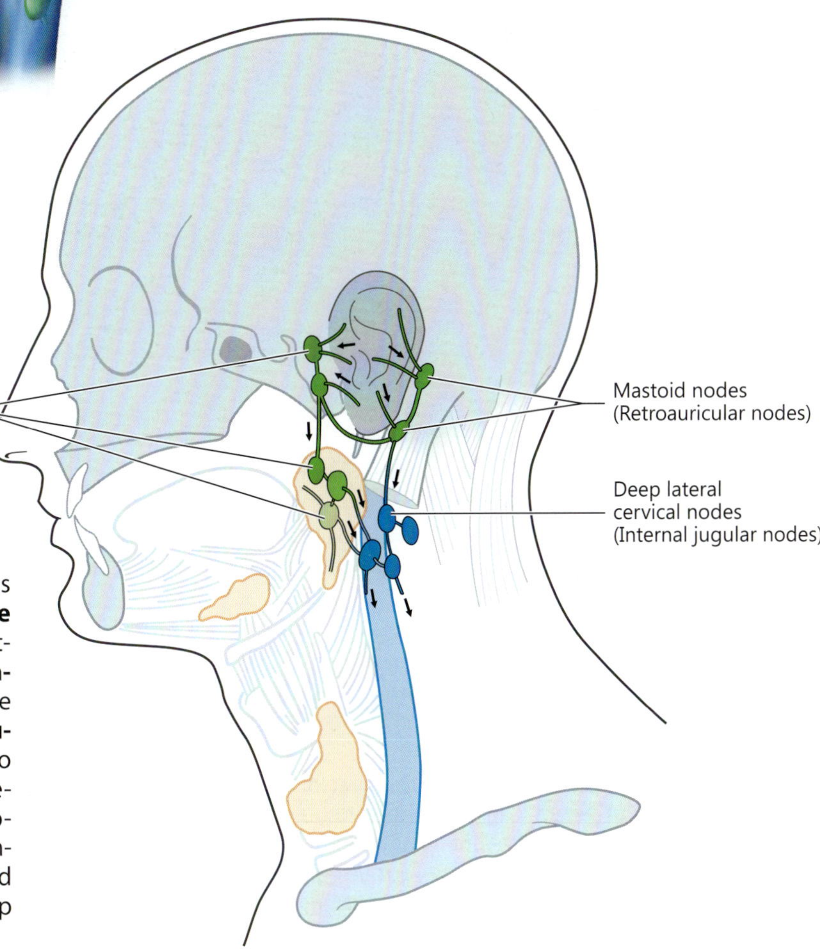

Schematic representation of the lymph nodes associated to the **lymphatic networks of the auricle**. The **superficial parotid nodes**, situated above the parotid fascia, and the **deep parotid nodes**, subfascial, are subdivided into the **preauricular**, **infra-auricular** and **intraglandular nodes**. The **mastoid nodes**, including also the retroauricular nodes, are located in correspondence to the origin of the sternocleidomastoid from the mastoid process of the temporal bone. The superficial and deep parotid nodes and mastoid nodes drain into the deep lateral cervical, or internal jugular, nodes.

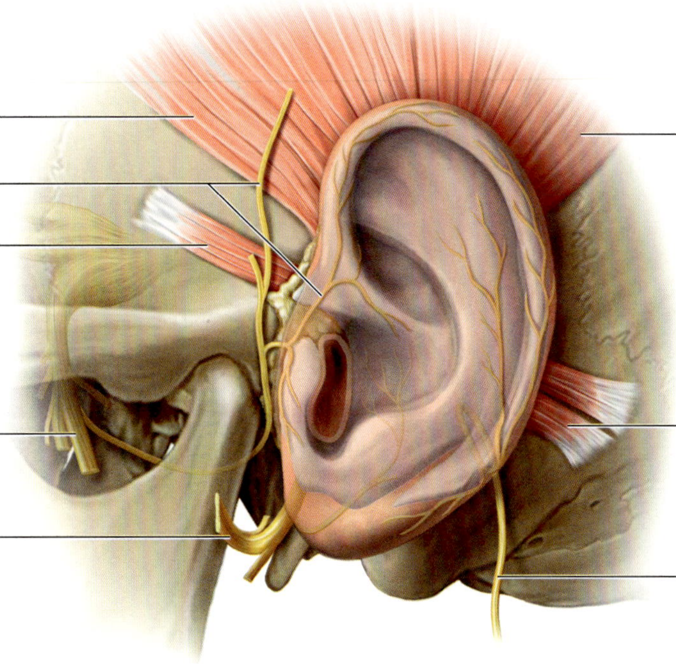

The **auriculotemporal nerve**, a branch of the mandibular nerve [V$_3$], after passing completely through the parotid gland, exchanging anastomoses with the parotid plexus of the facial nerve, runs upwards between the external acoustic meatus and superficial temporal vessels, supplying the anterior part of the auricle and skin of the temporal region.

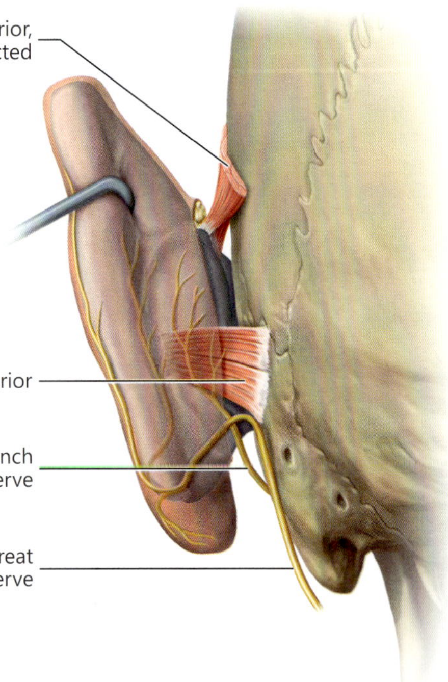

The **great auricular nerve** [C2, C3] is a cutaneous branch of the cervical plexus that runs behind and below the sternocleidomastoid and then winds around the posterior margin and ascends on its lateral surface up to the auricle, whose skin it innervates. Along its course it gives off sensory branches that anastomose with the facial nerve [VII] and cutaneous branches for the parotid region.

➤

Schematic representation showing the **innervation of the auricle**. In addition to the **auriculotemporal** and **great auricular nerves**, also the **facial nerve** [VII], with the auricular branch of the posterior auricular nerve, innervates the auricle through fibers that reach, in particular, the concha and initial part of the external acoustic meatus. The skin of the concha of the auricle is innervated not only by the facial nerve but also by the **vagus** [X] and **glossopharyngeal** [IX] **nerves**, through the auricular branch of the vagus nerve and the communicating branch of the glossopharyngeal nerve with the auricular branch of the vagus nerve.

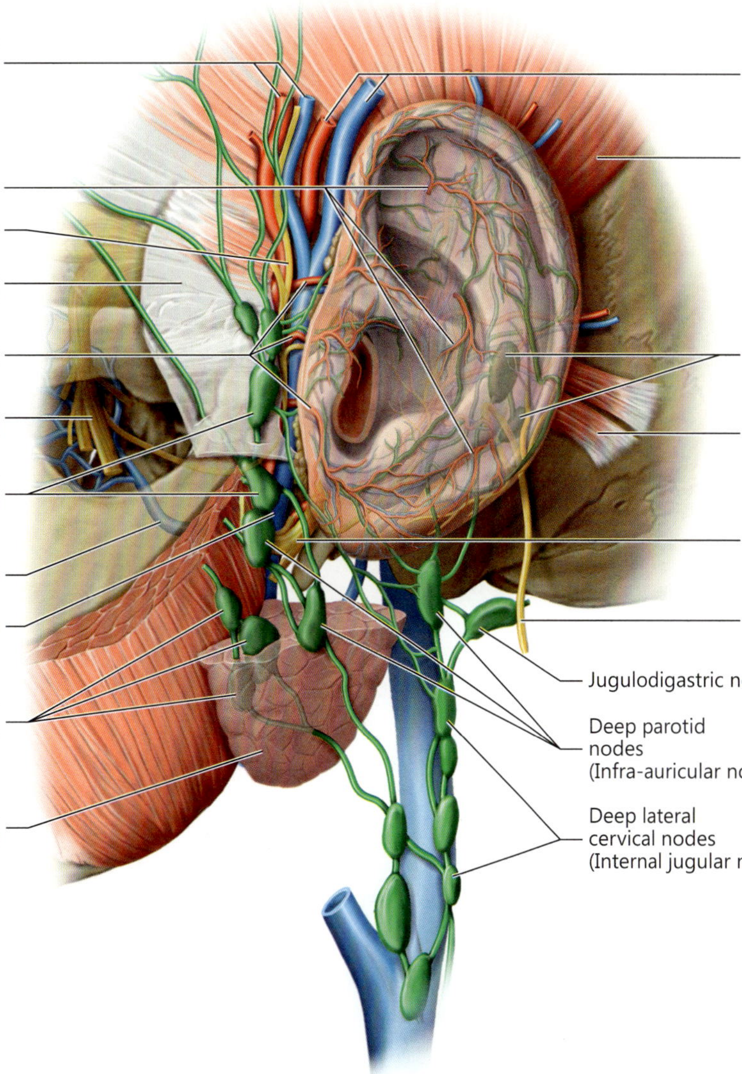

Vascularization, innervation and lymphatic drainage of the **external ear**, left lateral view of the lateral surface of auricle. The arterial supply of the auricle is provided principally by the superficial temporal and posterior auricular arteries; the veins are satellites of the arteries, and lymphatic drainage is towards the parotid and mastoid nodes. Sensory innervation is provided by the great auricular and auriculotemporal nerves, the latter a branch of the mandibular nerve [V_3], with contributions from the facial [VII], vagus [X] and glossopharyngeal [IX] nerves.

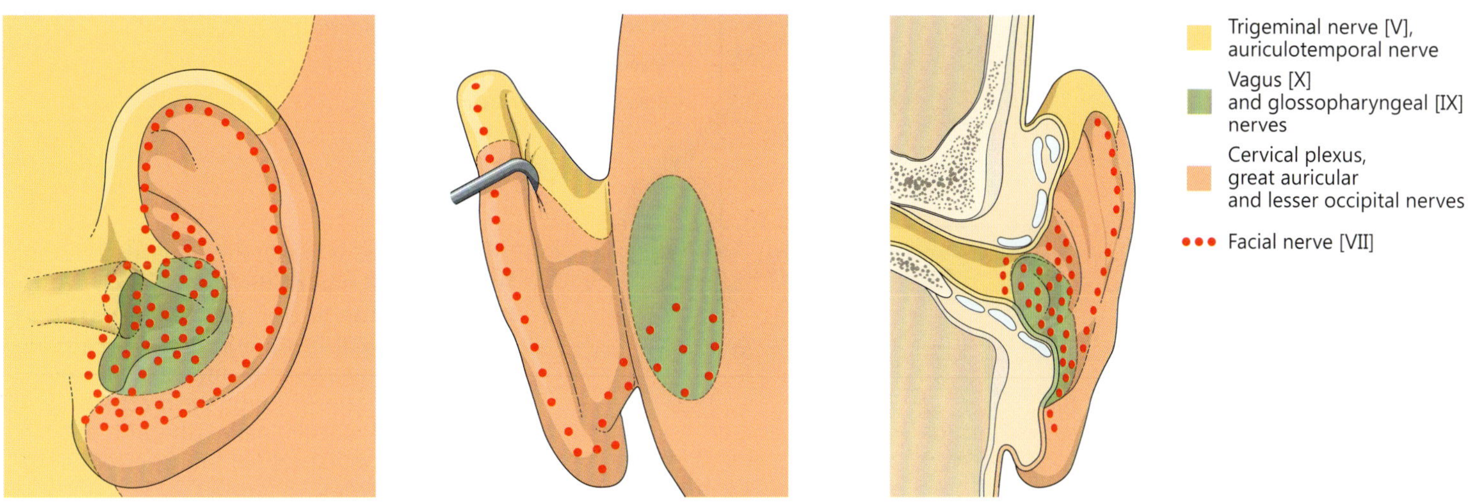

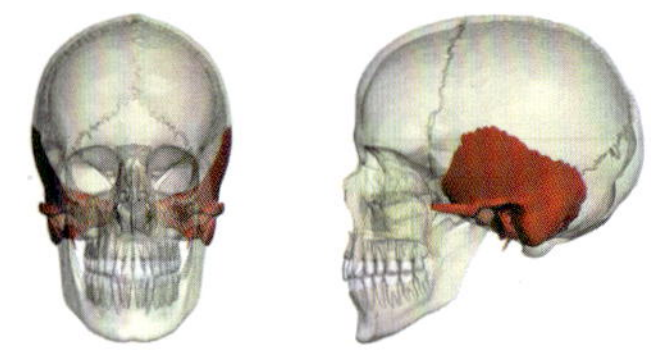

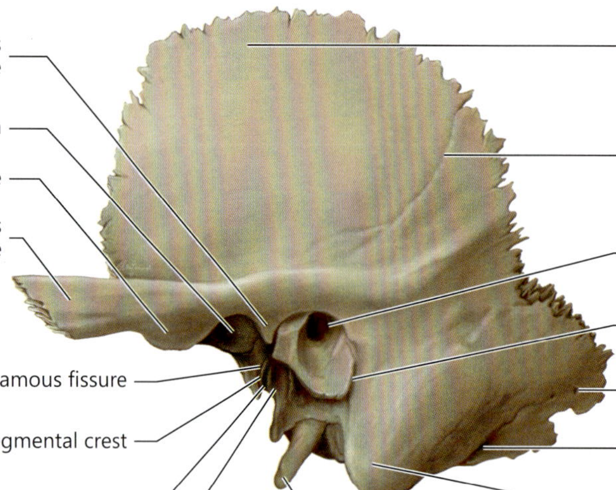

Left **temporal bone**, lateral surface of the extracranial surface.

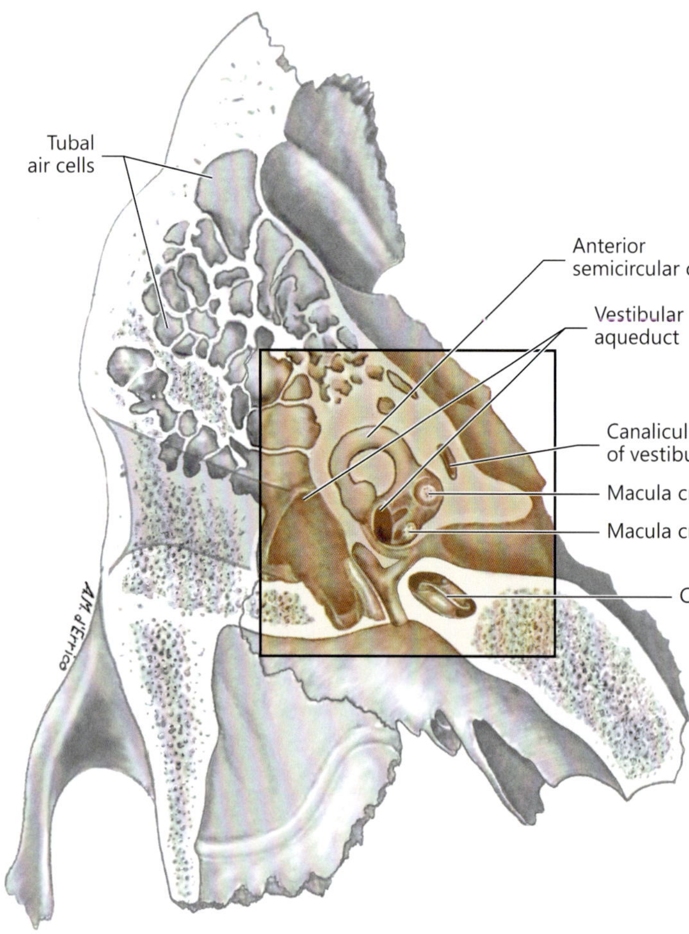

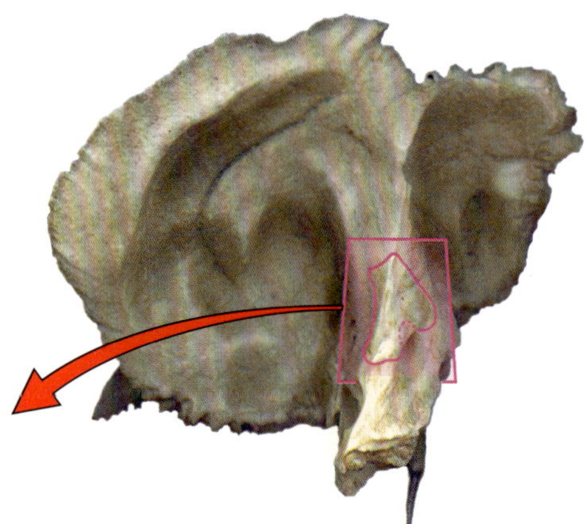

Transverse section of the **petrous part of the temporal bone** at the level of the **vestibule**. The medial wall has a cribriform appearance due to the passage of filaments of the utriculoampullary nerve (through the macula cribrosa superior) and saccular nerve (through the macula cribrosa media), and of branches of the vestibular nerve [VIII].

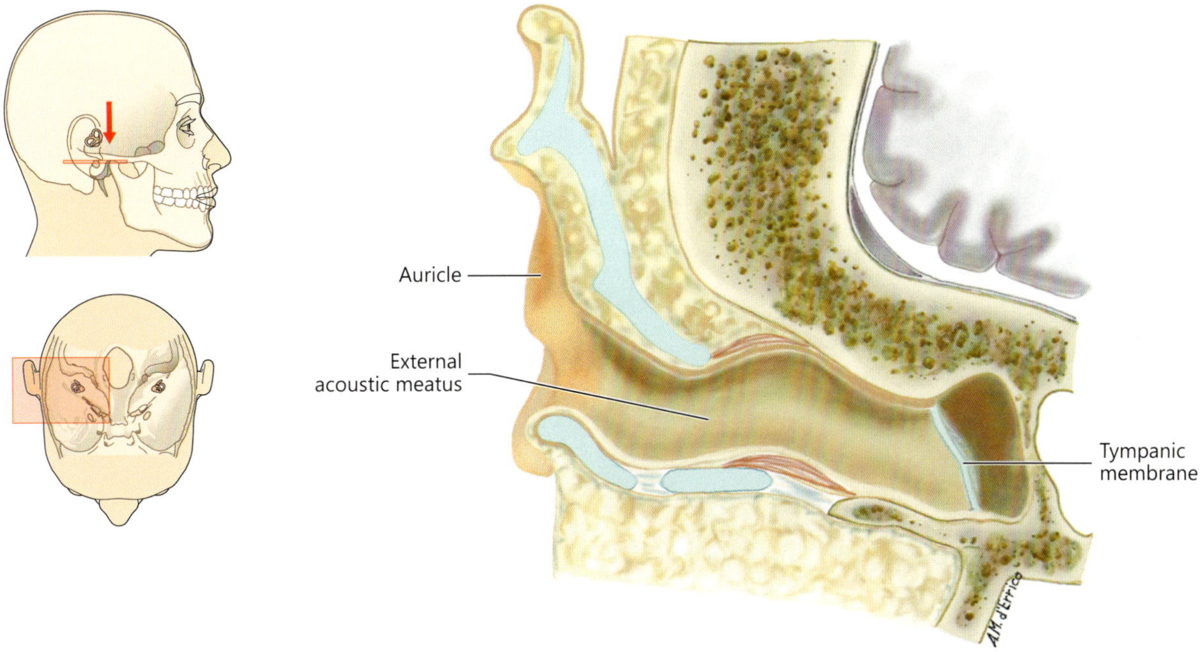

External acoustic meatus of the right ear in transverse section.

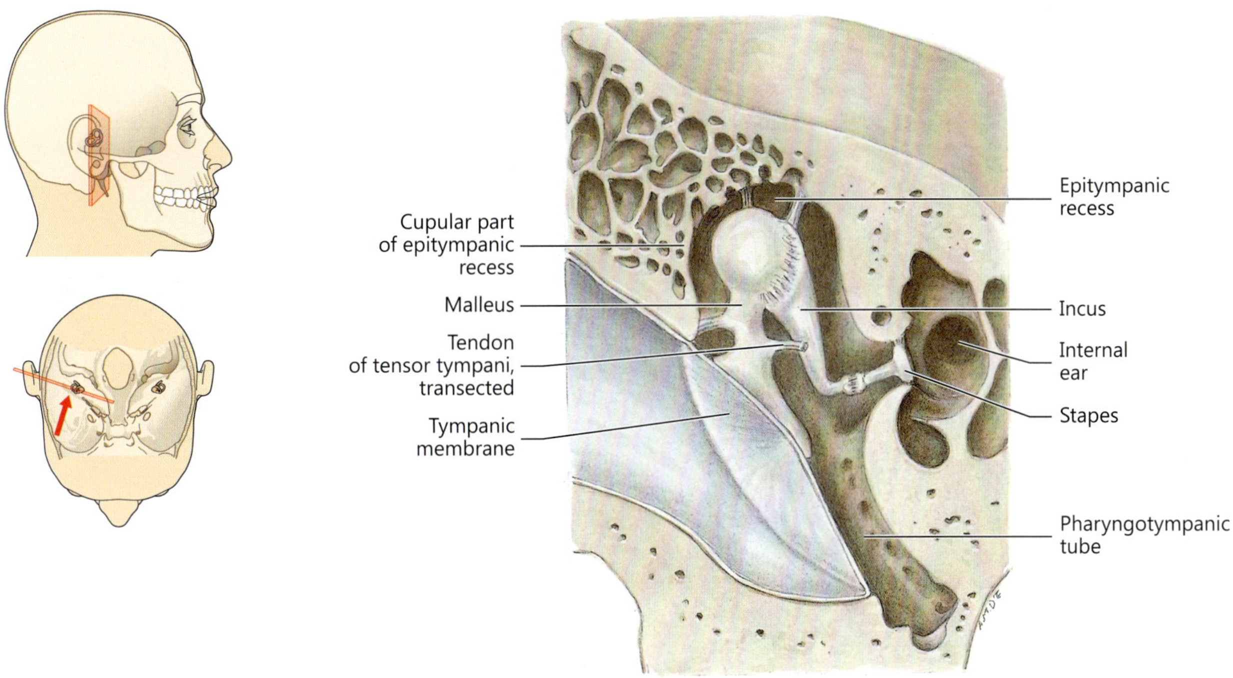

Right middle ear viewed from in front, in an oblique frontal section. The **tympanic cavity** is occupied in part by the ossicles.

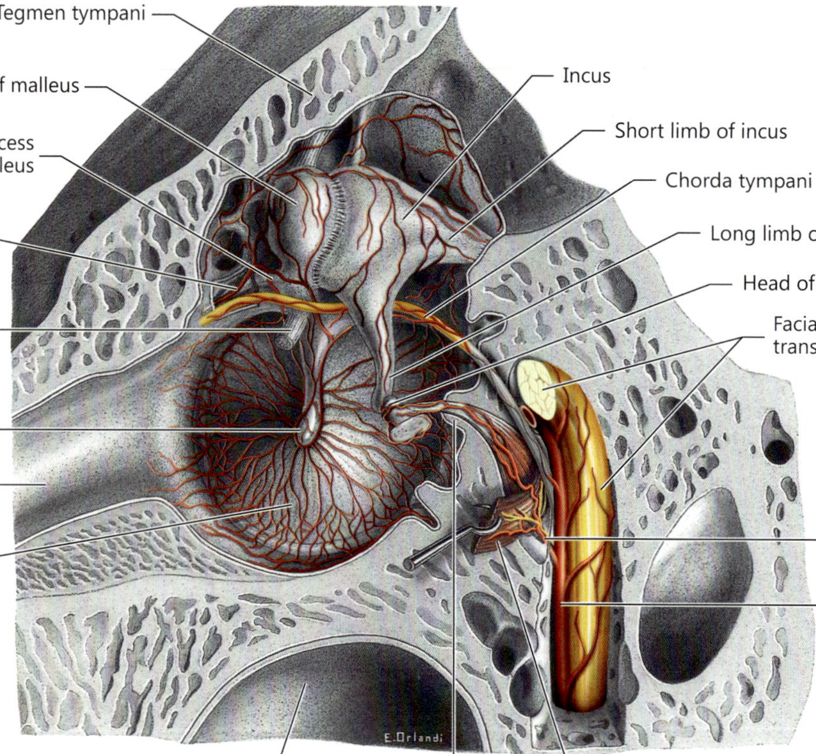

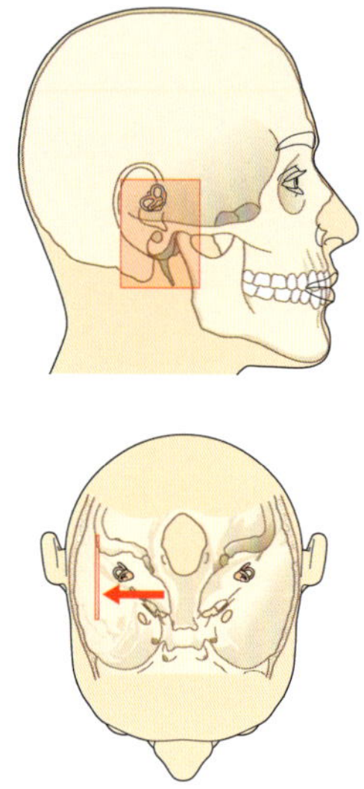

Right tympanic cavity transected sagittally: lateral half of the section viewed from the interior. Blood is supplied to the mucous surface of the tympanic membrane by branches of the **anterior tympanic artery**, a branch of the maxillary artery, and of the **stylomastoid artery**, a branch of the posterior auricular artery.

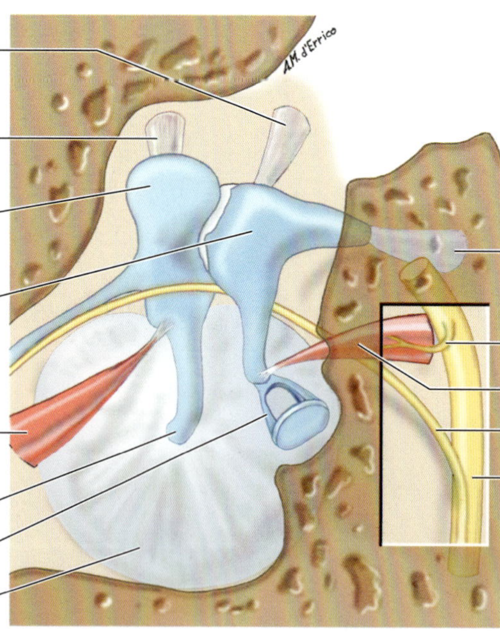

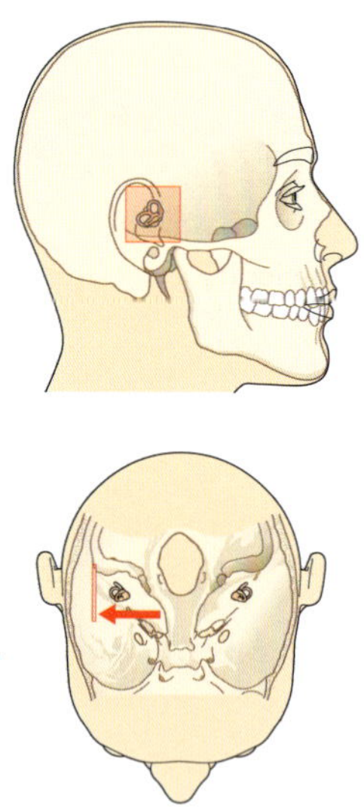

Schematic representation showing the right **tympanic cavity** viewed from the interior.

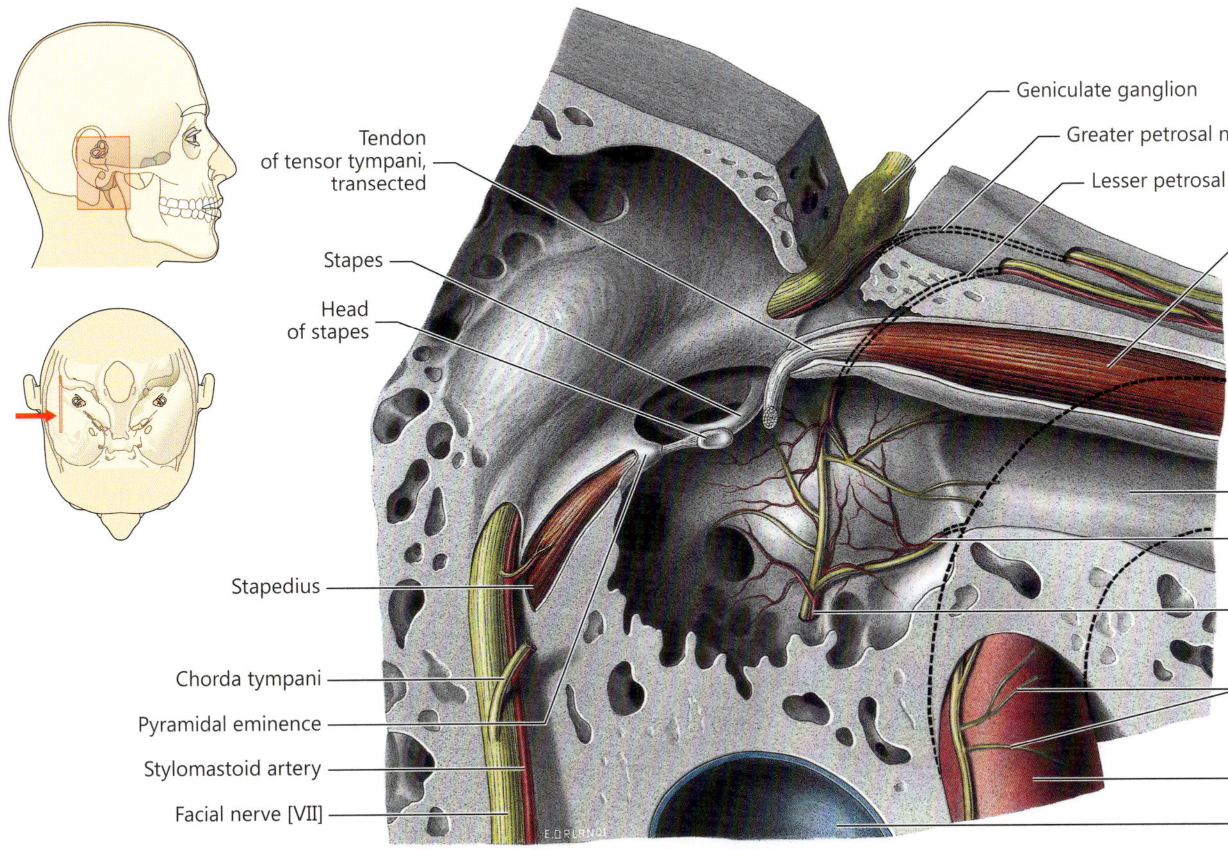

Arterial blood supply of the right **tympanic cavity**. The medial part of the cavity is viewed in a sagittal section of the middle ear. One can see the distribution of the various arterial branches that supply the mucosa of the tympanic cavity.

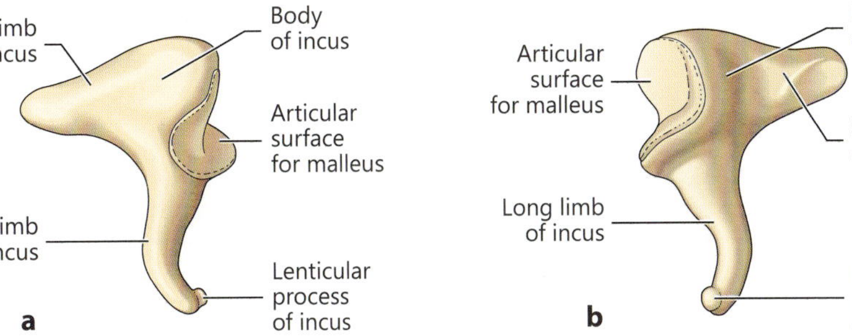

Incus of the auditory ossicles of the right middle ear, lateral (**a**) and medial (**b**) views.

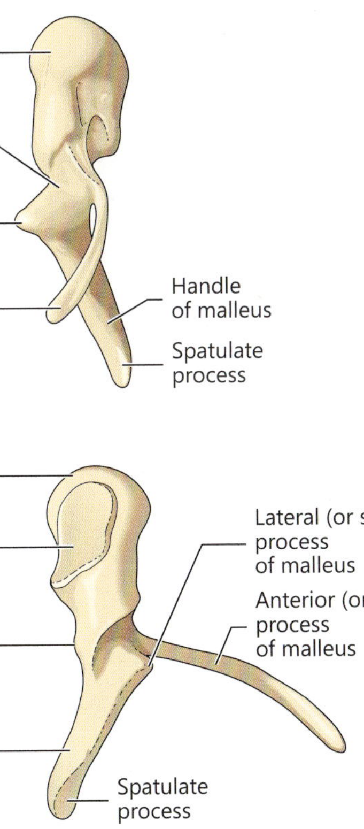

Malleus of the auditory ossicles of the right middle ear, anterior (**a**) and lateral (**b**) views.

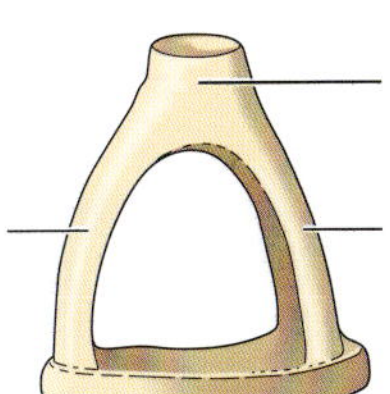

Stapes of the auditory ossicles of the right middle ear, viewed from above.

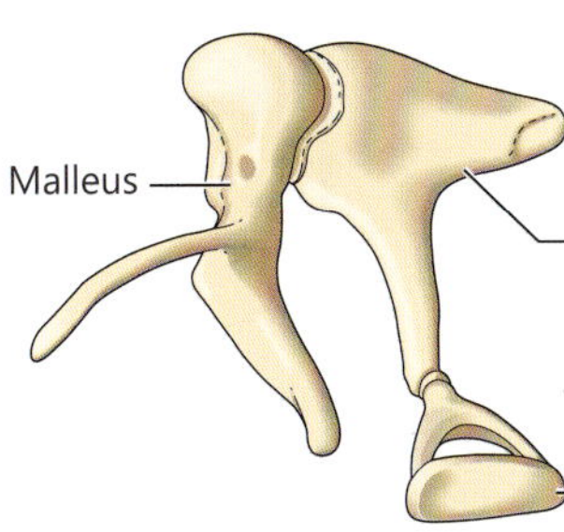

Auditory ossicles of the right middle ear, medial view. One can see the relationship between the three ossicles when they are placed in reciprocal articulation.

Muscles of the auditory ossicles					
MUSCLE	**ORIGIN**	**INSERTION**	**INNERVATION**	**ACTION**	**OBSERVATIONS**
Stapedius	Pyramidal eminence of the mastoid wall of the tympanic cavity	Posterior part of the head of the stapes	Facial nerve [VII]	Retracts the head of the stapes with a consequent slight inclination of its base. Function: reduces tension of the tympanic membrane	Smallest skeletal muscle in the human body
Tensor tympani	Bony canal above the pharyngotympanic tube, cartilaginous part of the pharyngotympanic tube and greater wing of the sphenoid	Root of the handle of the malleus	Facial nerve [VII]	Pulls the handle of the malleus medially. Function: increases tension of the tympanic membrane	

For the functional anatomy of the mechanisms of sound transmission ☞ page 391, volume 1

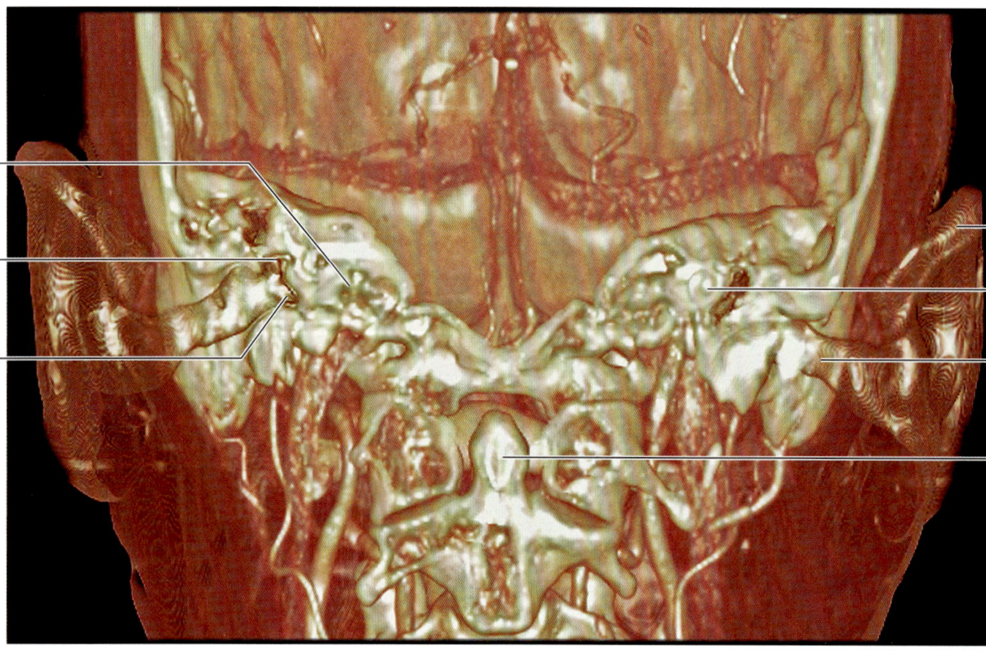

Three-dimensional image of a living human body, obtained by CT scan using a 3D volume rendering technique, showing, in a coronal section of the head viewed posteriorly, the structures of the **external**, **middle** and **internal ear**.

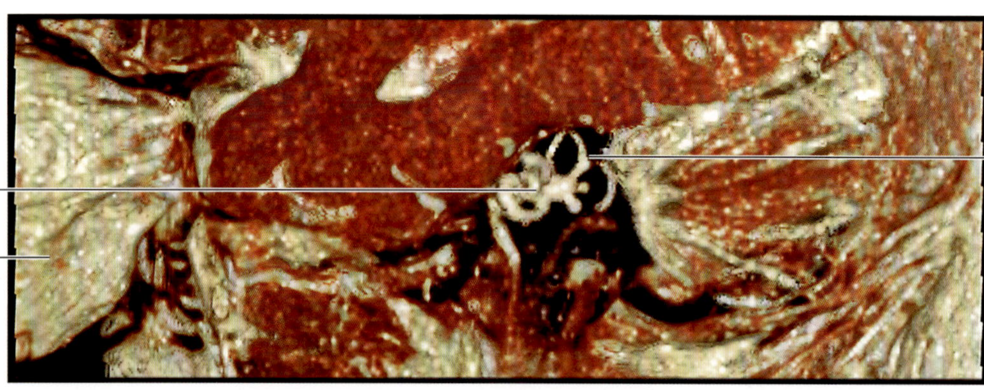

Three-dimensional image of a living human body, obtained by CT scan using a 3D volume rendering technique showing, in a tangential parasagittal section lateral to the eyeball, the **semicircular ducts** and **cochlear duct**.

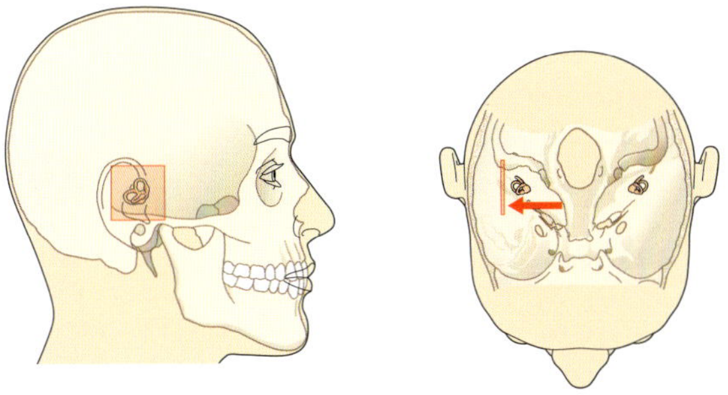

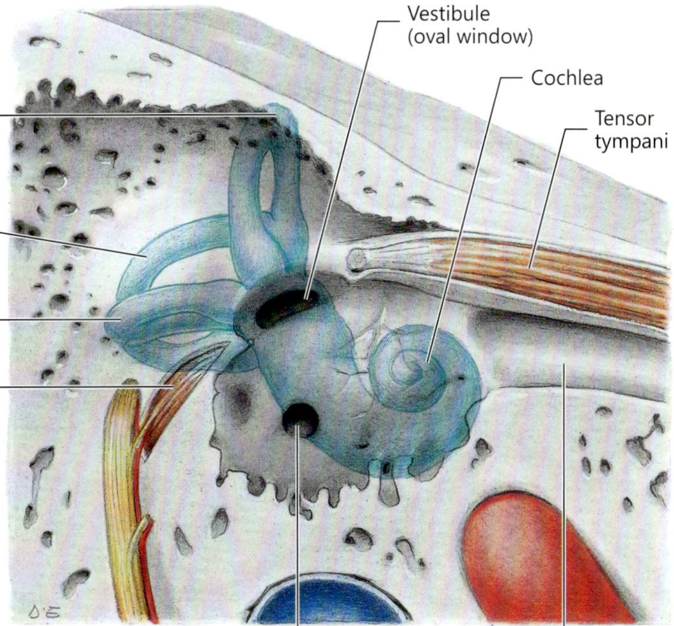

Transparent diagram showing the **bony labyrinth cavity** of the right ear in relation to the medial wall of the tympanic cavity. The lateral wall of the vestibule corresponds to the oval window.

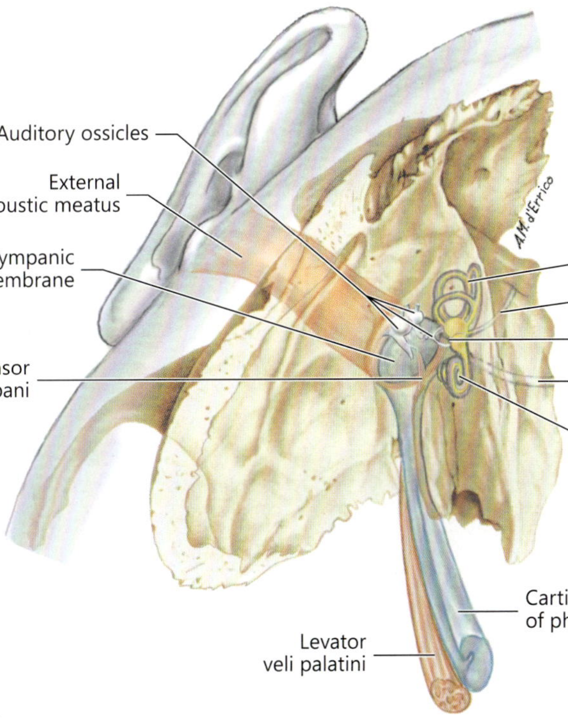

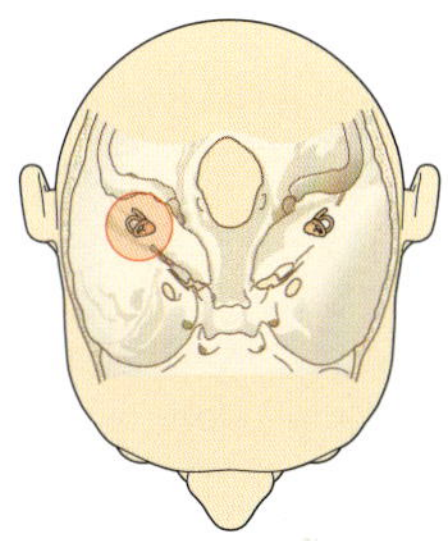

Components of the bony labyrinth of the right ear seen in relation to the **middle ear**, in superomedial view.

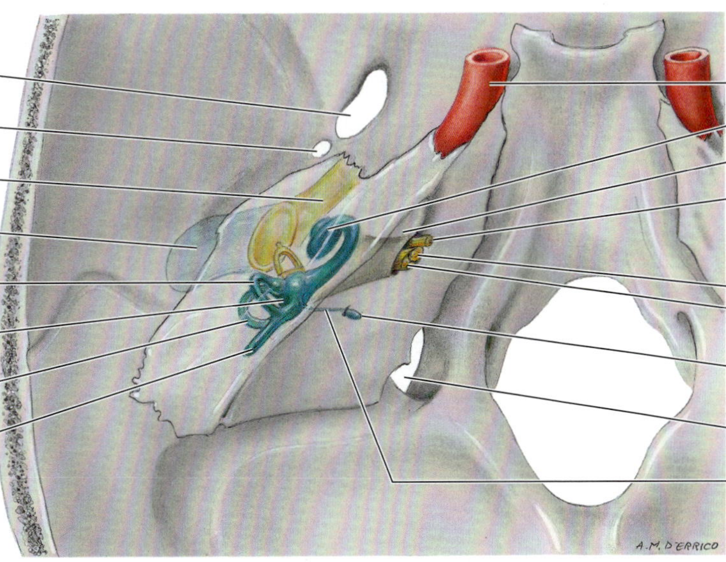

Topography of the anterior and posterior formations of the **internal ear** and their relationships with the other parts of the auditory system. Medially to the bony labyrinth one finds the internal acoustic meatus, which provides a passage for the vestibulocochlear [VIII] and facial [VII] nerves. For a three-dimensional image, see volume 1, page 381.

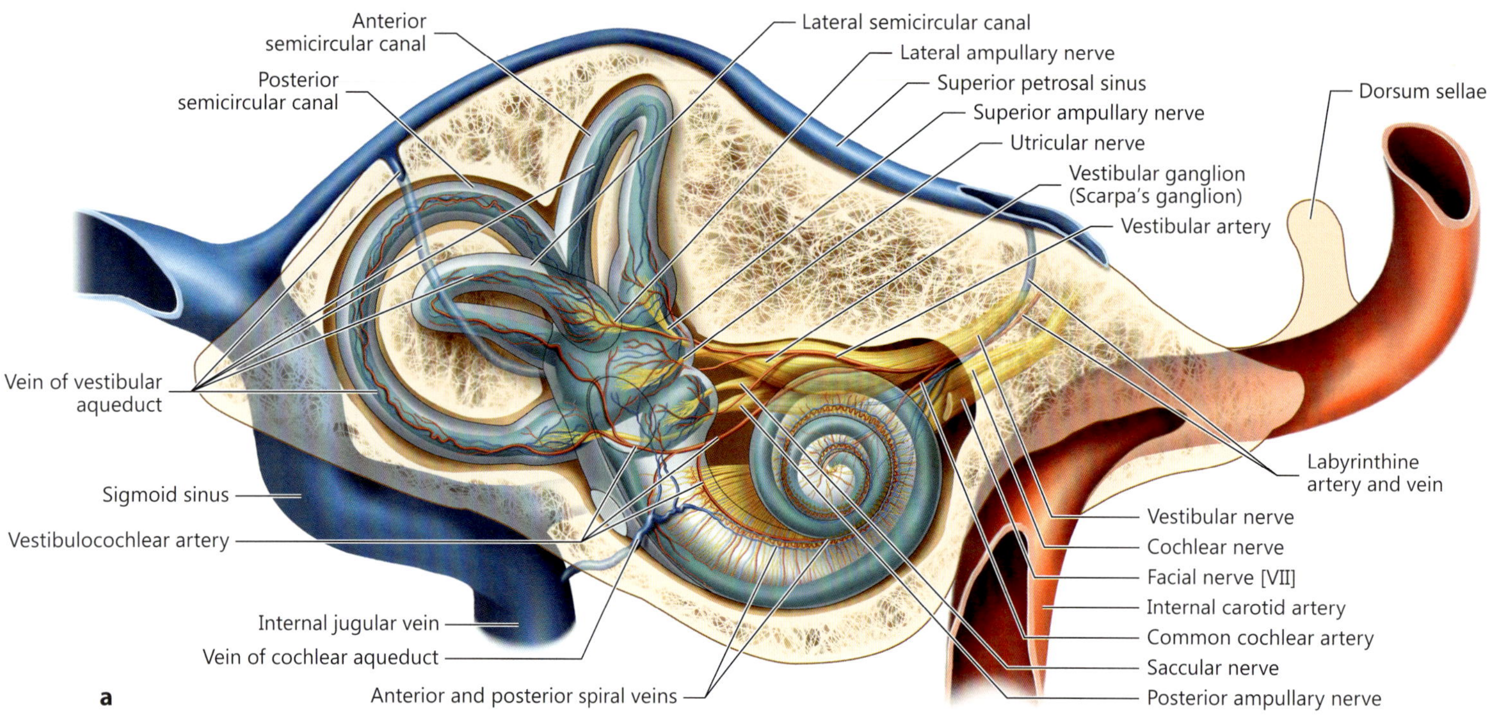

a

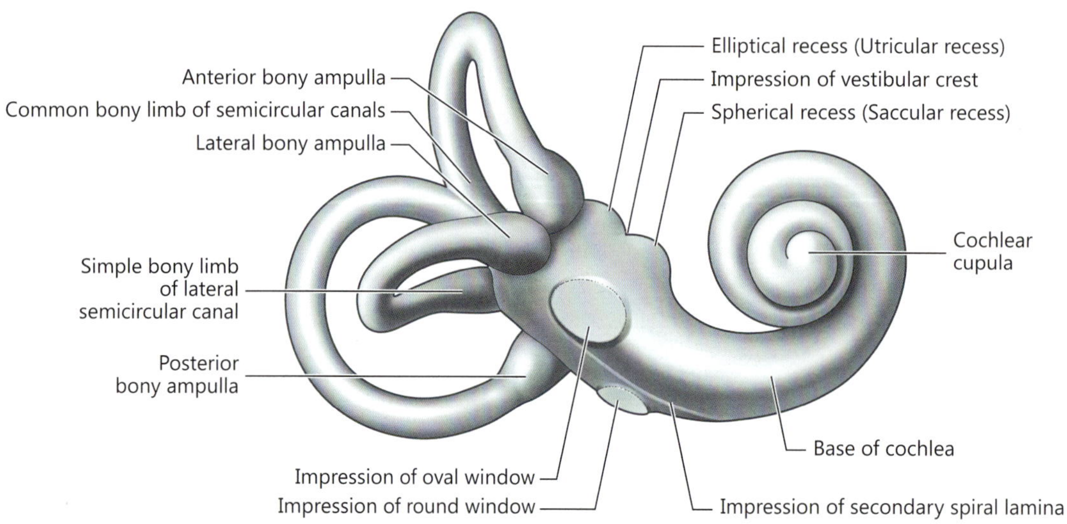

b

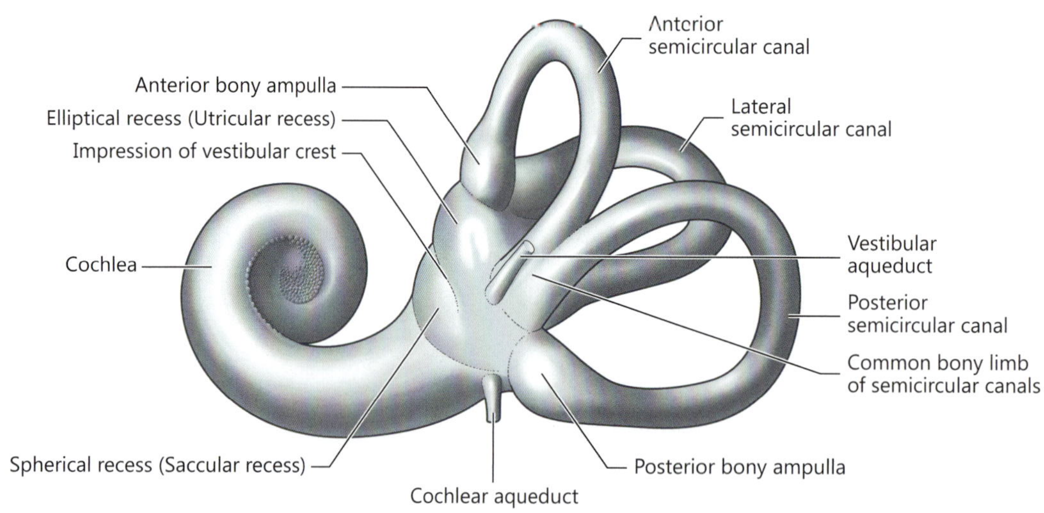

c

Right **bony labyrinth**. **a**, View from the exterior. Part of the bony structure has been demolished to display the vestibular and cochlear labyrinths. **b**, Lateral view. The cochlea, vestibule and semicircular canals follow one another in an anteroposterior succession. **c**, Medial view, showing the position of the vestibular and cochlear aqueducts.

Vestibular and cochlear labyrinths of the right **internal ear**. **a**, View from the external side, **b**, view from the internal side.

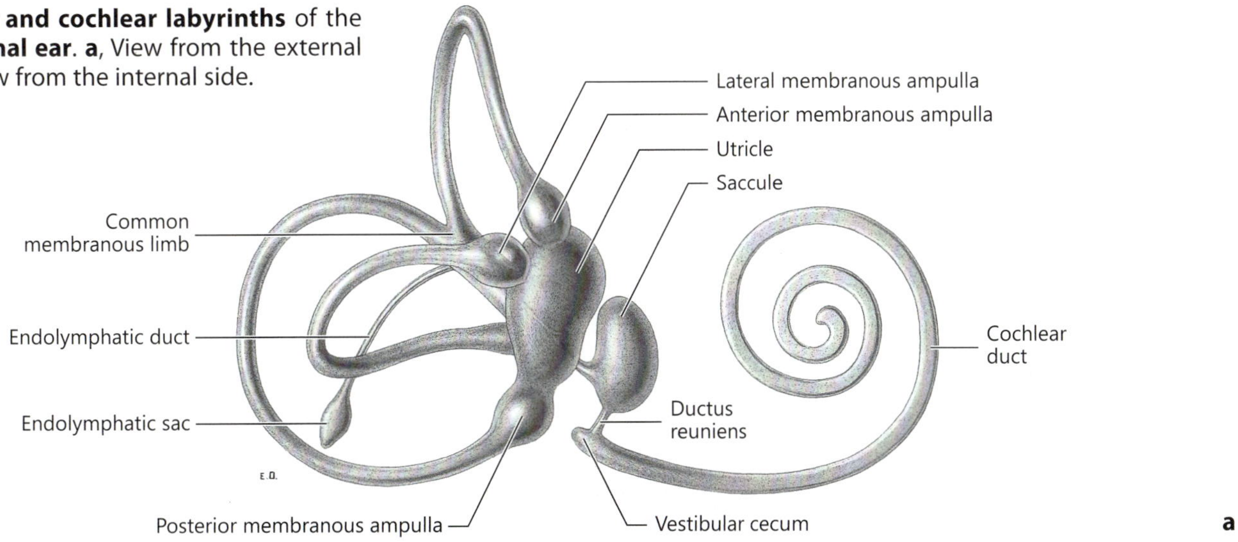

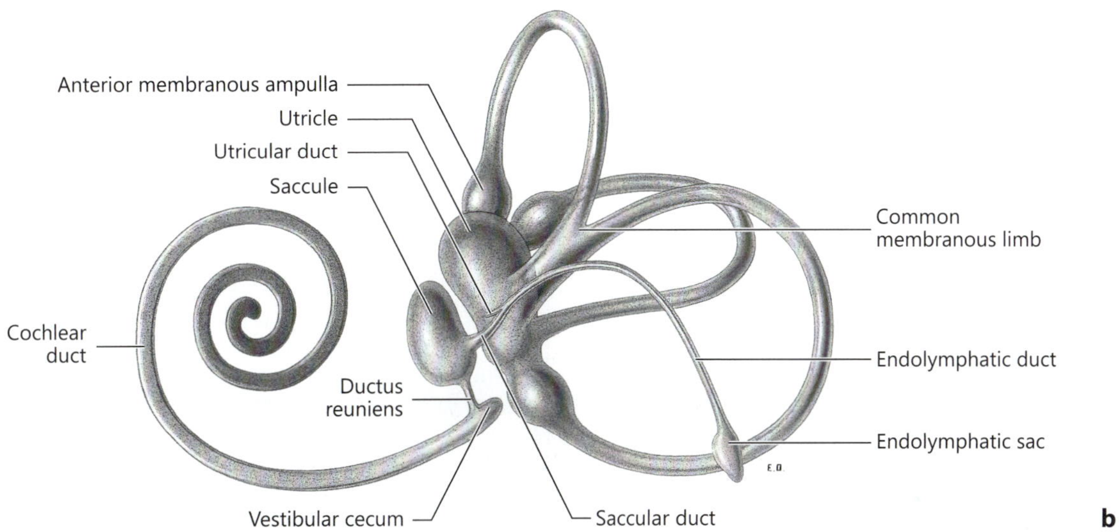

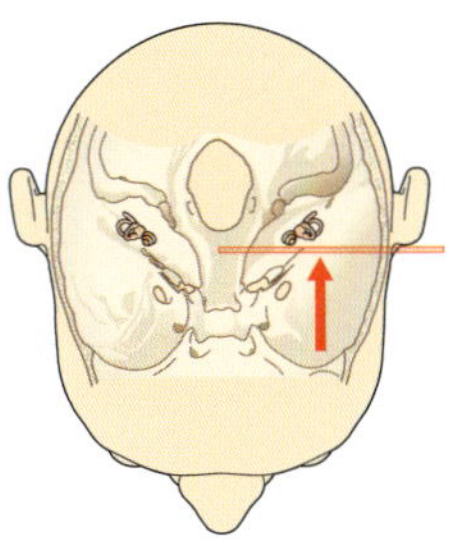

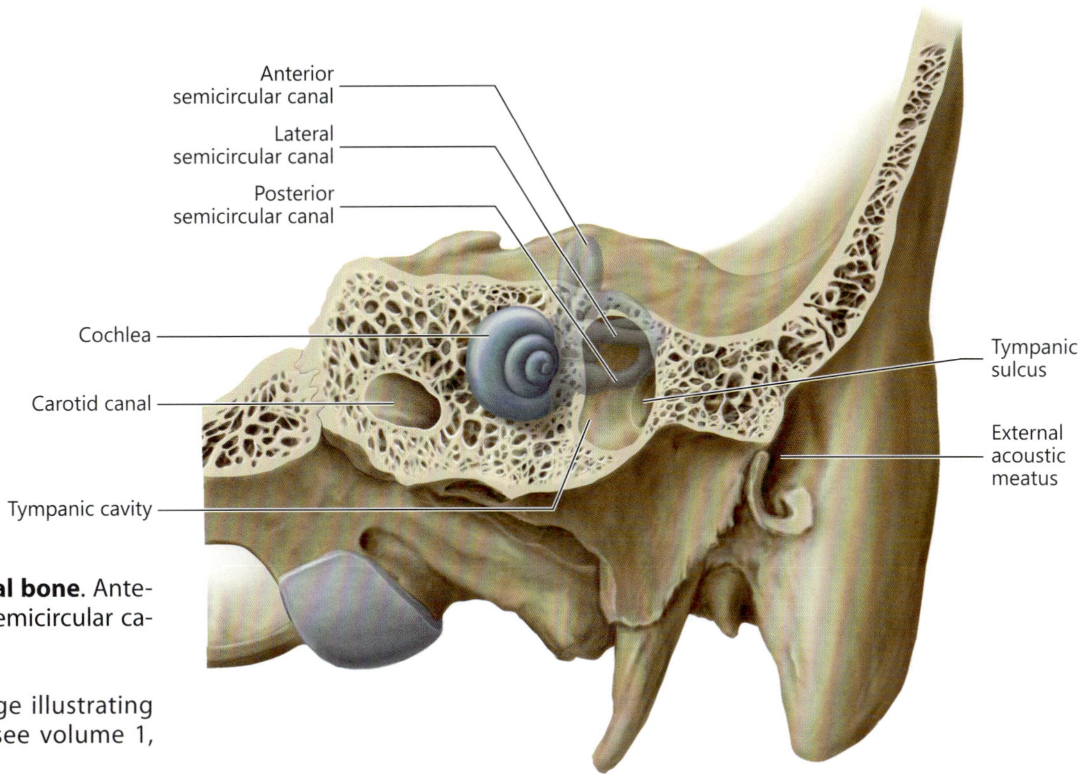

Frontal section of the **temporal bone**. Anterior view of the cochlea and semicircular canals, in transparency.

For a three-dimensional image illustrating the membranous labyrinth, see volume 1, page 383.

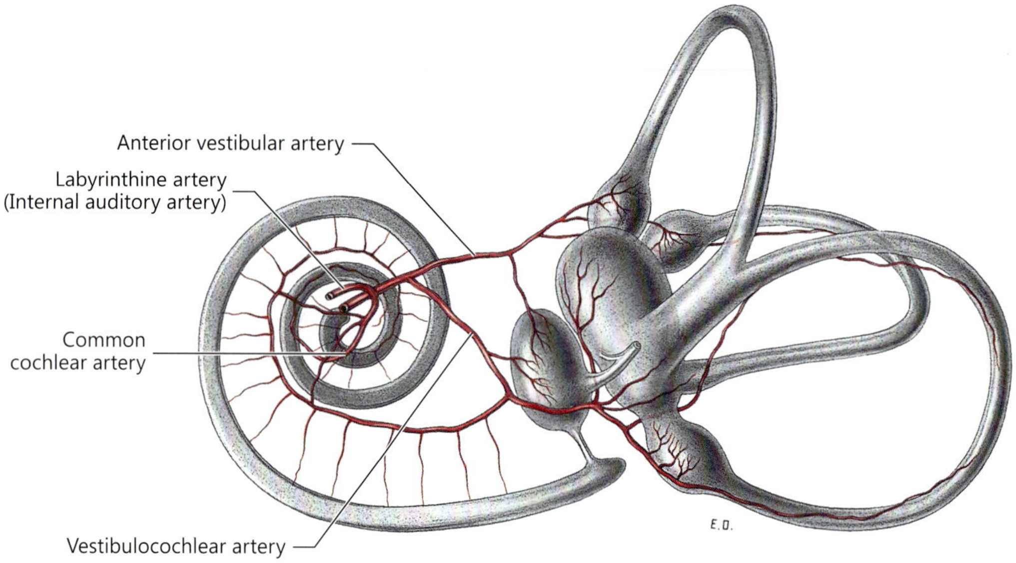

a

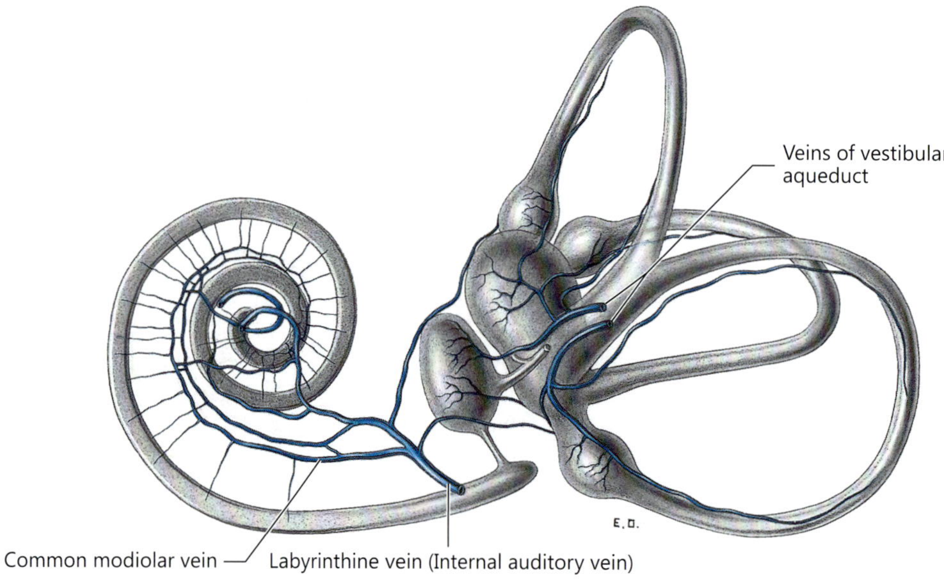

b

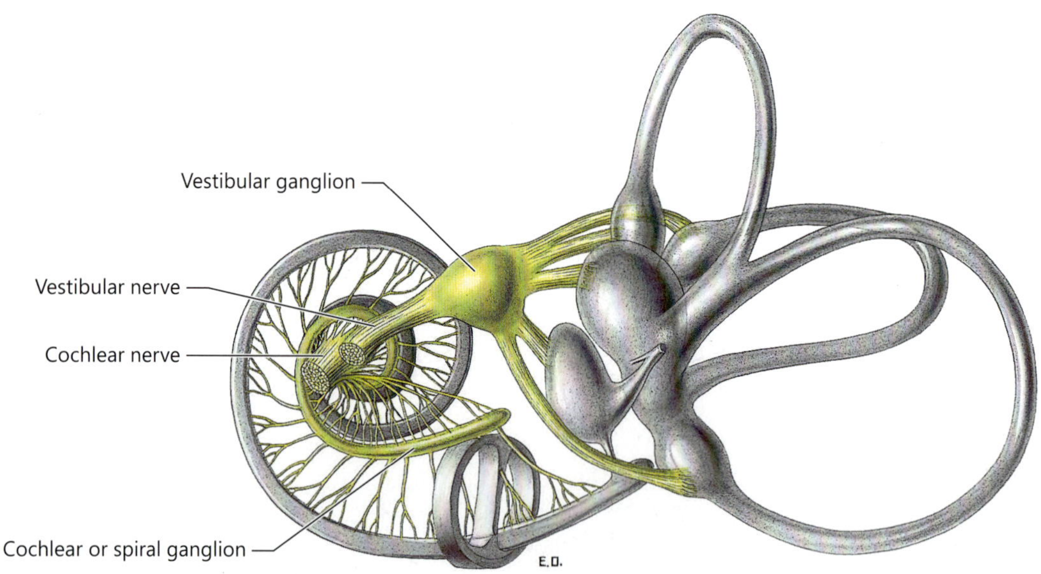

c

a, Arterial blood supply of the **vestibular** and **cochlear labyrinths**. **b**, Venous drainage of the **vestibular** and **cochlear labyrinths**. **c**, Territory of innervation of the vestibulocochlear nerve [VIII]. Peripheral branches of the vestibular and of the cochlear nerves are shown at their point of departure from, respectively, the vestibular ganglion (or Scarpa's ganglion) and the spiral ganglion (or Corti's ganglion).

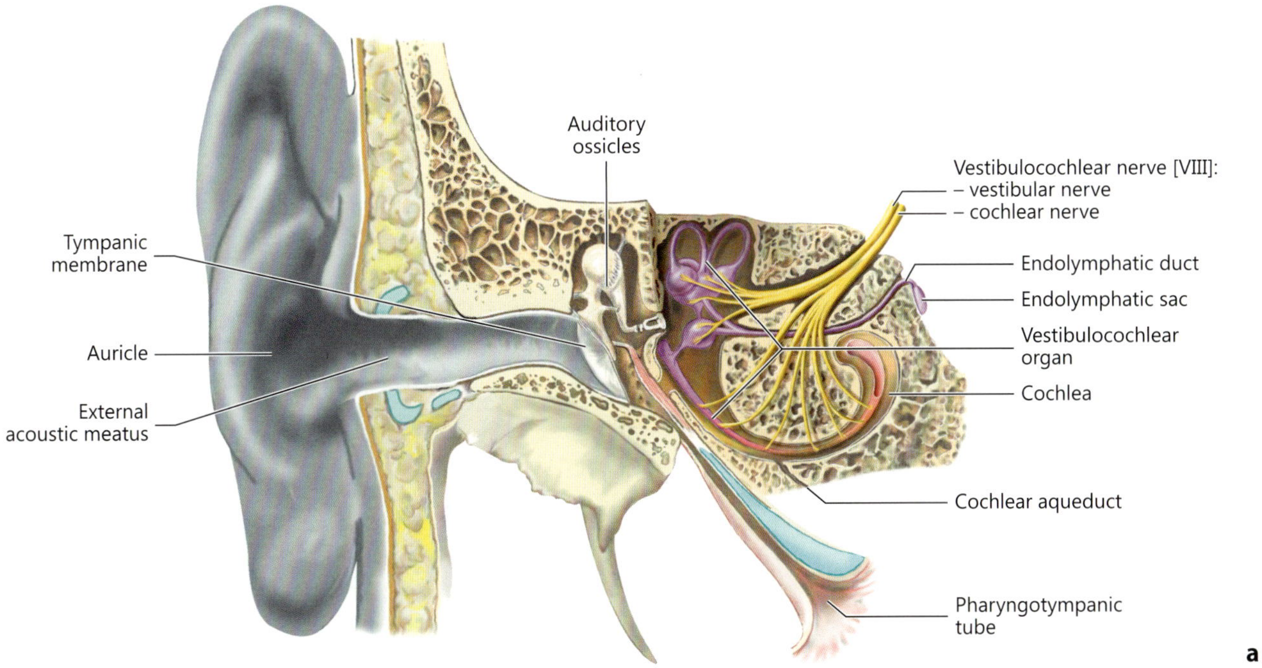

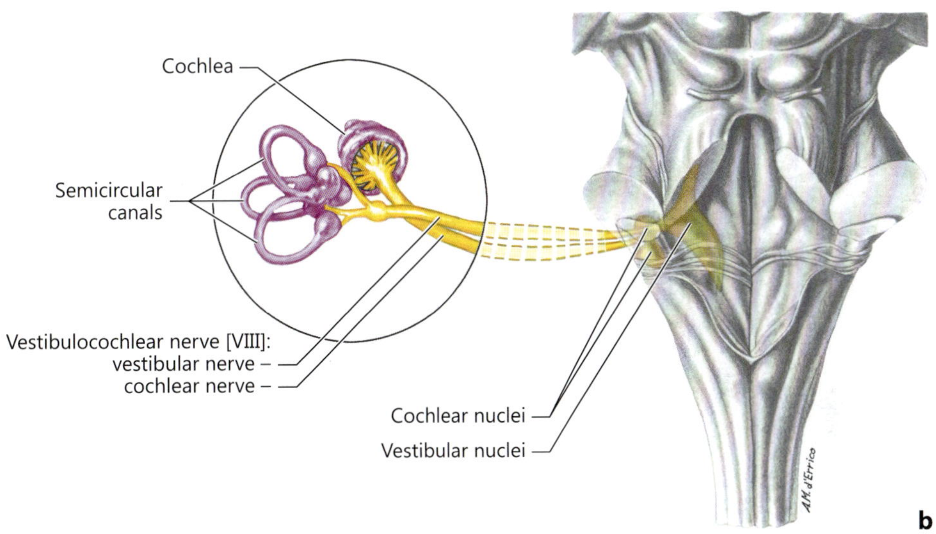

a, Peripheral distribution of the **vestibulocochlear nerve** [VIII]. Branches of the nerve penetrate into the labyrinth through the fundus of the internal acoustic meatus (☞ page 142, volume 1) and are distributed to the macula receptors of the utricle and saccule, to the ampullary crests of the semicircular ducts (vestibular nerve), and to the acoustic receptors of the cochlear duct (cochlear nerve). **b**, The site of the terminal nuclei of the **vestibular** and **cochlear nerves** in the bulbopontine tegmentum is indicated. The two nerves originate from their respective ganglia: the vestibular ganglion (Scarpa's ganglion), and the cochlear, or spiral, ganglion (Corti's ganglion).

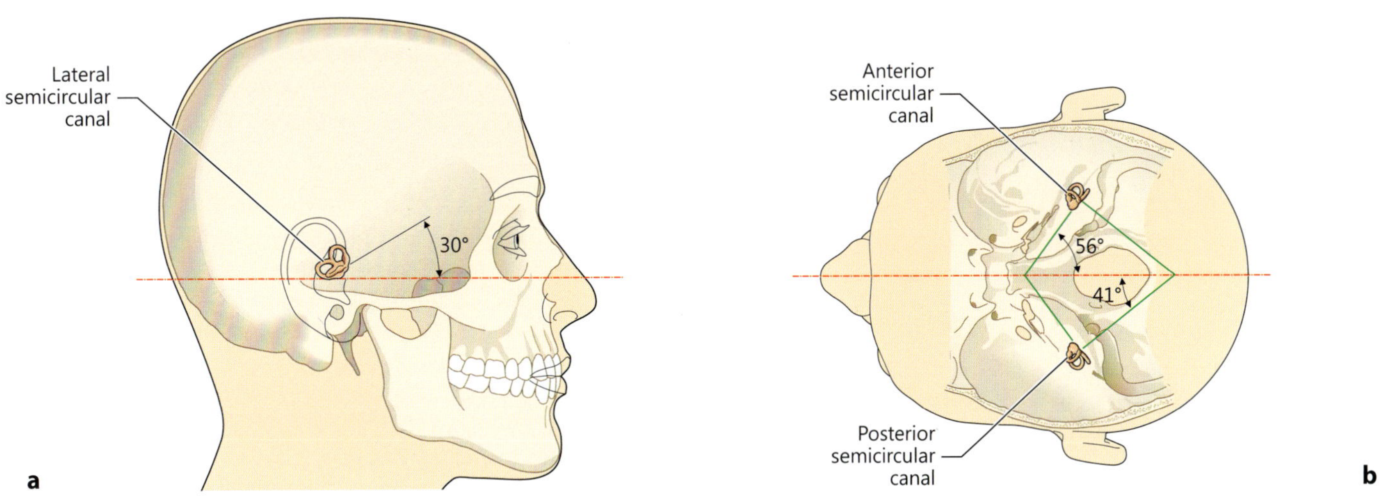

Orientation and angles formed by the **semicircular canals**. The anterior, posterior and lateral semicircular canals are located on the two sides in an orthogonal position (at right angles) to each other. The lateral semicircular canal is almost on a horizontal plane, inclined 30° forward and toward the top (**a**); the other canals are vertical, and oriented with respect to the sagittal plane at 56° (posterior canal) and 41° (anterior canal) (**b**).

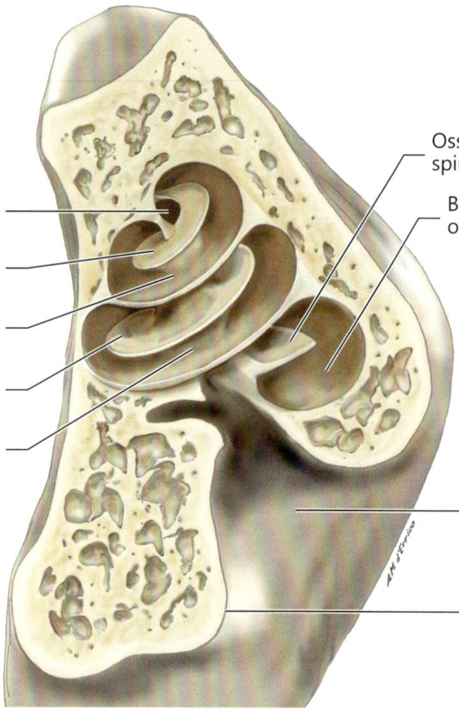

Cochlea, partially open, of the bony labyrinth of the right internal ear. The compact bone tissue of the wall is bounded by spongy bone of the petrous part of the temporal bone.

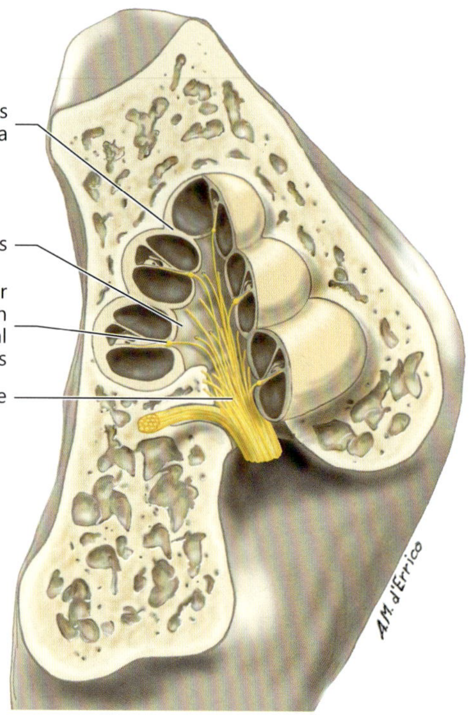

Section of the **cochlea** illustrating the modes of termination of the **cochlear nerve** and the position of the **cochlear**, or spiral, **ganglion** (Corti's ganglion) in the spiral canal of the modiolus.

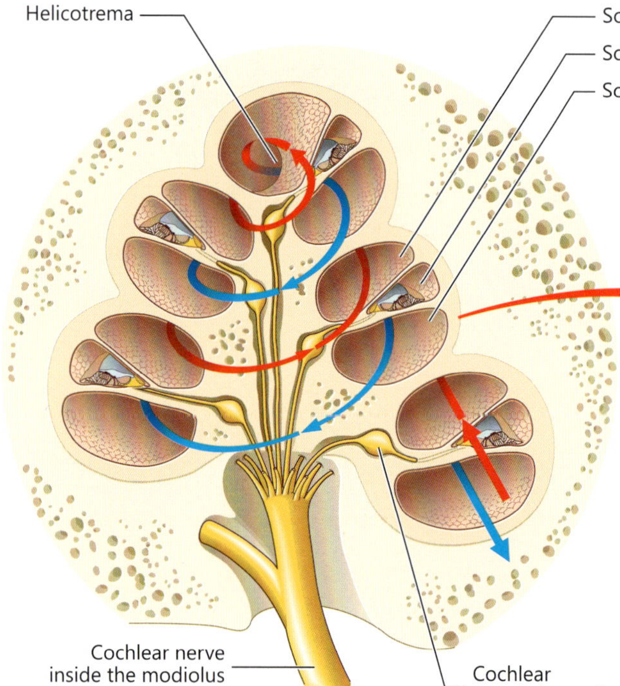

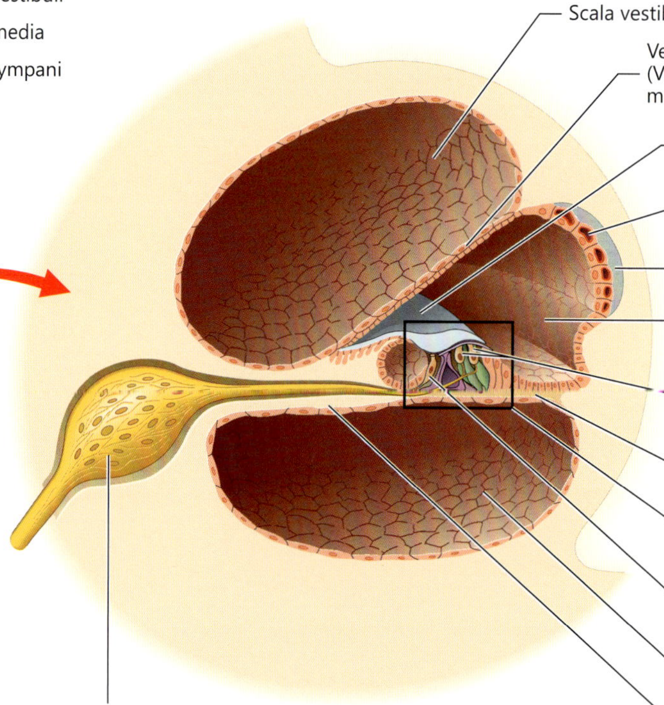

Structure of the **internal ear**. The cochlea is a spiraliform canaliculus that completes two and a half spirals over a length of approximately 35 mm. In its interior, the structures of the cochlear labyrinth demarcate three ducts, or scalae, that run parallel for the whole length. In the enlargement, the relative disposition of the three ducts is illustrated: the scala vestibuli, scala tympani and scala media. The scala media, which has a triangular cross-section, is bordered by three membranes: the basal lamina, on which the spiral organ (or organ of Corti) is found, separates it from the scala tympani; the vestibular surface (vestibular, or Reissner's, membrane) separates it from the scala vestibuli; the stria vascularis forms the boundary with the external surface of the cochlea. Lastly, the scala tympani and scala vestibuli continue, one into the other, through the helicotrema, situated at the apex of the cochlear duct.

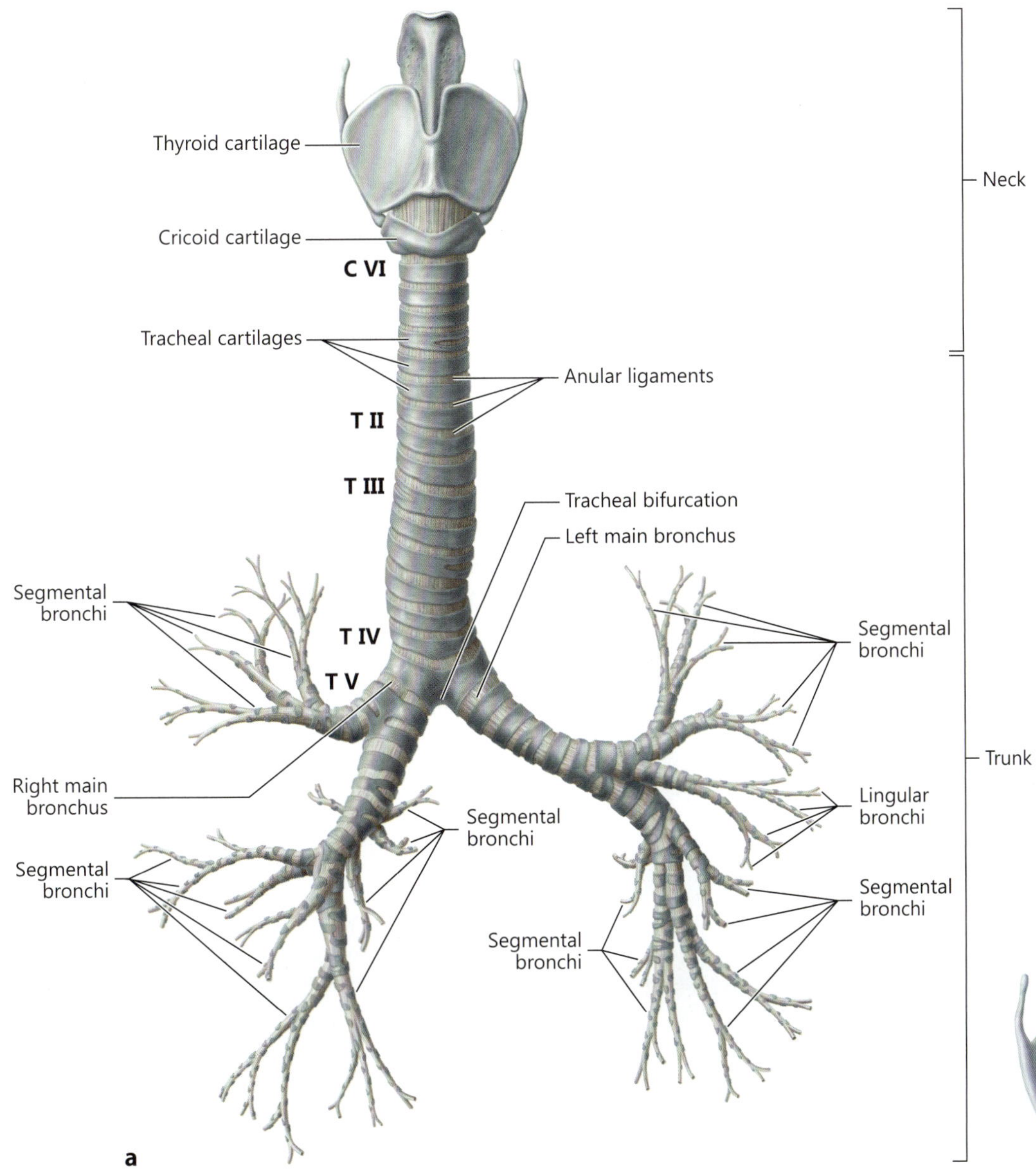

a

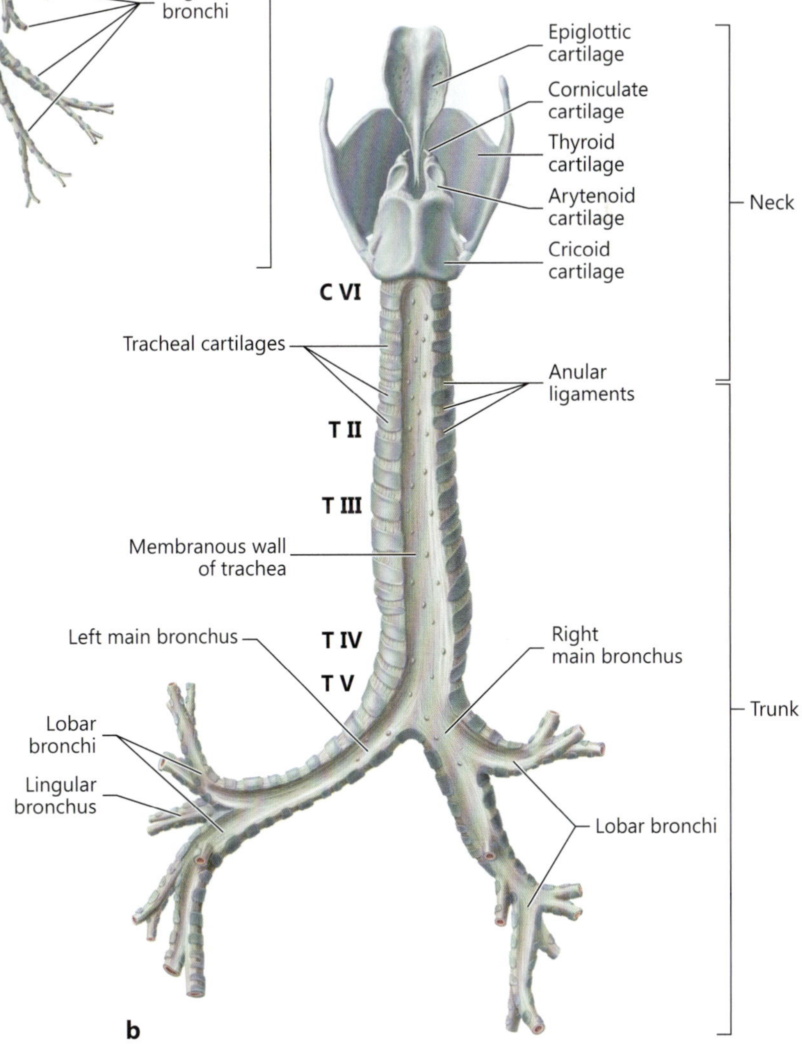

b

a, Anterior projection of the **trachea** and bronchial subdivisions. The trachea extends from the cricoid cartilage of the larynx, at the level of C VI, to the superior margin of T V, at which point it divides into the two main bronchi. The right main bronchus has a more vertical path than the left. **b**, Posterior projection of the **trachea**. The tracheal rings are incomplete posteriorly and continuity of the wall is provided by the membranous part of the trachea.
For more detail on the trachea, see chapter on the thorax.

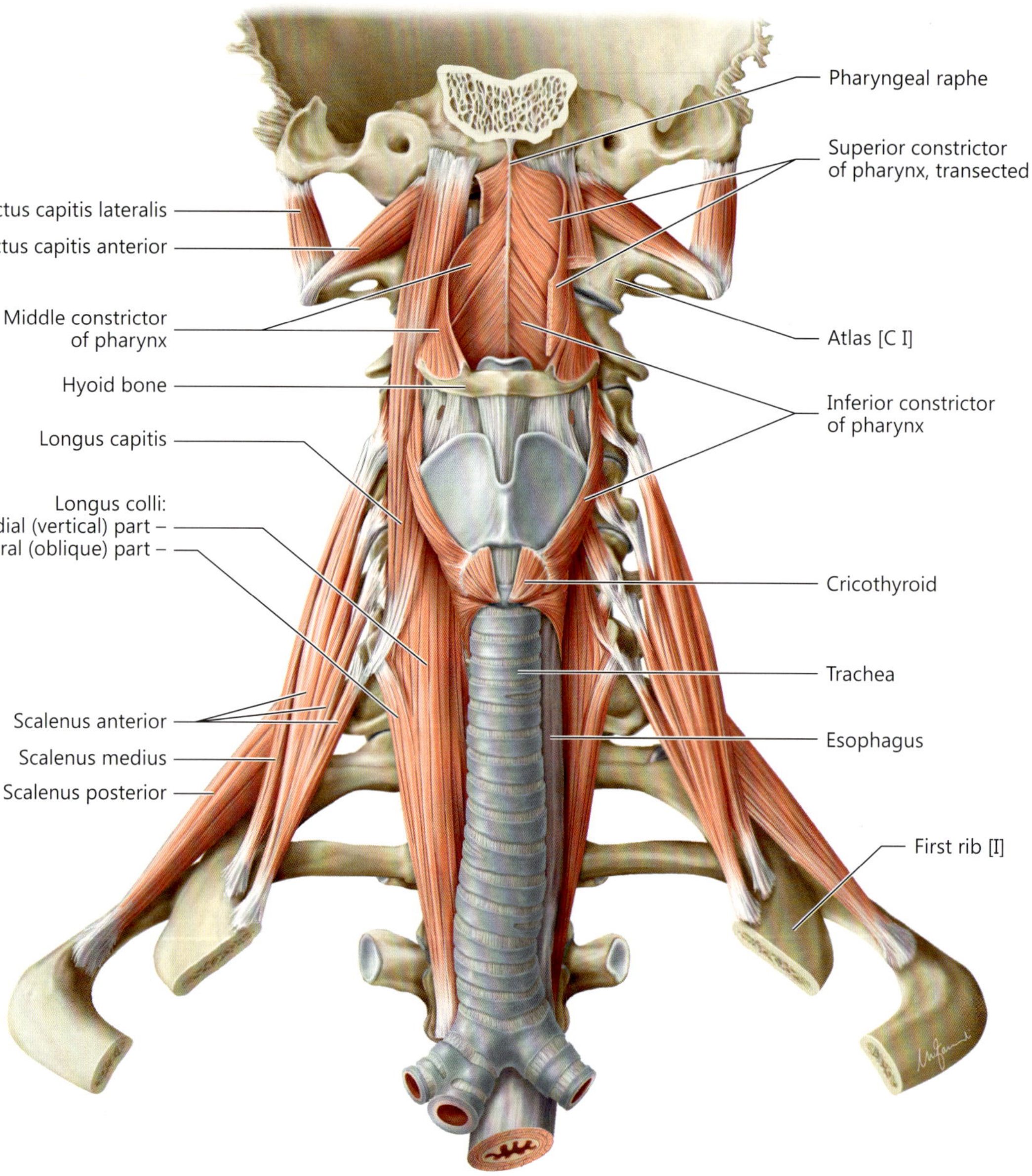

Diagram illustrating the relations of the pharynx, trachea and esophagus with the **prevertebral muscles** of the neck, viewed from the front. The prevertebral muscles of the neck are long muscles that are attached to the ventrolateral surface of the column, and covered by the prevertebral layer of cervical fascia; at the side of the prevertebral muscles are displayed the scalene muscles (scalenus anterior, scalenus medius and scalenus posterior). The prevertebral muscles stretch from the cranial base to the cervical column, whereas the scalene muscles go from the cervical column to the superior part of the thorax.
For a further description of the pharynx, see pages 145-147.

Infrahyoid muscles in relation to the larynx, anterior view. The sternohyoid and omohyoid are located on a more superficial plane, the sternothyroid and thyrohyoid are situated more deeply in direct contact with the larynx.

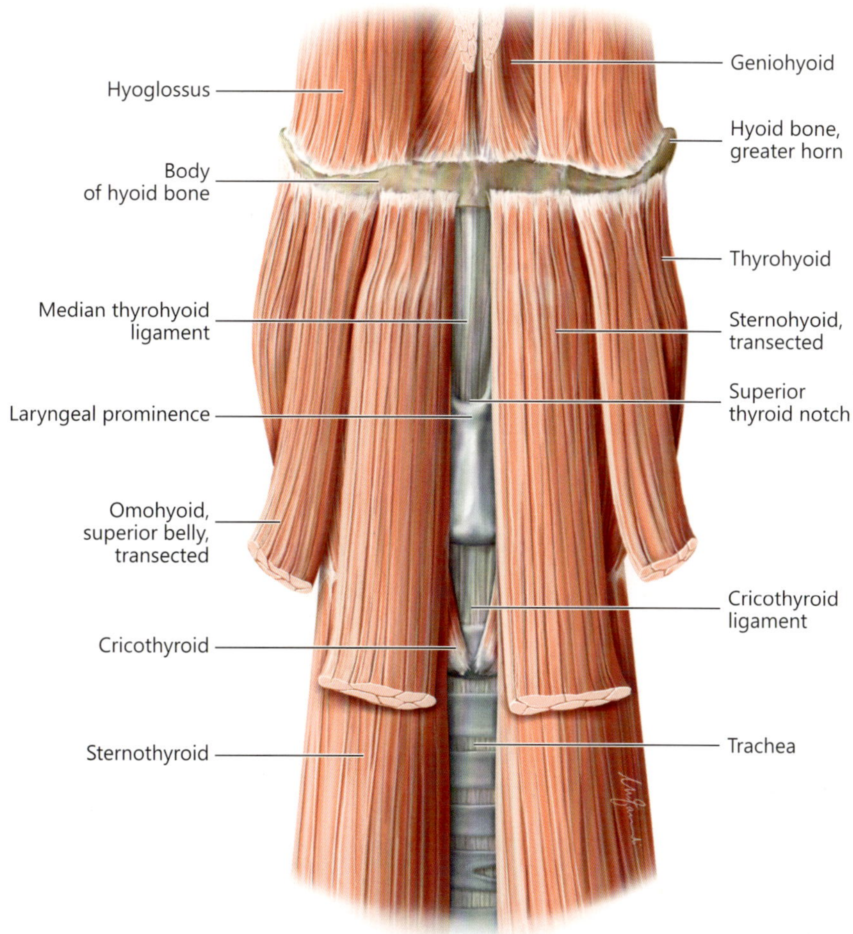

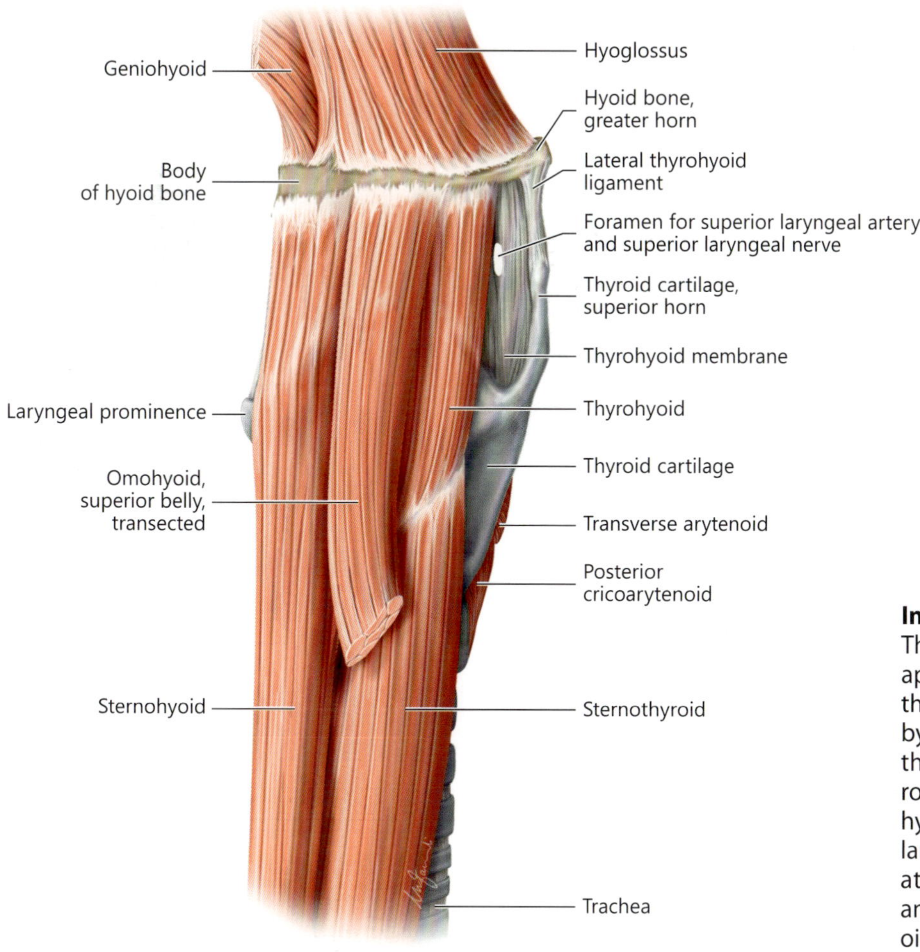

Infrahyoid muscles, left lateral view. The laryngeal prominence, or Adam's apple, is the most protuberant part of the angle formed on the median line by the two laminae, right and left, of the thyroid cartilage. The sternothyroid is situated deeply to the sternohyoid and unites the sternum to the larynx. The thyrohyoid is the continuation upwards of the sternothyroid and, situated deeply to the sternohyoid, it extends to the hyoid bone.

After removal of the infrahyoid muscles, one can see the **thyroid cartilage** of the larynx with the ligaments that connect it to the hyoid bone (**thyrohyoid membrane**, **median** and **lateral thyrohyoid ligaments**), and the **median cricothyroid ligament** of the cricothyroid joint. When the **cricothyroid** contracts it tends to elongate the vocal ligament, and is hence also called the tensor muscle of the vocal cords.

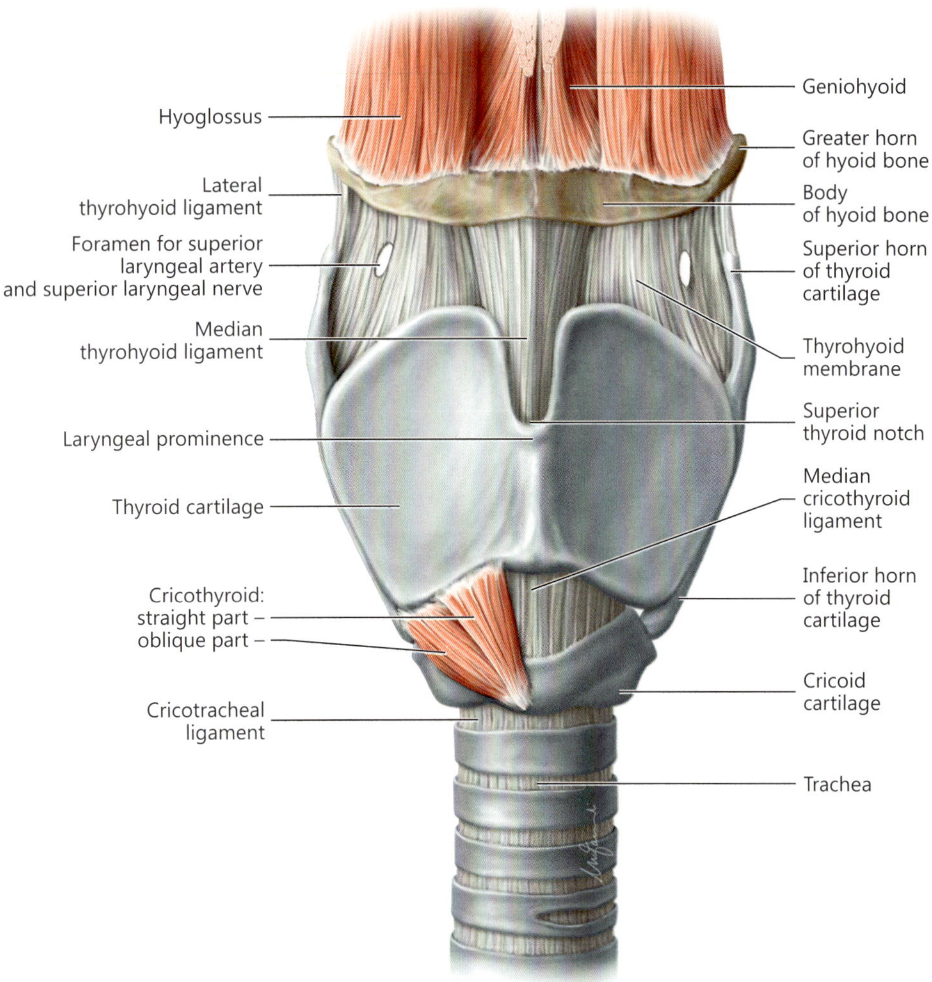

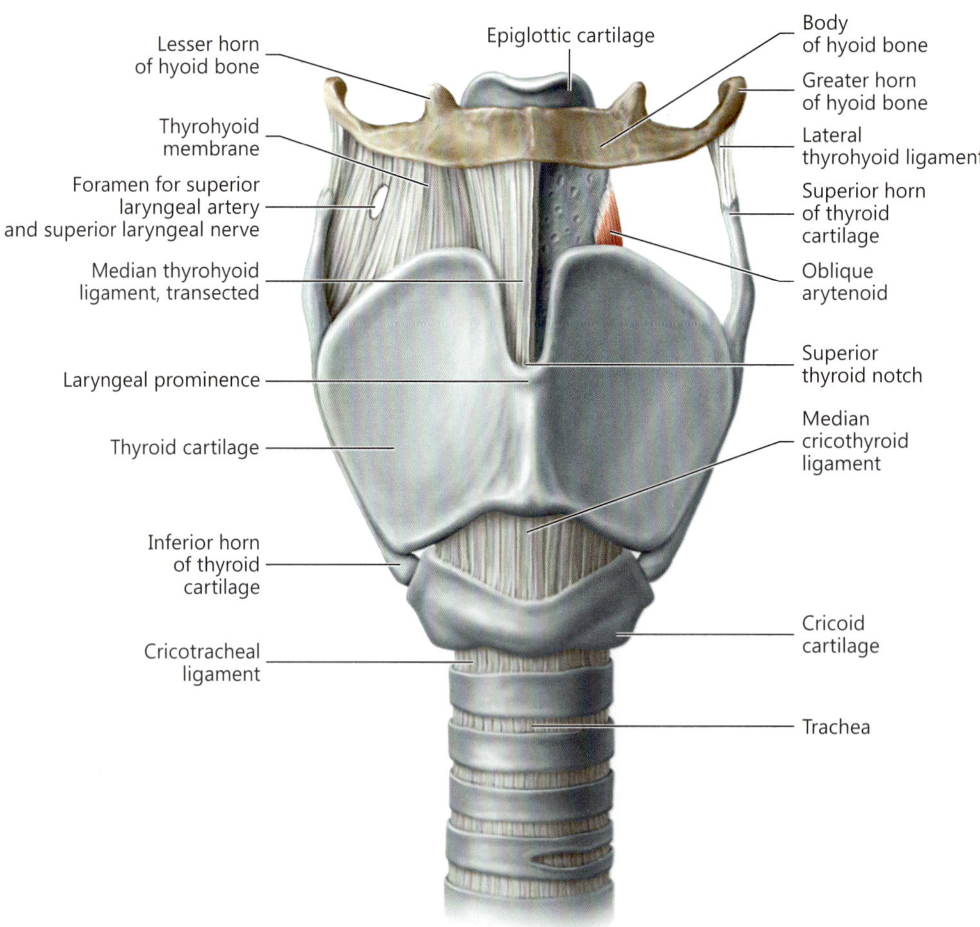

External configuration of the larynx, anterior view. One can see the relation of the organ to the hyoid bone, superiorly, and to the trachea, inferiorly. In the left part of the larynx, the thyrohyoid membrane and median thyrohyoid ligament have been removed so as to display the **oblique arytenoid**.

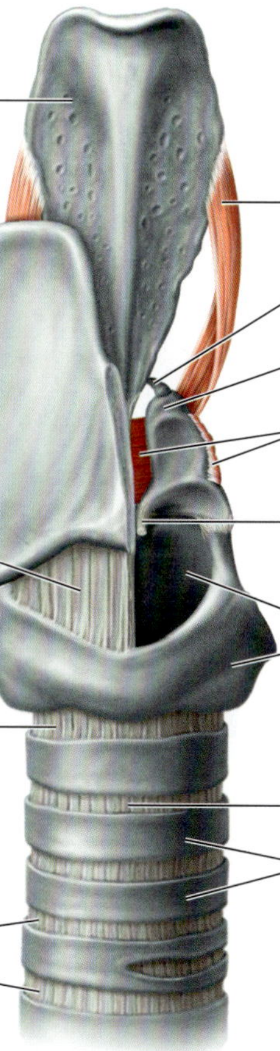

Larynx, anterior view. In the right half of the larynx, the thyroid cartilage and median cricothyroid ligament can be seen; in the left half, they have been transected to expose the arytenoid and corniculate cartilages, the **oblique and transverse arytenoid**, and the arch of the cricoid cartilage.

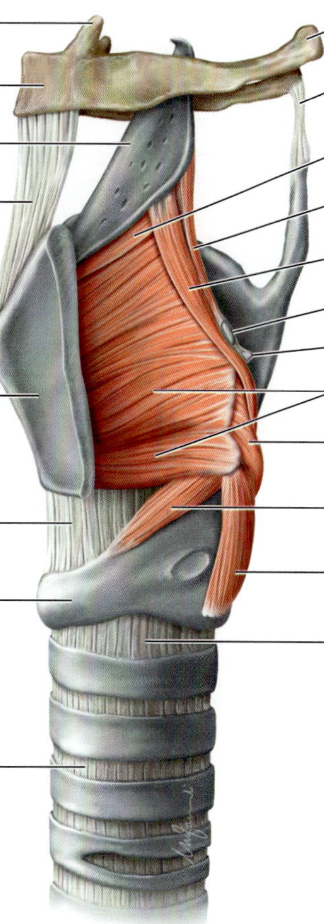

Muscles of the larynx, left lateral view, after demolition of the left lamina of the thyroid cartilage. The thyroarytenoid (above) and lateral cricoarytenoid (below) form part of the lateral wall of the larynx.

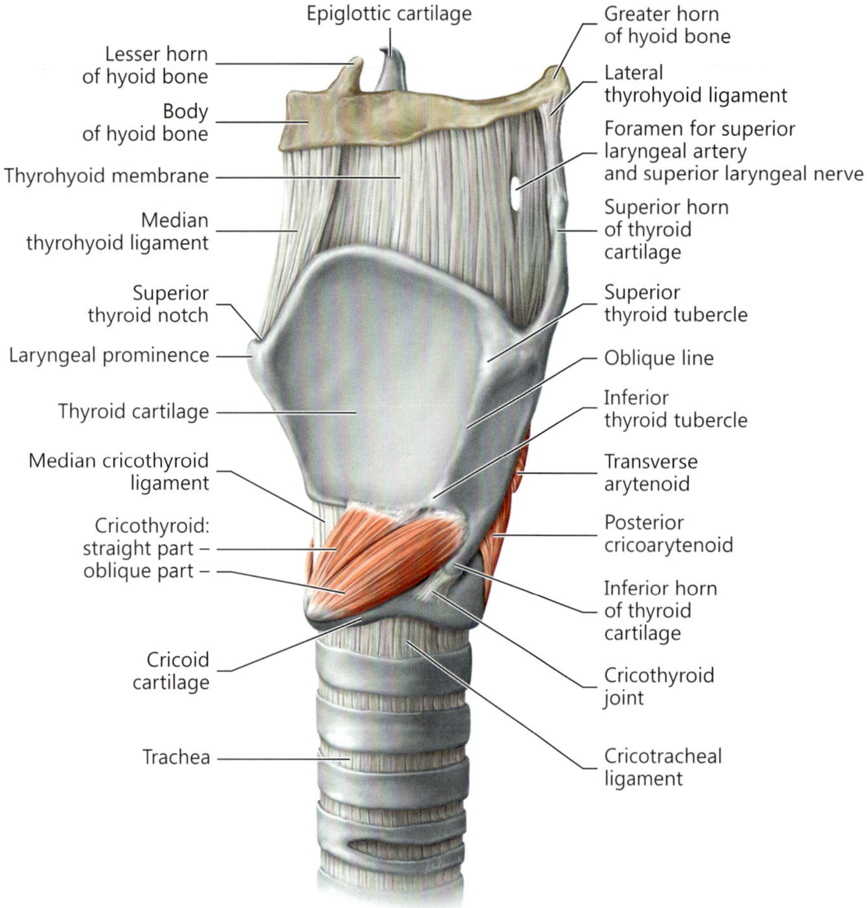

Cricothyroid, left lateral view. One can distinguish the two parts of the muscle: the straight part (medial) and the oblique part (lateral).

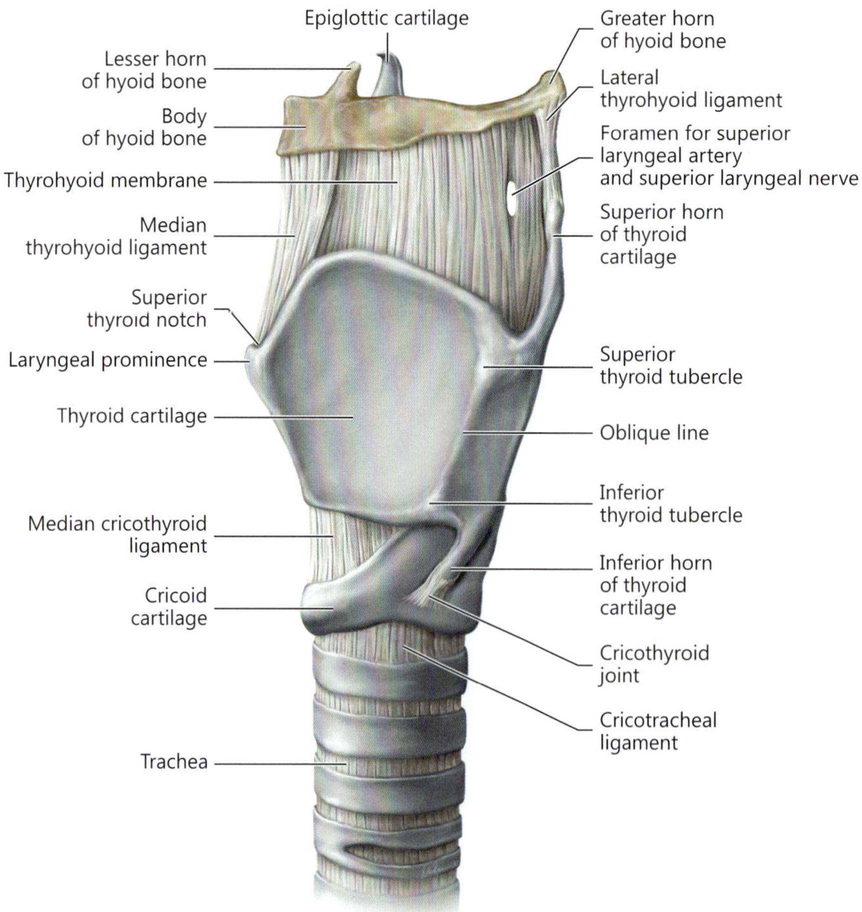

Principal means of union of the **laryngeal cartilages**, left lateral view. One can also see the connections and relations of the larynx with the hyoid bone (above) and trachea (below).

Larynx and **trachea**, posterior view. The arytenoid cartilages provide attachment for all the intrinsic laryngeal muscles except the cricothyroid muscles. Here one can see the **posterior cricoarytenoid muscles**, the **oblique arytenoid** (or aryepiglottic) **muscles** with their aryepiglottic parts, and the **transverse arytenoid**.

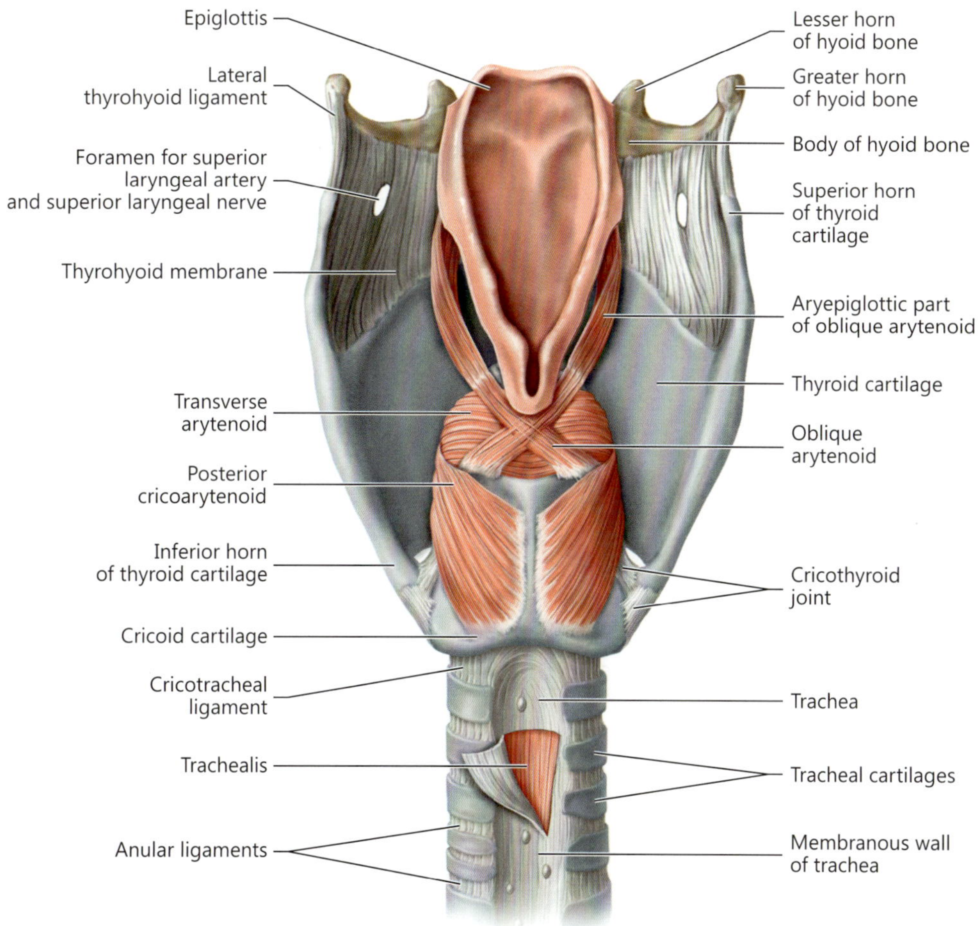

Larynx and **trachea**, posterior view. One can see the unpaired cartilages of the larynx: the thyroid, cricoid, and epiglottic cartilages. The corniculate cartilages, hook-like in form, surmount the apices of the arytenoid cartilages, which have the form of a triangular pyramid whose posterior concave surface corresponds to the **transverse arytenoid**, stretching between the lateral borders of the two arytenoid cartilages. The **posterior cricoarytenoid muscles** are situated behind the cricoid cartilage, below the mucosa of the pharynx. The cervical part of the trachea includes the first 5 to 6 tracheal rings. The tracheal rings are incomplete posteriorly, where they are continuous with the membranous wall of the trachea.

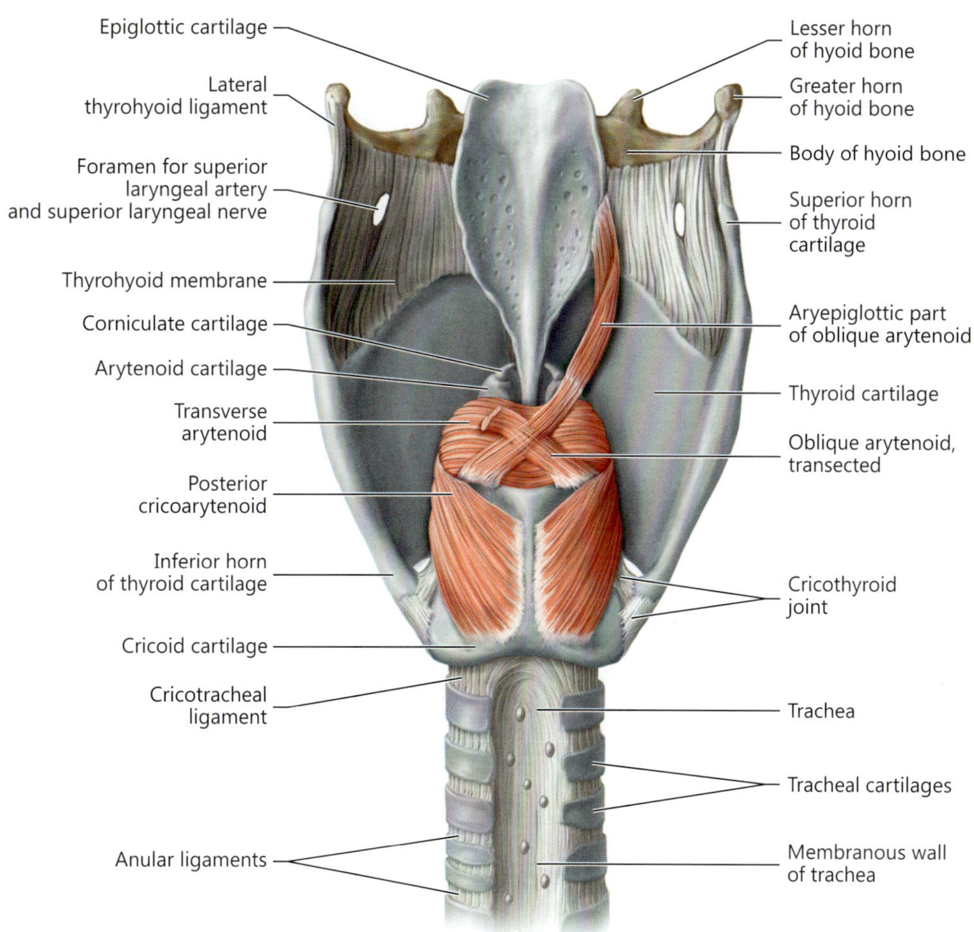

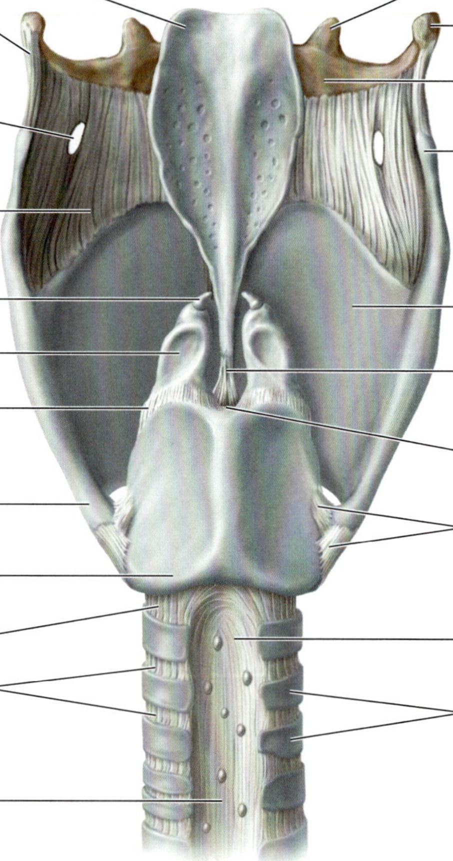

Larynx and **trachea**, posterior view. After removal of the intrinsic muscles of the larynx, one can see the laryngeal cartilages: the epiglottic cartilage, which unites with the thyroid cartilage through the thyroepiglottic ligament; the thyroid cartilage, which articulates with the cricoid cartilage through the inferior horns; the arytenoid cartilages, which sit on the arytenoid articular surfaces of the lamina of the cricoid cartilage; the corniculate cartilages, which are connected to the apices of the arytenoid cartilages; and the cricoid cartilage which, besides articulating with the thyroid and arytenoid cartilages, is united by means of the cricotracheal ligament to the first tracheal ring.

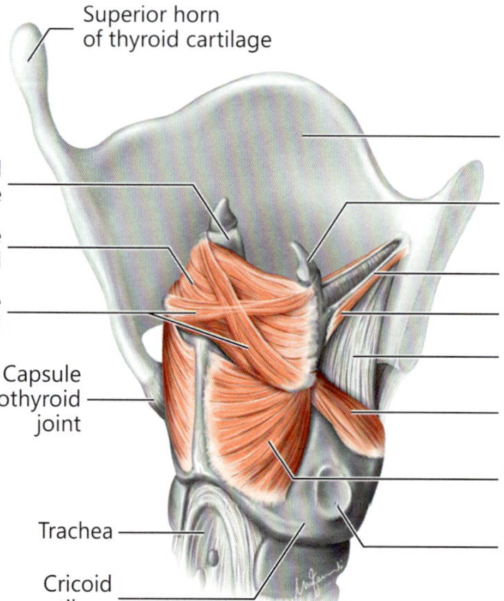

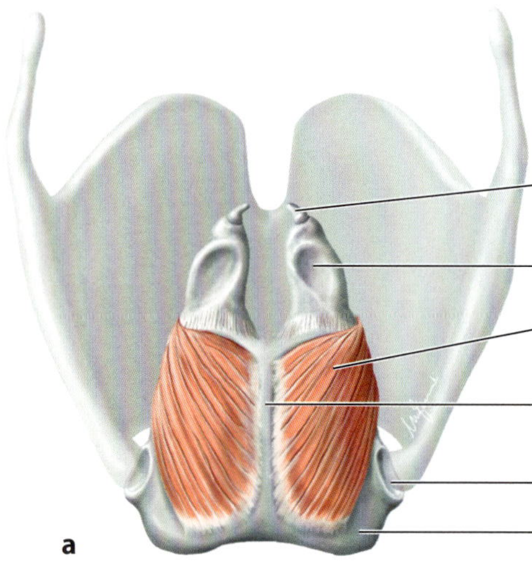

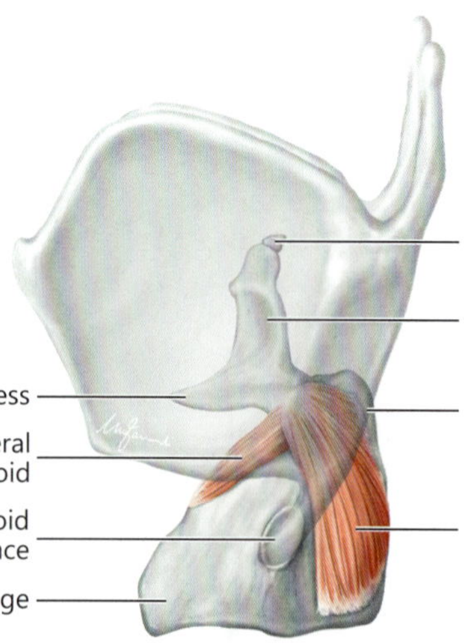

Cricoarytenoid muscles. **a**, Posterior view of the larynx showing the posterior cricoarytenoid. **b**, Posterolateral projection. The epiglottic cartilage has been removed and the right lamina of the thyroid cartilage transected. One can see the conus elasticus and the vocal ligament, which together with the vocalis constitutes the vocal fold, or true vocal cord, stretching from the internal surface of the thyroid cartilage, immediately under the notch, to the vocal process of the arytenoid cartilage. **c**, The left lateral projection enables one also to see the characteristic position of the lateral cricoarytenoid.

Larynx, view looking down from behind. The thyroarytenoid has been transected in the right half to expose the vocalis. Also visible are the straight and oblique parts of the cricothyroid and the lateral cricoarytenoid. Posteriorly, one can see the transverse arytenoid, covered by the oblique arytenoid muscles, and, behind the cricoid cartilage, the posterior cricoarytenoid muscles.

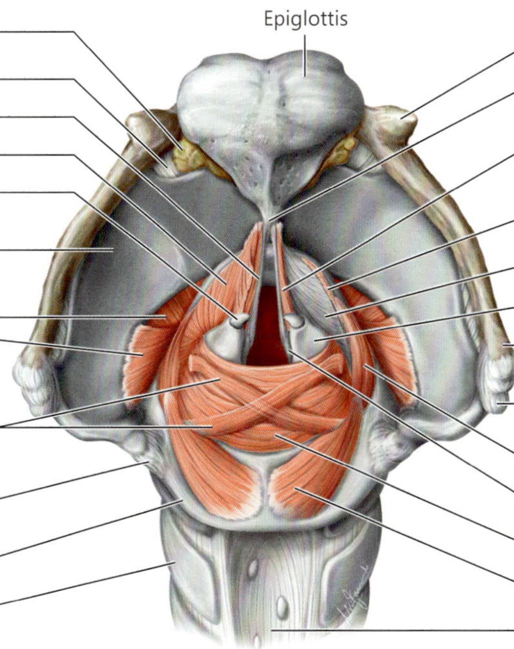

Larynx, view looking down from behind. After removal of the posterior cricoarytenoid muscles, transverse arytenoid and oblique arytenoid muscles, one can see the lamina of the cricoid cartilage and the arytenoid cartilages, whose vocal processes with their apices continue in the vocal ligaments.

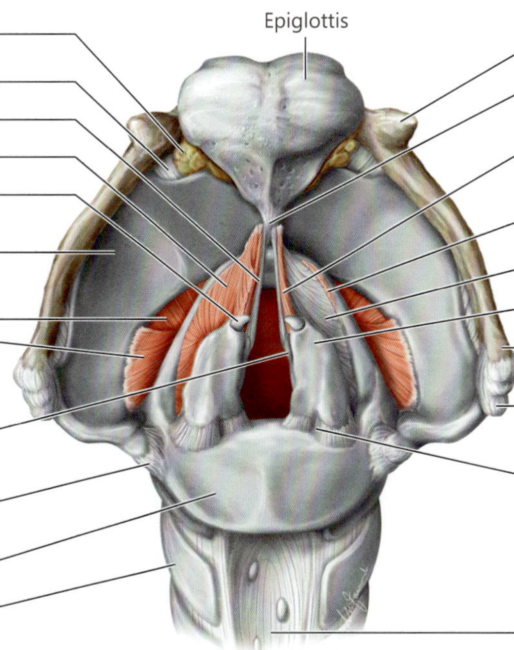

Larynx, superior view. With the muscles of the larynx removed, one can clearly see the conus elasticus, which, inferiorly, inserts on the superior circumference of the ring of the cricoid cartilage, while, at the top, it narrows and flattens into two laminae that terminate with the vocal ligament. Also visible are the vocal and muscular processes at the base of the arytenoid cartilages.

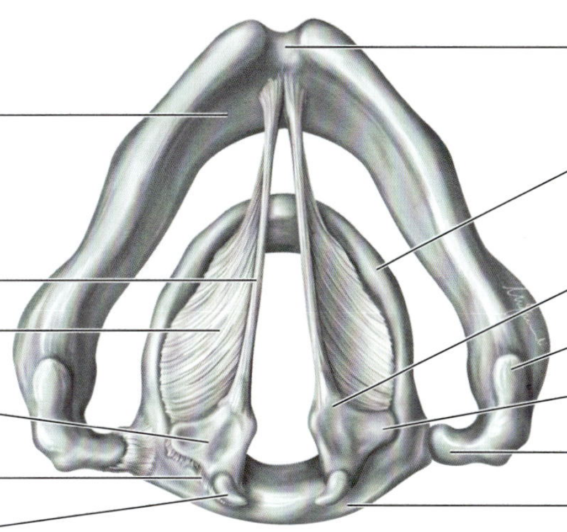

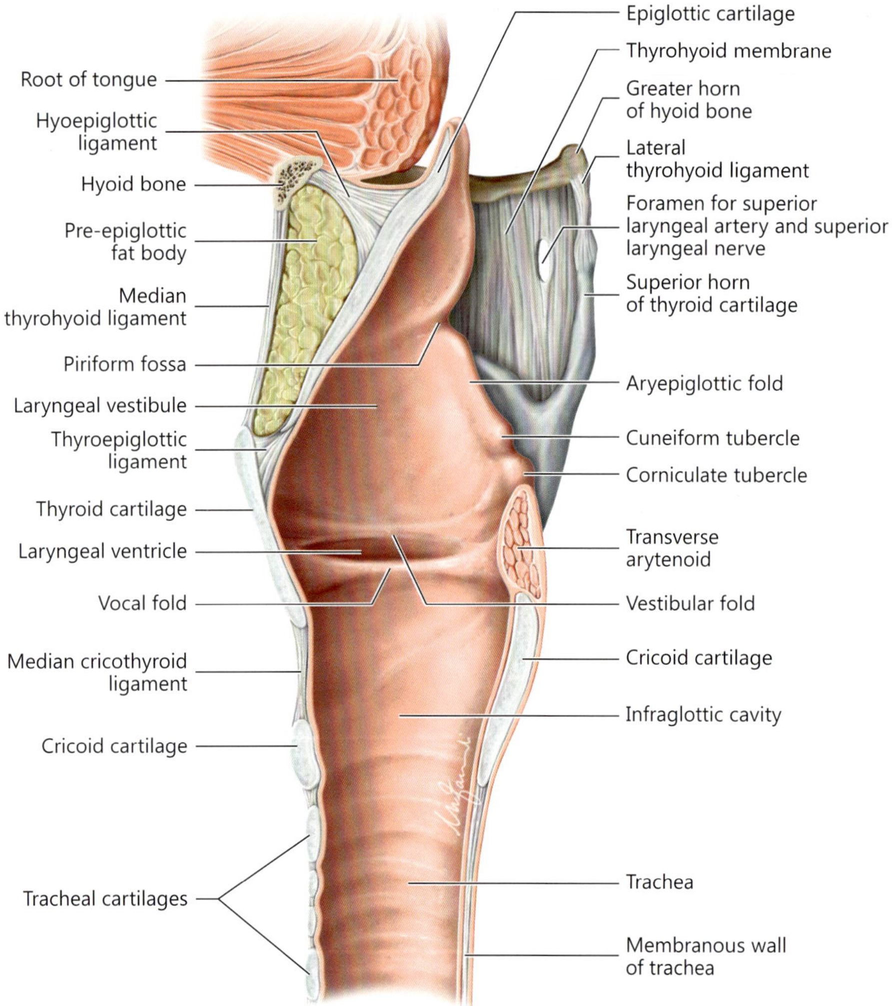

Median sagittal section of the **larynx**. One can see the laryngeal cavity, whose intermediate portion presents a sagittal fissure due to the presence, on each side, of two horizontal anatomical features oriented anteroposteriorly: the *vestibular folds*, above, and the *vocal folds*, below.

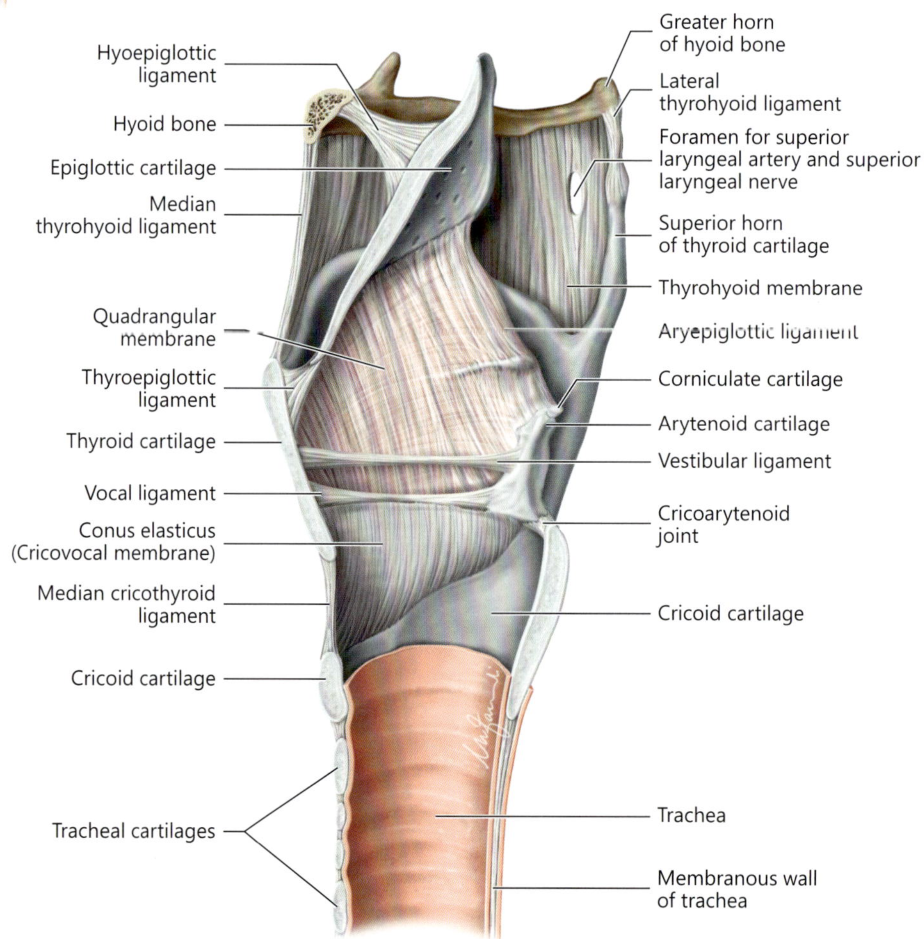

Median sagittal section of the **larynx**. One can see, in particular: the vestibular ligament, which represents the scaffold supporting the vestibular fold, or false vocal cord; the conus elasticus, whose free edge, thickened, is the vocal ligament, which together with the vocalis constitutes the vocal fold, or true vocal cord; and the quadrangular membrane, whose posterosuperior margin, free and thickened, forms the aryepiglottic ligament, while its inferior one, also thickened, constitutes the vestibular ligament.

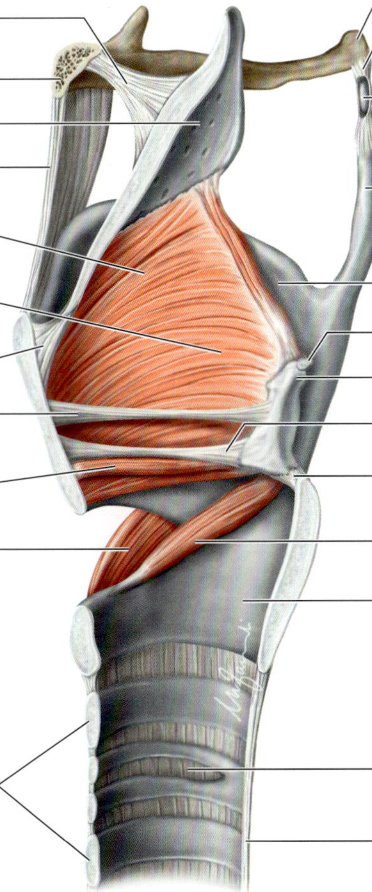

Median sagittal section of the **larynx**. The following muscles can be seen: the vocalis, the isometric contraction of which places the vocal ligament under tension (the vocal ligament and vocalis together constitute the vocal fold, or true vocal cord); the lateral cricoarytenoid; the cricothyroid, also known as the tensor muscle of the vocal cords because, contracting, it tenses and elongates the vocal ligament; and the thyroarytenoid, of which one can distinguish, besides the thyroepiglottic part or thyroepiglottic muscle, also a lateral bundle and a medial bundle or, as otherwise known (the latter), the vocalis.

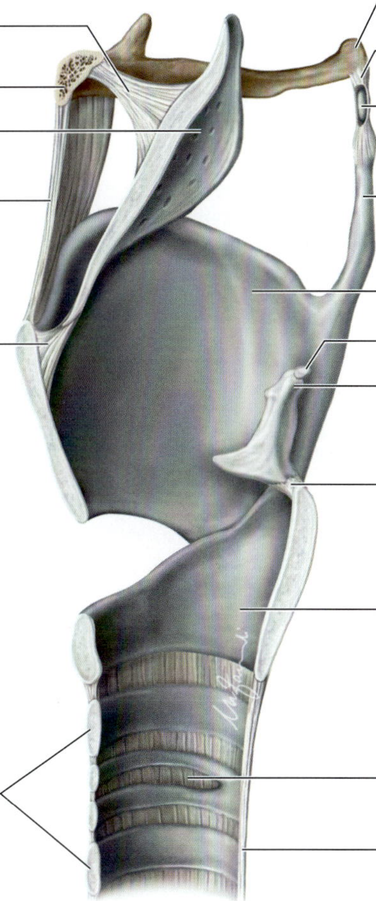

Median sagittal section of the **larynx**. One can distinguish the various cartilaginous elements articulated one to another for contiguity and united at a distance by means of ligaments. Here are shown the thyroepiglottic ligament and the hyoepiglottic ligament, which connects the epiglottic cartilage of the larynx to the hyoid bone, contributing to the return of the epiglottis after swallowing.

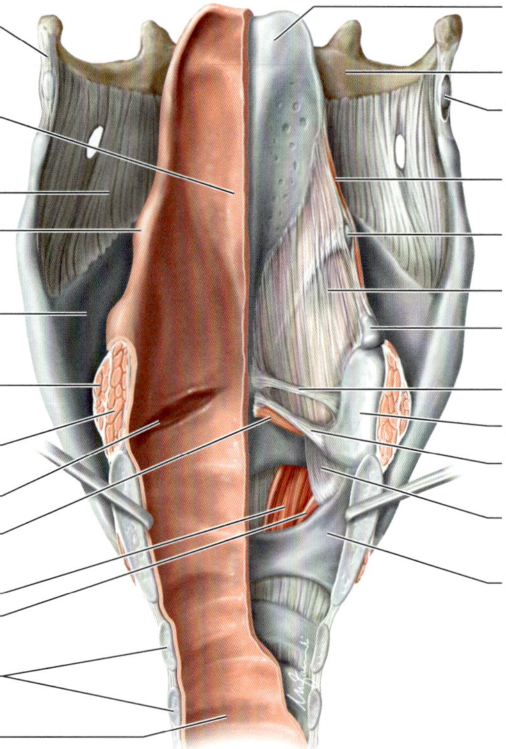

Larynx, posterior view after transecting the arytenoid muscles and cricoid cartilage. In the left half, one can see the laryngeal cavity covered by the mucosa of the larynx with, in succession from top to bottom, the laryngeal inlet, laryngeal vestibule, laryngeal ventricle, glottis and infraglottic cavity. In the right half, with the mucosa removed, the quadrangular membrane with the vestibular ligament is visible as well as the conus elasticus with the vocal ligament.

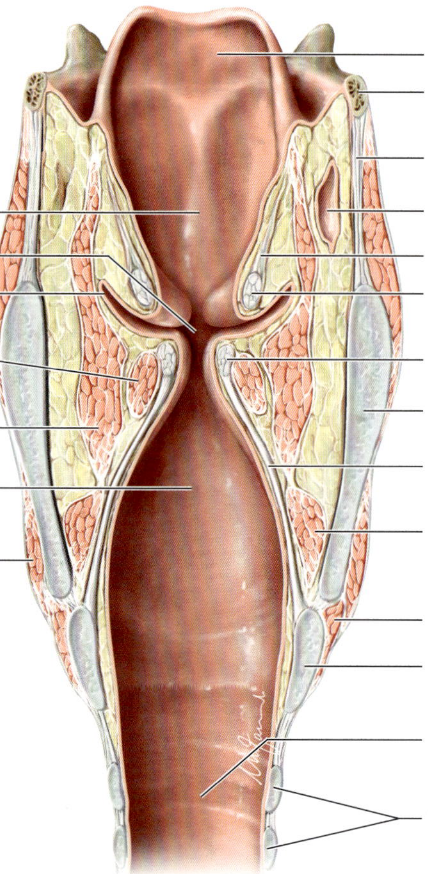

Frontal section of the **larynx**, posterior view of the anterior part. One can see the laryngeal vestibule, between the laryngeal inlet and the rima vestibuli, situated among the vestibular folds, which contain in their thickness the vestibular ligament. The vocal folds are situated below the vestibular folds and delimit the rima glottidis, the narrowest point of the laryngeal cavity. They contain in their anterior part the vocal ligament and the vocalis. The infraglottic cavity extends between the glottis and a plane passing through the inferior margin of the cricoid cartilage, narrowing as it descends.

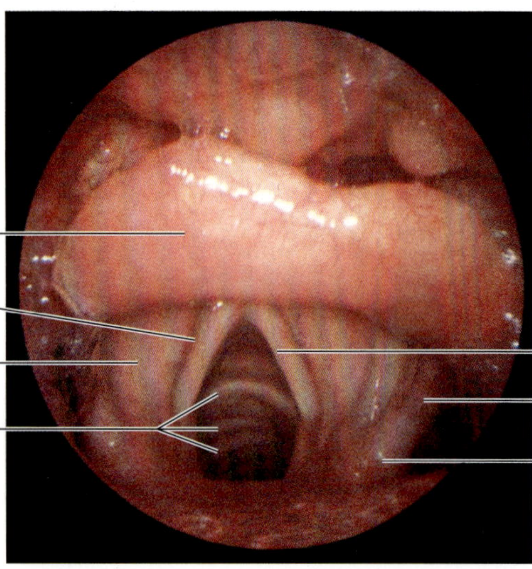

Rima glottidis observed with the laryngoscope. The vocal folds (true vocal cords) are found below the vestibular folds (ventricular folds or false vocal cords). The free edge of each true vocal cord protrudes toward the laryngeal cavity and delimits, with that of the other side, the rima glottidis, triangular in shape with its apex in front, corresponding to the apex of the thyroid cartilage, and its base behind, between the arytenoid cartilages.

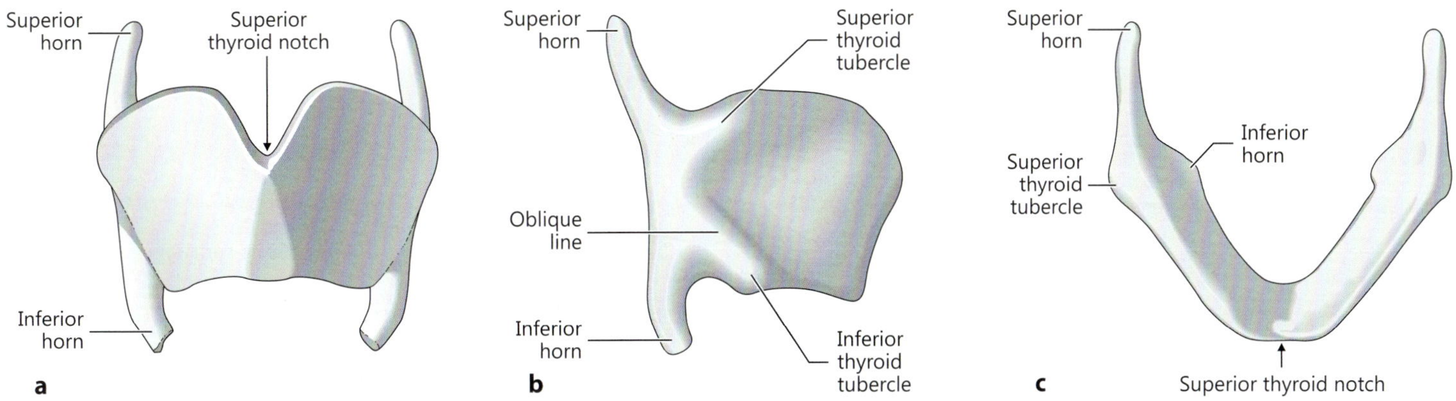

Thyroid cartilage in the male, viewed in anterior (**a**), lateral (**b**) and superior (**c**) projection.

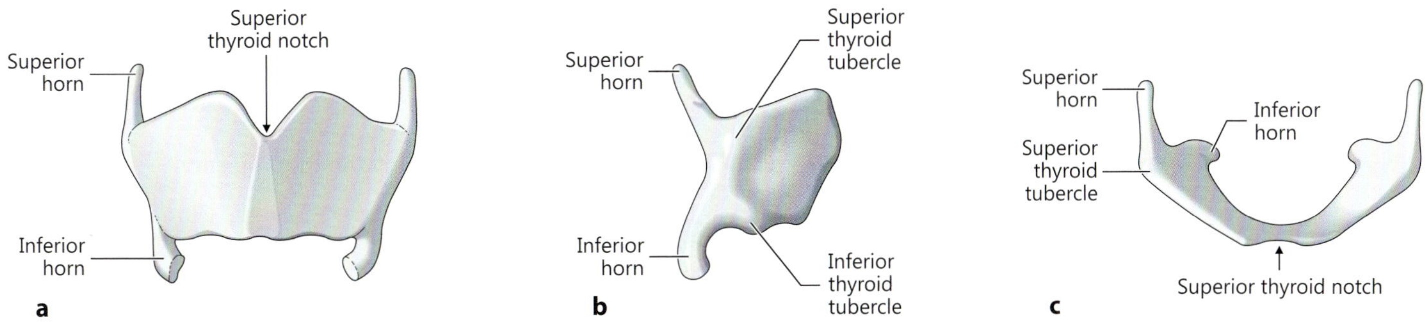

Thyroid cartilage in the female, in anterior (**a**), lateral (**b**) and superior (**c**) projection. Compared to the male larynx, numerous differences can be seen in the conformation of the thyroid cartilage. In particular, the angle formed by the two laminae of the thyroid cartilage, right and left, at the point where they meet in the laryngeal prominence is much wider in the female than in the male.

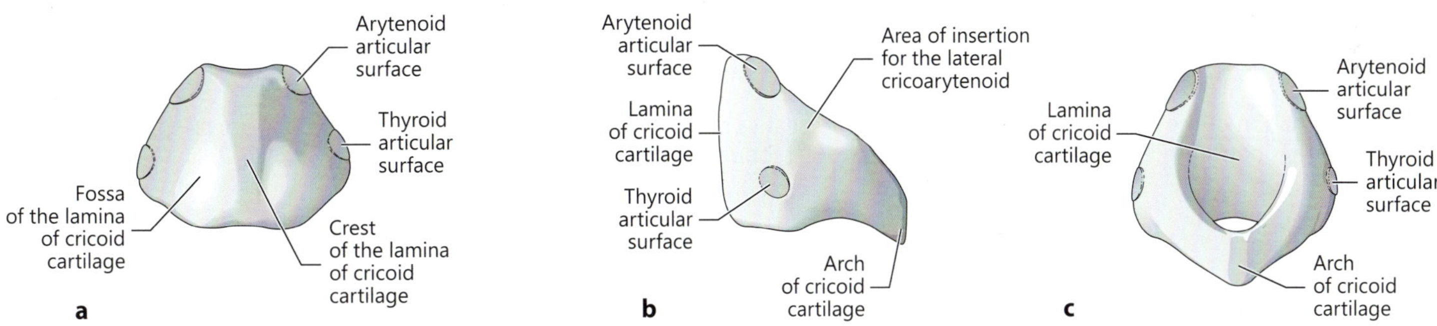

Cricoid cartilage in the male, viewed in dorsal (**a**), lateral (**b**) and anterior (**c**) projection. The areas indicated in *darker gray* correspond to the articular surfaces.

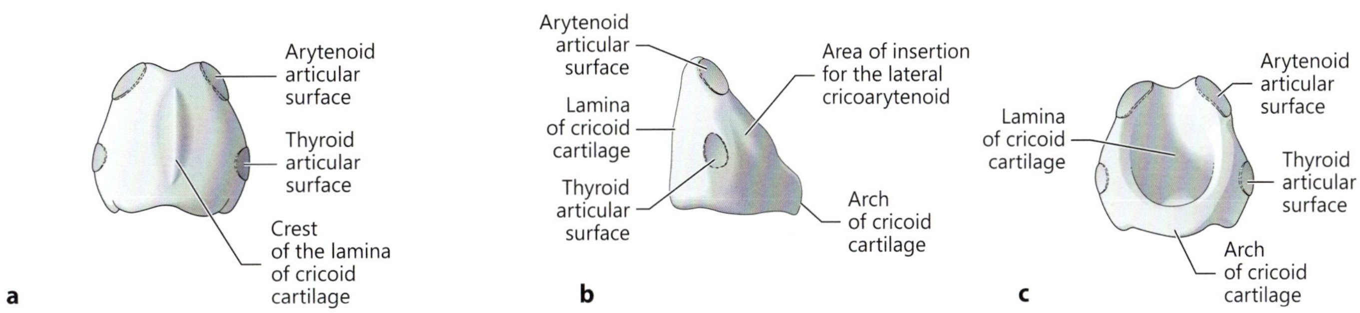

Cricoid cartilage in the female, viewed in dorsal (**a**), lateral (**b**) and anterior (**c**) projection. The cavity demarcated by the cartilaginous ring is more rounded compared to the male larynx.

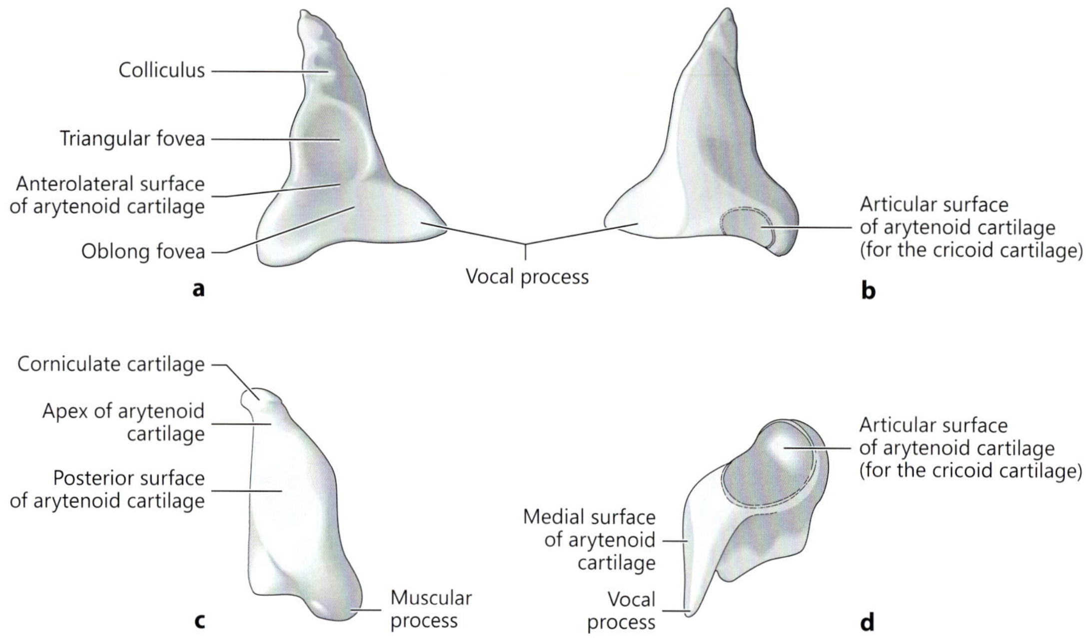

Right arytenoid cartilage of a male, in lateral (**a**), medial (**b**), posterior (**c**) and inferior (**d**) projection.

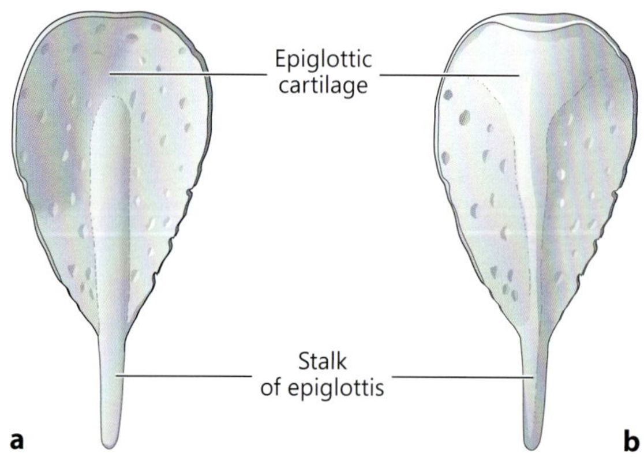

Conformation of the **epiglottic cartilage** and characteristics of its dorsal (**a**) and ventral (**b**) surfaces. The dorsal surface of the cartilage is perforated by small pits that lodge glandular lobules.

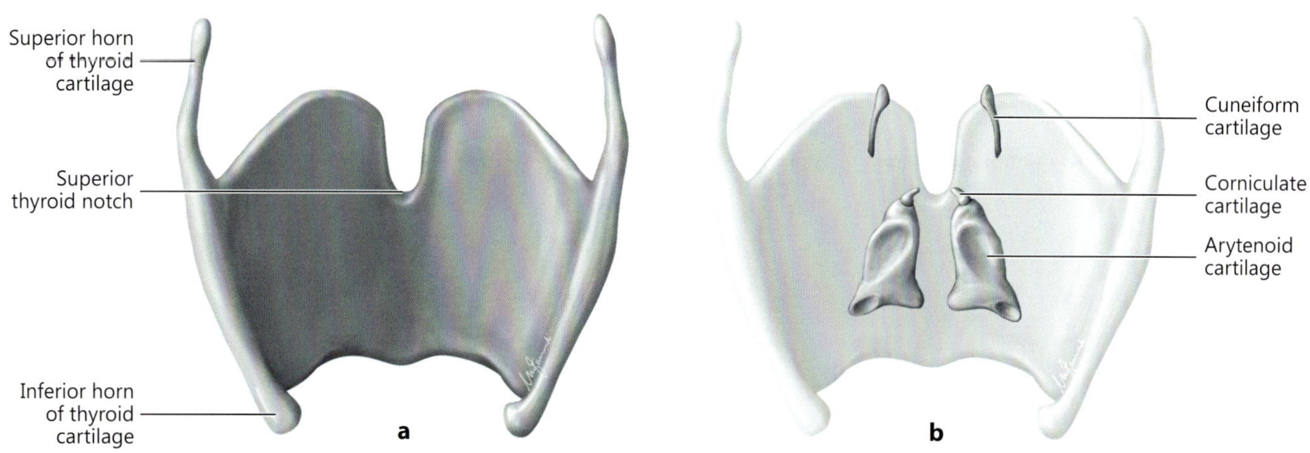

Cartilages of the larynx. **a**, Posterior view of the thyroid cartilage, which is located in the anterior, lateral and superior part of the larynx. **b**, The arytenoid cartilages, connected to which are the corniculate cartilages, are located in the superior and posterior part of the larynx. The cuneiform cartilages, parallel to the anterior margin of the arytenoid cartilages, are considered to be detached fragments of the epiglottic cartilage that run in the thickness of the quadrangular membrane. The posterior pole of the cuneiform cartilage, facing backwards and upwards, is responsible for the formation of the cuneiform tubercle that can be seen in the aryepiglottic fold.

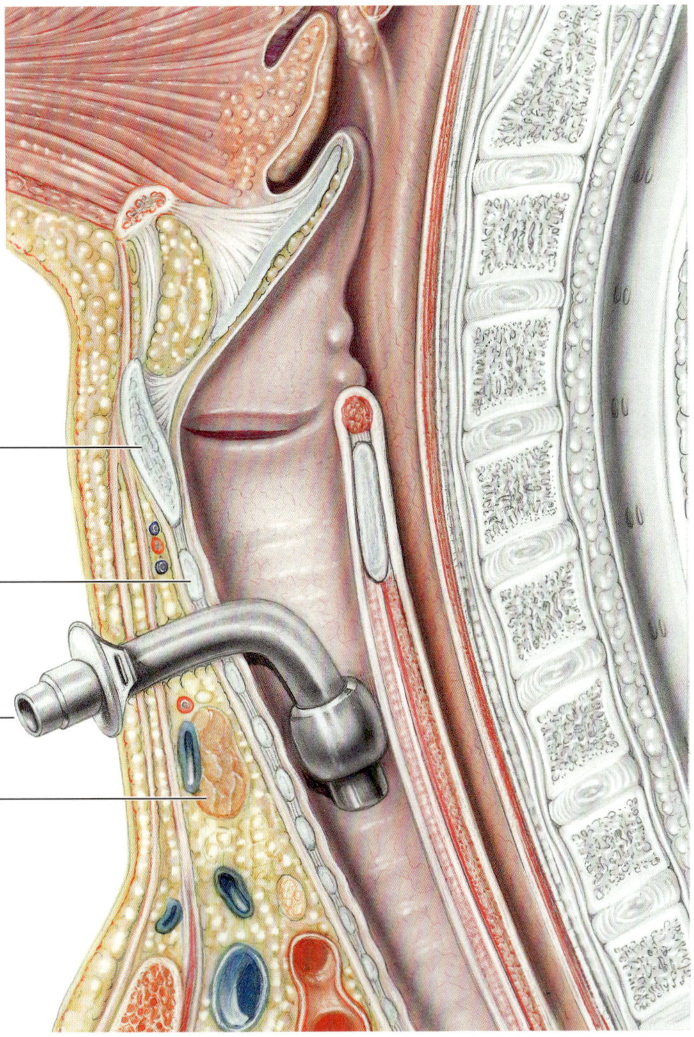

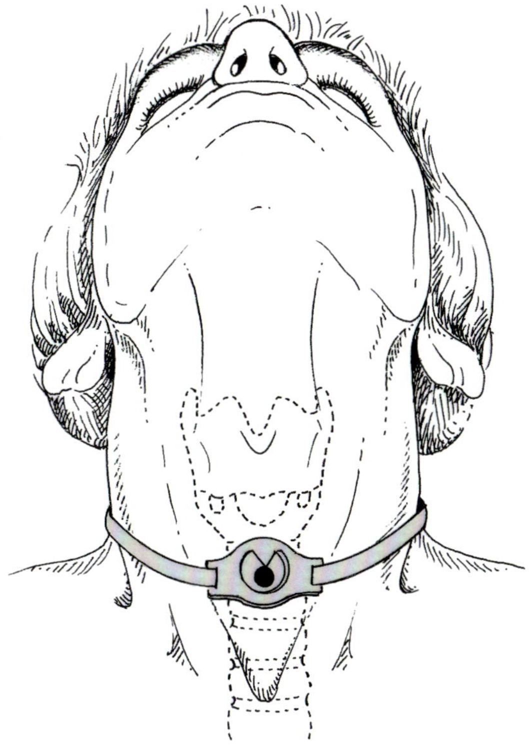

A **tracheotomy** consists of an incision of the trachea made in the neck, to connect the trachea itself with the exterior. Through the incision a cannula is introduced which allows air to reach the lungs.

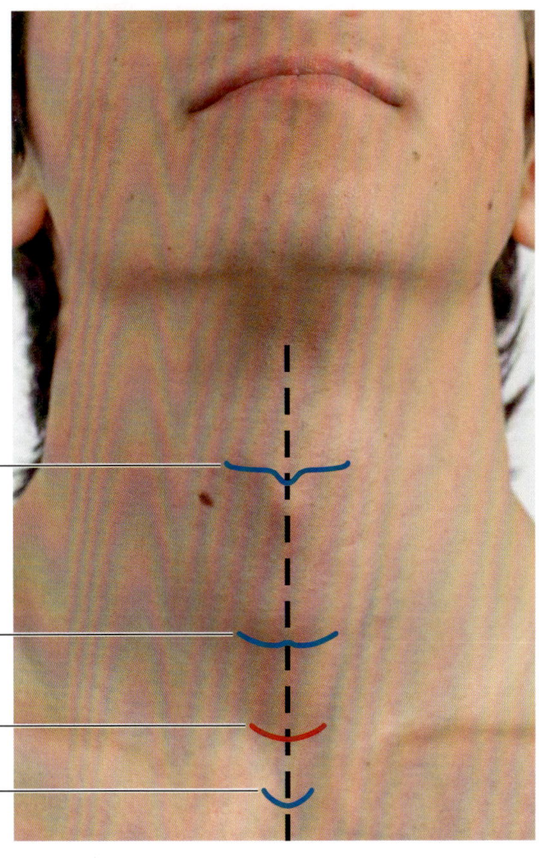

Landmarks for the tracheotomy. By palpation one can identify the two laminae and the superior notch of the thyroid cartilage. The location of the jugular notch corresponds to the superior border of the manubrium of the sternum between the clavicular notches.

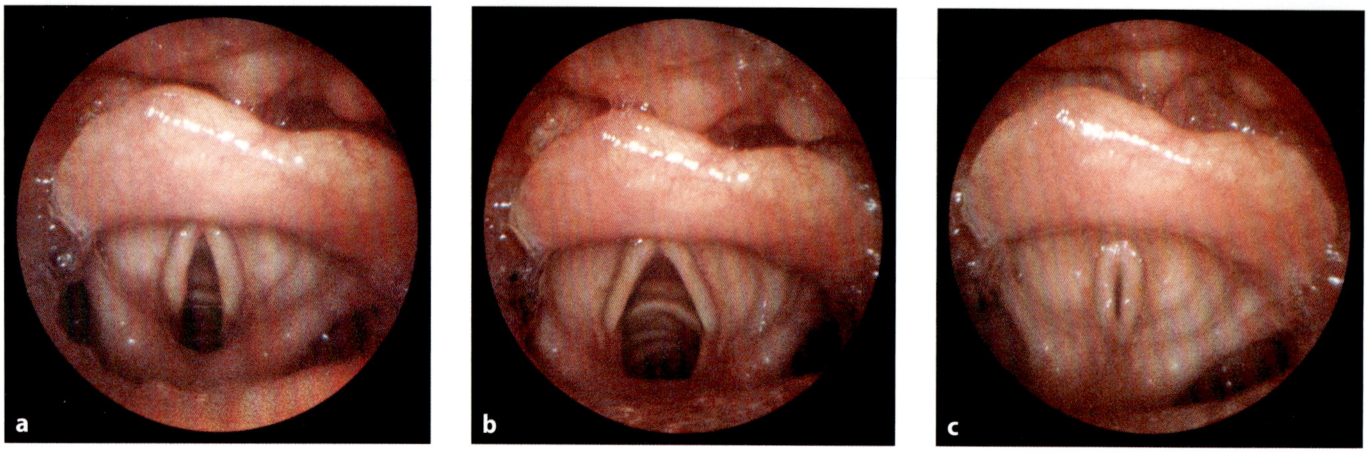

Rima glottidis observed with the laryngoscope. **a**, Open during respiration; **b**, open to maximum extent during a forced inspiration; **c**, closed during phonation.

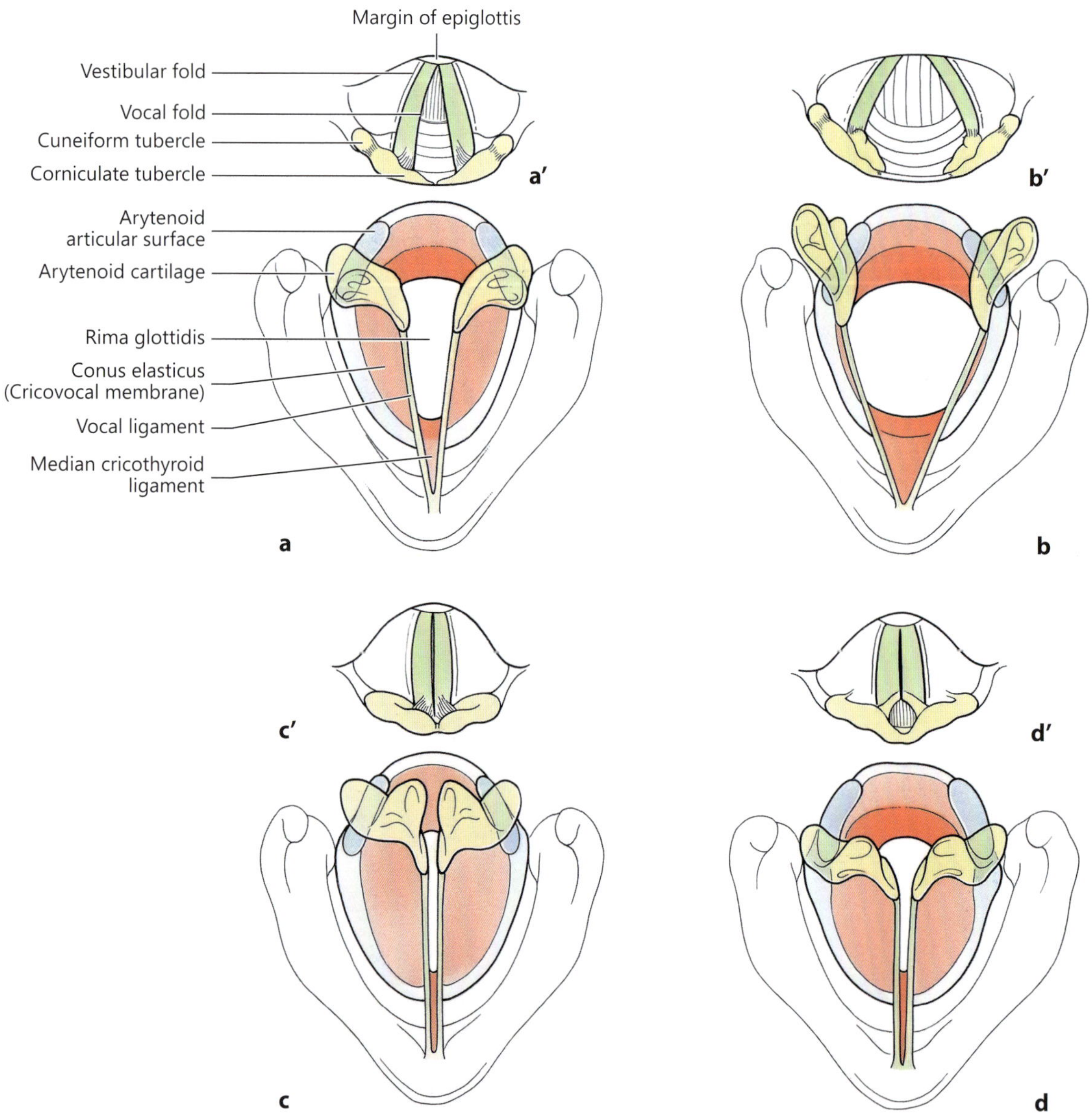

Characteristics of the **rima glottidis** and its variations in preparations of the laryngeal skeleton (**a**, **b**, **c**, **d**) and in laryngoscope images (**a′**, **b′**, **c′**, **d′**). **a-a′**, In vocal rest position; **b-b′**, during a normal phase of breathing; **c-c′**, during phonation with normal vocal tone; **d-d′**, during whisper phonation.

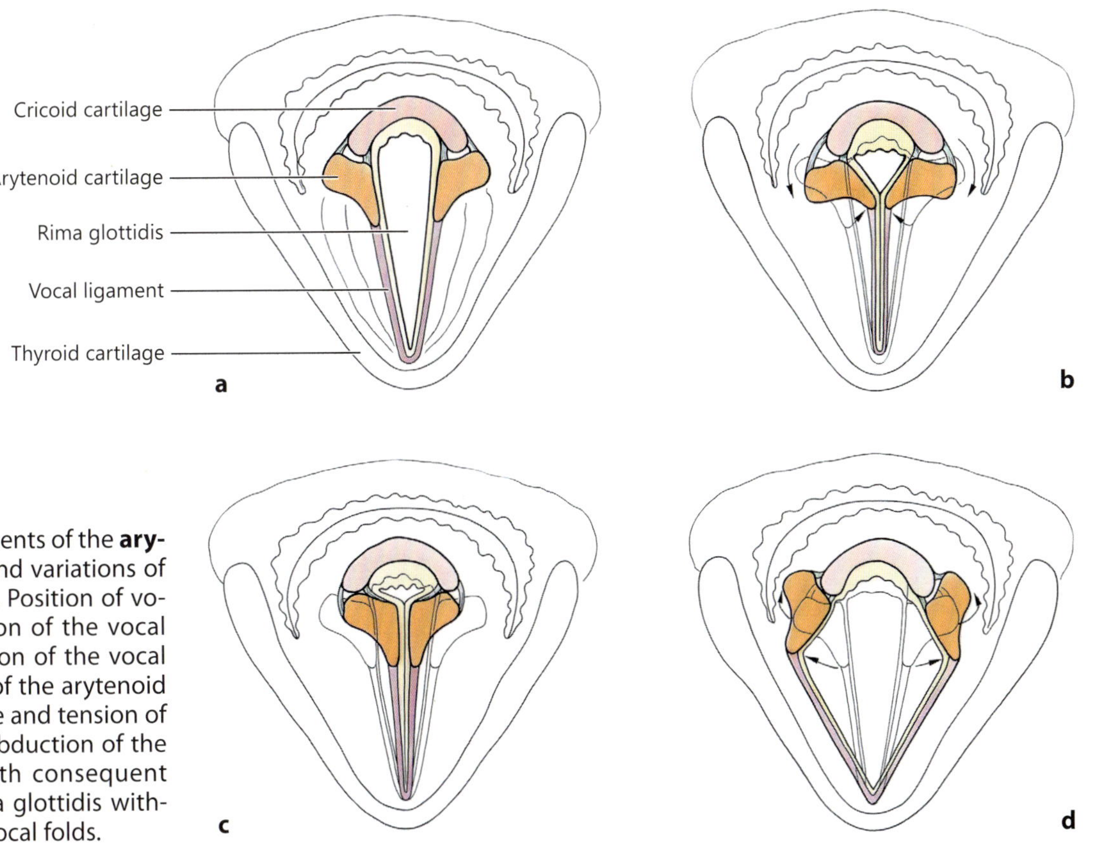

Position and movements of the **arytenoid cartilages** and variations of the rima glottidis. **a**, Position of vocal rest. **b**, Adduction of the vocal processes and tension of the vocal folds. **c**, Adduction of the arytenoid cartilages as a whole and tension of the vocal folds. **d**, Abduction of the vocal processes with consequent opening of the rima glottidis without tension of the vocal folds.

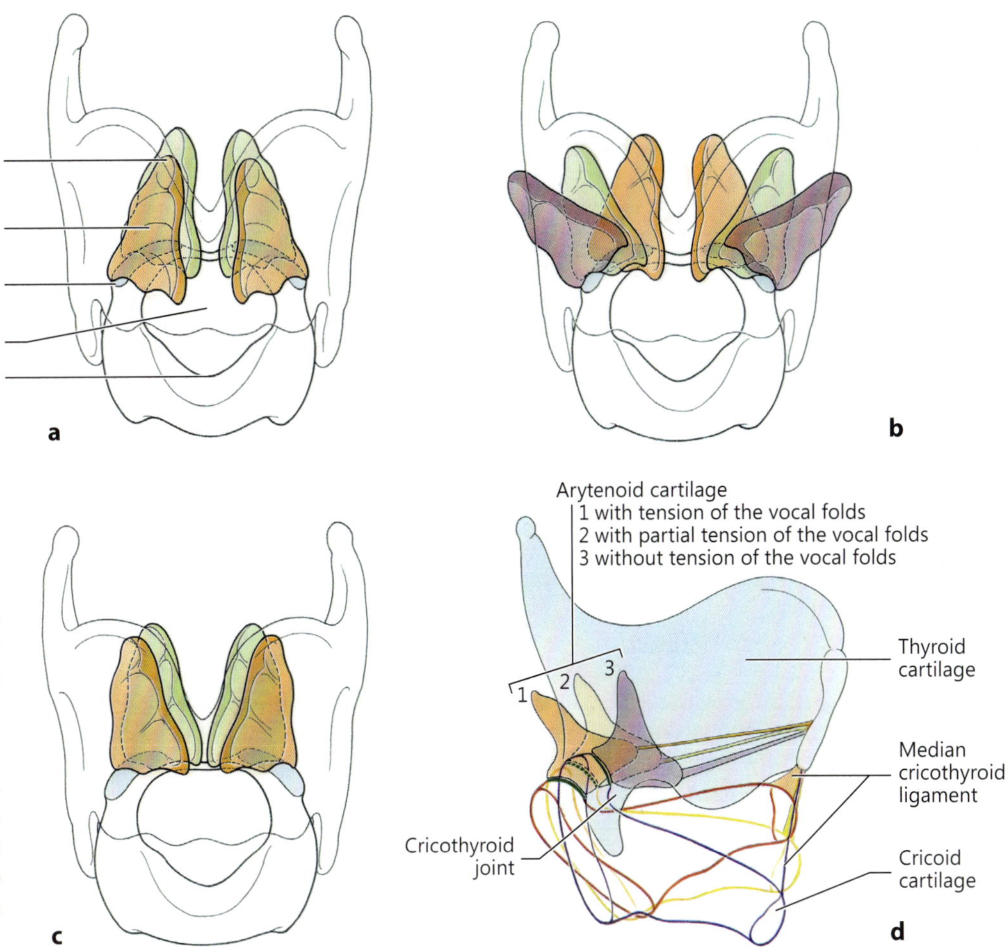

Diagram illustrating the movements of the **arytenoid cartilages** with respect to the **cricoid cartilage**. **a**, Movement in anteroposterior direction; **b**, movement in lateromedial direction with inclination; **c**, movement in lateromedial direction without inclination; **d**, relative movements of the arytenoid cartilages and cricoid cartilage in relation to the different length of the vocal folds.

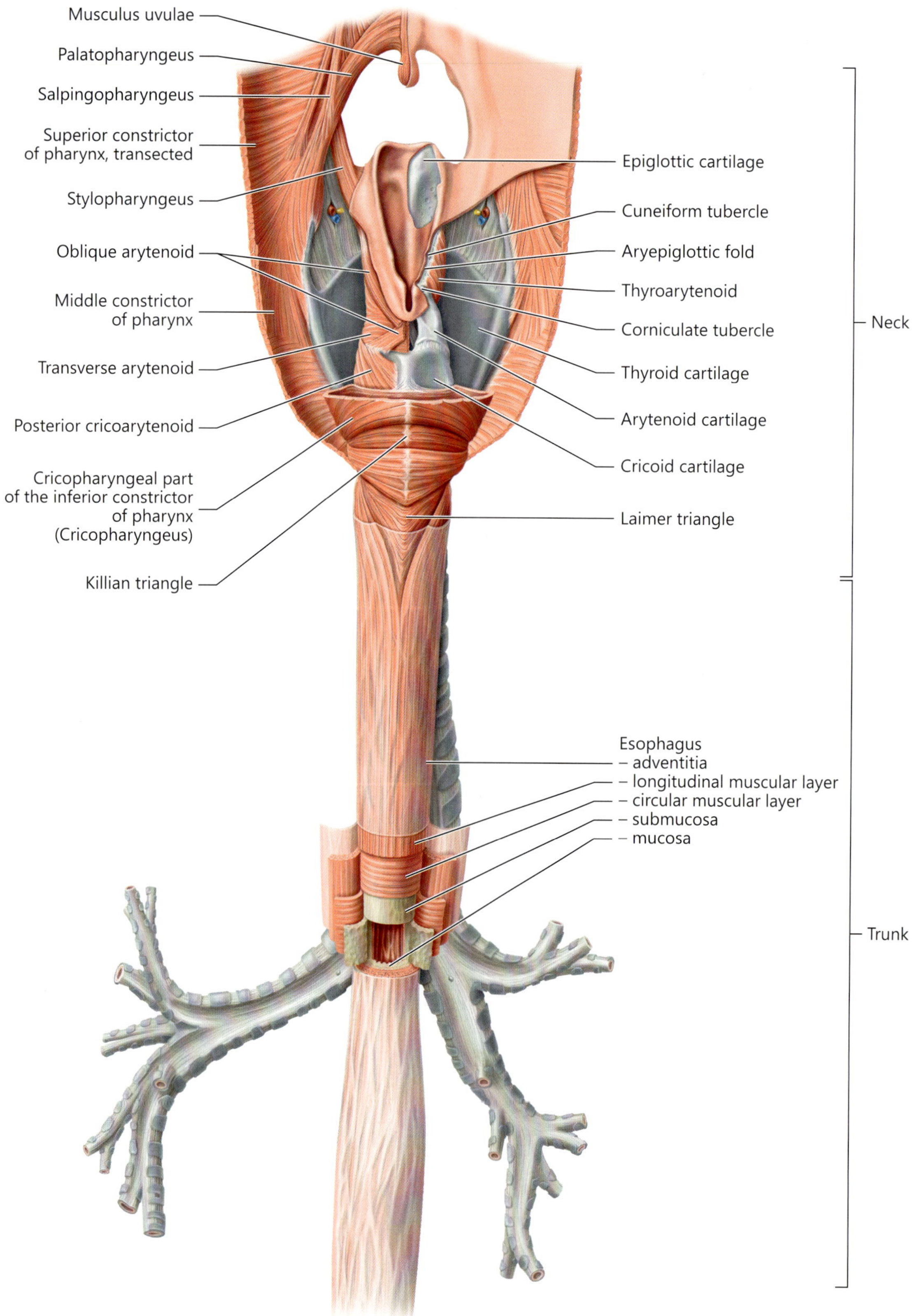

The **esophagus**, approximately 25 cm long, extends from C VI to T XI. It starts from the pharynx in the neck, at the level of the cricoid cartilage of the larynx, and proceeds into the thorax, running in the posterior mediastinum. It terminates in the abdominal cavity at the level of the cardia with the abdominal part of the esophagus.
The superior third of the esophagus presents a striated muscular layer, which plays a role in the swallowing process. In the inferior two-thirds, the muscular coat is composed of two layers of smooth muscle, an inner circular one and an outer longitudinal one (transected in the figure). The anterior surface of the esophagus adheres to the posterior surface of the trachea by means of small bundles of loose connective tissue and smooth muscle (tracheoesophageal muscle).

The structure of the esophagus is represented on page 314 (Thorax - Esophagus)

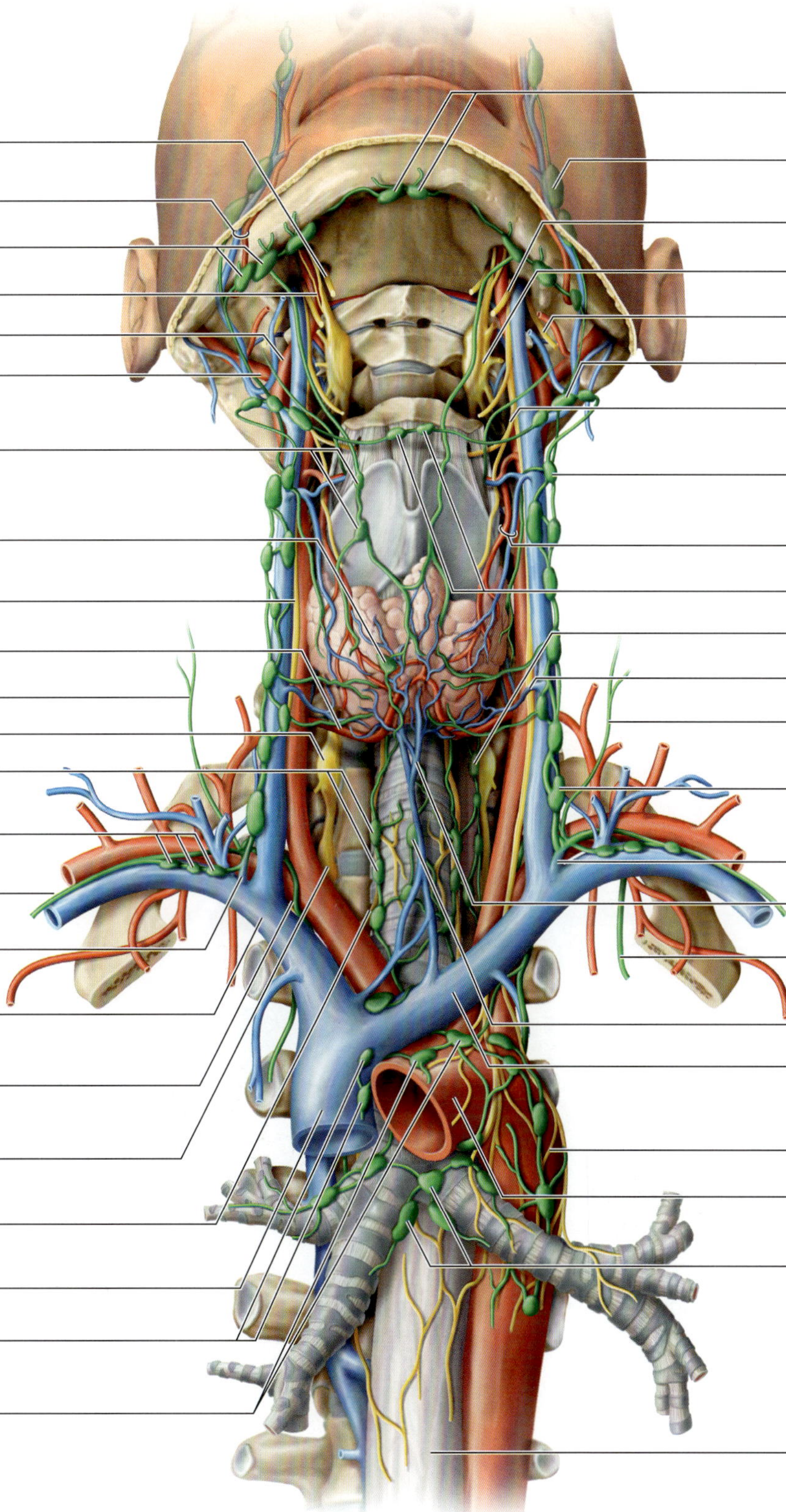

Neck, anterior view. The two common carotid arteries run vertically from the sternoclavicular joint to the point halfway between the angle of the mandible and mastoid process of the temporal bone. The two vessels are separated by a space occupied by the trachea at the base of the neck and, superiorly, by the thyroid gland, larynx and pharynx. The internal jugular veins descend in the neck externally and posteriorly to the internal carotid arteries and then laterally to the common carotid arteries.

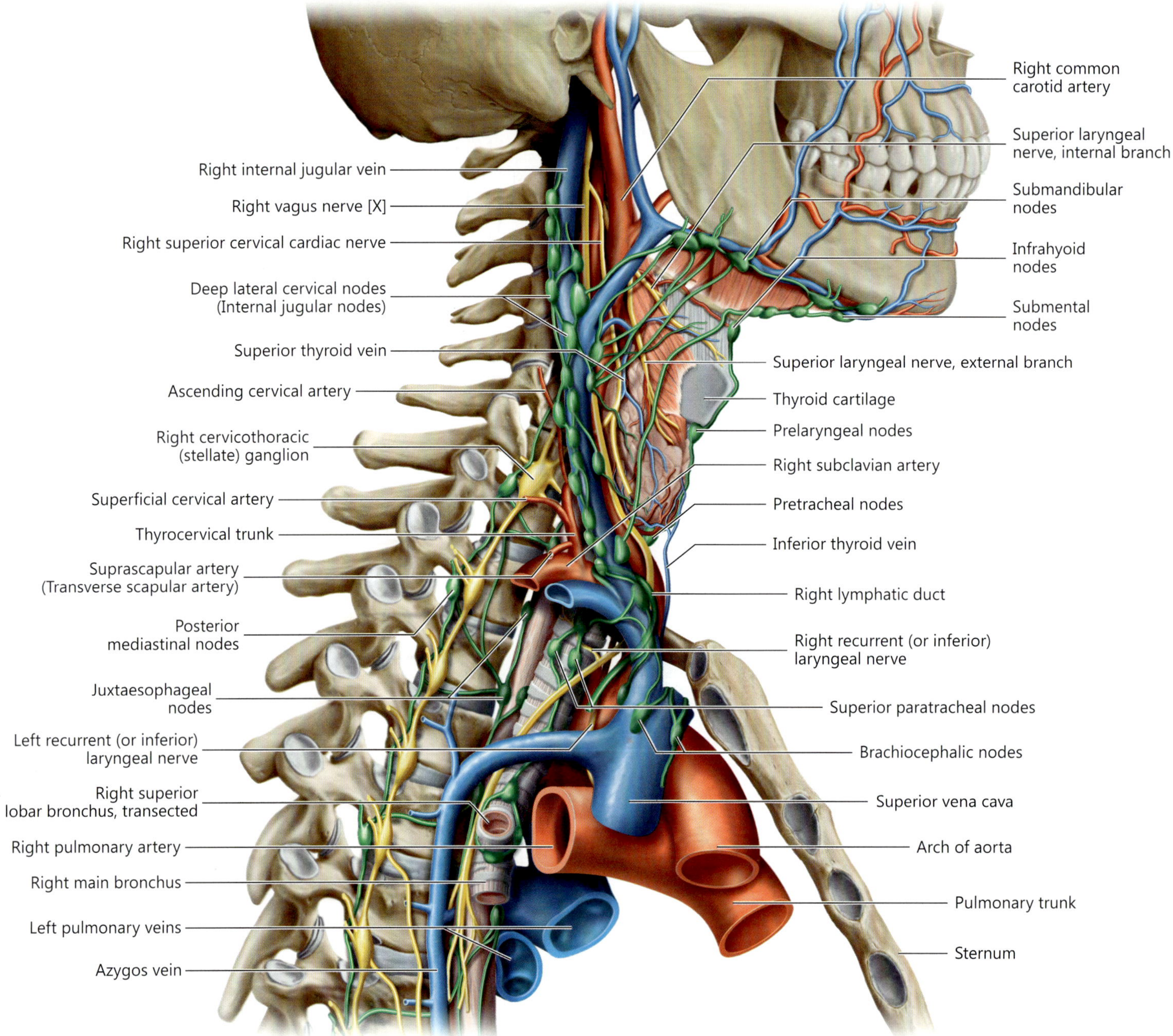

Vessels and nerves of the neck, right lateral view. One can see, in particular, the internal jugular vein, the vagus nerve [X] with the superior and the recurrent (or inferior) laryngeal nerves, the superior cervical cardiac nerve, which arises from the superior cervical ganglion of the sympathetic trunk, the cervicothoracic (or stellate) ganglion, the superior thyroid vein, an affluent of the internal jugular vein, and the inferior thyroid vein, an affluent of the brachiocephalic vein.

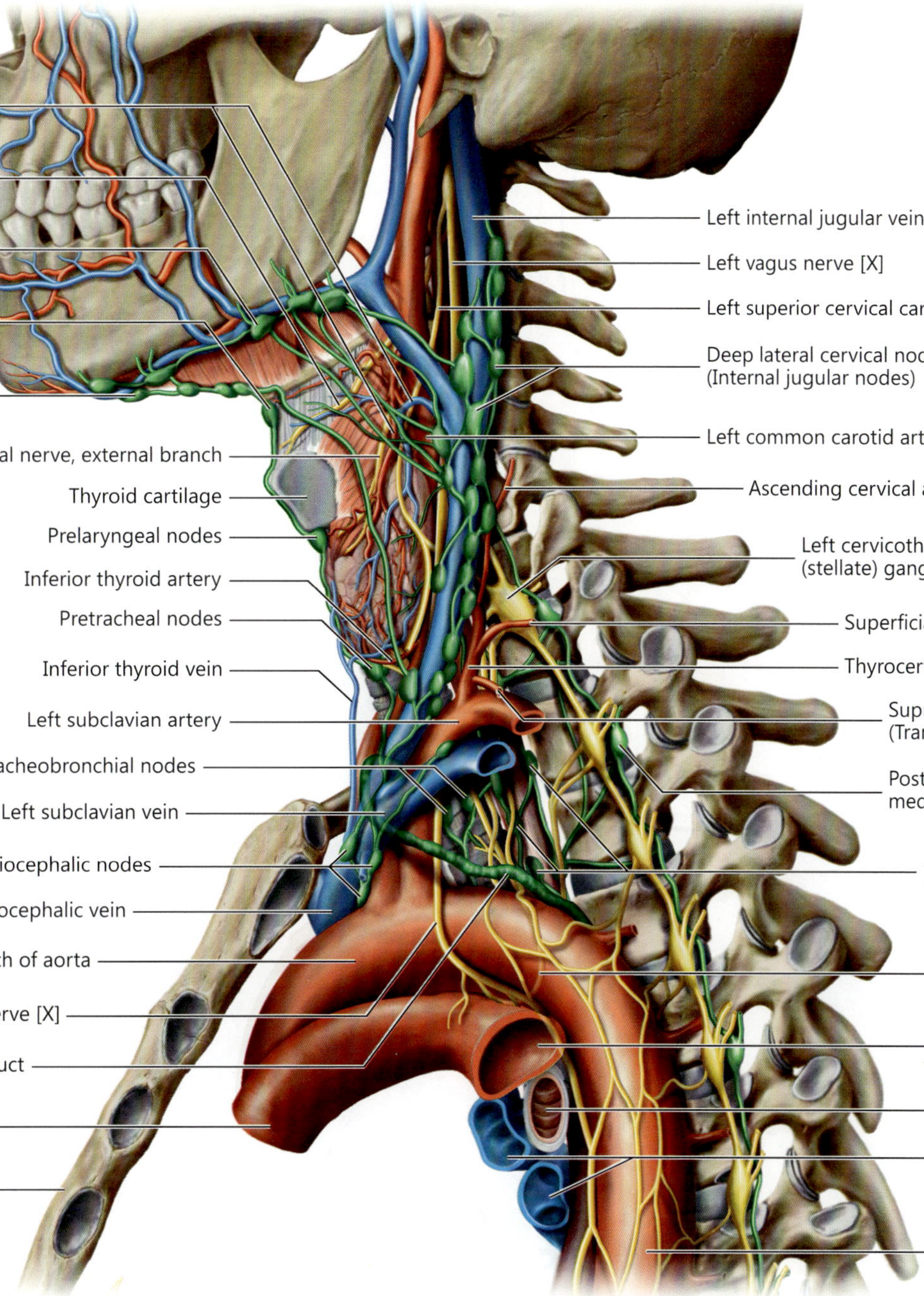

Vessels and nerves of the neck, left lateral view. One can see, in particular: the common carotid artery; the superior and inferior thyroid arteries, which stem, respectively, from the external carotid artery and thyrocervical trunk; the thyrocervical trunk, from which arise also the ascending cervical artery (which otherwise can originate from the inferior thyroid artery); the suprascapular (or transverse scapular) artery, and the superficial cervical artery (which can otherwise originate from the transverse cervical artery, itself a branch of either the thyrocervical trunk or the subclavian artery).

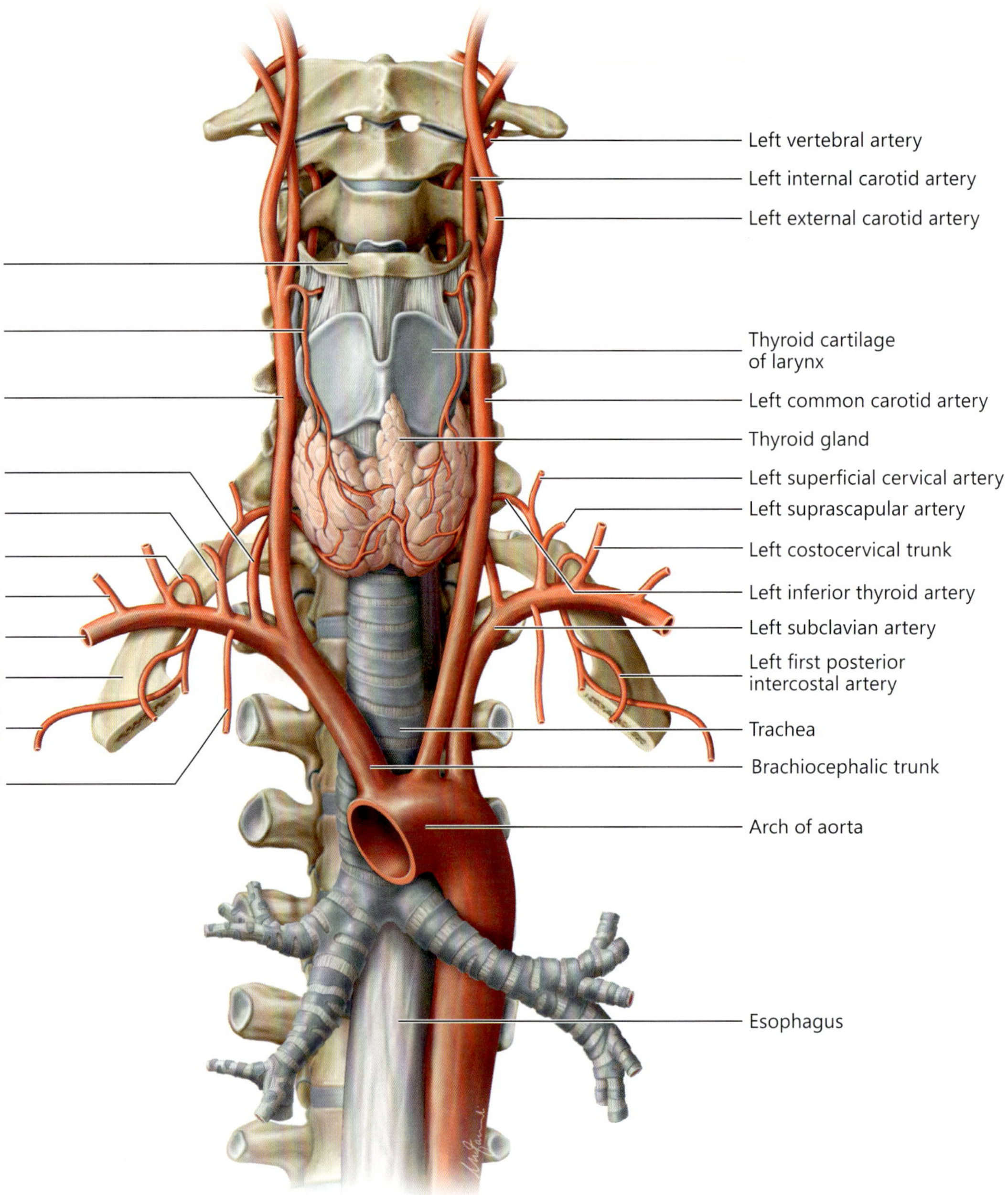

Arteries of the neck, anterior view. The **common carotid artery** originates on the right side from the brachiocephalic trunk, behind the sternoclavicular joint, while on the left it arises directly from the arch of the aorta. At the level of the superior border of the thyroid cartilage of the larynx, it divides into the internal and external carotid arteries. The **subclavian artery**, that originates on the right from the brachiocephalic trunk and on the left from the arch of the aorta, can be subdivided into three portions: the first, from its origin to the medial border of the scalenus anterior; the second, posterior to this muscle; and the third, from the lateral border of the scalenus anterior to the external border of the first rib. From the first part arise: superoposteriorly, the **vertebral artery**, which passes through the foramina transversaria of all cervical vertebrae except the seventh; inferiorly, the **internal thoracic artery**; and, anteriorly, the **thyrocervical trunk**, which divides into the **suprascapular** (or transverse scapular), **superficial cervical** and **inferior thyroid arteries**. From the second part of the subclavian artery (on the right) and from the first part (on the left), the **costocervical trunk** arises posteriorly, which then divides into the **supreme intercostal** and **deep cervical** (here not visible) **arteries**. The third portion of the subclavian artery gives rise to the **transverse cervical artery** and to the posterior scapular artery. In one-third of cases, the superficial cervical and posterior scapular arteries originate as superficial and deep branches of the transverse cervical artery. The **superior thyroid artery** originates anteriorly from the external carotid artery at the level of the greater horn of the hyoid bone.

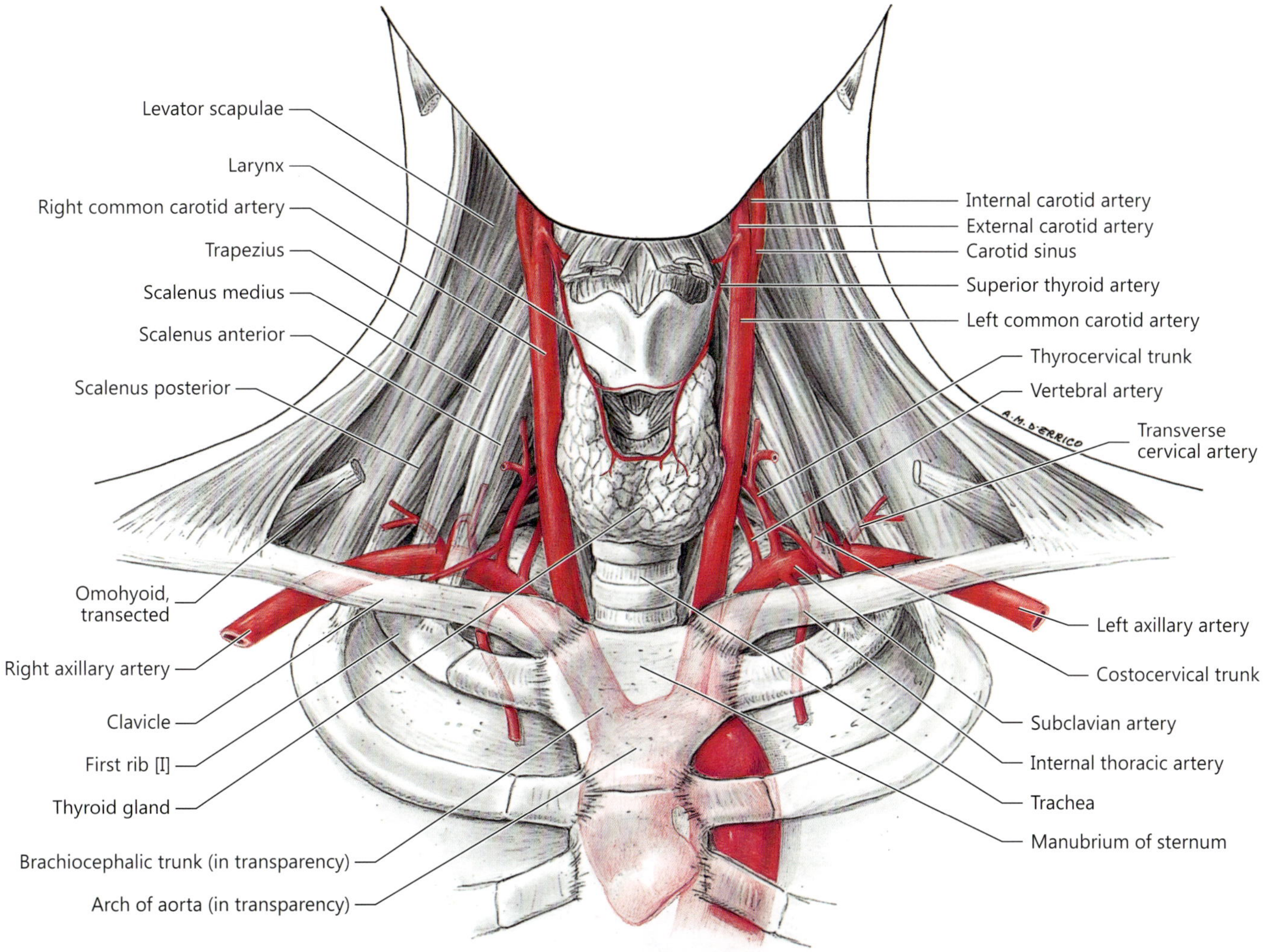

Branches of the **arch of the aorta**. To highlight the position of the arteries and their relations, the anterior, cutaneous and muscular planes of the thorax and neck have been amply demolished. The **brachiocephalic trunk** and the thoracic portion of the **common carotid** and left **subclavian arteries** are visible in transparency. One can see the collateral branches of the subclavian artery (resected at a short distance from their origin) and the **superior thyroid artery**, first collateral branch of the external carotid artery.

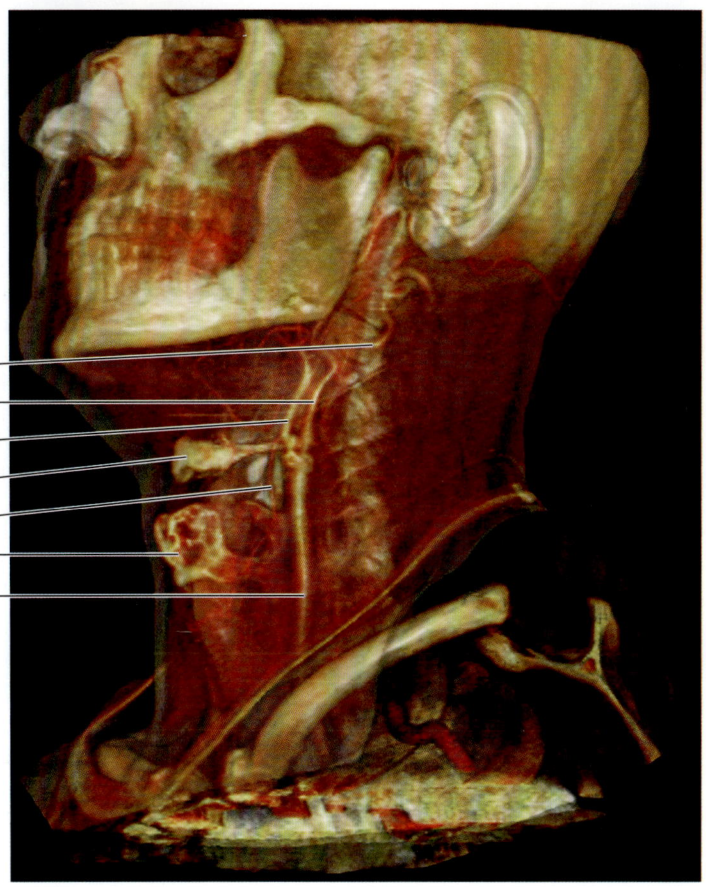

Three-dimensional image of a living human body, obtained by CT scan using a 3D volume rendering technique, showing the **vessels passing through the neck** in relation to the bony structures, in left lateral view.

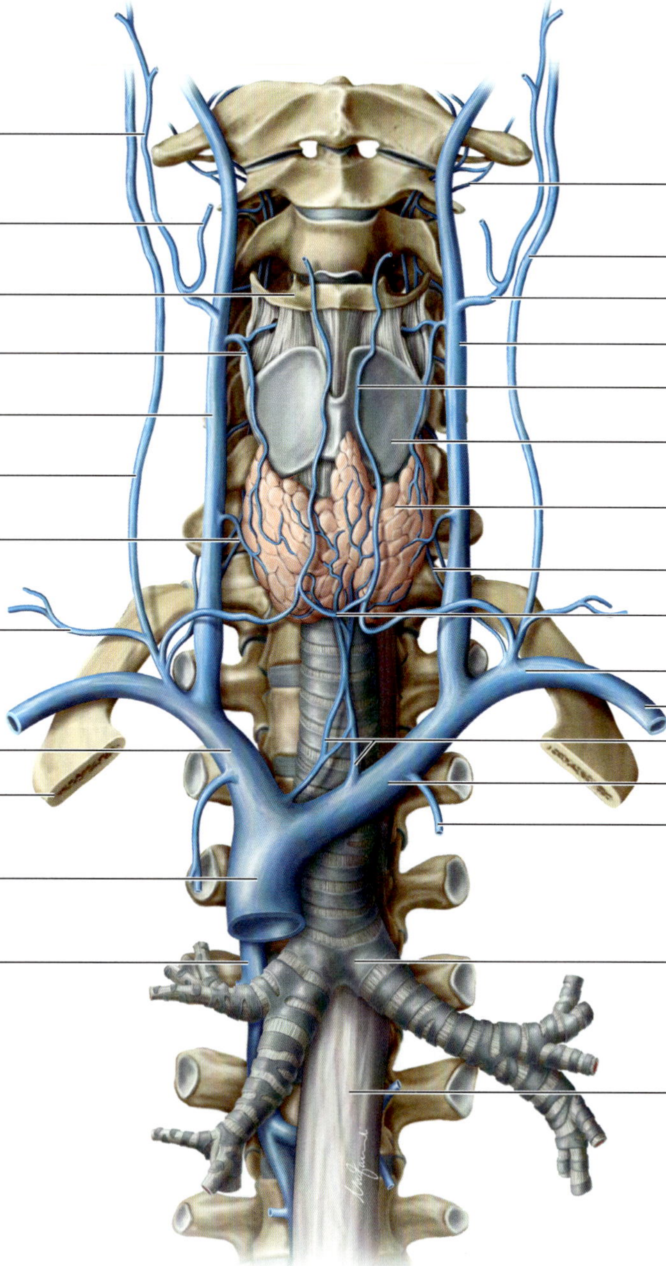

Veins of the neck, anterior view. The **internal jugular vein**, which drains blood from the cranium, brain, superficial parts of the face and much of the neck, descends in the neck and unites with the **subclavian vein** posteriorly to the sternal end of the clavicle, forming the **brachiocephalic vein**. The **external jugular vein** collects blood principally from the scalp and face and is formed by the union of the posterior division of the **retromandibular vein** (or **posterior facial vein**) with the **posterior auricular vein**. It descends in the lateral part of the neck and empties into the subclavian vein at a short distance from its confluence with the internal jugular vein. The **anterior jugular vein**, which drains blood from the skin and muscles of the anterior cervical region, descends anteriorly in the neck to its base and then heads laterally to unite with the termination of the external jugular vein or with the subclavian vein. The two anterior jugular veins are united, just above the manubrium of the sternum, by the jugular venous arch. The **common facial vein**, formed by the union of the anterior branch of the retromandibular vein with the facial vein (or anterior facial vein), is not always present. The facial vein can, in fact, drain directly into the internal jugular vein, while the retromandibular vein can connect to the external jugular vein, through an anastomotic branch, before uniting with the facial vein.

➤

Schematic representation showing the **superior vena cava** and large affluent veins. The drainage territories of the principal vessels are indicated. The superior vena cava collects venous blood from the territories of the body above the diaphragm, with the exception of the heart. It is formed by the confluence of the right and left brachiocephalic veins and the only affluent branch it receives during its course is the azygos vein. It has an almost vertical path and terminates in the posterosuperior part of the right atrium of the heart. The azygos, hemiazygos, accessory hemiazygos and, in part, subclavian and brachiocephalic veins drain territories of the thorax and of the upper limbs.

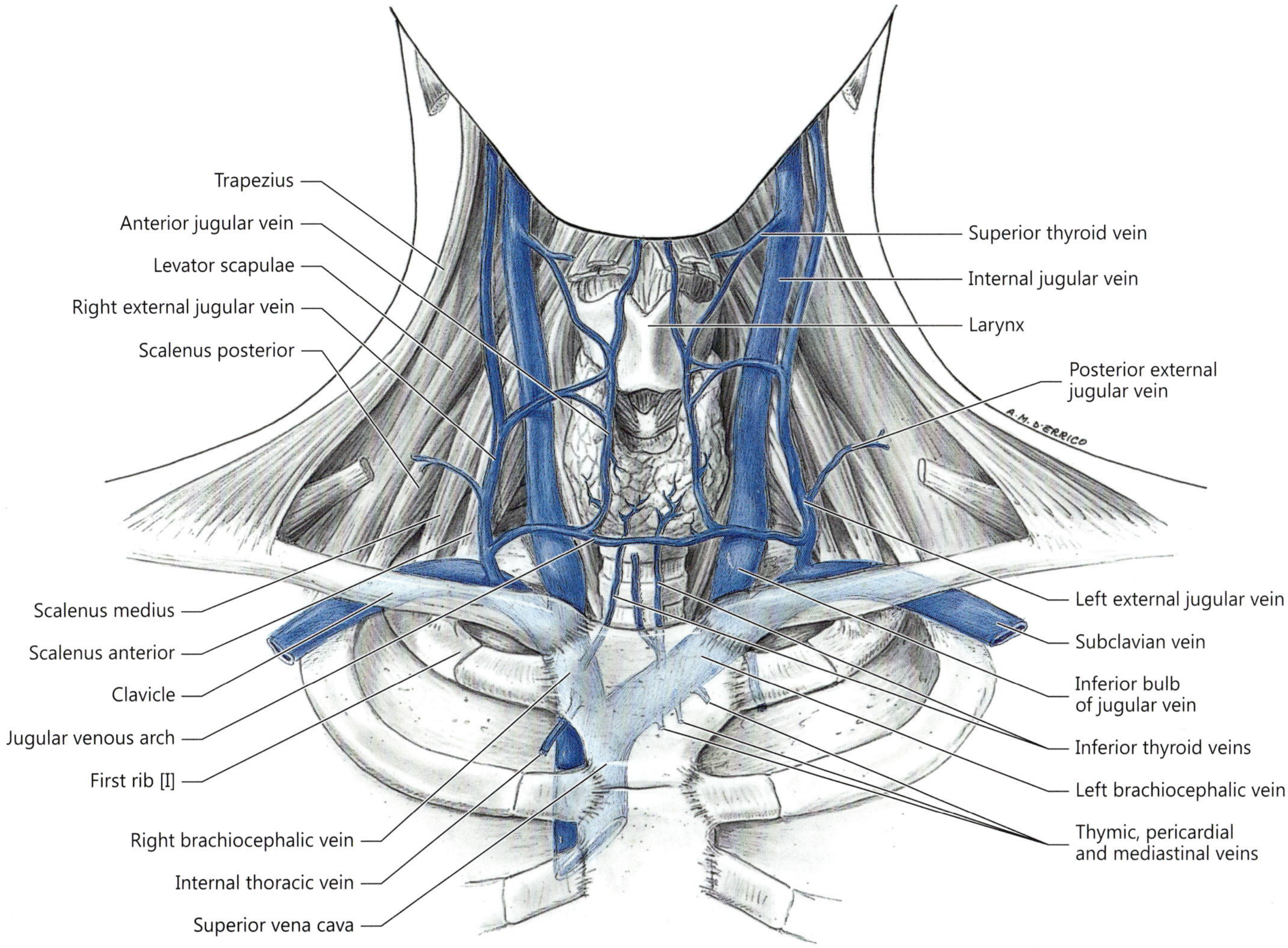

Diagram of the **internal jugular veins**, **subclavian veins** and of their affluent branches. Through the thoracic wall, in transparency, one can see the two **brachiocephalic veins**, right and left, from their origin to the point of their confluence into the **superior vena cava**.

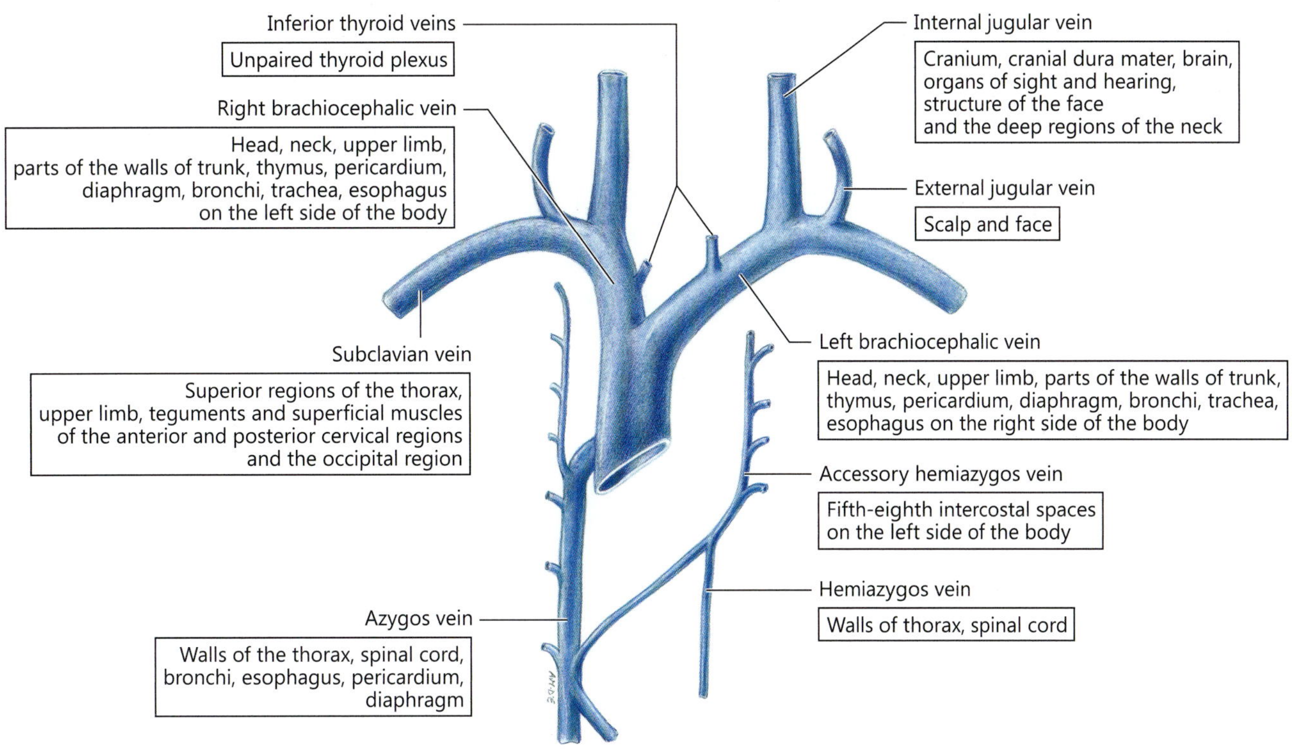

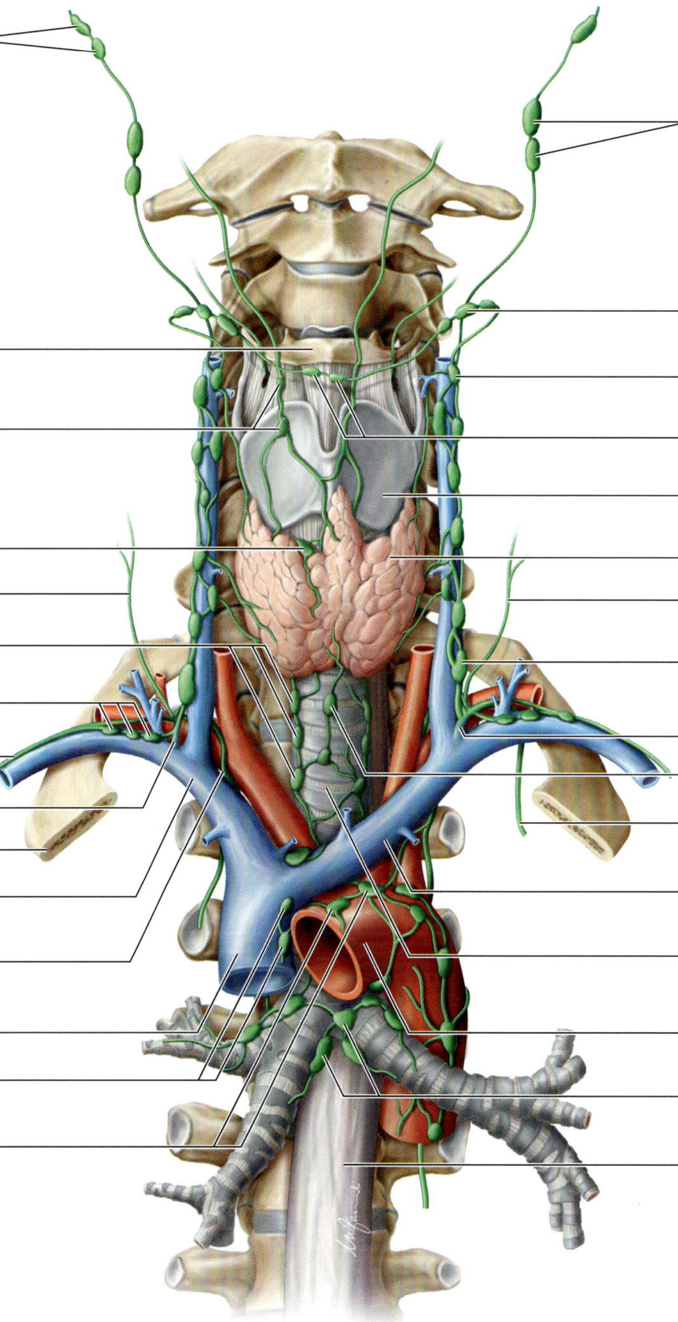

Deep lymph nodes of the neck, anterior view. The **deep anterior cervical nodes** (**anterior visceral nodes**) below the hyoid bone in relation with the larynx (**prelaryngeal infrahyoid nodes**), thyroid gland (**thyroid nodes**) and trachea (**pretracheal and paratracheal nodes**) are represented. Also represented are the **deep lateral cervical nodes** located along the course of the internal jugular vein (**internal jugular nodes**) as well as the **supraclavicular nodes** (**transverse cervical artery nodes**), situated in the supraclavicular fossa, which are related to the transverse cervical artery. The **brachiocephalic nodes**, situated in the superior mediastinum and related to the large vessels, the para-aortic nodes, situated anteriorly and laterally to the ascending aorta and arch of the aorta, and the **inferior tracheobronchial nodes**, situated in correspondence to the tracheal bifurcation, are classified as lymph nodes of the thorax.

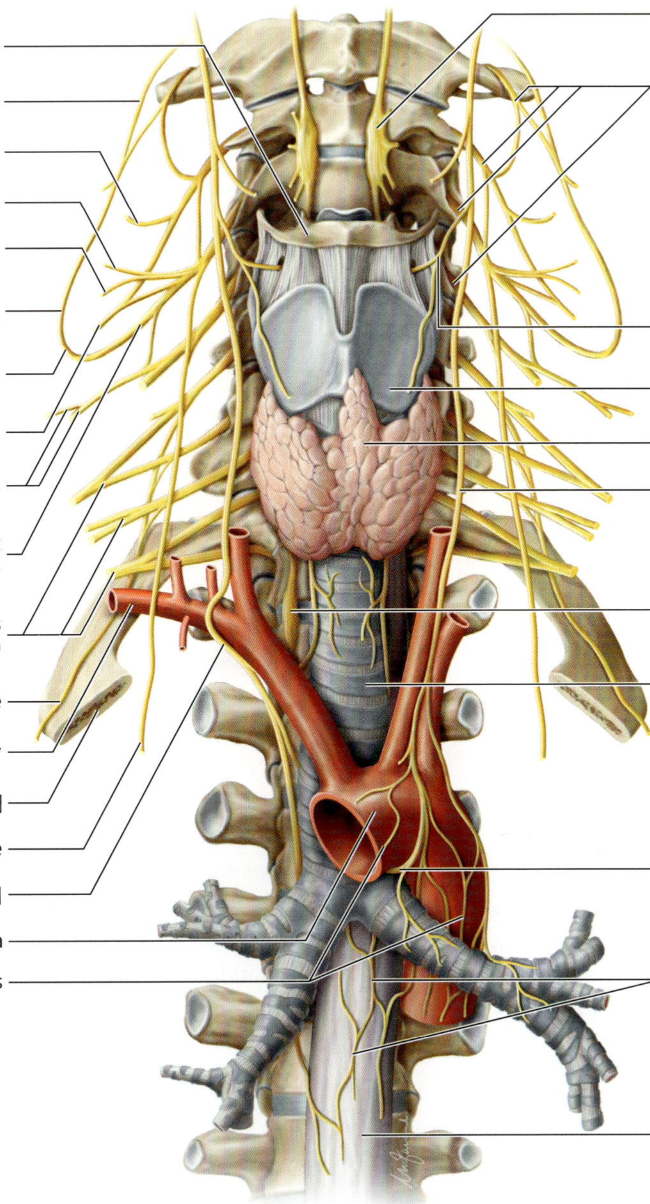

Nerves of the neck, anterior view. The anterior rami of the first four cervical nerves [C1-C4] divide into branches that unite forming anastomotic loops constituting the **cervical plexus**, situated in front of the transverse processes of the cervical vertebrae. The cutaneous branches of the cervical plexus are exclusively sensory nerves: the **lesser occipital**, **great auricular**, **transverse cervical** and **supraclavicular nerves**. The **ansa cervicalis** (or **ansa of the hypoglossal nerve**, cranial nerve XII) is formed by two roots: a superior one, derived from the union with the hypoglossal nerve of an anastomotic branch coming from the anterior ramus of C1, and an inferior one, derived from the union of anastomotic branches coming from the anterior rami of C2 and C3. The **phrenic nerve**, the largest branch of the cervical plexus, originates with a principal root from C4 and with two accessory, inconstant, roots from C3 and C5. The primary trunks of the **brachial plexus**, formed by the anterior rami of C5, C6, C7, C8 and T1, occupy the supraclavicular space, while the cords (secondary trunks) are contained in the axilla. The **vagus nerve** [X] gives rise to numerous branches in the neck, including the **recurrent** (or inferior) **laryngeal nerve** which on the right forms a loop around the subclavian artery, while on the left it loops around the arch of the aorta, as it ascends in the neck. The cervical segment of the sympathetic trunk, which extends from the cranial base to the superior thoracic aperture, includes three ganglia, one of which is visible here: the **superior cervical ganglion**, in front of the transverse processes of the second and third cervical vertebrae.

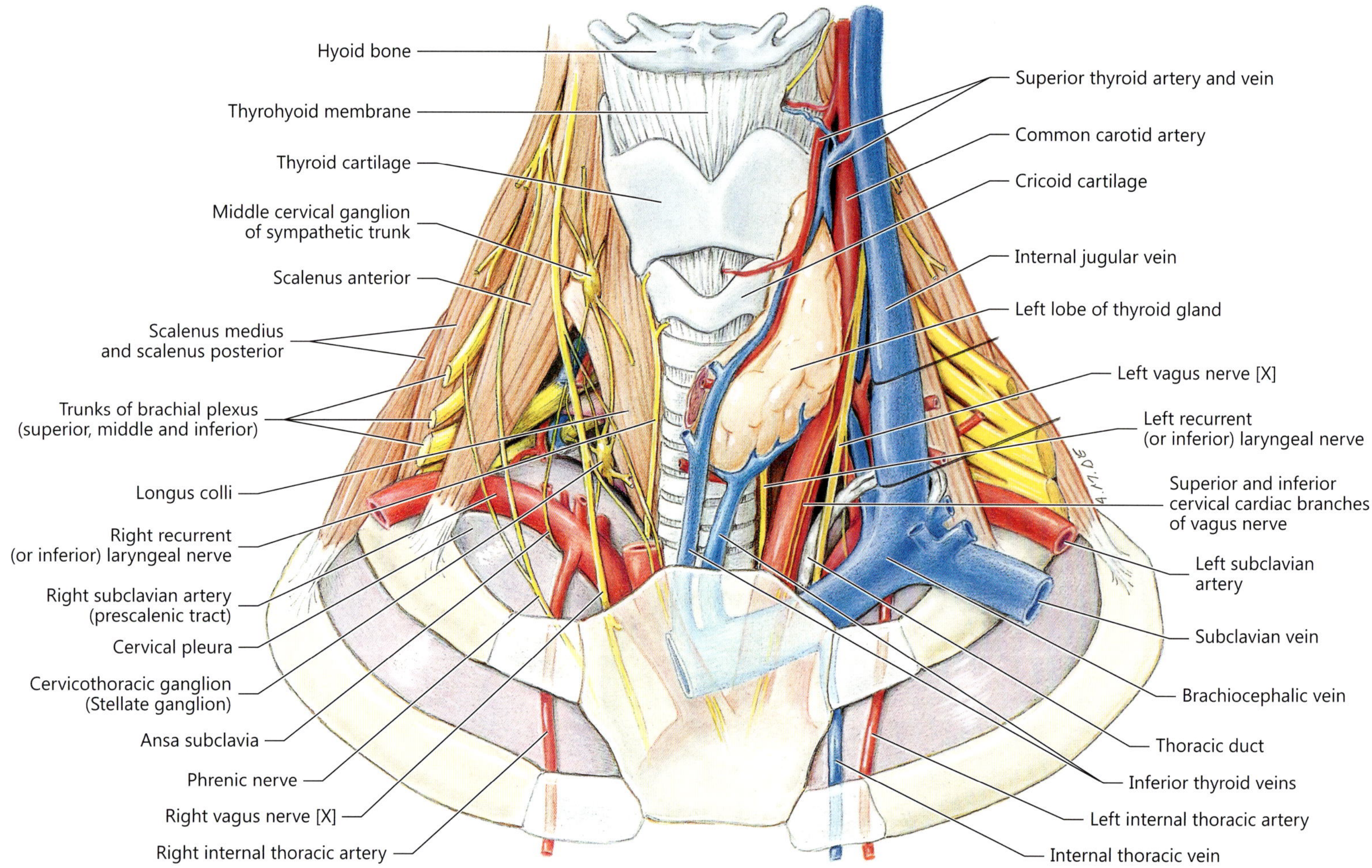

Schematic representation showing the course and relations of the **common carotid** and **subclavian arteries** and of the **subclavian** and **internal jugular veins**. The anterior thoracic wall and anterior cervical region have been amply demolished to highlight the organs and the vascular and nerve formations located behind.

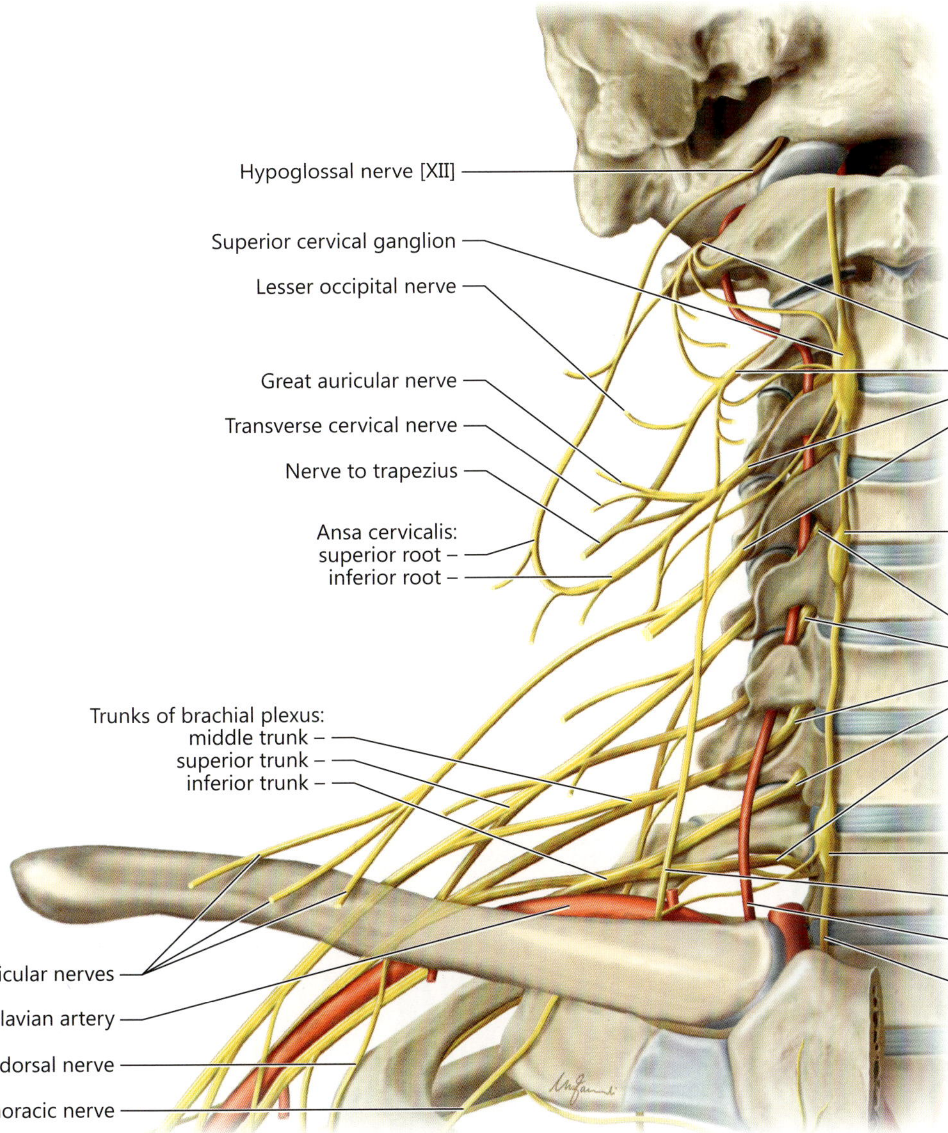

Cervical plexus, **trunks of the brachial plexus**, **ansa cervicalis** and **cervical segment of the sympathetic trunk**, anterior view. The cervical plexus is formed by the anterior rami of the first four cervical nerves that unite to form anastomotic loops, or arches, superimposed in a vertical direction. The anterior ramus of the first cervical nerve anastomoses with the hypoglossal nerve [XII]: part of the anastomotic fibers unite for a brief tract with the hypoglossal nerve, then separate as a descending branch that constitutes the superior root of the ansa cervicalis, or ansa of the hypoglossal nerve, whose inferior root (descending cervical nerve) is formed instead of branches originating from the anterior rami of the second and third cervical nerves which unite, continuing in the superior root. The brachial plexus, formed by anterior rami of the last four cervical nerves and first thoracic nerve, is characterized by anastomoses and subdivisions that form three (primary) trunks above the clavicle (supraclavicular part of the cervical nerves), from which arise the cords of the plexus (or secondary trunks).

For a lateral view and schematic representation of the cervical plexus ☞ page 76.
The brachial plexus is illustrated on page 77.

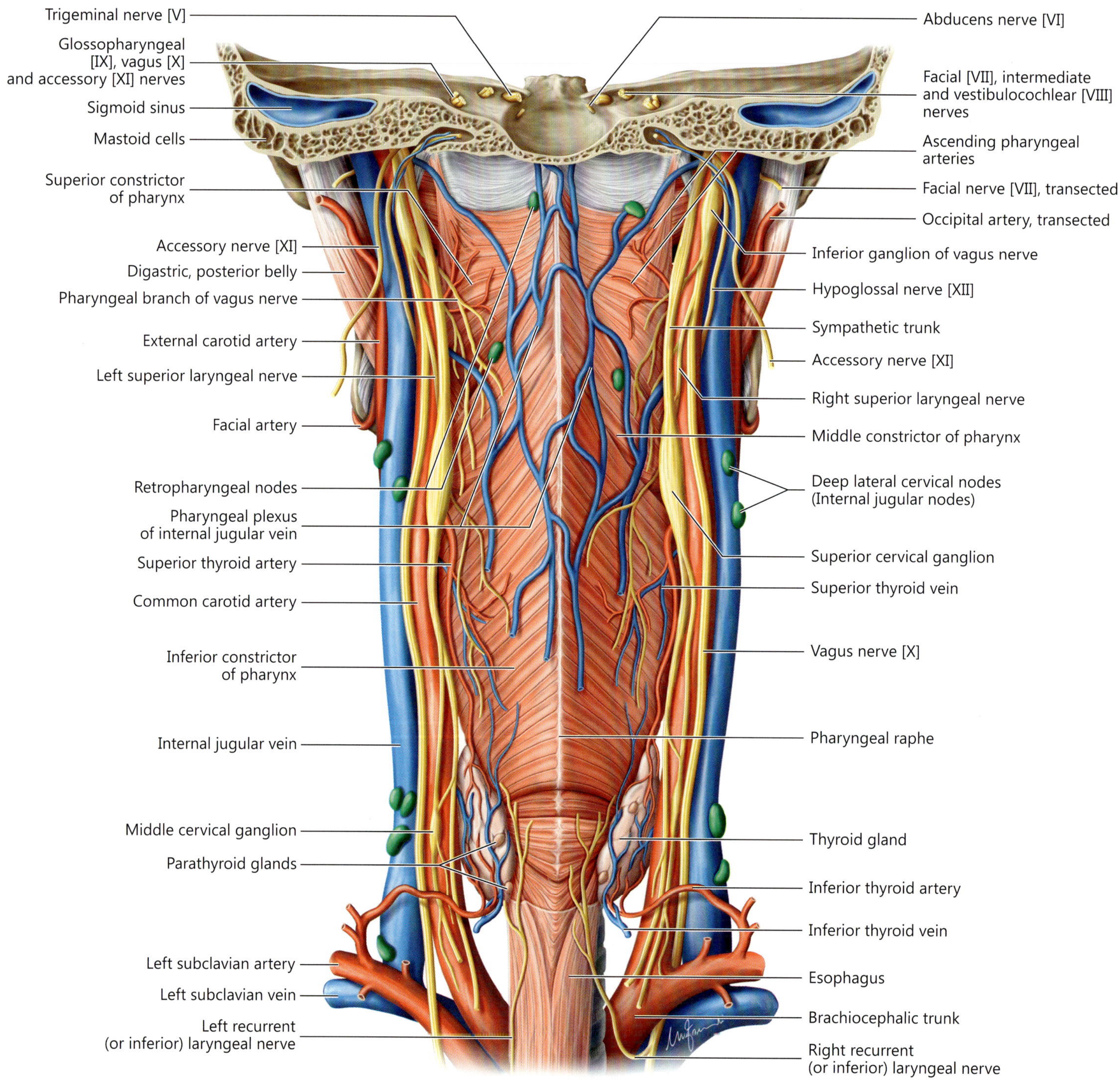

Vessels and nerves in the **parapharyngeal** (**lateral pharyngeal**) **space**, posterior view after removal of the vertebral column and muscles of the back. The **common carotid artery** ascends in the neck up to the superior border of the thyroid cartilage of the larynx where it divides into the **external and internal carotid arteries**. Together with the **internal jugular vein**, which descends in the neck along the lateral wall of the pharynx, at first posteriorly to the internal carotid artery and then laterally to the common carotid artery, and with the **vagus nerve**, in the posteriorly open dihedral angle that the two vessels form alongside each other, it constitutes the *neurovascular bundle of the neck* inside the carotid sheath, which here has been removed. The cervical segment of the sympathetic trunk extends from the cranial base to the superior thoracic aperture, posteriorly to the neurovascular bundle of the neck.

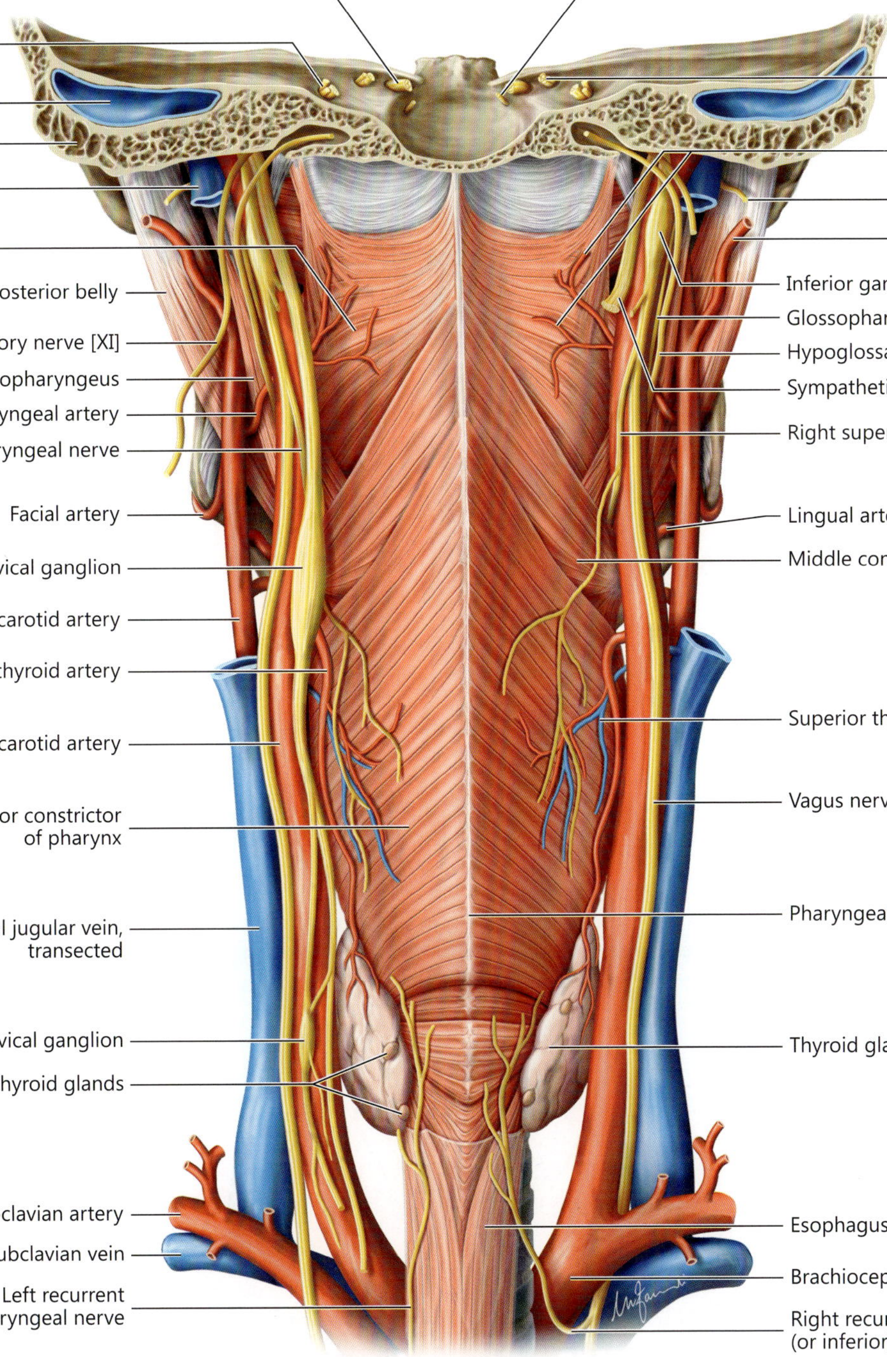

Vessels and nerves in the **parapharyngeal (lateral pharyngeal) space**, posterior view after removal of the vertebral column and muscles of the back. The internal jugular vein has been transected revealing the **external carotid artery**, and the origins of its collateral branches such as the **superior thyroid artery**, the **facial artery**, the **lingual artery**, the **ascending pharyngeal artery** and the **occipital artery**. The **superior laryngeal nerve** departs from the inferior, or nodose, ganglion of the vagus nerve or slightly below. The **recurrent laryngeal**, or inferior, **nerve** is so defined because of the loop that it makes, first descending into the thorax and then re-ascending in the neck to reach the larynx.

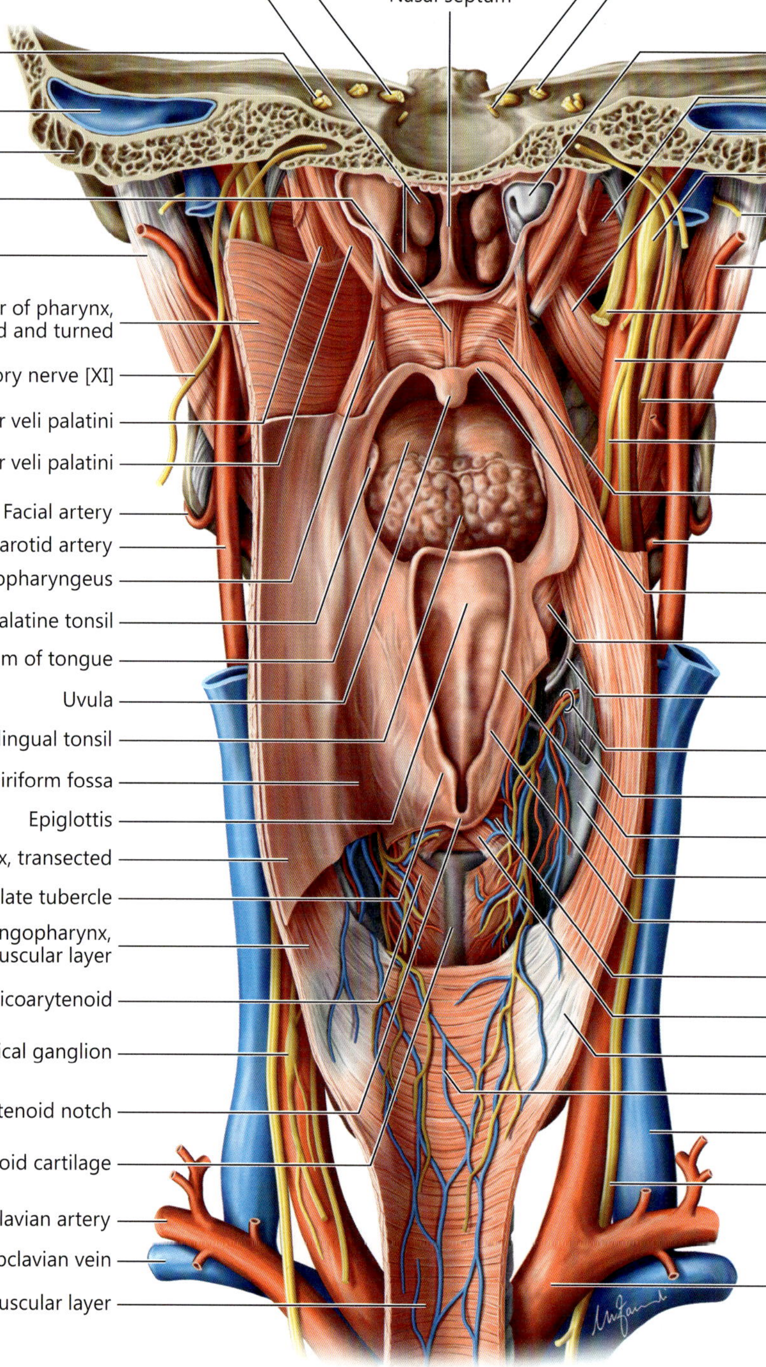

Posterior view of the **pharynx** after opening its posterior wall. One can see the anterior wall of the pharynx, which is complete only in correspondence to the posterior surface of the larynx. Above it, one finds, from bottom to top: the **laryngeal inlet**, an oval opening bounded anteriorly by the free border of the epiglottis and laterally and posteriorly by the aryepiglottic folds; the posterior surface of the **epiglottis**; the **isthmus of the fauces**, formed by the root of the tongue with the **lingual tonsil** on its dorsal surface, by the free border of the soft palate with the **uvula** and by the **palatoglossal and palatopharyngeal arches**; the posterior surface of the **soft palate** and the **choanae**, quadrangular openings bounded superiorly by the body of the sphenoid, laterally by the medial plates of the pterygoid processes of the sphenoid, medially by the posterior border of the vomer and inferiorly by the posterior border of the horizontal plate of the palatine bone.

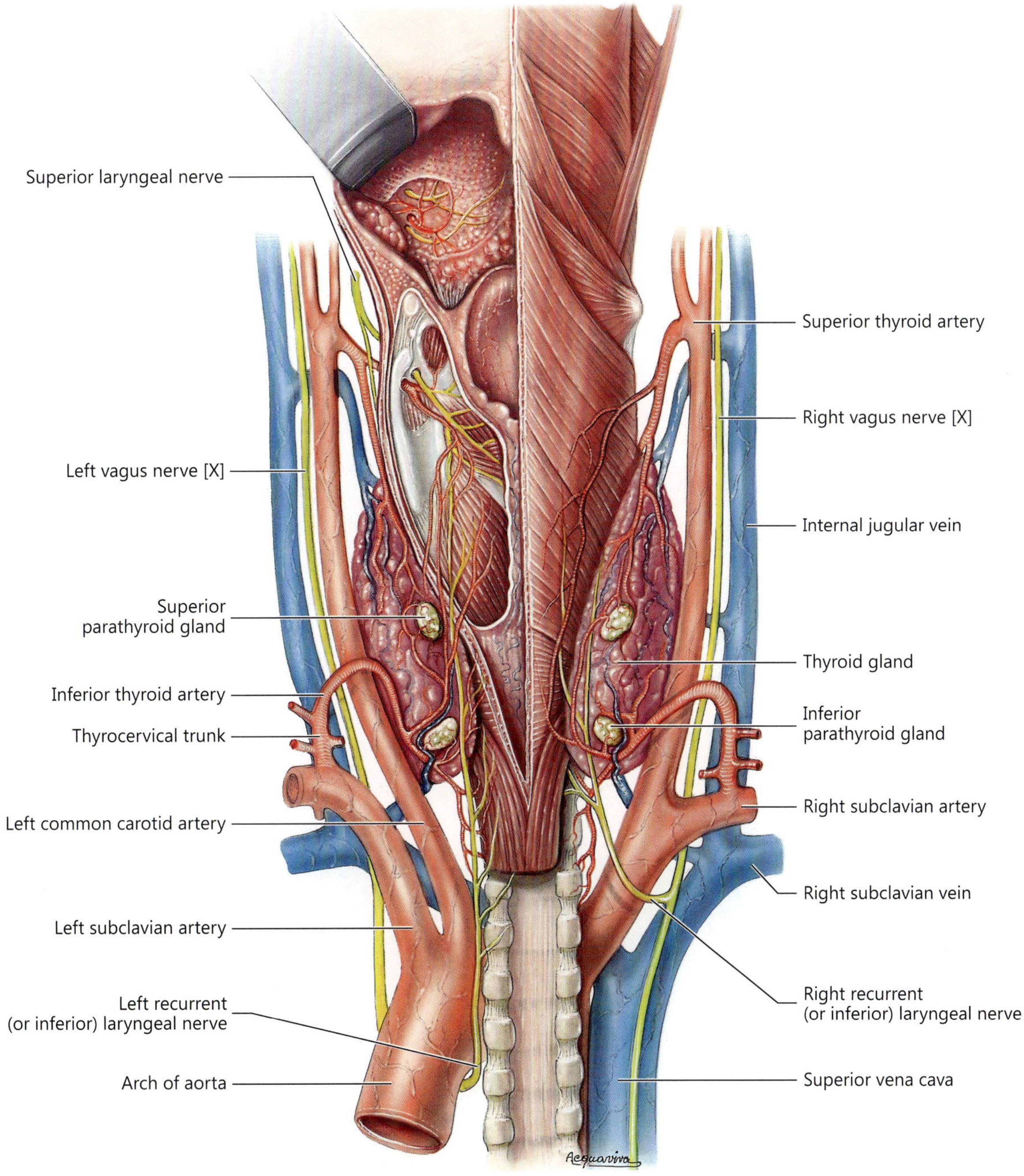

Configuration and relations of the **thyroid** and **parathyroid glands**, posterior view. On the left side, the posterolateral wall of the pharynx has been demolished in order to display the **superior laryngeal nerve** and the posterior wall of the larynx.

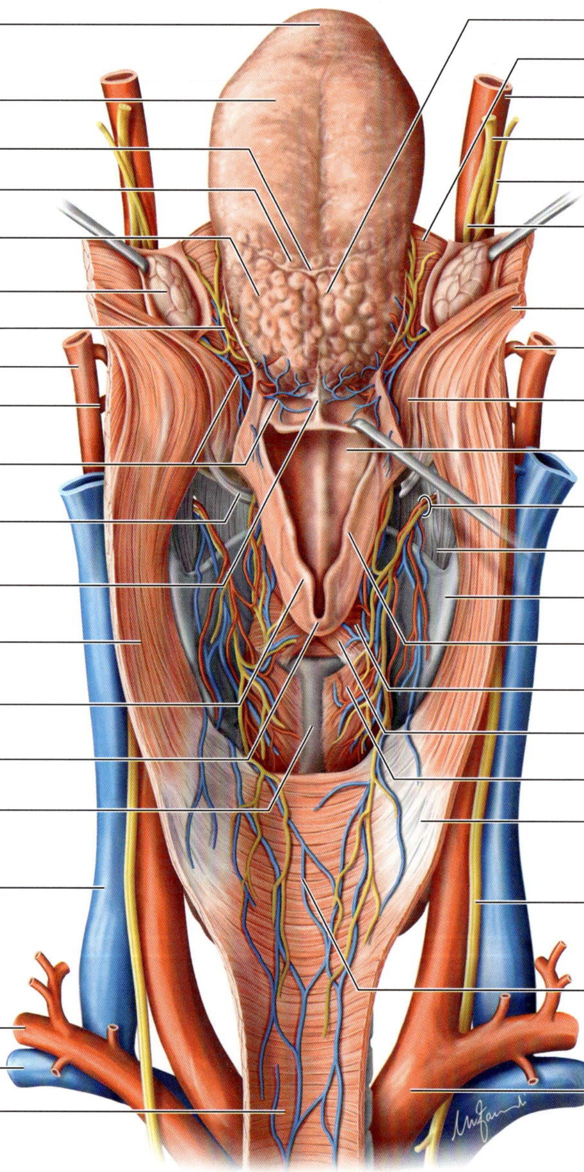

Dorsum of the tongue, **laryngeal inlet** and **laryngopharynx**, posterior view. Much of the pharynx has been removed, conserving only the anterior wall of the laryngopharynx and a small part of the lateral walls of the oropharynx. One can see the **lingual and palatine tonsils** and **branches of the hypoglossal nerve** [IX] that penetrate transversally into the posterior third of the tongue, the so-called territory of the terminal sulcus of the tongue. The vallate papillae, 7-11 in number, are situated in front of the terminal sulcus that marks the border between the body and the root of the tongue. Below the laryngeal inlet, through which the epiglottis is visible, one can see the **thyroid and cricoid cartilages** of the larynx with the posterior crico-arytenoid and oblique and transverse arytenoid.

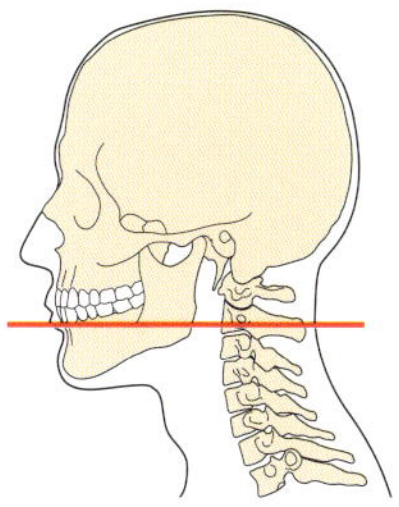

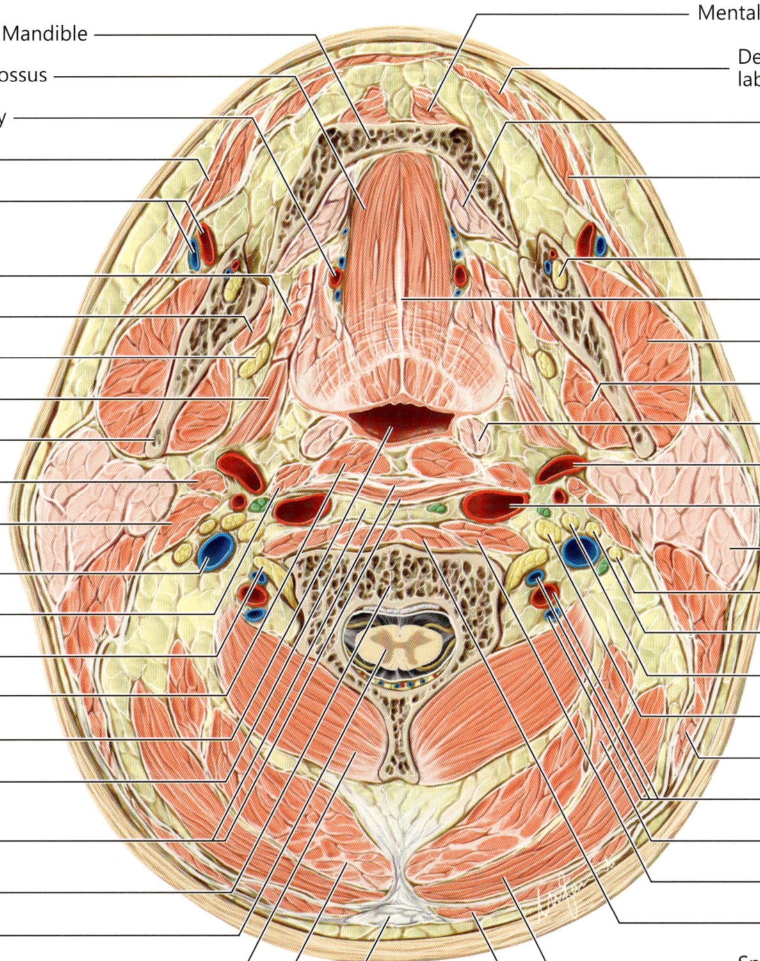

Transverse section of the **neck** passing through the second cervical vertebra (axis [C II]). One can see the **internal and external carotid arteries**, which arise from the bifurcation of the common carotid artery at the level of the disc between the third and fourth cervical vertebra, the **glossopharyngeal** [IX], **vagus** [X] and **accessory** [XI] **nerves**, which exited the cranium through the anteromedial part of the jugular foramen, the **hypoglossal nerve** [XII], which exited the posterior cranial fossa through the hypoglossal canal at the base of the occipital condyle, and the **internal jugular vein**, whose origin is at the level of the postero-lateral part of the jugular foramen. Note also: the **inferior alveolar nerve**, a branch of the mandibular nerve [V_3] during its passage through the mandibular canal; the **lingual nerve**, another offshoot of the mandibular nerve [V_3] which, after passing between the medial pterygoid and the ramus of the mandible, enters in contact with the tongue on the lateral surface of the hyoglossus; the **facial artery and vein**, which pass in front of the masseter; and the **lingual artery**, which becomes the deep artery of the tongue as it runs between the genioglossus and the anterior border of the hyoglossus.

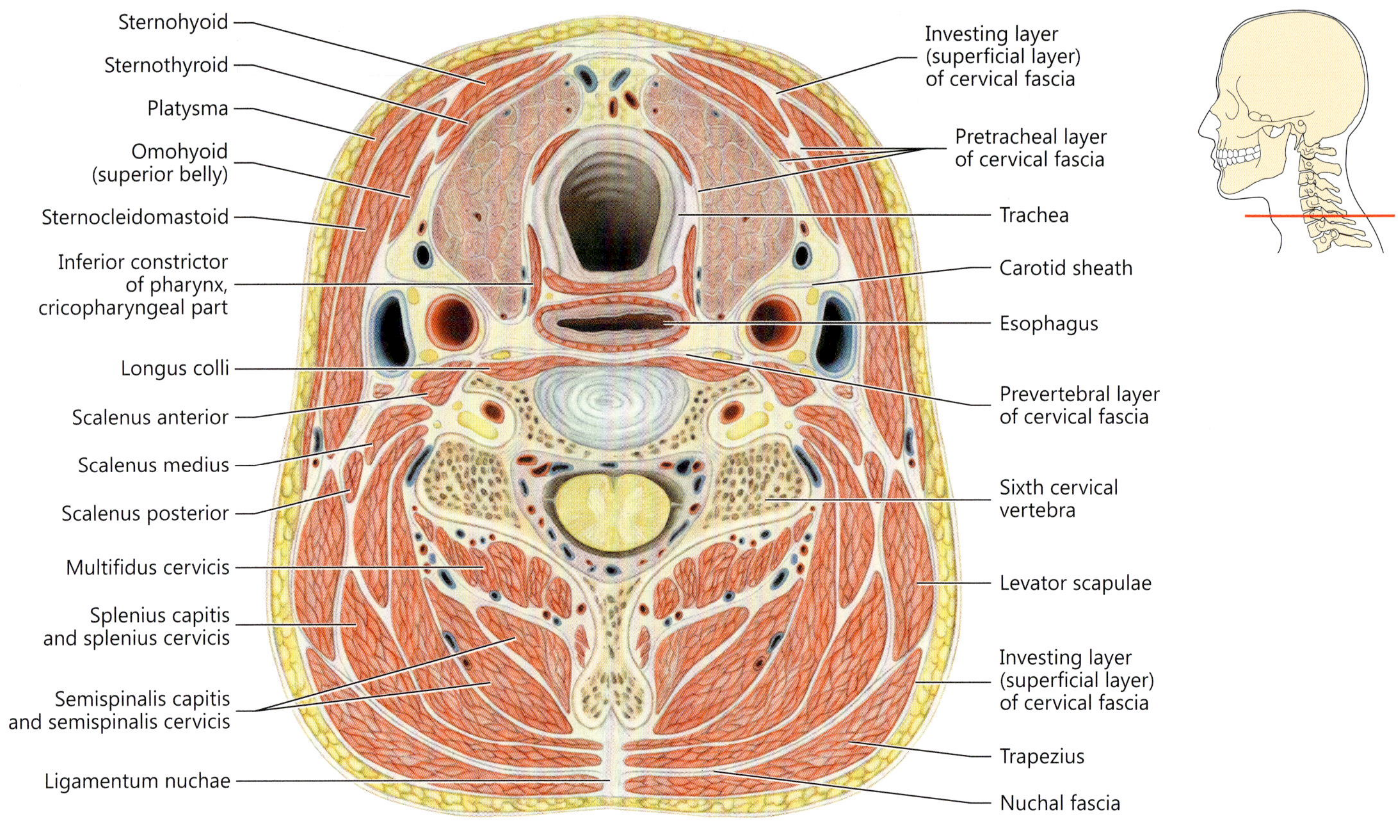

Transverse section of the neck at the level of the **6th cervical vertebra**, showing the layers of the **cervical fascia** and the structures contained within them.

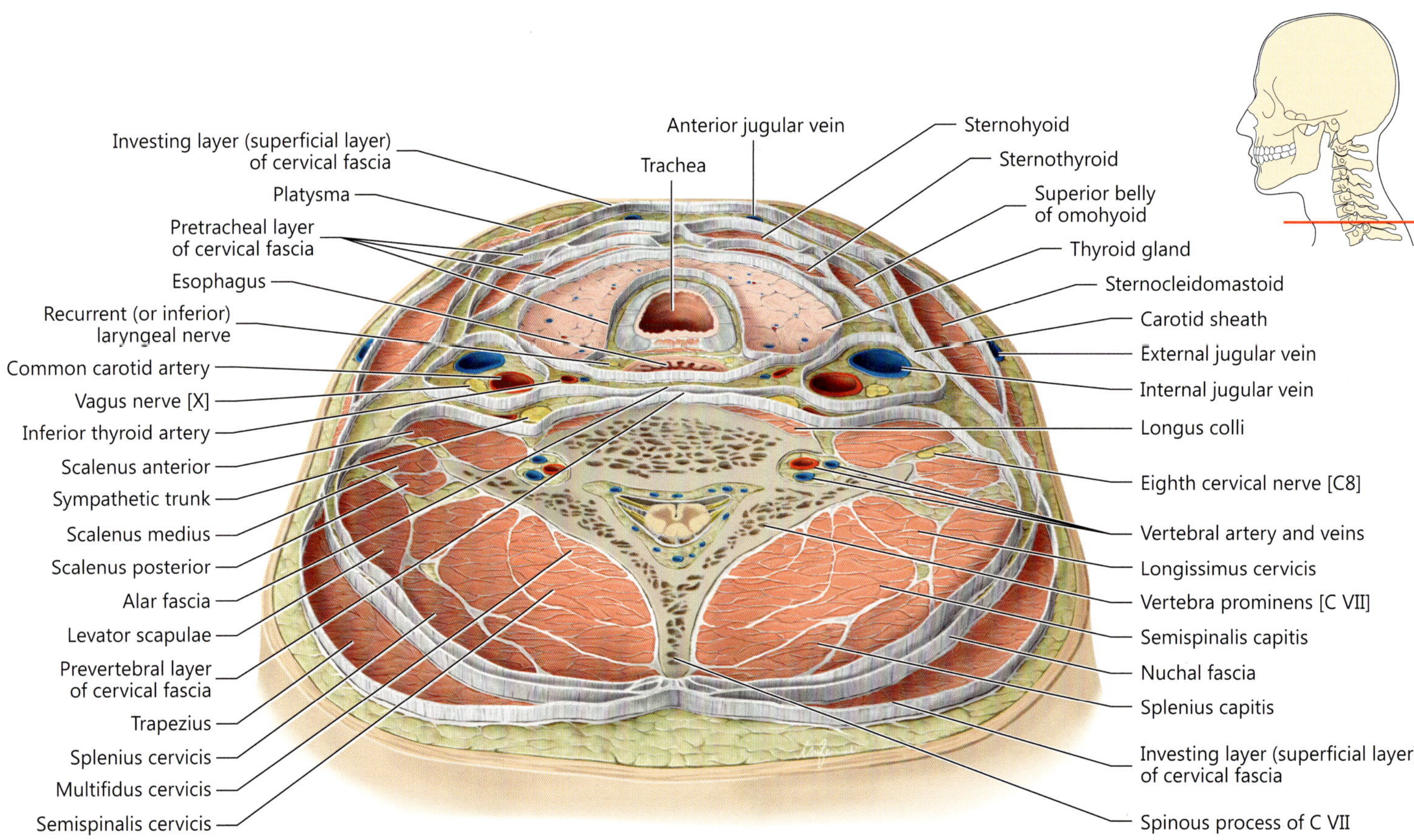

Fasciae of the neck. Schematic representation showing their organization in a transverse section of the neck at the level of the **7th cervical vertebra**.

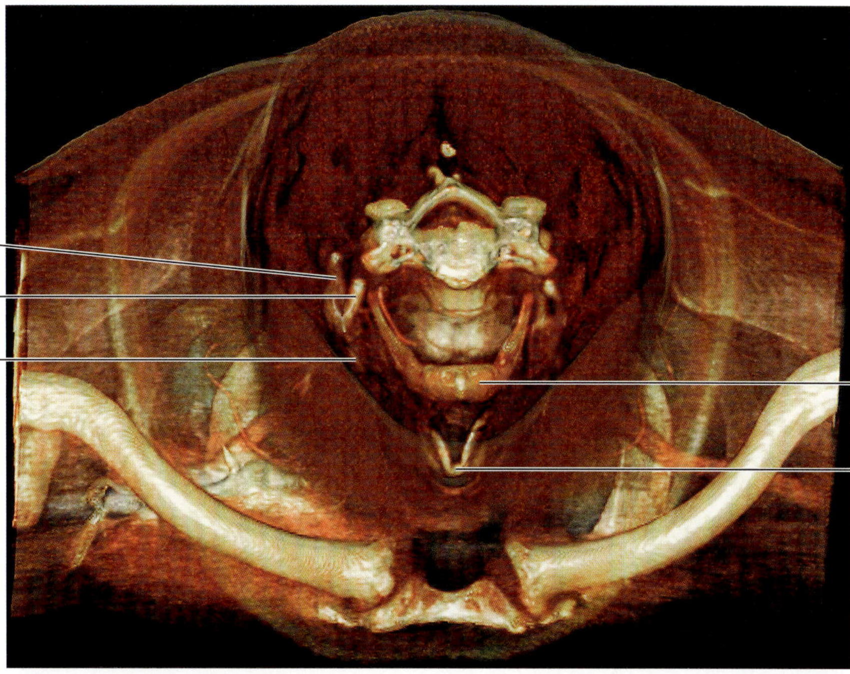

Three-dimensional image of a living human body, obtained by CT scan using a 3D volume rendering technique, showing the **vessels passing through the neck** in relation to the bony structures, in a transverse section immediately above the hyoid bone.

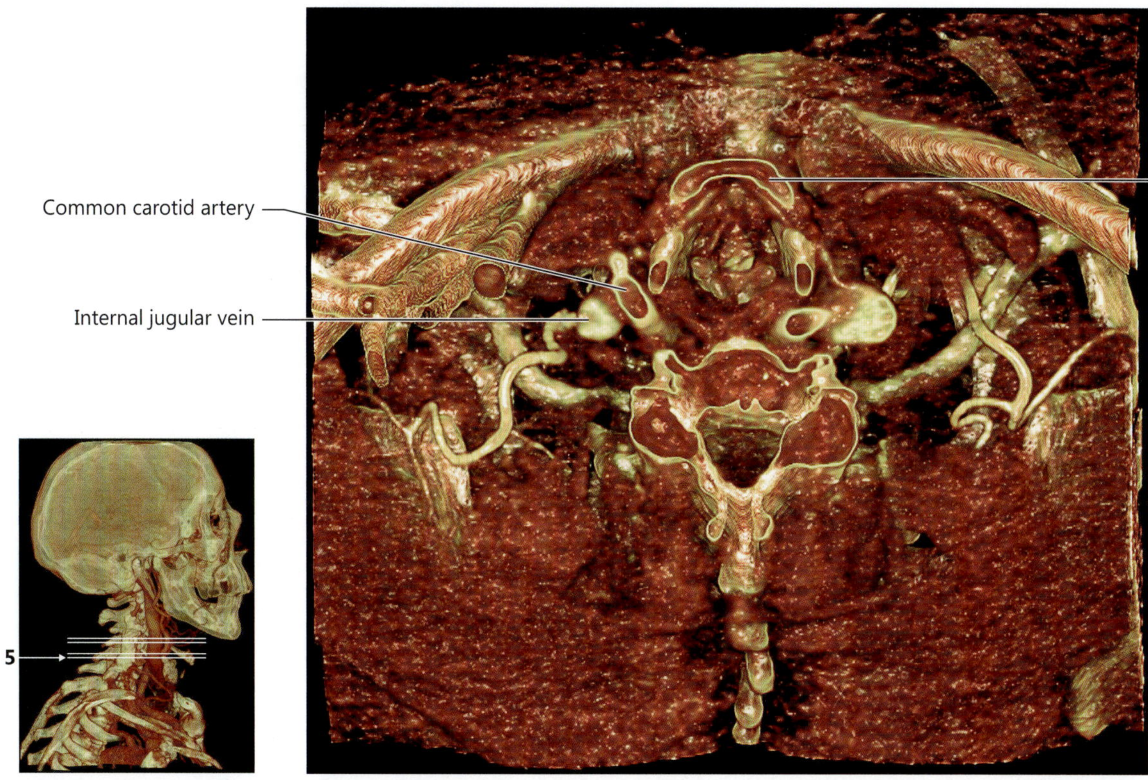

Three-dimensional image of a living human body, obtained by CT scan using a 3D volume rendering technique, showing the **vessels passing through the neck**, in a transverse section immediately below the inferior margin of the mandible before the bifurcation of the common carotid artery, on a plane (5) that passes through the fifth cervical vertebra.

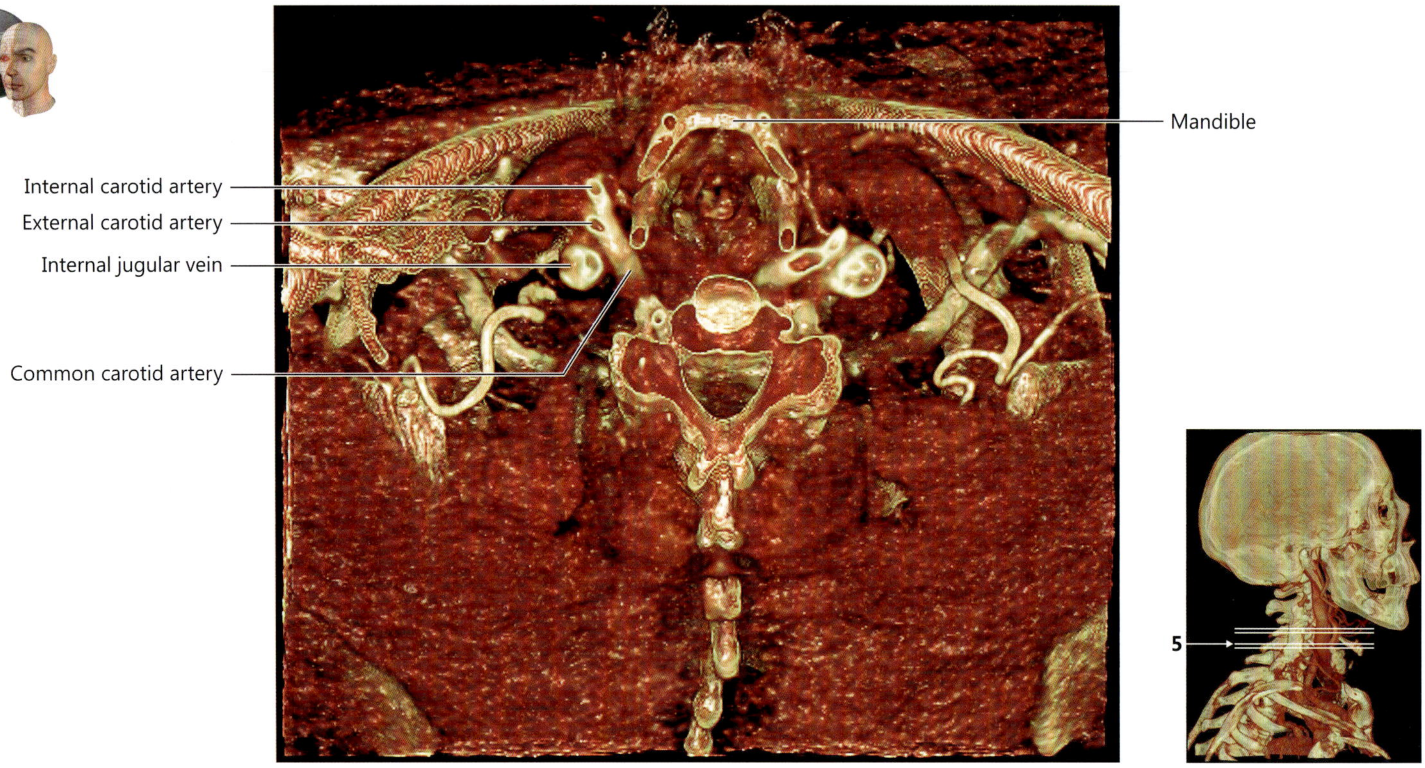

Three-dimensional image of a living human body, obtained by CT scan using a 3D volume rendering technique, showing the **vessels passing through the neck**, in a transverse section immediately above the bifurcation of the common carotid artery, on a plane (5) that passes through the fifth cervical vertebra.

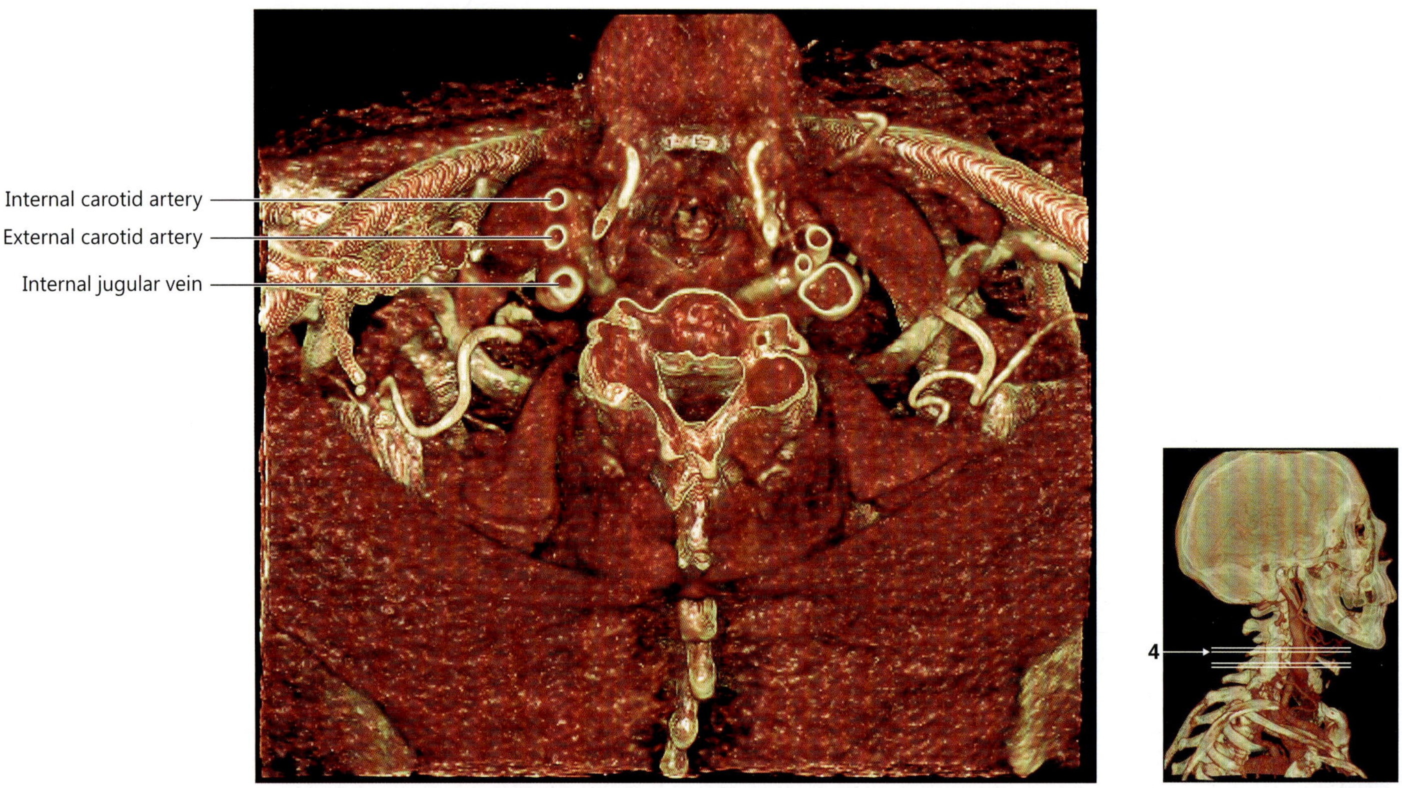

Three-dimensional image of a living human body, obtained by CT scan using a 3D volume rendering technique, showing the **vessels passing through the neck**, in a transverse section immediately above the bifurcation of the common carotid artery, on a plane (4) that passes through the fourth cervical vertebra.

THORAX

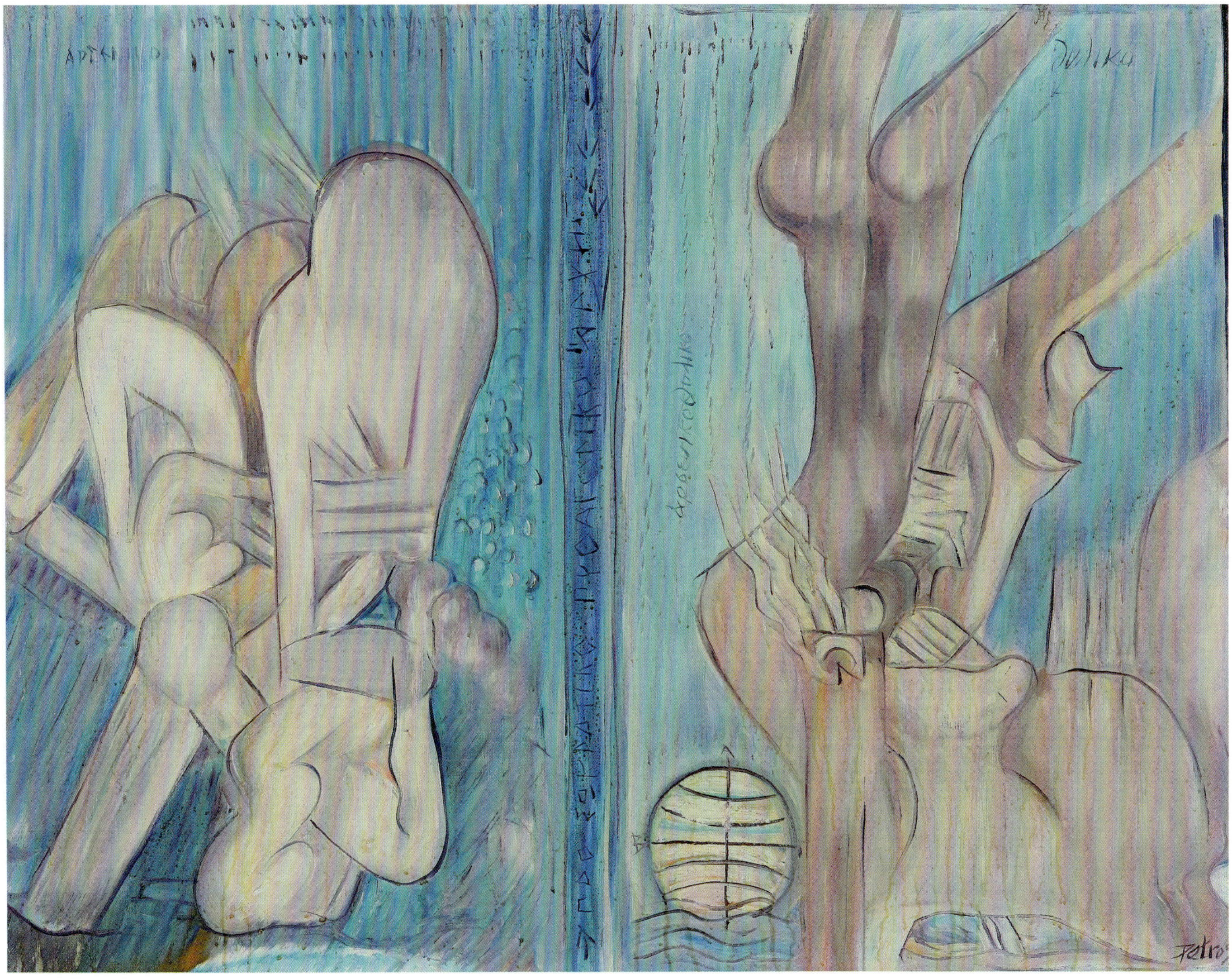

Petros (Athens, 1928 - Milan, 2014), *Pitagoro archi*, oil on canvas, cm 80 × 60, 1991

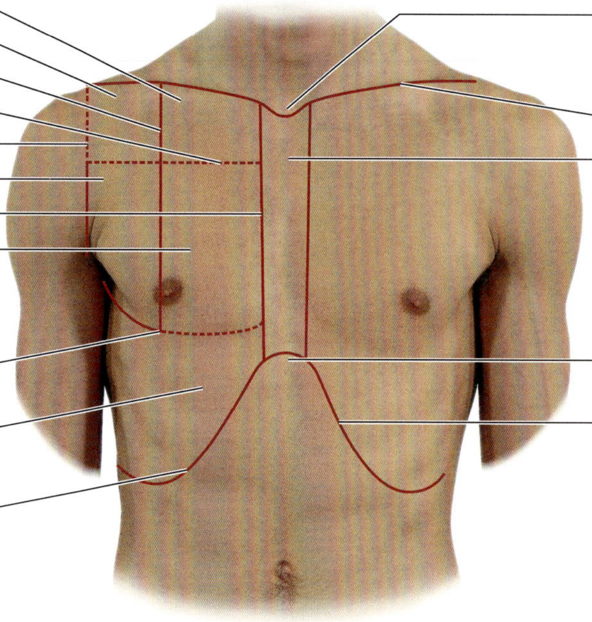

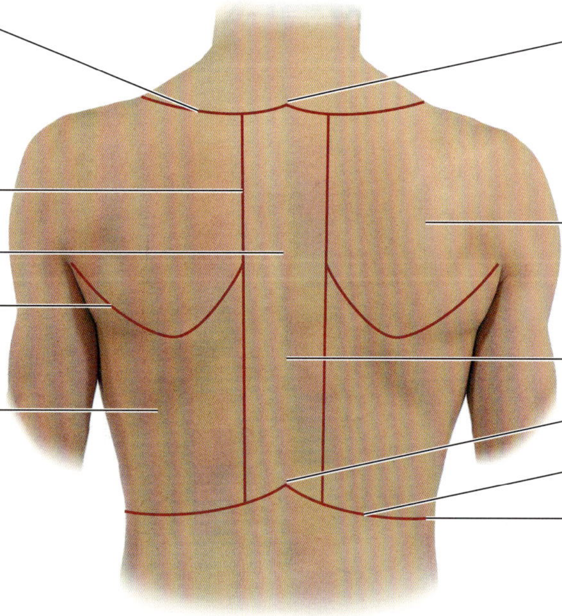

THORACIC REGIONS	***BOUNDARIES OR LOCATION***
Infraclavicular region and infraclavicular fossa (clavipectoral or deltopectoral triangle)	Infraclavicular fossa: depression of the skin between the clavicle (superiorly), deltoid (laterally) and pectoralis major (medially), to which the clavipectoral triangle corresponds at deep level. Superior, inferior, medial and lateral boundaries of the infraclavicular region: inferior border of the neck, line passing over the third rib, sternal line and anterior axillary line
Costal	Superficial area of the thorax between the inframammary sulcus and costal margin, including, posteriorly, the infrascapular region. Inferior boundary: thoracoabdominal line. Note: the diaphragmatic cupula is situated at a higher level than the thoracoabdominal line and some abdominal organs are located in a zone belonging superficially to the thorax, but deeply to the abdomen (hypochondrium)
Pectoral	Area overlying the pectoralis major
– inframammary	Area of the pectoral region underlying the mammary region. Inferior boundary: inframammary sulcus
– lateral pectoral	Area of the pectoral region between the midclavicular (medially) and anterior axillary (laterally) lines, including the anterior and medial walls of the axilla (pectoralis major, pectoralis minor and serratus anterior)
– mammary	Area of the pectoral region corresponding to the breast
Presternal (or sternal)	Area in front of the sternum, between the jugular notch (superiorly), xiphoid process (inferiorly) and sternal lines (laterally)
Vertebral (at the thoracic level)	Region of the back, at the thoracic level, between the spinous processes of the seventh cervical vertebra [C VII] (superiorly) and the twelfth thoracic vertebra [T XII] (inferiorly) and vertical lines passing through the medial border of the scapula or the angle of the rib
Infrascapular	Region of the back underlying the scapular region. Inferior and superior boundaries: twelfth rib [XII] and scapula
Interscapular	Region of the back between the two scapulae

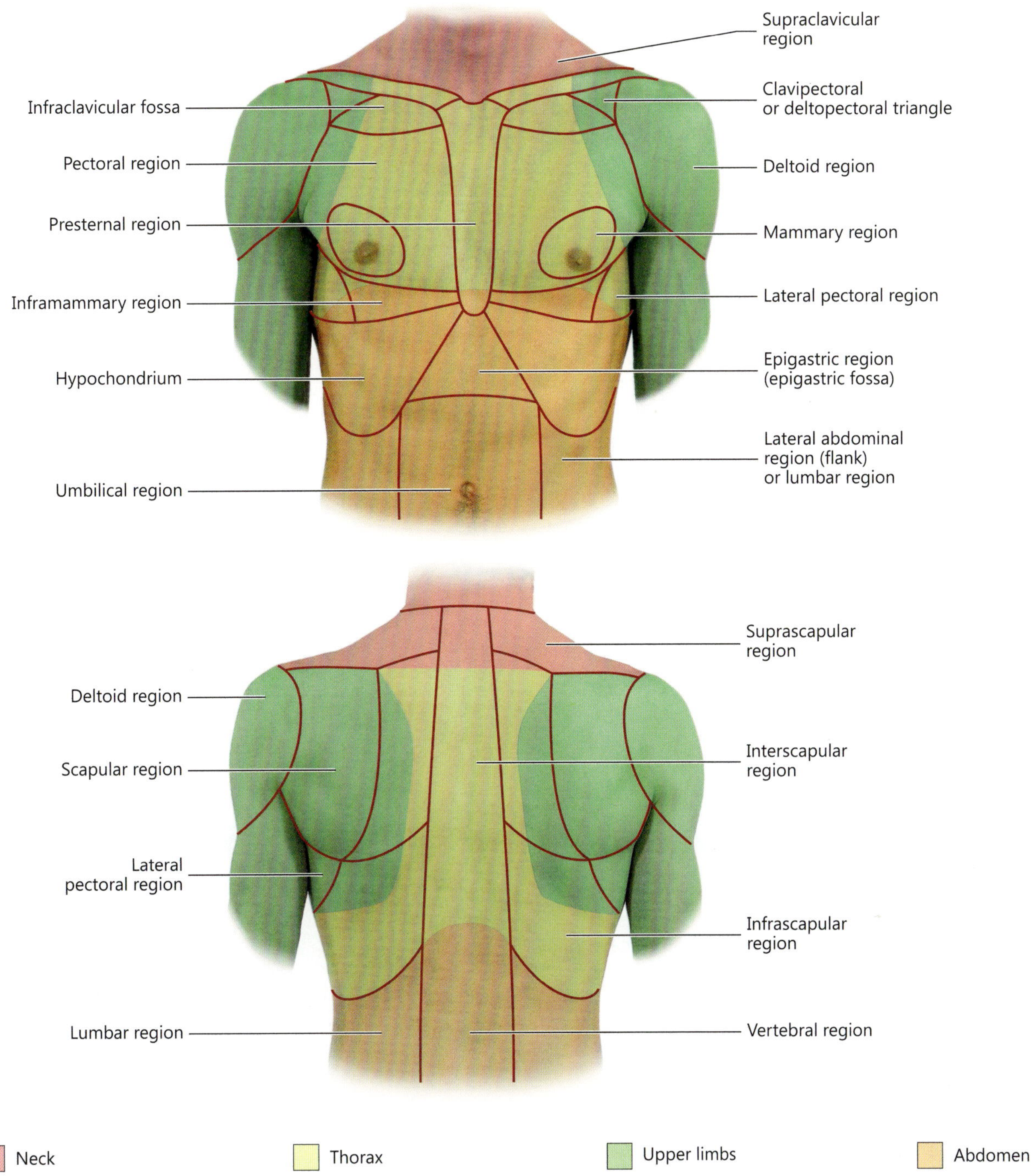

Projection of the thoracic cavity and regions of the thorax. The thoracic cavity has different boundaries from those of the wall. At the top it surpasses the inferior border of the neck reaching the supraclavicular fossae with the cervical pleurae and the apexes of the lung, while below it corresponds to the diaphragmatic cupula which is situated at a higher level than the thoracoabdominal line, so that some abdominal organs are located in a zone that, superficially, belongs to the thorax. Superficially this boundary corresponds approximately to the xiphoid line in front, while at the back it coincides with the thoracoabdominal line. The thorax is separated from the upper limb by a line that anteriorly passes medially to the glenohumeral joint and posteriorly along the medial border of the scapula.

➤

Boundaries of the thorax. The superficial boundaries of the thorax are represented by the **inferior border of the neck** – that separates the thorax from the neck – which starts from the jugular notch of the sternum and follows, on each side, the superior border of the clavicle and the acromion to reach the spinous process of the seventh cervical vertebra, and the **thoracoabdominal line** – that separates the thorax from the neck – which begins at the base of the xiphoid process of the sternum and follows, on each side, the costal margin and the inferior border of the twelfth rib to reach the spinous process of the twelfth thoracic vertebra.

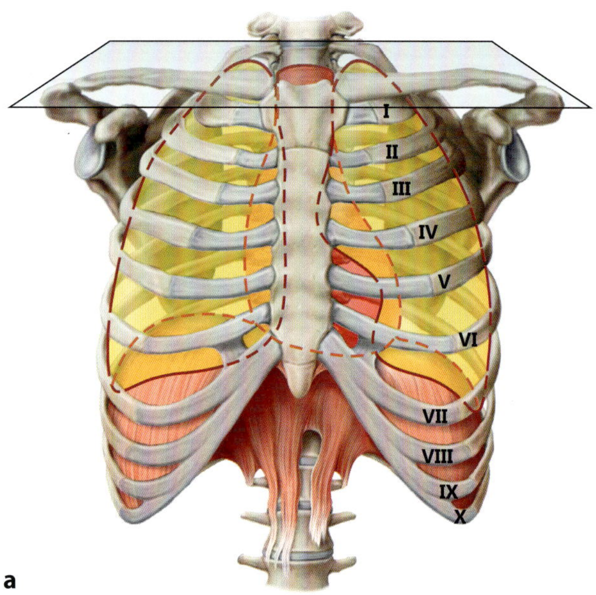

a

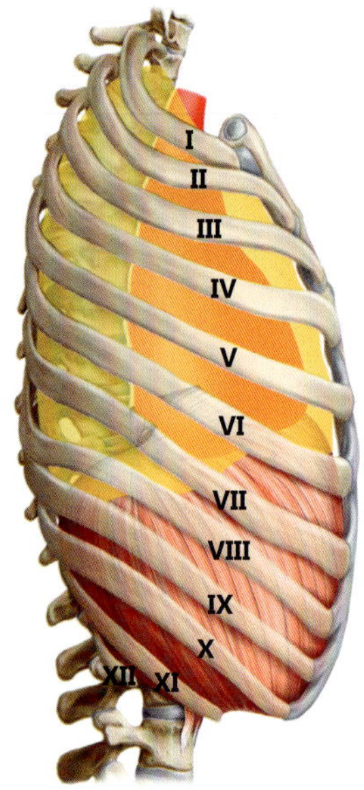

b

The **thoracic cavity** is contained within the thoracic cage. At the top, an imaginary transverse plane passing through the first rib separates it from the neck (**a**). At the bottom, the diaphragm separates it from the abdominal cavity (**a**, **b**). The concavity of the diaphragmatic cupula, convex at the top, encloses the superior part of the abdominal cavity (supramesocolic space and high part of the retroperitoneal space) and its contents. The thoracic cavity, thus, does not coincide with the boundaries of the thoracic cage (☞ Musculoskeletal System - General Anatomy) (**c**).

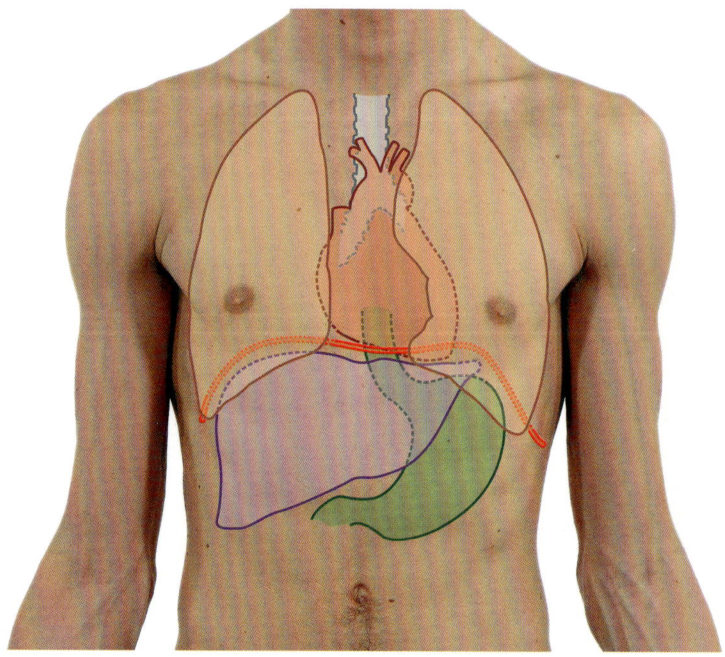

c

X-ray image of the **heart**, posteroanterior projection. In the thoracic cavity, two large lateral cavities can be detected, the pleural compartments, separated by a median space, the mediastinum. The pleural compartments house the lungs and the pleurae. The mediastinum contains numerous anatomical structures, the largest of which is the heart.

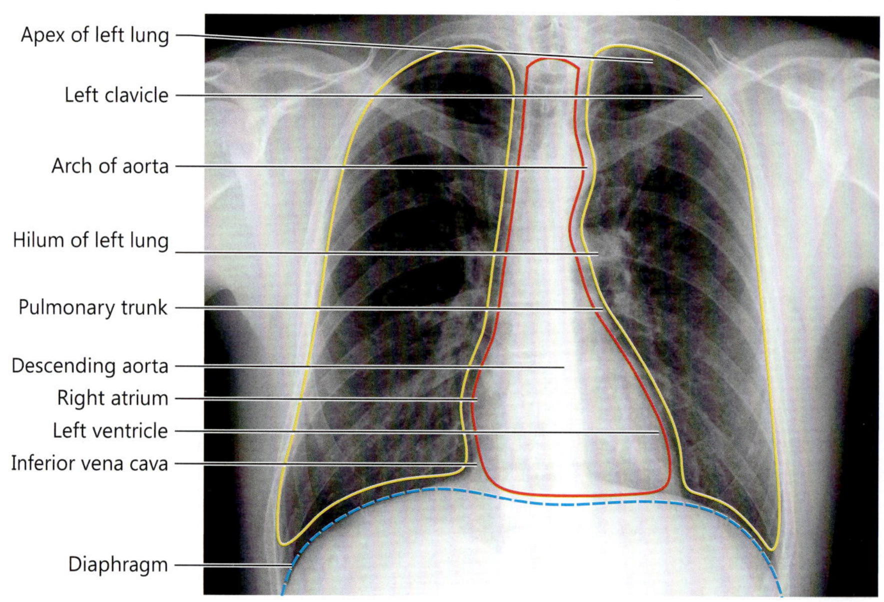

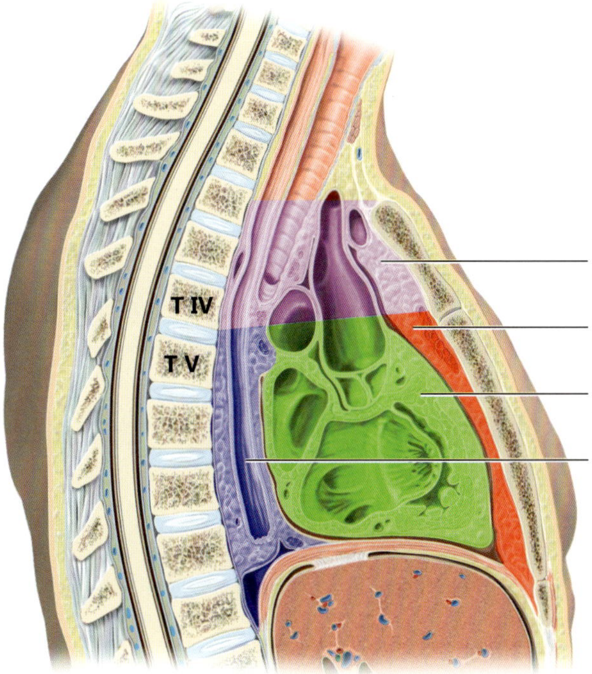

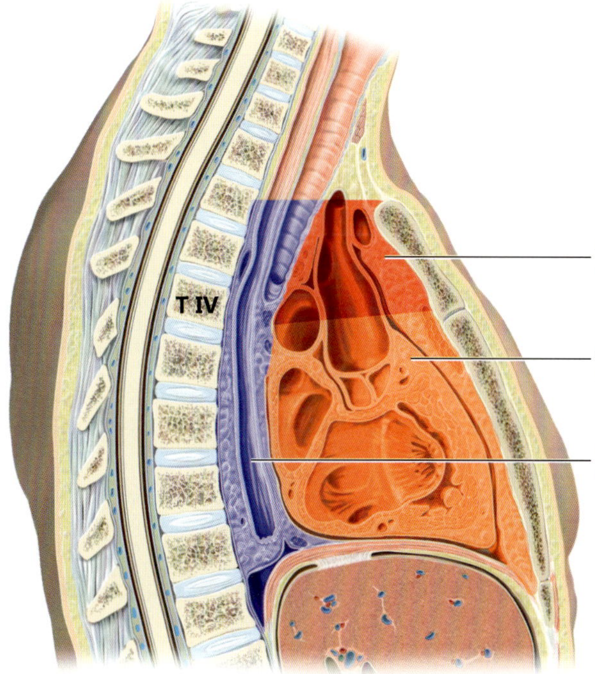

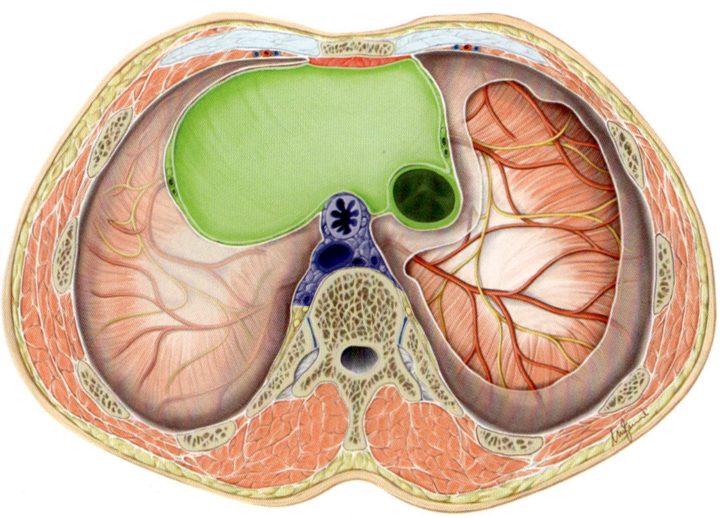

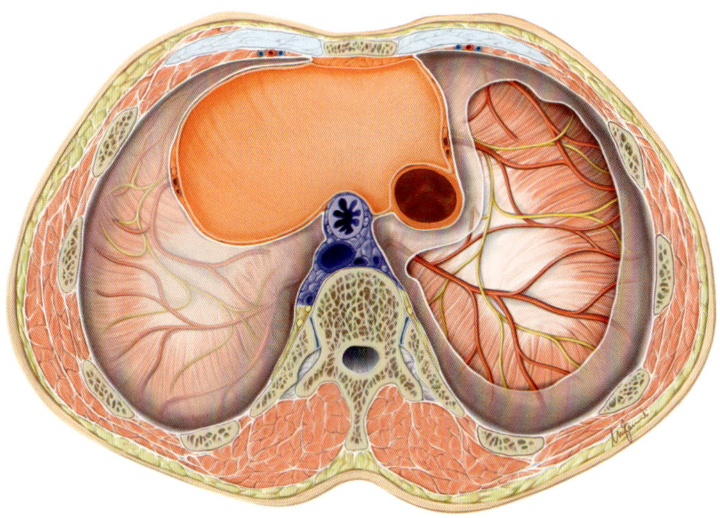

Subdivisions of the **mediastinum** according to the international anatomical nomenclature. The subdivisions are described in the table below. In the image above, the boundary between the superior and inferior mediastinum is represented by a plane passing through the intervertebral disc between T IV and T V and the sternal angle.

Subdivisions of the mediastinum according to the Latin school. The subdivision between anterior and posterior mediastinum is defined by the course of the posterior layer of the pretracheal layer of cervical fascia (☞ Head and Neck - Fasciae of the Neck), which extends downwards to the great vessels of the heart. The subdivision between superior and inferior mediastinum is limited to the anterior mediastinum.

SUBDIVISION	***BOUNDARIES***
Mediastinum	*Upper*: oblique plane passing through the superior border of the manubrium of sternum and first rib. *Lower*: central part of the diaphragm. *Front*: sternum and costal cartilages [I-VII]. *Back*: thoracic part of the vertebral column [T I-T XII]
Superior mediastinum	*Inferior boundary*: plane passing through intervertebral disc between T IV and T V and the sternal angle
Inferior mediastinum	*Inferior boundary*: diaphragm
• anterior	Between the sternum and the sternocostal surface of the pericardium
• middle	Between the sternocostal surface of the pericardium and a frontal plane passing through the posterior surface of the trachea and main bronchi and the posterior surface of the pericardium
• posterior	Between the posterior surfaces of the trachea, main bronchi and pericardium and the vertebral column (between T IV/T V and T XII, in according to the Anglo-saxon school, or T I-T XII, in according to the Latin school)

Contents of the mediastinum	
DENOMINATION	***CONTENTS***
Superior mediastinum	• Arch of aorta • Branches of the arch of aorta (brachiocephalic trunk, left common carotid artery, left subclavian artery) • Supreme intercostal artery (right and left) • Pericardiacophrenic artery (right and left) • Internal thoracic artery (right and left) • Thoracic duct • Esophagus • Pretracheal layer of cervical fascia • Thoracic ganglia of sympathetic trunk (right and left) • Insertions of sternohyoid and sternothyroid (right and left) • Insertions of longus colli on the first three thoracic vertebrae [T I-T III], medial and inferior lateral bundles (right and left) • Brachiocephalic nodes • Posterior intercostal nodes (right and left) • Paratracheal nodes (right and left) • Preaorticocarotid nodes • Prevascular nodes • Superior tracheobronchial nodes (right and left) • Upper half of the superior vena cava • Phrenic nerves • Vagus nerves (right and left) • Right and left recurrent (or inferior) laryngeal nerves • Cardiac plexus • Thymus or residual thymic tissue and fibroadipose tissue • Trachea • Bronchomediastinal trunks • Accessory hemiazygos vein (first tract) • Supreme intercostal vein (right and left) • Brachiocephalic vein (right and left) • Pericardiacophrenic vein (right and left) • Internal thoracic vein (right and left)
Posterior mediastinum	• Thoracic aorta • Branches of the thoracic aorta: mediastinal branches, bronchial branches, esophageal branches, pericardial branches • Right Intercostal arteries from 4th to 12th • Thoracic duct • Esophagus • Thoracic ganglia of sympathetic trunk (right and left) • Pulmonary (triangular) ligaments (right and left) • Vertebropericardial ligaments • Posterior intercostal nodes • Posterior mediastinal nodes (juxtaesophageal nodes, interaorticoesophageal nodes, juxta-aortic nodes, posterior superior diaphragmatic nodes) • Splanchnic nerves • Esophageal plexus • Azygoesophageal and interaortoesophageal pleural recesses • Anterior and posterior vagal trunks • Azygos vein on right side • Hemiazygos vein and accessory hemiazygos vein (last tract) on left side
Middle mediastinum	• Ascending aorta • Bronchial branches of thoracic aorta (right and left) • Pericardial branches of thoracic aorta • Pericardiacophrenic artery and vein (right and left) • Pulmonary arteries (right and left) • Tracheal bifurcation • Main bronchi (right and left) • Heart • Pericardiacophrenic ligaments • Middle superior diaphragmatic nodes (diaphragmatic anterior mediastinal nodes) • Superior and inferior tracheobronchial nodes • Lower half of the superior vena cava • Phrenic nerves • Pericardium • Cardiac plexus • Pulmonary plexus • Pulmonary trunk and ligamentum arteriosum (ligamentum of Botallo) • Opening of azygos vein into the superior vena cava • Bronchial veins (right and left) • Superior and inferior pulmonary veins (right and left)
Anterior mediastinum	• Sternopericardial ligaments (superior and inferior) • Prepericardial nodes, lateral pericardial nodes and anterior superior diaphragmatic nodes • Costomediastinal pleural recesses • Loose connective tissue • Thymus or residual thymic tissue

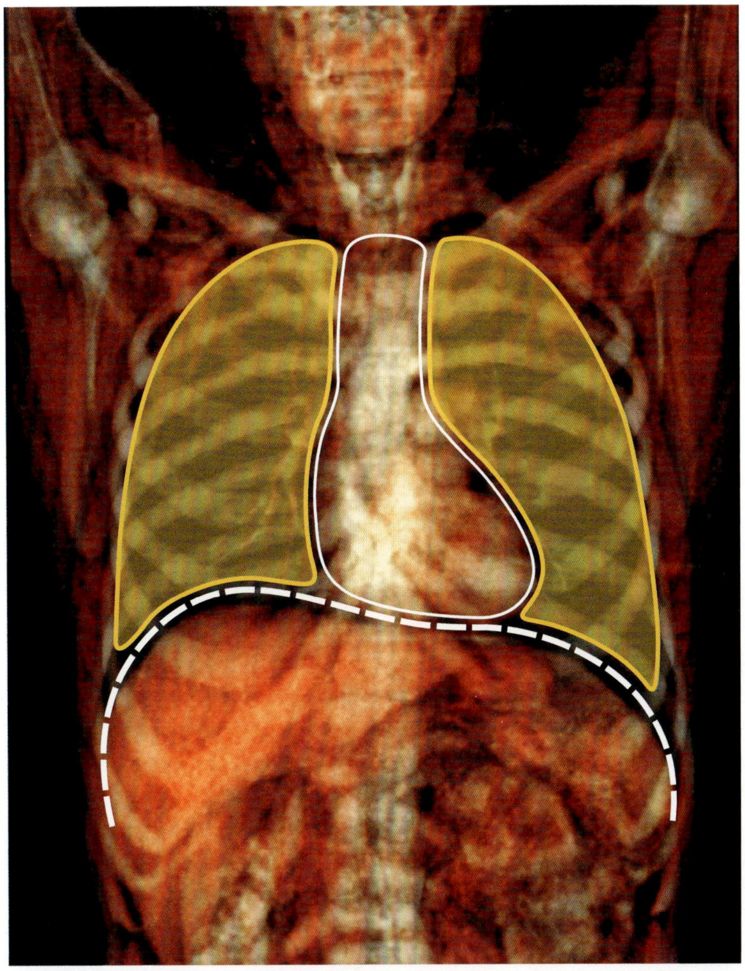

The lungs are housed in the **pleural compartments** inside the thoracic cavity (three-dimensional image of a living human body, obtained by CT scan using a 3D volume rendering technique).

Pleural compartments

DENOMINATION	*BOUNDARIES*	*CONTENT*	*BLOOD SUPPLY*	*INNERVATION*	*LYMPHATIC DRAINAGE*
Right and left pleural compartments	Superior: subclavian vessels, brachial plexus, scalenus anterior Inferior: diaphragm Medial: mediastinum Lateral: ribs and intercostal muscles	Right and left lungs	Lung: pulmonary artery, pulmonary veins; bronchial branches of thoracic aorta and bronchial veins	Lung: anterior and posterior pulmonary plexuses (branches of the vagus nerve and the sympathetic part)	Lung: superficial (subpleural) lymphatic plexus and deep lymphatic plexus (which accompanies the branches of the pulmonary and bronchial vessels) draining into the bronchopulmonary nodes (the deep lymphatic plexus, through the intrapulmonary nodes)
		Visceral pleura Pleural cavity	Visceral pleura: bronchial branches of thoracic aorta and pulmonary veins	Visceral pleura: pulmonary plexuses	Visceral pleura: subserosal lymphatic network connected to the lymphatic vessels which accompany the pulmonary veins and drain into the tracheobronchial nodes
		Parietal pleura	Parietal pleura: intercostal arteries (costal part of parietal pleura), superior phrenic arteries and inferior phrenic arteries (diaphragmatic part of parietal pleura), mediastinal branches of thoracic aorta (mediastinal part of parietal pleura), azygos vein and internal thoracic veins	Parietal pleura: intercostal nerves, vagus nerve, phrenic nerve, branches of the sympathetic part	Parietal pleura: intercommunicating lymphatic networks which drain into the parasternal, intercostal and diaphragmatic nodes

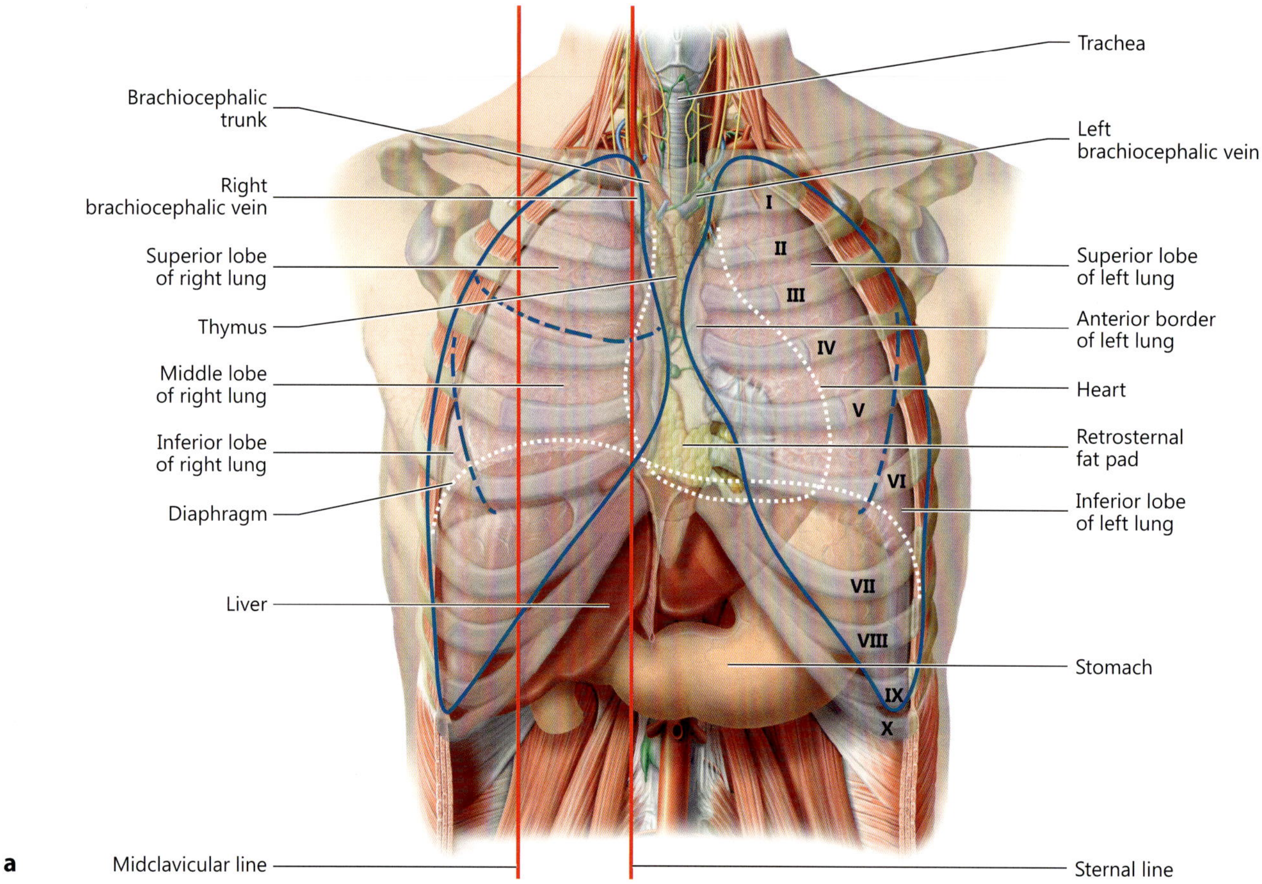

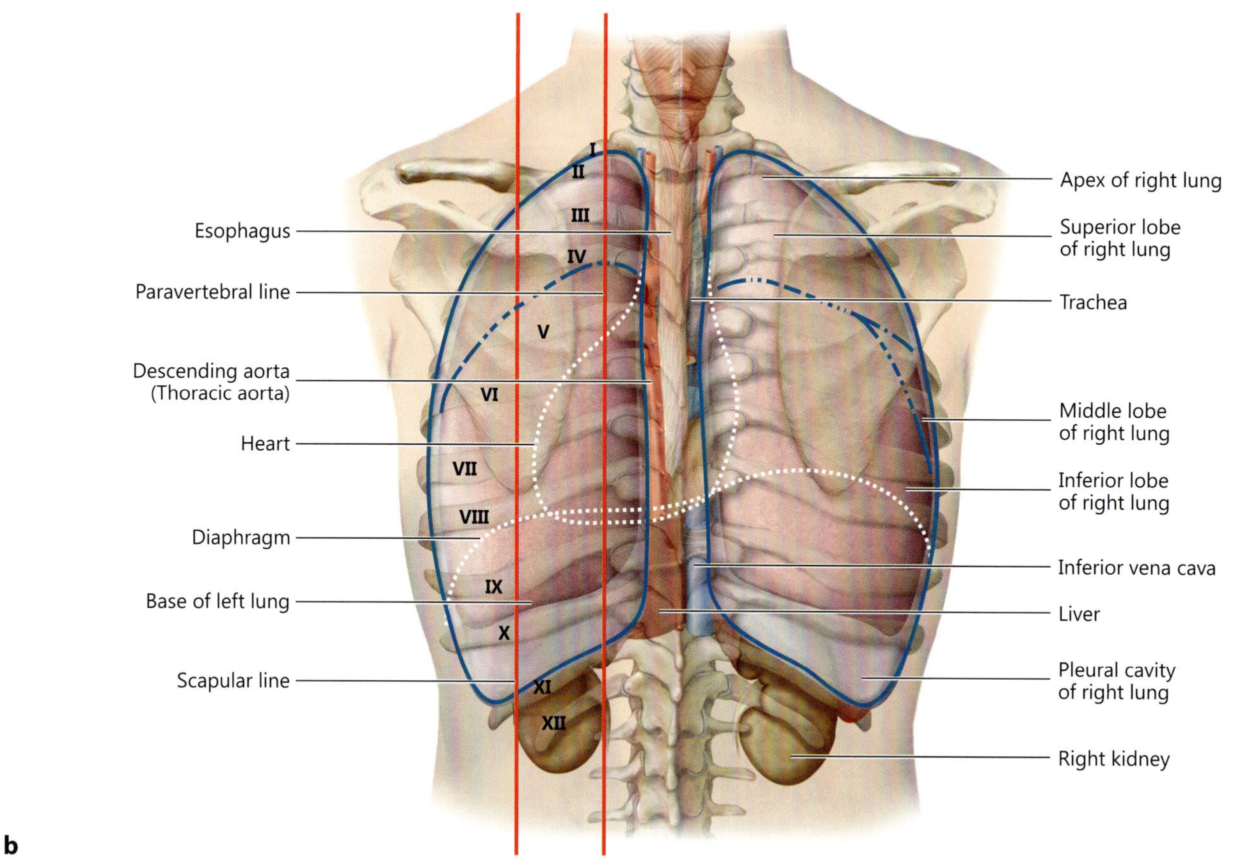

Projection onto the surface of the thoracic cage of the visceral and vascular formations of the **mediastinum** and of the **pleural compartments**. The *white* dotted lines define the contours of the diaphragm, heart and the great vessels. The *blue* lines define the boundaries of the parietal pleura. Within these boundaries one can see, in transparency, the lungs and the course of the pulmonary fissures (indicated by the dotted line). Also visible, in transparency, are some internal organs of the abdominal cavity on account of the latter's extension into the thoracic cage below the diaphragm. **a**, Anterior projection; **b**, posterior projection.

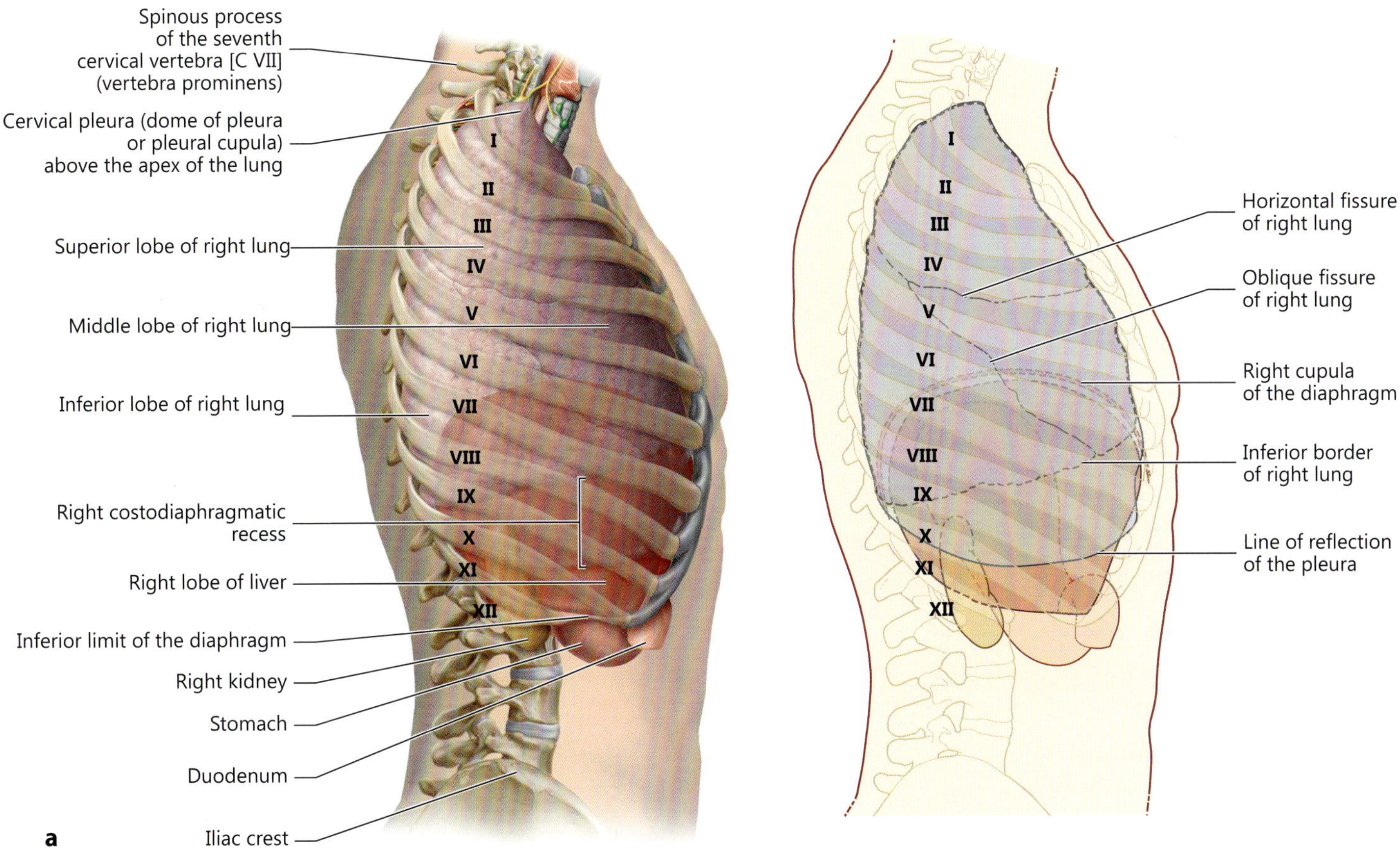

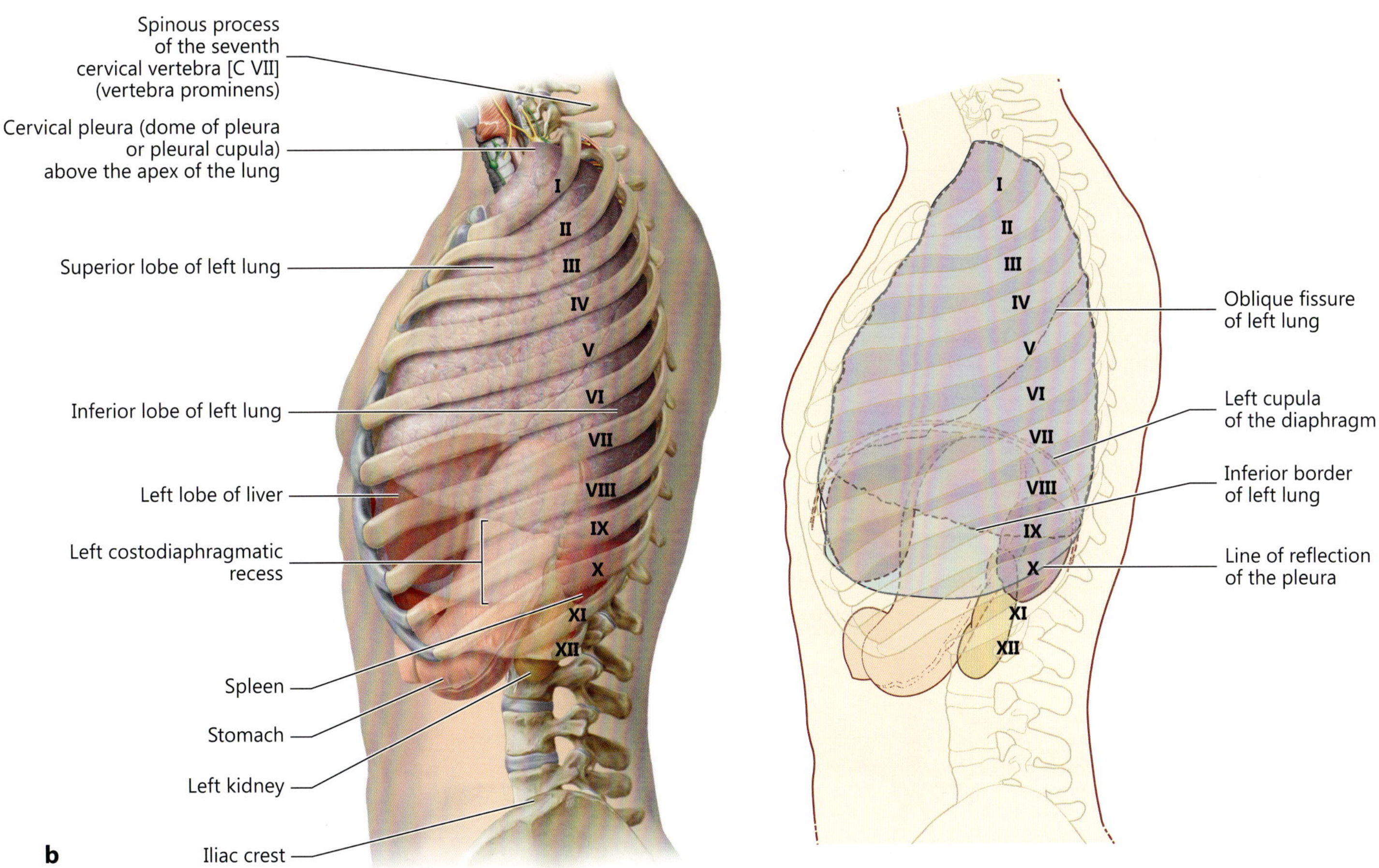

Projection onto the thoracic cage of the **lungs** and **supramesocolic** and **retroperitoneal organs** located in the thoracic cage. **a**, Right lateral projection. **b**, Left lateral projection.

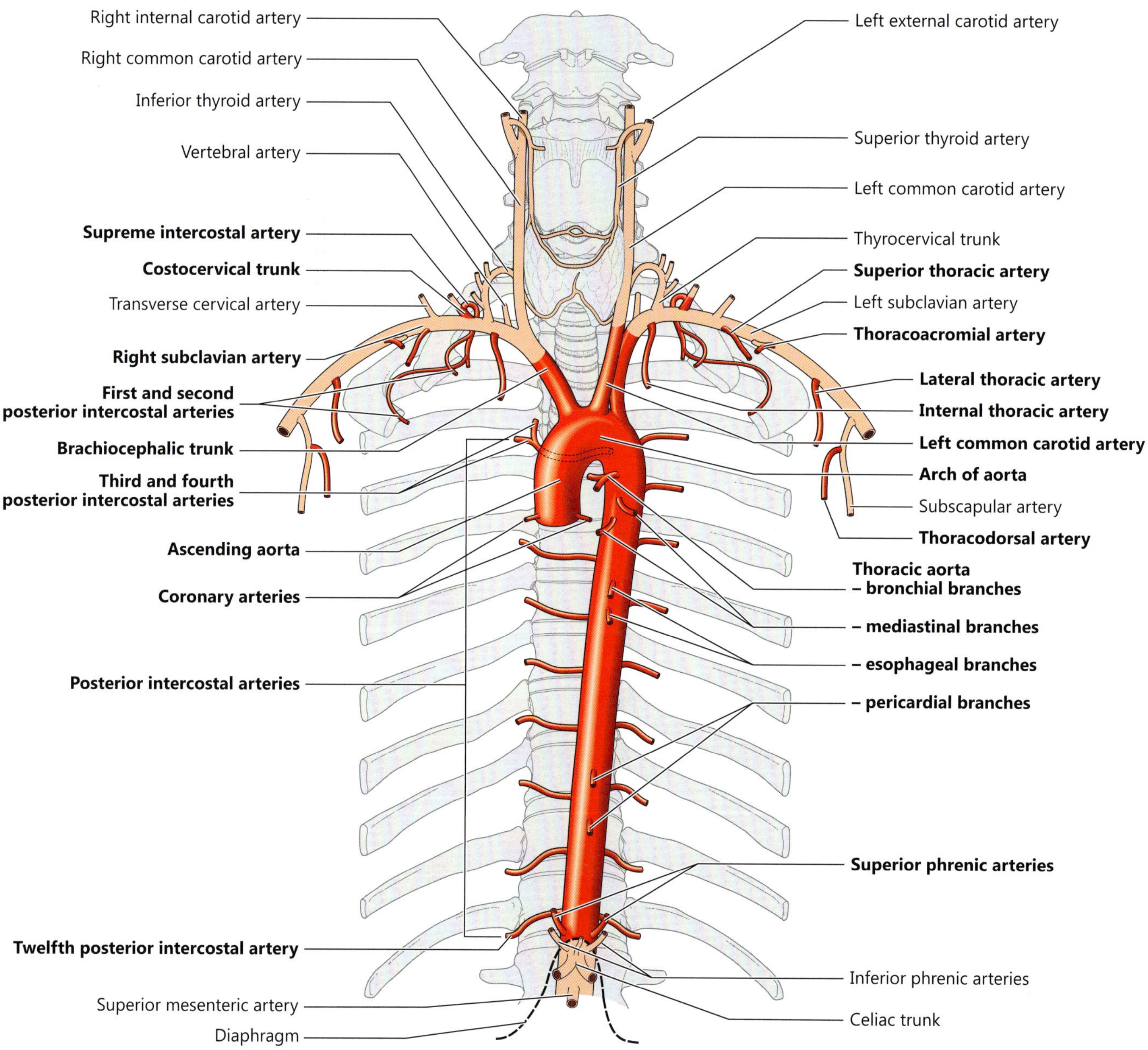

Schematic representation of the **arch of the aorta** and **thoracic aorta** with the arteries and branches involved in the visceral and parietal blood supply of the thorax.

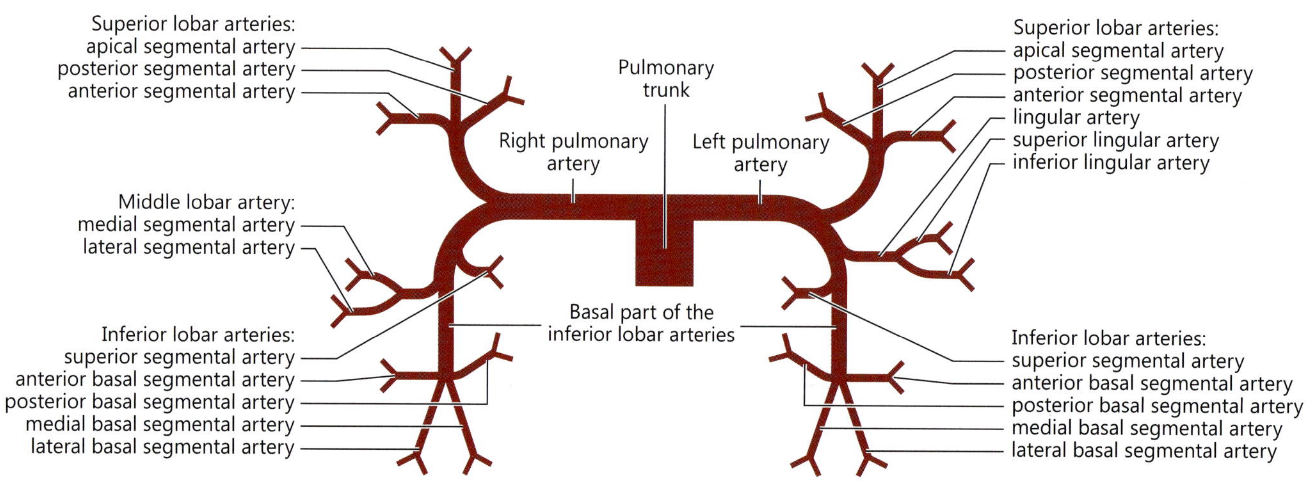

Schematic representation of the division of the **pulmonary trunk** into the **right and left pulmonary arteries**, which ramify attaching themselves to the bronchial branches and following their subdivisions.

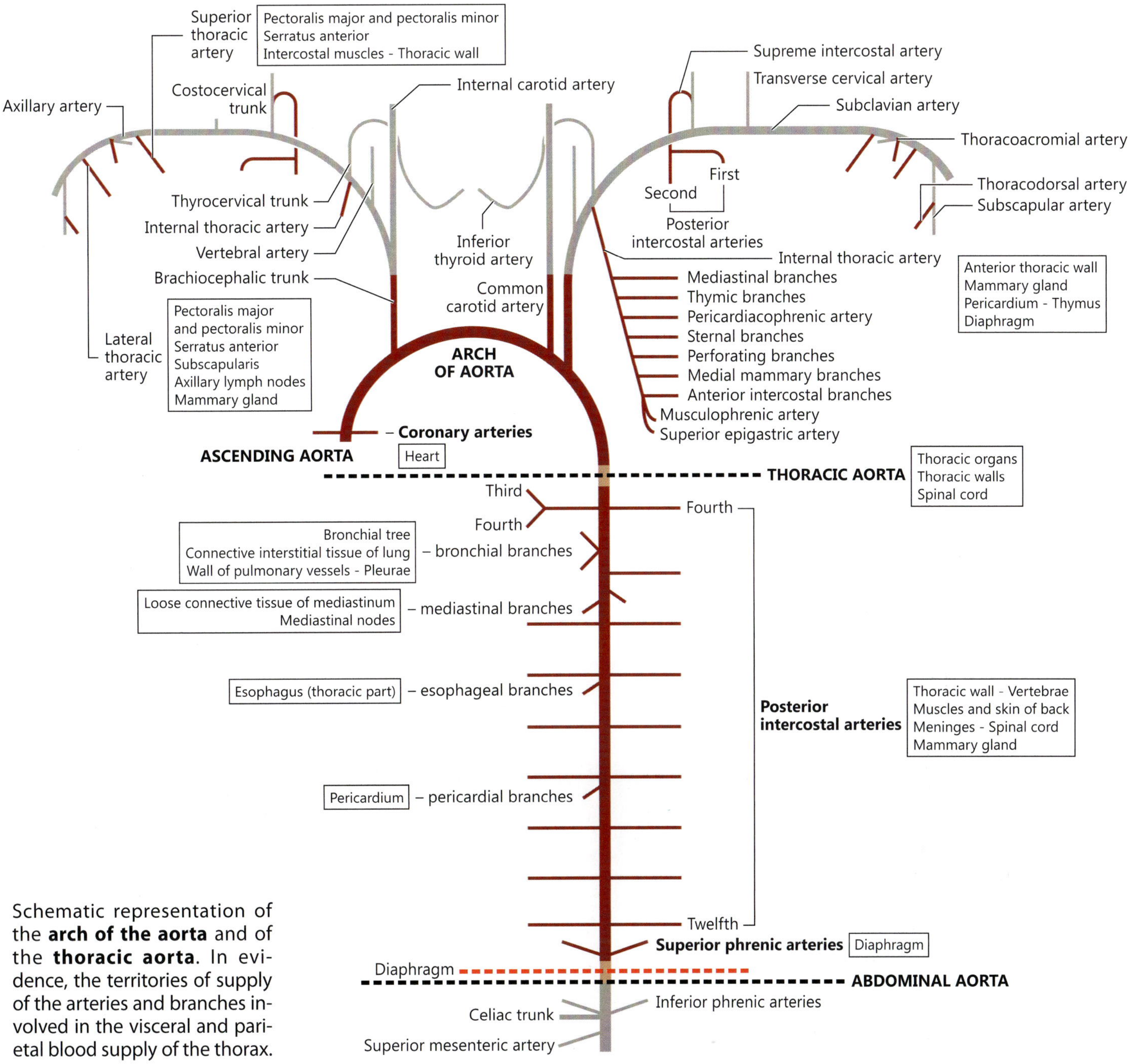

Schematic representation of the **arch of the aorta** and of the **thoracic aorta**. In evidence, the territories of supply of the arteries and branches involved in the visceral and parietal blood supply of the thorax.

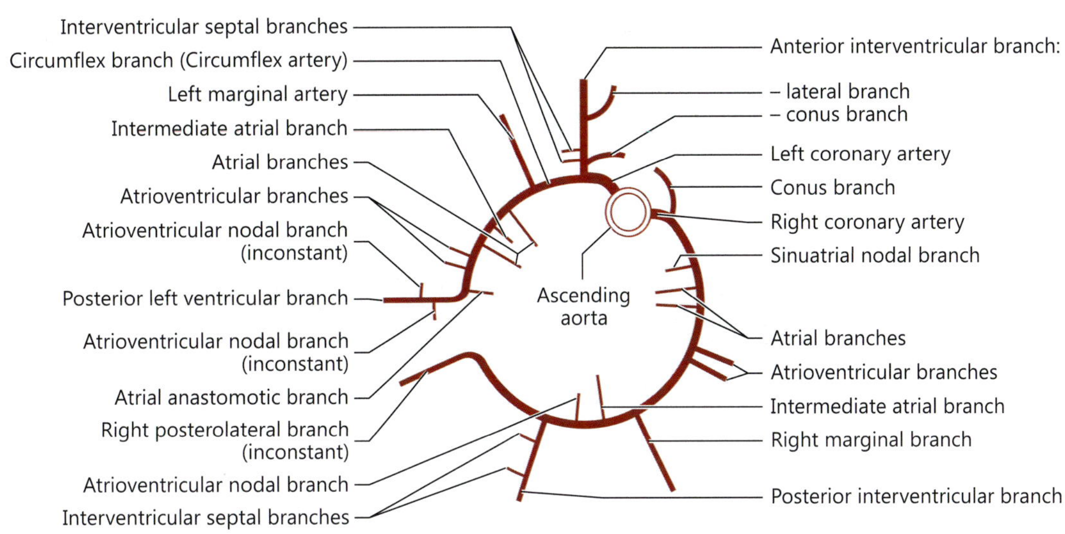

Schematic representation of the **coronary circulation**. The coronary arteries and their principal branches run on the external surface of the heart, in the coronary and interventricular sulci.

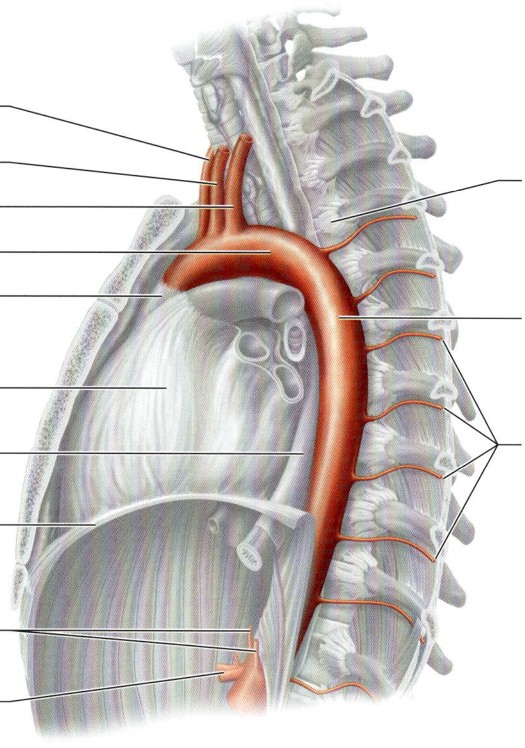

Course and relations of the **aorta** in the mediastinum and in the passageway between the **thoracic part** and **abdominal part**. The ascending aorta is partially covered by pericardium. The arch of the aorta can be seen in relation to the root of the left lung, and the thoracic aorta in relation to the esophagus. From the posterolateral surface of the thoracic aorta branch off the posterior intercostal arteries.

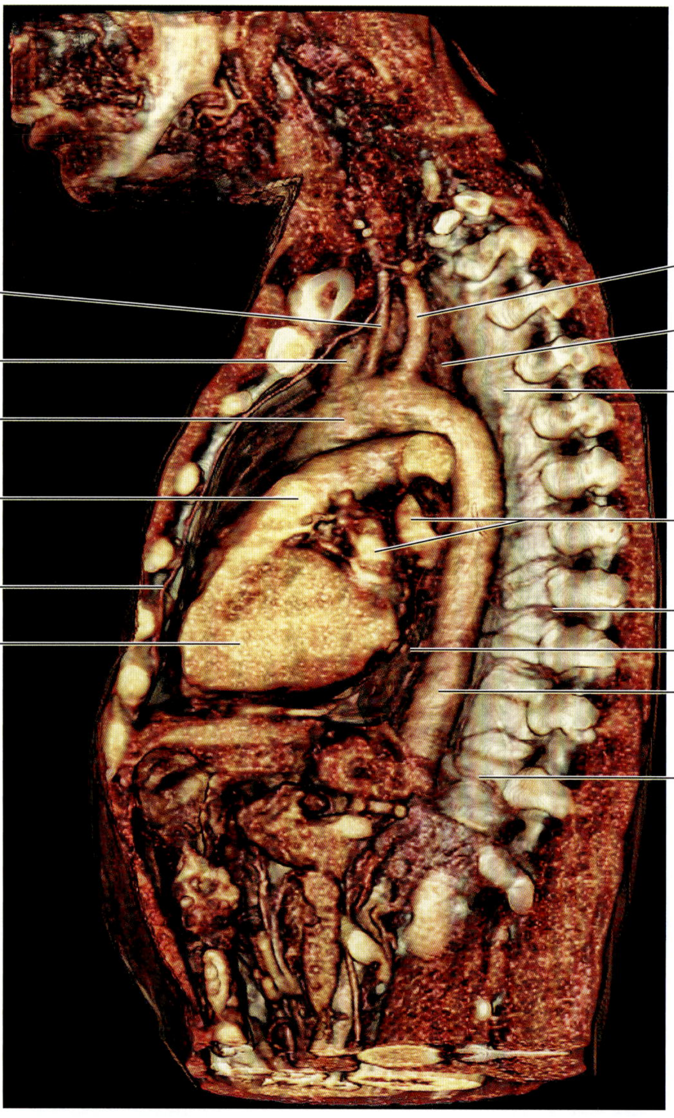

Three-dimensional image of a living human body, obtained by CT scan using a 3D volume rendering technique, showing the **thorax**, in sagittal section, at the level of the **aorta**.

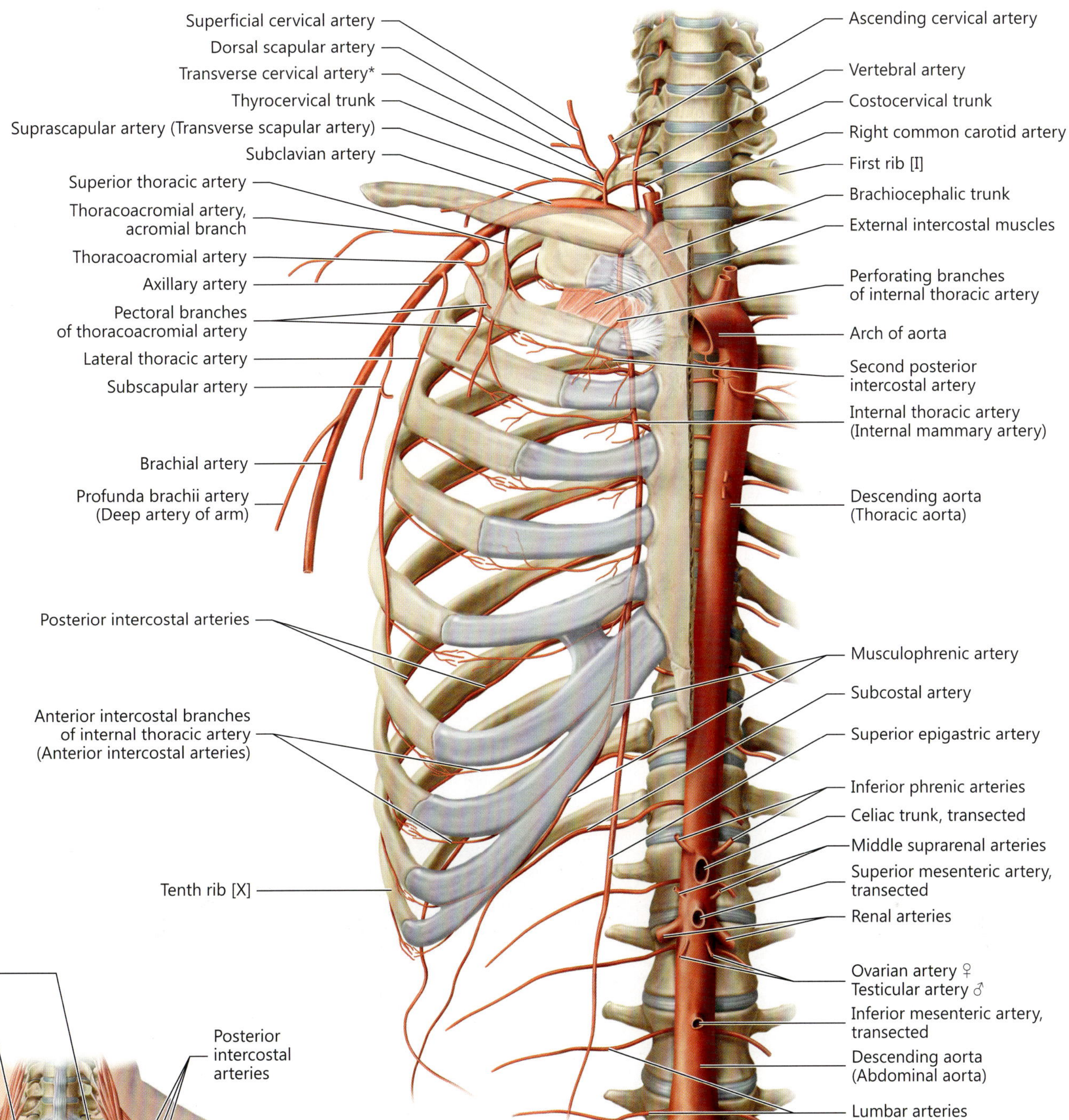

a

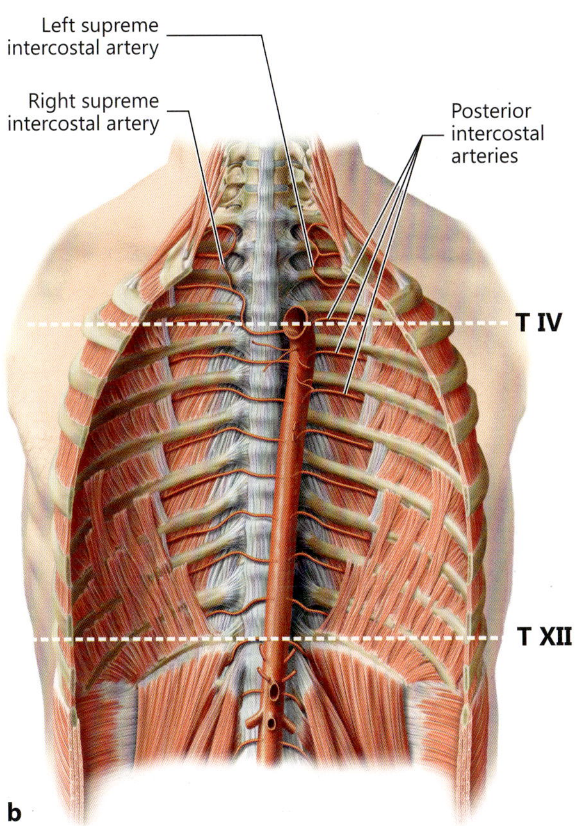

b

The **parietal blood supply of the thorax** has a metameric arrangement and receives branches of the descending aorta (thoracic aorta) and subclavian artery. The posterior intercostal arteries run in their respective intercostal spaces, against the superior border. The first two originate from the supreme intercostal artery (a branch of the costocervical trunk of the subclavian artery); the last nine pairs, from the descending aorta (thoracic aorta) (**a**, **b**). The subcostal artery completes the series, taking its position under the twelfth rib (**b**). The right intercostal arteries, which originate from the aorta, and the right subcostal artery pass in front of the vertebral column to reach their respective intercostal spaces, taking a longer route than the contralateral ones (**a**). Once past the angle, the posterior intercostal arteries proceed along the body of the ribs and anastomose with the corresponding anterior intercostal branches of the internal thoracic artery (a branch of the subclavian artery), or of its musculophrenic branch. The last two arteries anastomose instead with the superior epigastric artery (a branch of the internal thoracic artery) and with the first lumbar artery (a branch of the descending abdominal aorta). Also the superior thoracic, thoracoacromial and lateral thoracic branches of the axillary artery are part of the parietal circulation (**b**).

* Here it is represented the origin of the thyrocervical trunk and not directly of the subclavian artery.

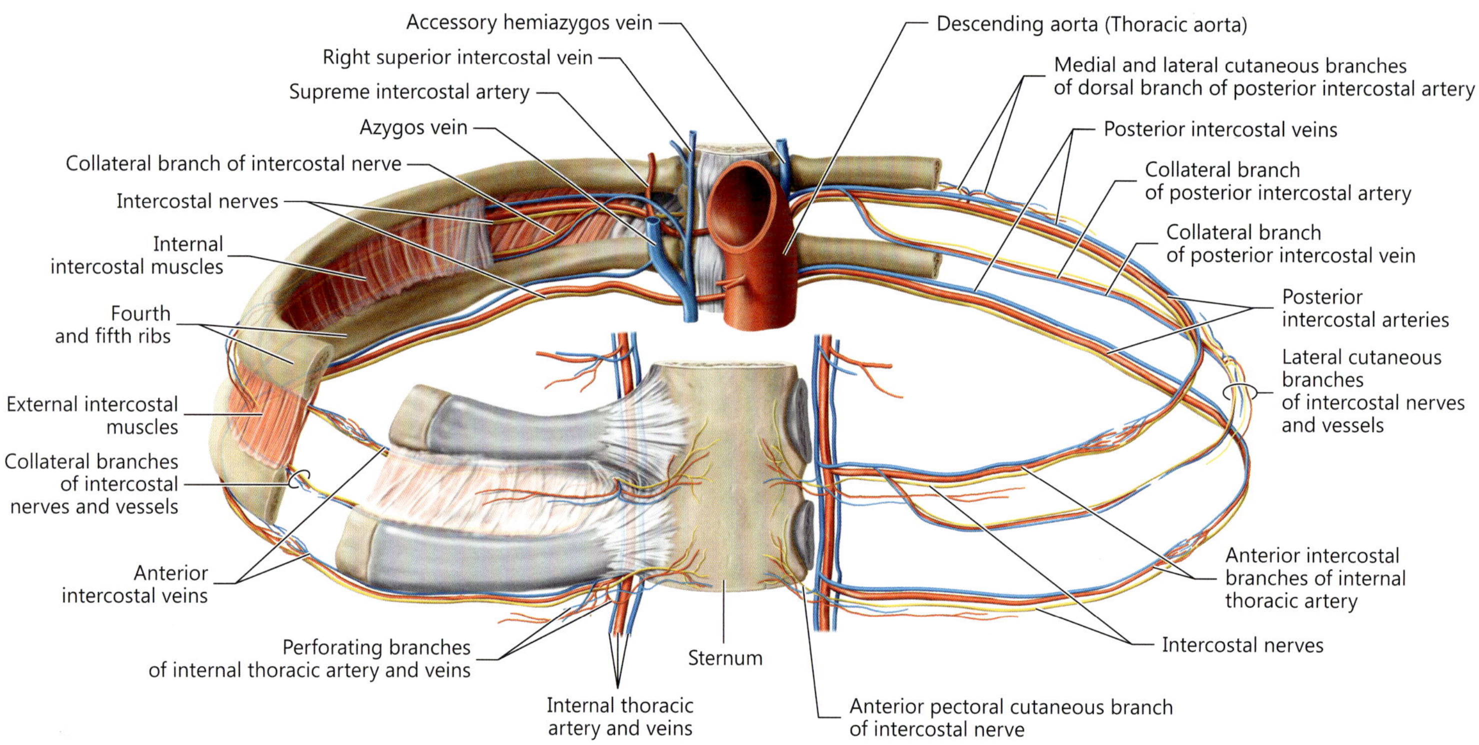

Pathway of the **intercostal blood vessels** and **nerves** at the level of T IV-T V.

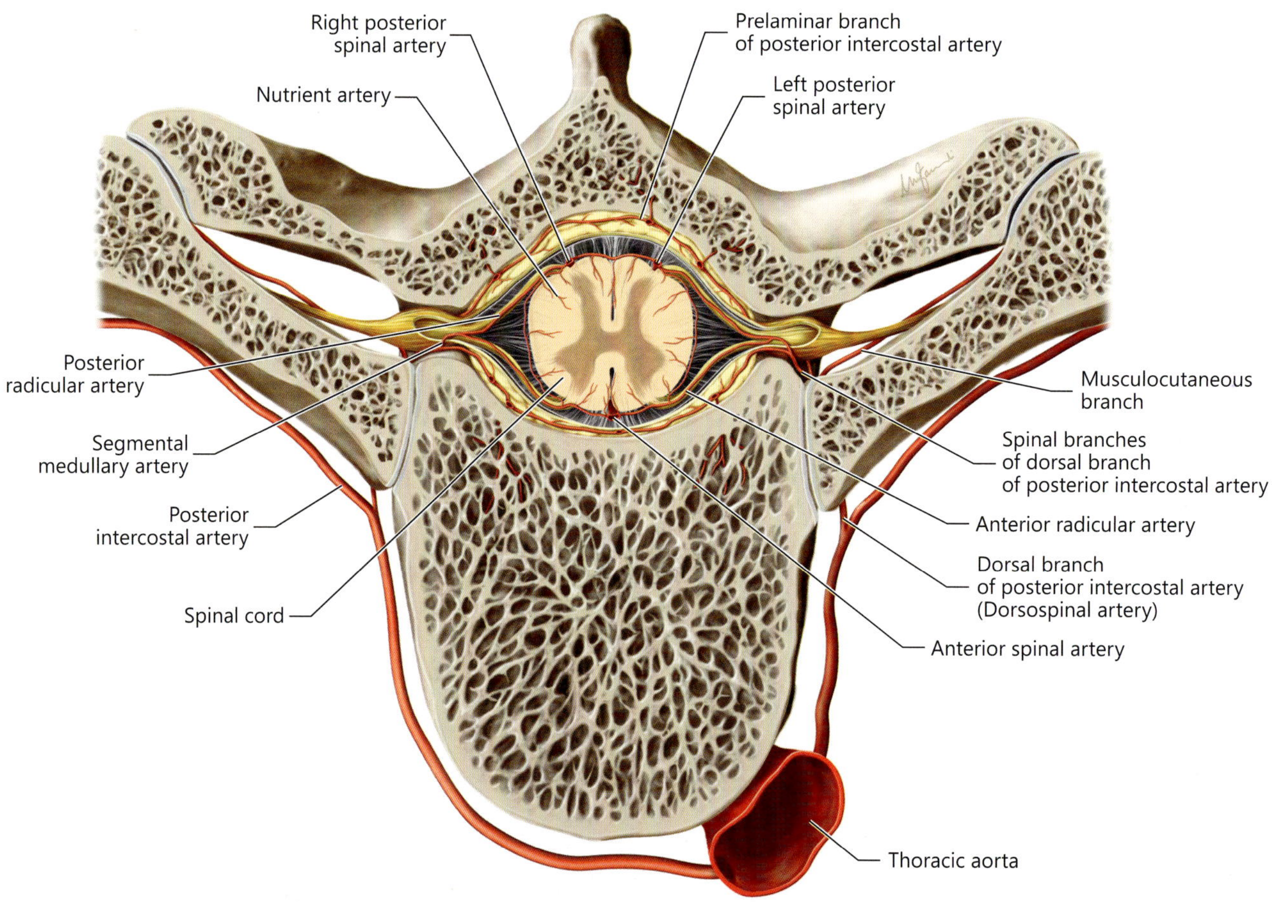

Transverse section of the dorsal vertebral column; representation of the **arterial circulation of the spinal cord**. The segmental branches of the spinal arteries reach the spinal cord after passing through the intervertebral foramina together with the medullary nerves. Each spinal artery is linked to those situated above and below it by longitudinal anastomoses, one anterior and two posterior, which extend from the interior of the neurocranium to the conus medullaris. From the anastomotic tracts and from the perimedullary network which they create arise the nutrient arteries of the spinal cord.

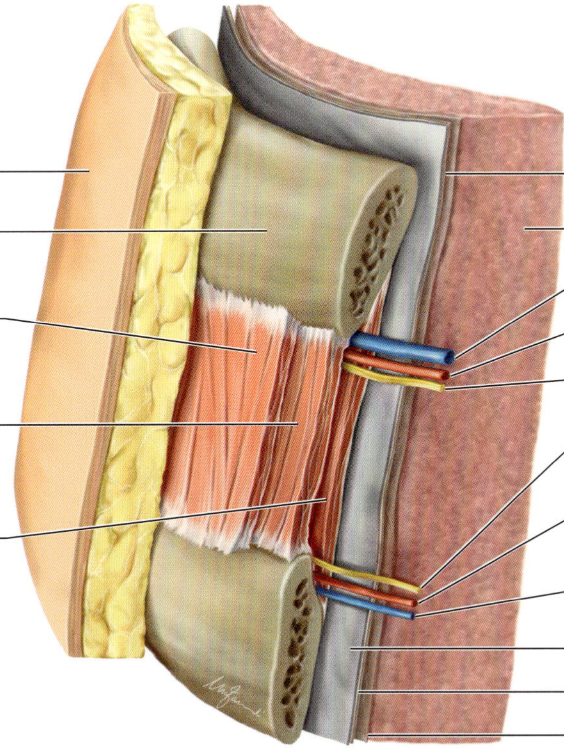

Dissection of the **thoracic wall** at the level of an intercostal space, displaying the passage of the intercostal blood vessels and nerves.

Images of the **internal wall** of the **thoracic cavity** obtained during a thoracoscopy. The endoscope is positioned, within the pleural cavity, between the parietal and visceral layers of pleura.

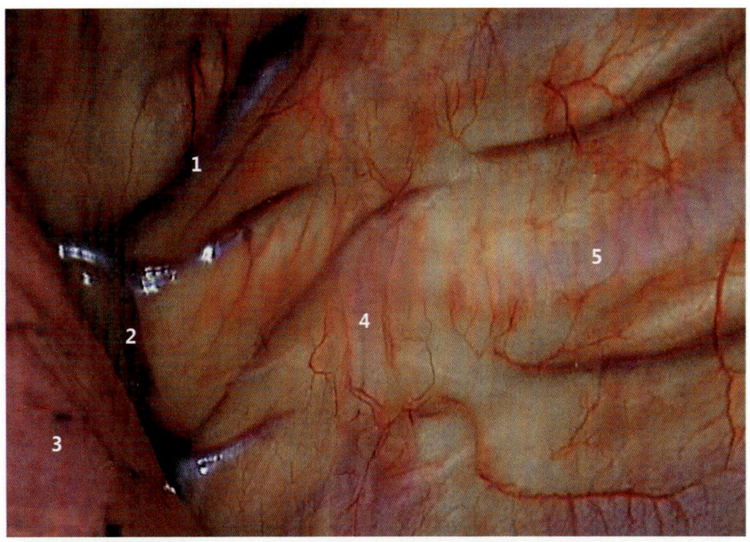

1, Posterior intercostal vein
2, Accessory hemiazygos vein
3, Lung invested by the visceral layer of pleura
4, Thoracic ganglia of sympathetic trunk covered by the parietal layer of pleura
5, Rib covered by the endothoracic fascia and parietal layer of pleura

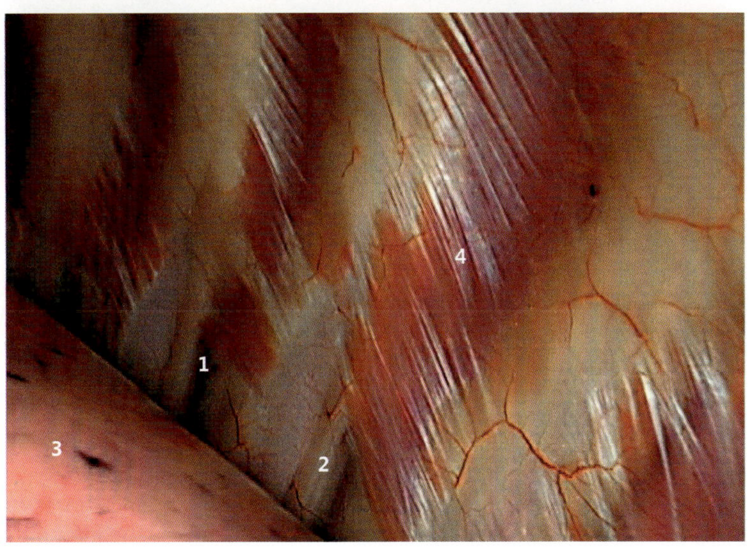

1, Intercostal vessels
2, Rib
3, Lung invested by the visceral layer of pleura
4, Internal intercostal muscles covered by the parietal layer of pleura and endothoracic fascia

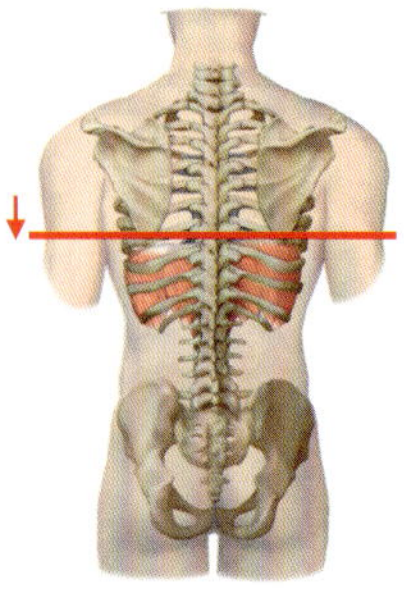

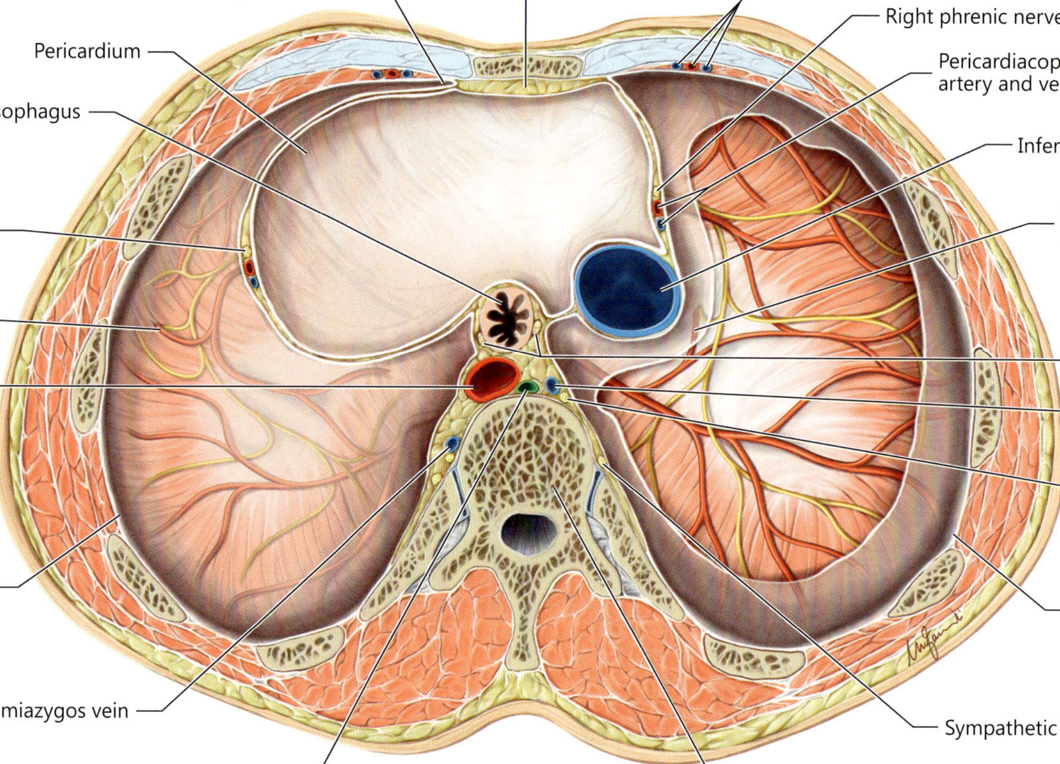

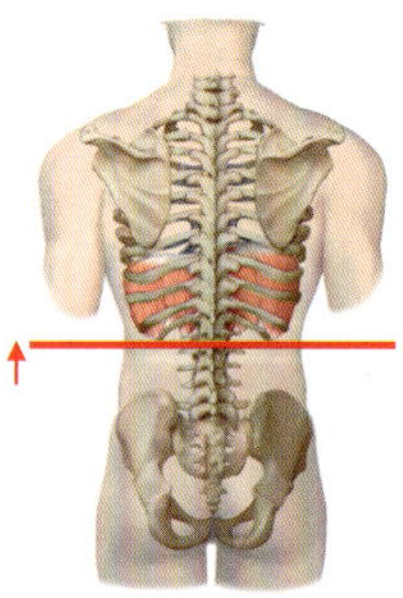

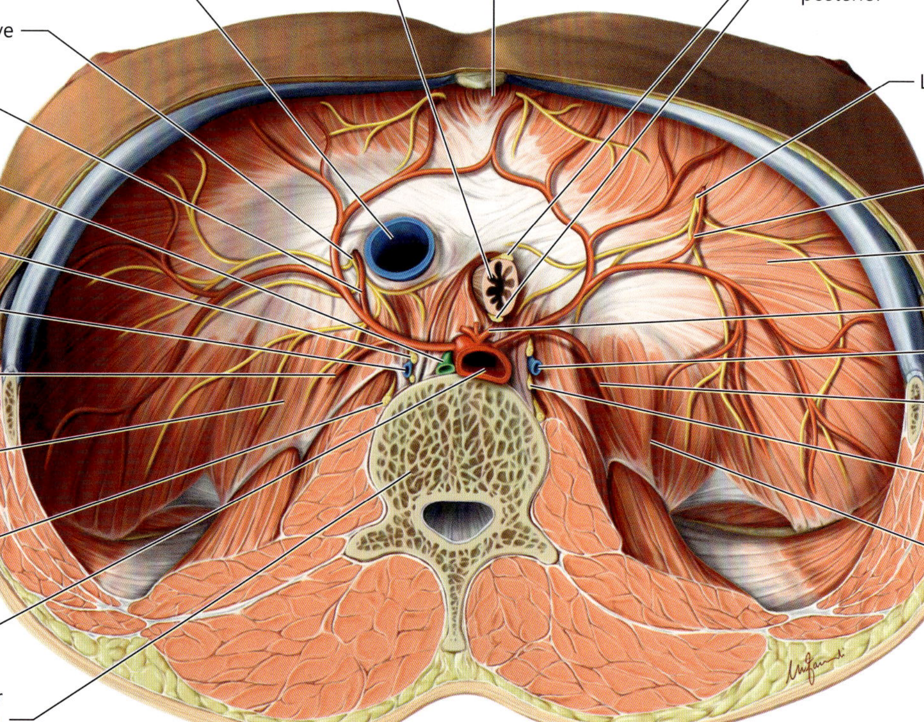

Superior (**a**) and inferior (**b**) view of the **diaphragm**. The parietal vascularization of the thorax is completed by the blood supply to the diaphragm, carried out by the superior phrenic arteries (branches of the descending thoracic aorta) and the pericardiacophrenic artery (a branch of the internal thoracic artery) on the superior surface of the diaphragm (**a**) and by the inferior phrenic arteries (branches of the descending abdominal aorta) (**b**).

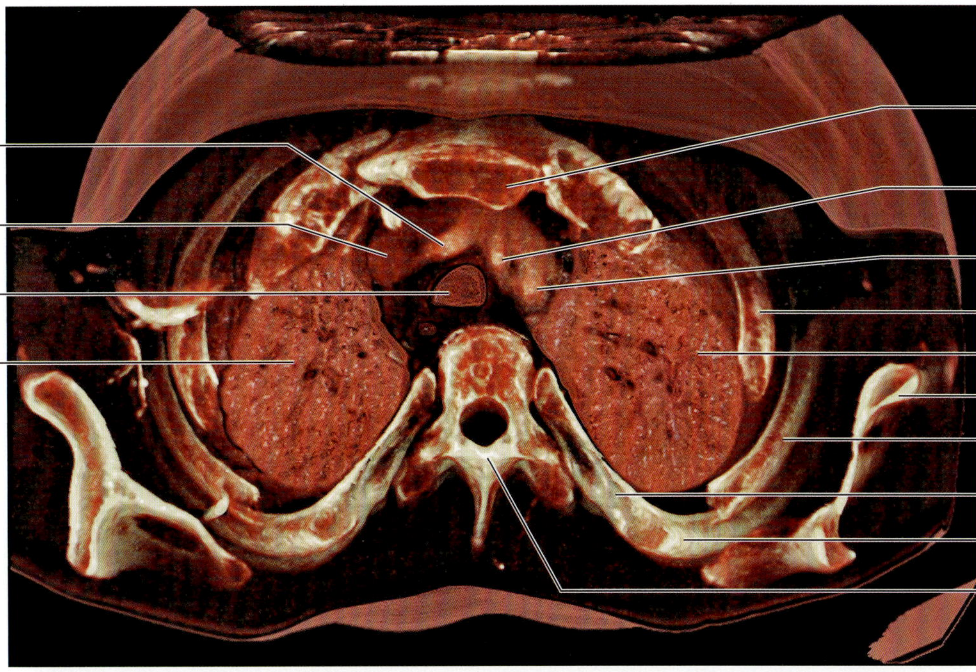

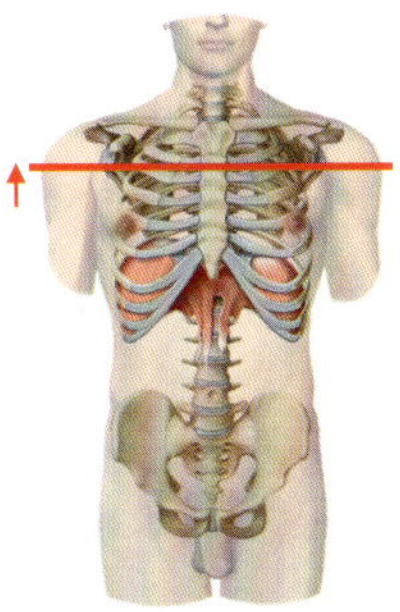

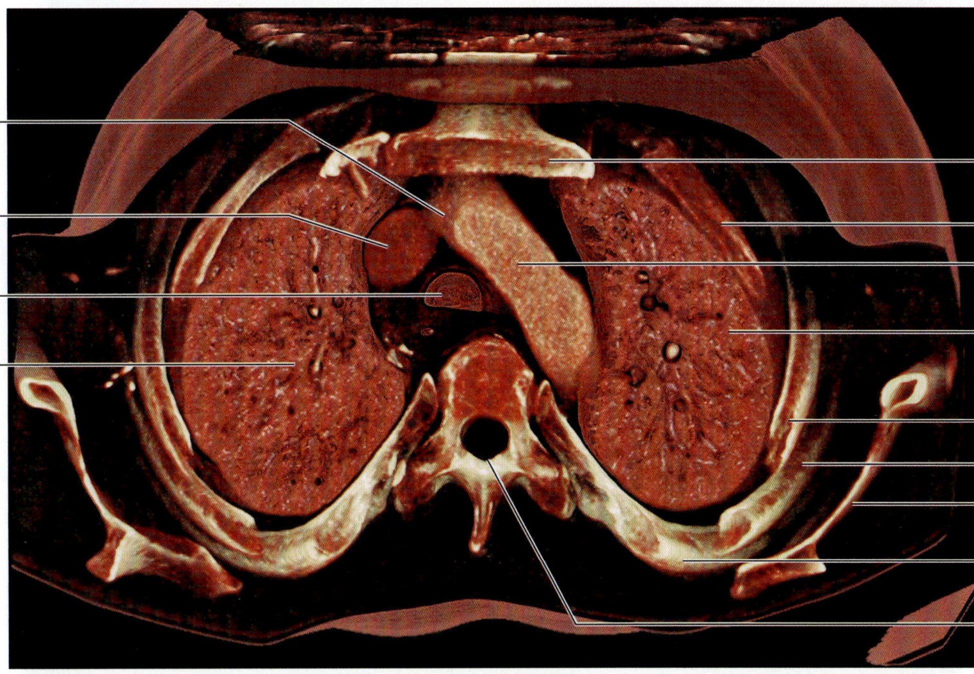

The thorax contains, besides the vessels of the large circle, also the vessels of the small circle of pulmonary circulation. In this series of three-dimensional images of a living human body, obtained by CT scan using a 3D volume rendering technique, featuring transverse sections at the level of the vertebrae T IV and T V, one can see the **pulmonary vessels** (arteries and veins) viewed from below, in radiological position.

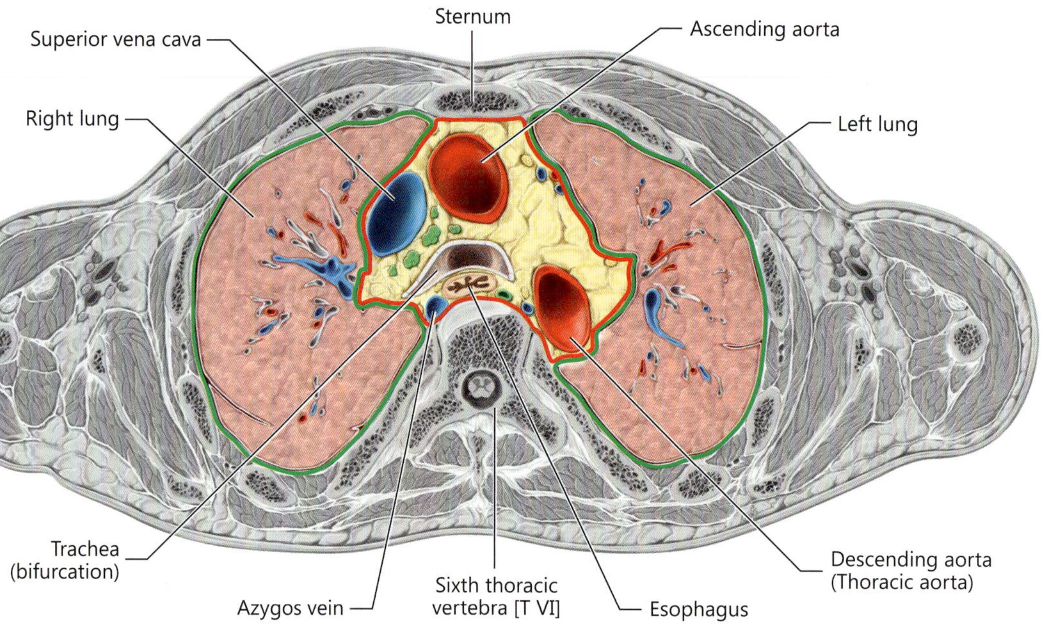
Sternum
Superior vena cava
Ascending aorta
Right lung
Left lung
Trachea
(bifurcation)
Azygos vein
Sixth thoracic
vertebra [T VI]
Esophagus
Descending aorta
(Thoracic aorta)

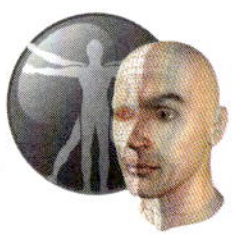

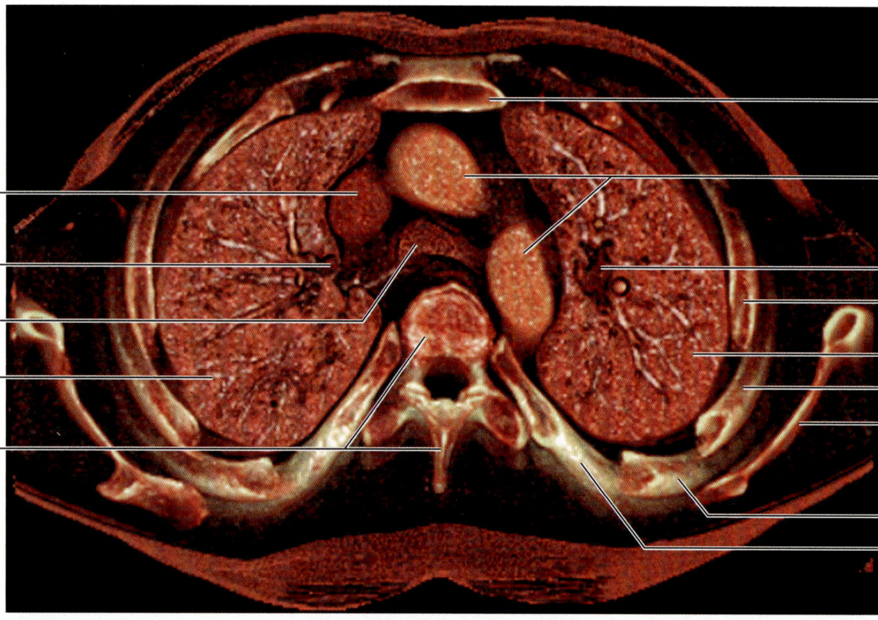
Sternum
Superior vena cava
Arch of aorta
Hilum of right lung
Hilum of left lung
Third rib [III]
Trachea
Left lung
Right lung
Fourth rib [IV]
Scapula
Sixth thoracic
vertebra [T VI]
Fifth rib [V]
Sixth rib [VI]

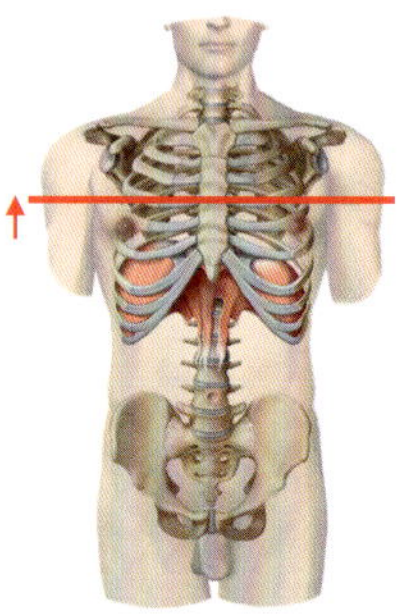

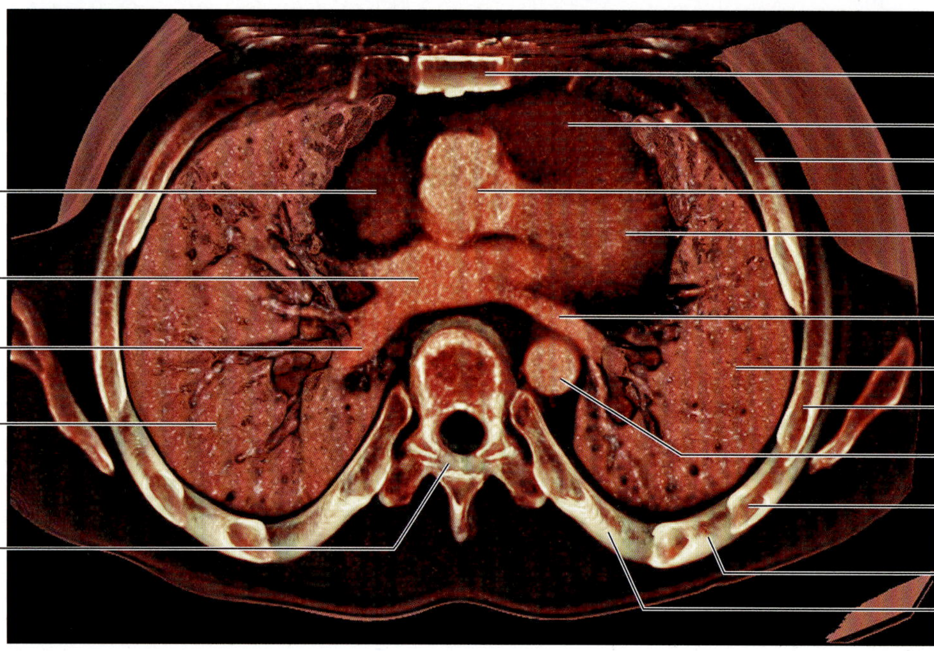
Sternum
Right ventricle
Fourth rib [IV]
Right atrium
Aortic valve
Left ventricle
Left atrium
Left inferior
pulmonary vein
Right inferior
pulmonary vein
Left lung
Fifth rib [V]
Right lung
Descending aorta
(Thoracic aorta)
Sixth rib [VI]
Seventh thoracic
vertebra [T VII]
Seventh rib [VII]
Eighth rib [VIII]

Summary table of the arteries of the thorax

ARTERY	*ORIGIN*	*BRANCHES*	*TERRITORIES OF SUPPLY*
anterior spinal (in the tract that runs along the anterior median fissure in the thoracic part of the spinal cord)	Vertebral artery		Anterior surface of the myelencephalon (medulla oblongata or bulb) spinal cord, filum terminale, meninges
aorta			See specific branches
ascending aorta	Left ventricle	Right and left coronary arteries	Sinuatrial node, atrioventricular node, right and left atria, interventricular septum and right and left ventricles
arch of aorta	Ascending aorta at the level of the superior border of the second right sternocostal joint	Brachiocephalic trunk, left common carotid artery, left subclavian artery; continues as the thoracic aorta	Thoracic organs, thoracic walls, spinal cord, head, neck, upper limb, thyroid gland and thymus, muscles of the arm and shoulder, brain
descending aorta			
– thoracic (thoracic aorta)	Arch of aorta at the level of the fourth thoracic vertebra	*Visceral*: pericardial, bronchial, esophageal and mediastinal branches; *parietal*: posterior intercostal, subcostal and superior phrenic arteries; continues as the abdominal aorta	Thoracic organs, thoracic walls, spinal cord
– – bronchial branches (bronchial arteries)	Thoracic aorta		Bronchi, lung parenchyma, tracheobronchial nodes, esophagus
– abdominal (abdominal aorta)	Descending aorta at the level of the aortic hiatus (in correspondence to the inferior border of T XII)		☞ Territories of supply of the arteries of the abdomen
brachiocephalic trunk	Arch of aorta	Right common carotid, right subclavian, thyroid ima (inconstant) arteries	Right side of the head, neck and upper limb, thyroid gland, thymus
costocervical trunk (at the origin of the thoracic tract of the subclavian artery, on the left)	Subclavian artery	Deep cervical and supreme intercostal arteries	Deep muscles of the neck, first and second intercostal spaces, spinal cord
first and second posterior intercostal	Supreme intercostal artery	Dorsal (or dorsospinal), medial and lateral cutaneous, spinal (or vertebromedullary artery), postcentral, prelaminar; posterior and anterior radicular arteries, segmental medullary artery; collateral (intercostal or supracostal), lateral cutaneous, lateral mammary	Superior part of the thoracic wall, vertebrae, spinal cord, meninges, muscles and skin of the back, mammary gland
internal thoracic	Subclavian artery	Mediastinal, thymic, bronchial (inconstant) and tracheal (inconstant); pericardiacophrenic artery; sternal, perforating, medial mammary, lateral costal (inconstant), anterior intercostal; musculophrenic and superior epigastric arteries	Anterior thoracic wall, diaphragm, pericardium, thymus, mammary gland
– anterior intercostal branches (anterior intercostal arteries)	Internal thoracic artery		First five or six intercostal spaces, pectoralis major and pectoralis minor

continued

➤
The thorax contains, besides the vessels of the large circle, also the vessels of the small circle of pulmonary circulation. On the page beside, two three-dimensional serial images of a living human body, obtained by CT scan using a 3D volume rendering technique, show transverse sections at the level of the vertebrae T VI and T VII, viewed from below, in radiological position. In the first, one can see the initial and final tracts of the arch of the aorta, and the position of the arch with respect to the trachea and its left bifurcation. In the second, the **pulmonary vessels** (arteries and veins) are visible, viewed from below, in radiological position. Also evident are the relations of these structures with the origin of the aorta (one can see the aortic valve at the level of the vertebra T VII) and the thoracic aorta.
At the top, a graphic representation, shown for comparative purposes, of a section at the level of the superior border of the vertebra T VI.

Summary table of the arteries of the thorax *(continued)*

ARTERY	*ORIGIN*	*BRANCHES*	*TERRITORIES OF SUPPLY*
lateral thoracic	Thoracoacromial, subscapular or axillary arteries	Lateral mammary	Pectoralis major and pectoralis minor, serratus anterior and subscapularis; axillary lymph nodes, mammary gland
left common carotid (in the thoracic tract)	Arch of aorta		Head and neck
left coronary	Ascending aorta, left aortic sinus (of Valsalva)	Anterior interventricular (or anterior interventricular or anterior descending artery), conus branch, lateral branch of anterior interventricular branch, interventricular septal, circumflex (or circumflex artery), atrial anastomotic, atrioventricular, left marginal, intermediate atrial, posterior left ventricular branch, sinuatrial nodal and atrioventricular nodal (inconstant), atrial	Interventricular septum, left atrium, left and right ventricles
left pulmonary	Pulmonary trunk	Superior lobar arteries: anterior and posterior apical segmental arteries and inferior and superior lingular arteries; inferior lobar arteries: superior segmental artery and anterior, lateral, medial and posterior basal segmental arteries	Left lung
musculophrenic	Internal thoracic artery		Diaphragm, seventh, eighth and ninth intercostal spaces, pericardium
pericardiacophrenic	Internal thoracic artery		Diaphragm, pericardium, pleura
posterior spinal (in the tract that runs along the posterolateral sulcus in the thoracic part of the spinal cord)	Posterior inferior cerebellar artery and vertebral artery		Myelencephalon (medulla oblongata or bulb), posterior part of the spinal cord, cauda equina, meninges, fourth ventricle
pulmonary trunk	Conus arteriosus	Right and left pulmonary arteries	Lungs
right coronary	Ascending aorta, right aortic sinus (of Valsalva)	Atrioventricular, conus branch, sinuatrial nodal, atrial, right marginal, intermediate atrial, posterior interventricular (or posterior interventricular or posterior descending artery), interventricular septal, atrioventricular nodal, right posterolateral (inconstant)	Sinuatrial node, atrioventricular node, right atrium, interventricular septum, right and left ventricles
right pulmonary	Pulmonary trunk	Superior lobar arteries: anterior and posterior apical segmental arteries; middle lobar artery: medial and lateral segmental arteries; inferior lobar arteries; superior segmental artery and anterior, lateral, medial and posterior basal segmental arteries	Right lung
subclavian (from the origin to the superior thoracic aperture, on the right side; thoracic tract, on the left)	*Right side*: brachiocephalic trunk; *left side*: arch of aorta	Vertebral artery, thyrocervical trunk, internal thoracic artery, costocervical trunk, dorsal scapular artery (originating more often from the thyrocervical trunk); becomes the axillary artery in correspondence to the outer border of the first rib	Neck, thoracic wall, muscles of the shoulder and the arm, spinal cord and brain
subcostal (in the tract that passes behind the lateral arcuate ligament)	Thoracic aorta	Dorsal and spinal	Superior abdominal wall; anastomoses with the superior epigastric, eleventh posterior intercostal and first lumbar arteries

continued

Summary table of the arteries of the thorax *(continued)*

ARTERY	ORIGIN	BRANCHES	TERRITORIES OF SUPPLY
superior epigastric (in the part that runs between the sternal and costal insertions of the diaphragm)	Internal thoracic artery		Diaphragm, xiphoid process, rectus abdominis, liver, peritoneum; anastomoses with the inferior epigastric artery which creates a connection between the system of the subclavian artery and that of the external iliac artery
superior phrenic	Thoracic aorta		Diaphragm
superior thoracic	Axillary or thoracoacromial arteries		Pectoralis major and pectoralis minor, serratus anterior and intercostal muscles, thoracic wall
supreme intercostal	Costocervical trunk	First and second posterior intercostal arteries	First and second intercostal spaces
third to eleventh posterior intercostal	Thoracic aorta	Dorsal (or dorsospinal), medial and lateral cutaneous, spinal (or vertebromedullary artery), postcentral, prelaminar; posterior and anterior radicular arteries, segmental medullary artery; collateral (intercostal or supracostal), lateral cutaneous, lateral mammary, bronchial (or bronchial artery; can originate from the third right posterior intercostal artery)	Thoracic wall, vertebrae, spinal cord, meninges, muscles and skin of the back, mammary gland
thoracoacromial	Axillary artery	Acromial, clavicular, deltoid, pectoral	Pectoralis major and pectoralis minor, deltoid and subclavius, mammary gland, sternoclavicular joint, coracoid process, acromion
thoracodorsal	Subscapular artery		Subscapularis, latissimus dorsi, serratus anterior and intercostal muscles
thyroid ima	Arch of aorta or brachiocephalic trunk		Thyroid gland, thymus
vertebral (at its origin from the subclavian artery)	Subclavian	*Cervical part*: spinal and muscular branches; *intracranial part*: meningeal branches; posterior and anterior spinal arteries, posterior inferior cerebellar artery; medial and lateral medullary branches	Vertebral body, deep muscles of the neck, falx cerebelli, spinal cord, cerebellum, brainstem

ARTERY	
abdominal	☞ abdominal aorta
acromiothoracic	☞ thoracoacromial artery
dorsal spinal	☞ posterior spinal artery
innominate	☞ brachiocephalic trunk
internal mammary	☞ internal thoracic artery
long thoracic or **external mammary**	☞ lateral thoracic artery
twelfth thoracic	☞ subcostal artery
ventral spinal	☞ anterior spinal artery

The table alongside lists some arteries by their name normally used or eponym, with the corresponding reference to the official term.

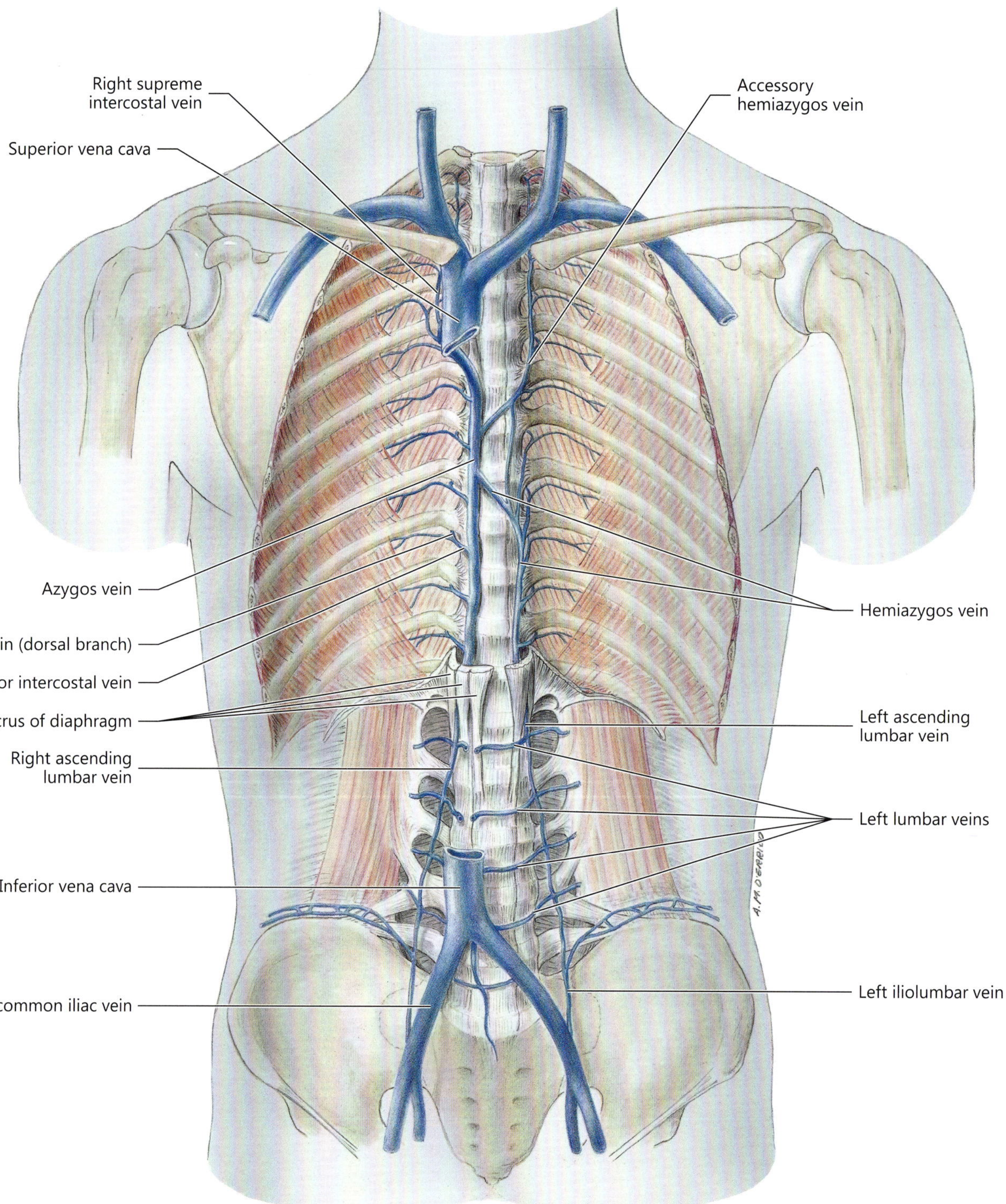

The **azygos**, **hemiazygos** and **accessory hemiazygos veins** viewed from the front after demolition of the thoracic and abdominal walls and removal of the splanchnic organs. Note the dorsospinal branches of the intercostal veins which drain the vertebral plexuses. The system of the azygos veins constitutes an important deep anastomotic system between the superior vena cava and the inferior vena cava through the ascending lumbar veins.

Schematic representation of the superior vena cava and of the major affluent veins ☞ page 222 (Neck - Veins).

➤

Schematic representation showing the affluent branches of the **superior vena cava**, **coronary sinus** and **veins of the pulmonary circulation**. The superior vena cava, which is formed by the confluence of the right and left brachiocephalic veins, after receiving refluent blood from the walls of the thorax, spinal cord and some structures of the posterior mediastinum through the azygos vein, reaches the right atrium of the heart, into which also the coronary sinus opens, near the opening of the inferior vena cava. The pulmonary veins conduct arterial blood from the lungs to the left atrium of the heart.

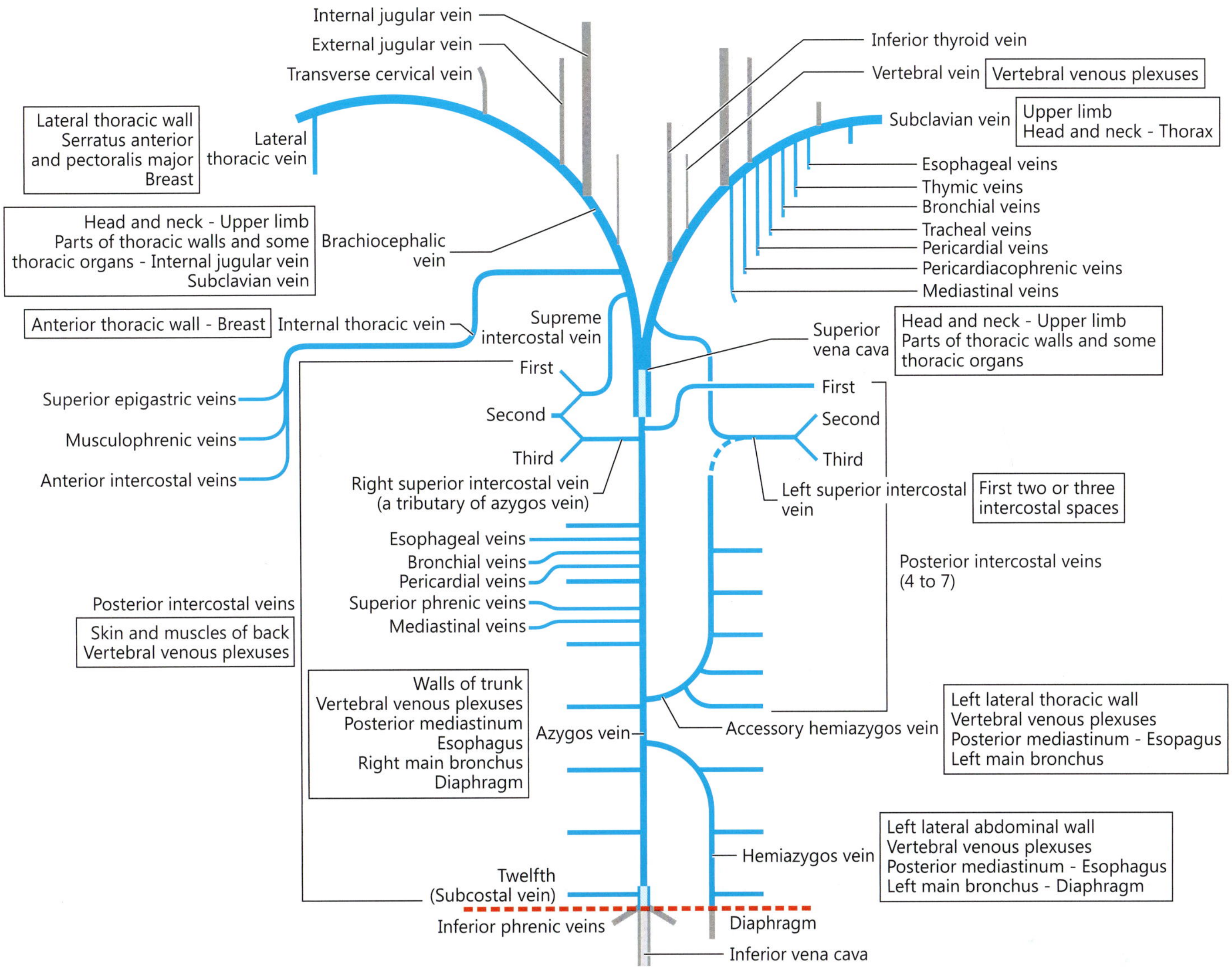

Internal jugular vein
External jugular vein
Transverse cervical vein
Lateral thoracic wall
Serratus anterior
and pectoralis major
Breast
Lateral thoracic vein
Head and neck - Upper limb
Parts of thoracic walls and some thoracic organs - Internal jugular vein
Subclavian vein
Brachiocephalic vein
Anterior thoracic wall - Breast
Internal thoracic vein
Supreme intercostal vein
First
Second
Third
Superior epigastric veins
Musculophrenic veins
Anterior intercostal veins
Right superior intercostal vein (a tributary of azygos vein)
Esophageal veins
Bronchial veins
Pericardial veins
Superior phrenic veins
Mediastinal veins
Posterior intercostal veins
Skin and muscles of back
Vertebral venous plexuses
Walls of trunk
Vertebral venous plexuses
Posterior mediastinum
Esophagus
Right main bronchus
Diaphragm
Azygos vein
Twelfth (Subcostal vein)
Inferior phrenic veins
Inferior thyroid vein
Vertebral vein
Vertebral venous plexuses
Subclavian vein
Upper limb
Head and neck - Thorax
Esophageal veins
Thymic veins
Bronchial veins
Tracheal veins
Pericardial veins
Pericardiacophrenic veins
Mediastinal veins
Superior vena cava
Head and neck - Upper limb
Parts of thoracic walls and some thoracic organs
First
Second
Third
Left superior intercostal vein
First two or three intercostal spaces
Posterior intercostal veins (4 to 7)
Accessory hemiazygos vein
Left lateral thoracic wall
Vertebral venous plexuses
Posterior mediastinum - Esopagus
Left main bronchus
Hemiazygos vein
Left lateral abdominal wall
Vertebral venous plexuses
Posterior mediastinum - Esophagus
Left main bronchus - Diaphragm
Diaphragm
Inferior vena cava

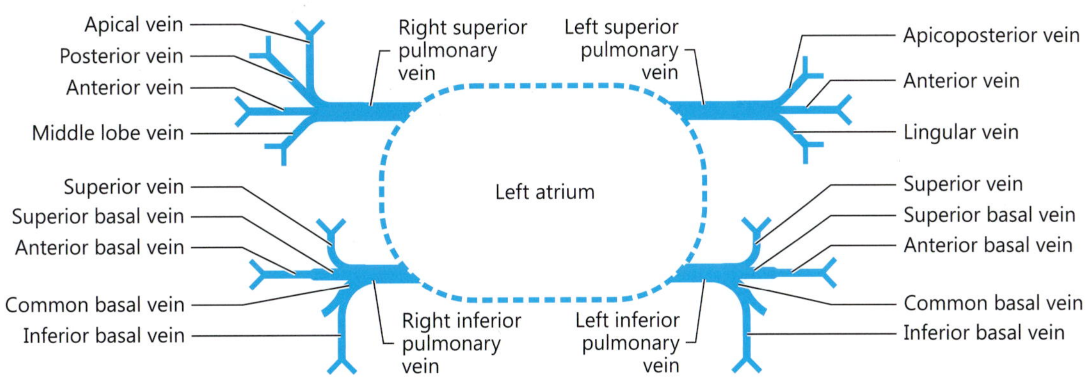

Apical vein
Posterior vein
Anterior vein
Middle lobe vein
Right superior pulmonary vein
Left superior pulmonary vein
Apicoposterior vein
Anterior vein
Lingular vein
Left atrium
Superior vein
Superior basal vein
Anterior basal vein
Common basal vein
Inferior basal vein
Right inferior pulmonary vein
Left inferior pulmonary vein
Superior vein
Superior basal vein
Anterior basal vein
Common basal vein
Inferior basal vein

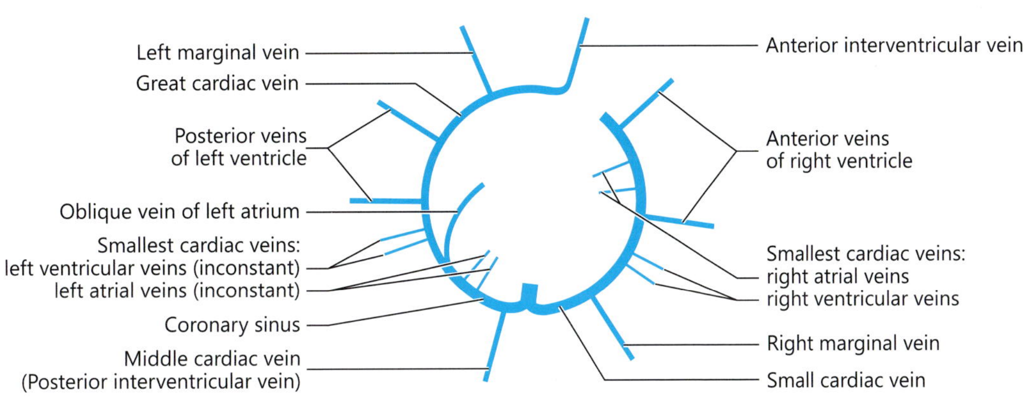

Left marginal vein
Great cardiac vein
Posterior veins of left ventricle
Oblique vein of left atrium
Smallest cardiac veins:
left ventricular veins (inconstant)
left atrial veins (inconstant)
Coronary sinus
Middle cardiac vein (Posterior interventricular vein)
Anterior interventricular vein
Anterior veins of right ventricle
Smallest cardiac veins:
right atrial veins
right ventricular veins
Right marginal vein
Small cardiac vein

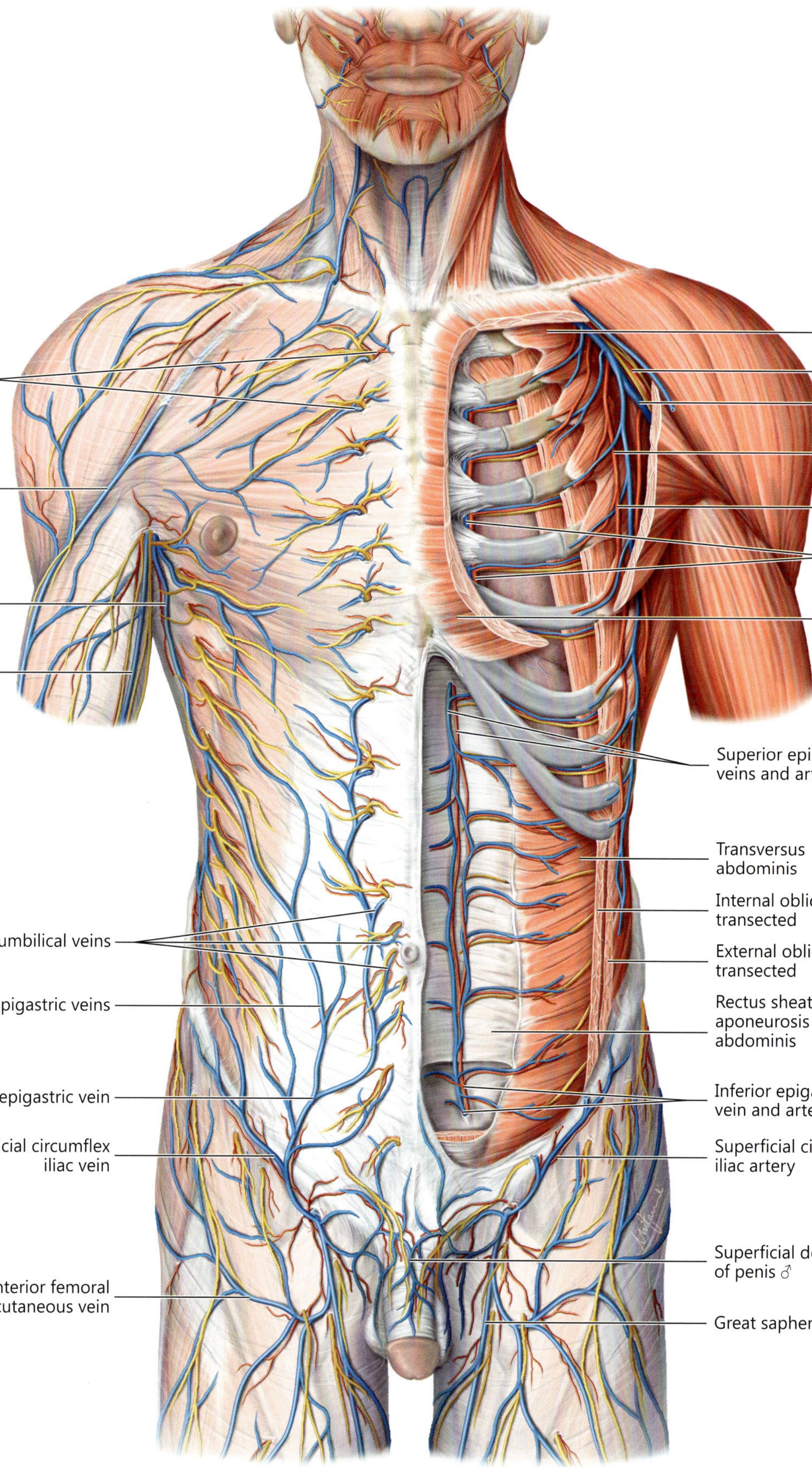

Parietal vascularization of the trunk: **cava-caval anastomoses**. The superficial and deep venous drainage of the thorax and of the abdomen are communicating. These anastomoses connect the circulation of the superior vena cava with that of the inferior vena cava. At superficial level, the lateral thoracic veins (affluents of the axillary veins) anastomose with the superficial epigastric veins (affluents of the femoral veins), through the thoracoepigastric veins. At deep level, in the context of the rectus sheath, the superior epigastric veins (affluents of the internal thoracic veins) anastomose with the inferior epigastric veins (affluents of the external iliac veins).

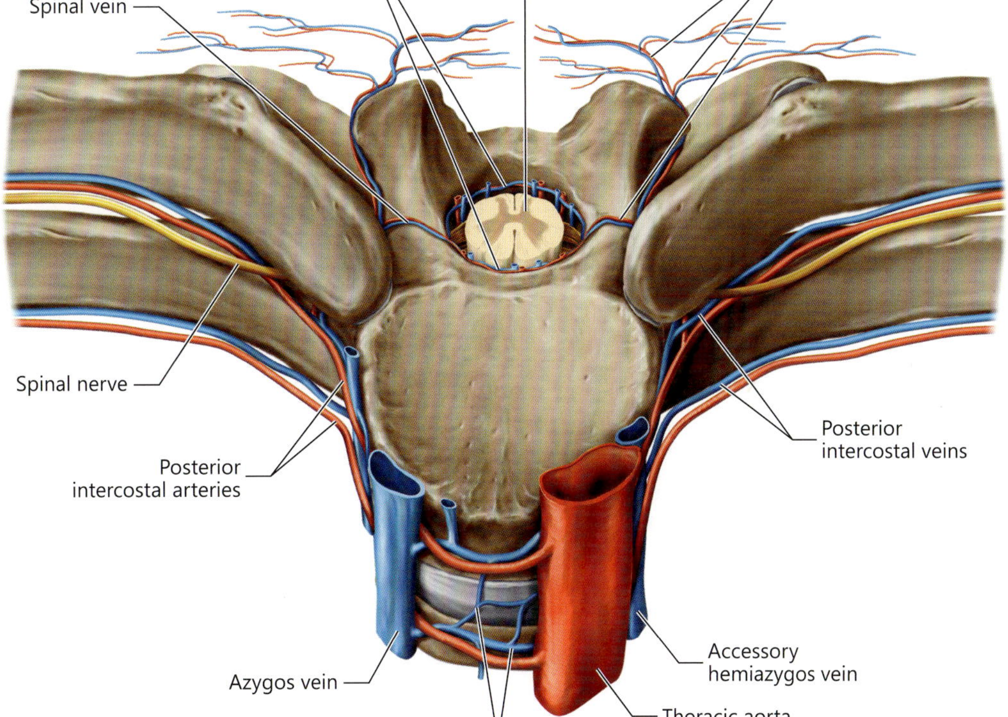

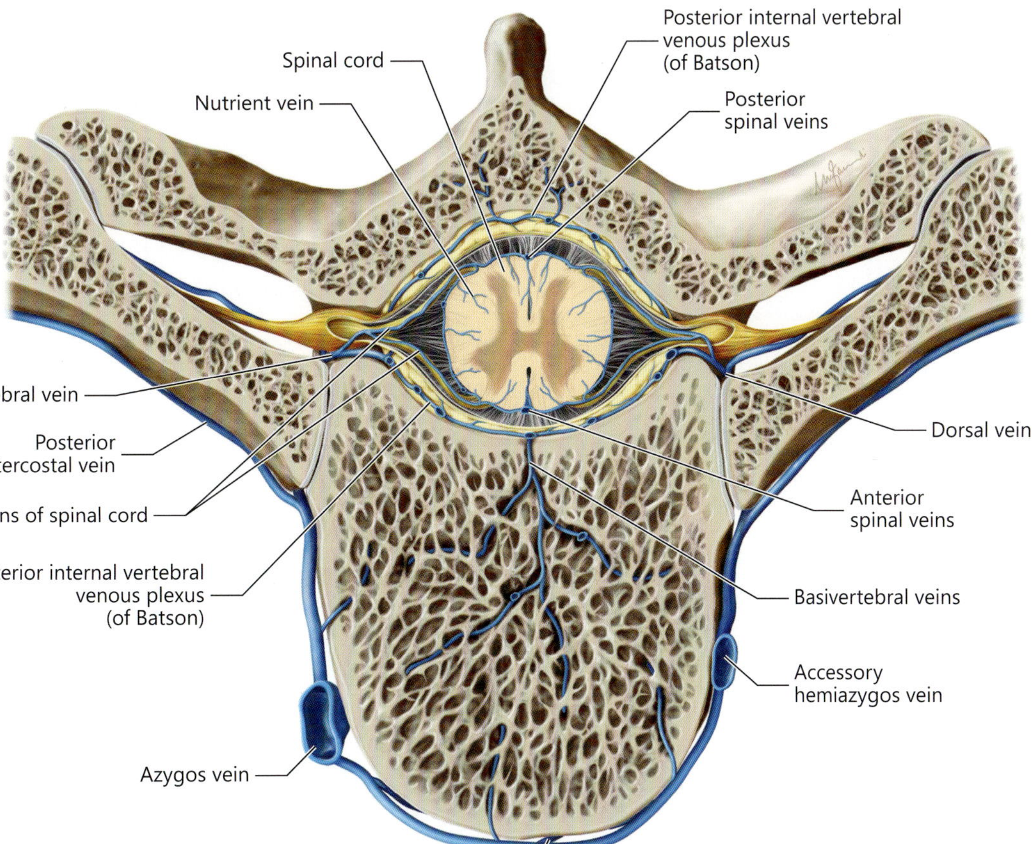

Transverse section of the dorsal vertebral column. Disposition of the **internal vertebral venous plexuses** of the epidural space. The plexuses extend longitudinally from the foramen magnum to the apex of the sacrum.

Summary table of the veins of the thorax			
VEIN	***ORIGIN/LOCATION***	***DRAINAGE***	***CONFLUENCE***
accessory hemiazygos	Left side of T II-T III; crosses T VII-T VIII moving rightwards	From four to seven posterior intercostal veins	Azygos vein
anterior and posterior spinal	Longitudinal venous plexus along the surface of the spinal cord	Meninges and spinal cord	Anterior internal vertebral venous plexus
anterior intercostal (12 pairs)	Inferior border of each rib	Ribs and intercostal muscles	Internal thoracic and musculophrenic veins
anterior veins of right ventricle or anterior cardiac veins (three or four in number; one of these ascends along the right margin and is known as the small coronary)	Anterior or sternocostal surface of the heart	Ventral side of the right ventricle	Small cardiac vein or right atrium
azygos	Anterior surface of L I; right side of T IV; anterior arch, passes over the top of the root of the right lung; opening into the superior vena cava	Ascending lumbar, right subcostal, posterior intercostal, hemiazygos, esophageal, mediastinal, pericardial and right bronchial veins	Superior vena cava
basivertebral	Anterior internal vertebral venous plexus; spongy bone of vertebral body	Vertebrae	Anterior internal and external vertebral venous plexuses
brachiocephalic	Origin behind the sternoclavicular joint through the confluence of the internal jugular and subclavian veins; termination behind the first sternocostal joint	Head, neck, upper limb, parts of thoracic walls, thymus, pericardium, diaphragm, bronchi, trachea, esophagus	Merge with each other to form the superior vena cava
bronchial	They follow the ramifications of the bronchi	Main bronchi and roots of the lungs	*Right side*: azygos vein; *left side*: left superior intercostal vein, accessory hemiazygos vein or left brachiocephalic vein
coronary sinus	Posterior part of the coronary sulcus	Great, middle and small cardiac veins, posterior vein of left ventricle, oblique vein of left atrium	Right atrium, between the opening of inferior vena cava and the right atrioventricular orifice
esophageal (varying in number)	Along the esophagus	Esophagus	*Right side*: azygos vein; *left side*: hemiazygos, left gastric and inferior thyroid or left brachiocephalic veins on left side
great cardiac	Anterior interventricular sulcus; coronary sulcus on the left	Tributary veins from the left atrium and from both ventricles; anterior interventricular and left marginal veins	Left extremity of the coronary sinus
hemiazygos	Left side of T XII; crosses T VIII-T IX moving rightwards	Left ascending lumbar, four or five posterior caudal intercostal, left subcostal, esophageal and mediastinal veins	Azygos vein
inferior vena cava	Anterior right surface of L IV; Right side of the lumbar segment of the vertebral column; diaphragmatic opening of the inferior vena cava at the level of the fifth costal cartilage	Both common iliac veins; lumbar, renal, right testicular (♂), right ovarian (♀), suprarenal, inferior phrenic and hepatic veins	Right atrium of the heart
internal thoracic	From the confluence of the musculophrenic and superior epigastric veins	Besides the musculophrenic and superior epigastric veins, other affluent branches are the anterior intercostal and subcutaneous abdominal veins	Brachiocephalic vein
intervertebral (in the thoracic segment of the vertebral column)	Internal vertebral venous plexuses; passes through the intervertebral foramen accompanied by the roots and initial tract of the spinal nerve	Superficial planes of the posterior regions of the trunk, erector spinae, vertebrae, meninges and spinal cord; in part, also the external vertebral venous plexuses	Vertebral, posterior intercostal, lumbar and lateral sacral veins

continued

Summary table of the veins of the thorax			(continued)
VEIN	**ORIGIN/LOCATION**	**DRAINAGE**	**CONFLUENCE**
lateral thoracic	Lateral thoracic wall	Lateral thoracic wall; anastomoses, through the costoaxillary veins, with the posterior intercostal veins	Axillary vein
left inferior pulmonary	From the left lung to the heart	Inferior lobe of left lung; receives the superior vein and common, superior (which receives the anterior basal vein) and inferior basal veins	Left atrium
left superior intercostal	From the confluence of the 2nd-3rd or 2nd-4th left posterior intercostal vein; in front of the left costovertebral joints	2nd-3rd or 2nd-4th intercostal space; left bronchial vein and, occasionally, left superior phrenic vein	Left brachiocephalic vein or accessory hemiazygos vein
left superior pulmonary	From the left lung to the heart	Superior lobe of left lung; receives the apicoposterior, anterior and lingular veins	Left atrium
mediastinal	Mediastinum	Areolar tissue and lymph nodes of the anterior mediastinum, pericardium	Azygos and brachiocephalic veins or superior vena cava
middle cardiac or **posterior interventricular**	Posterior interventricular sulcus	Tributary veins from both ventricles	Right extremity of the coronary sinus
musculophrenic	From the confluence of the 6th-9th anterior intercostal vein they follow the internal border of the thoracic cage until the sixth costal cartilage	Diaphragm and inferior intercostal spaces	Internal thoracic veins
oblique vein of left atrium	Posterior wall of the left atrium	Posterior part of the left atrium	Coronary sinus
pericardiacophrenic	Satellites of the pericardiacophrenic artery and phrenic nerve; they ascend from the superior surface of the diaphragm between the pleura and pericardium	Diaphragm; tributary veins from the pericardium	Brachiocephalic vein
pericardial (varying in number)	Fibrous pericardium	Pericardium	Azygos and brachiocephalic veins or superior vena cava
posterior intercostal (12 pairs)	Inferior border of each rib, from the neck to approximately half of the body of the rib	Skin and muscles of the back, vertebrae, meninges and spinal cord; dorsal vein or branch, intervertebral vein and spinal vein or branch	*Right side*: azygos and right superior intercostal veins; *left side*: left brachiocephalic and hemiazygos or accessory hemiazygos veins
posterior vein of left ventricle	Diaphragmatic or inferior surface of the heart near the apex	Posterior surface of the left ventricle	Coronary sinus
right inferior pulmonary	From the right lung to the heart	Inferior lobe of right lung; receives the superior vein and common basal vein, where the superior basal vein (which receives the anterior basal vein) and inferior basal vein drain	Left atrium
right superior intercostal	From the confluence of the 2nd-3rd or 2nd-4th right posterior intercostal vein; in front of the right costovertebral joints	2nd-3rd or 2nd-4th intercostal space	Azygos vein
right superior pulmonary	From the right lung to the heart	Superior and middle lobes of right lung; receives the apical, anterior, posterior veins and middle lobe veins	Left atrium
small cardiac vein	Right margin of the heart; coronary sulcus on the right	Posterior part of right atrium and ventricle; right marginal vein and anterior veins of right ventricle or anterior cardiac veins	Right extremity of the coronary sinus or right atrium
smallest cardiac veins	Thickness of the myocardium	Muscular wall of the heart; right atrial and ventricular veins; left atrial and ventricular veins (inconstant)	Majority in the atria, some in the ventricles

continued

Summary table of the veins of the thorax *(continued)*

VEIN	*ORIGIN/LOCATION*	*DRAINAGE*	*CONFLUENCE*
subclavian	From the external border of the first rib to the sternal end of the clavicle	Continuation of the axillary vein; external jugular vein and anterior jugular vein (occasionally)	Unites with the internal jugular vein to form the brachiocephalic vein
subcostal	Satellite of the subcostal artery along the inferior border of twelfth rib	Anterior abdominal wall	Azygos vein
superior epigastric	Satellites of the superior epigastric artery	Territory corresponding to the supply territory of the superior epigastric artery	Unite with the musculophrenic veins to form the internal thoracic veins
superior phrenic	Superior surface of the diaphragm; they ascend along the lateral surface of the pericardium	Diaphragm	*Right side*: azygos vein or confluence of the two brachiocephalic veins; *left side*: left brachiocephalic vein
superior vena cava	Superior mediastinum, at the level of the first costal cartilage, from the confluence of the brachiocephalic veins; in correspondence to the third costal cartilage	Supradiaphragmatic part of body	Roof of the right atrium
supreme intercostal	From the confluence of 1st-2nd posterior intercostal vein; in front of the costovertebral joints	1st intercostal space	Brachiocephalic vein or superior intercostal vein or vertebral vein of the corresponding side
thoracoacromial	Satellite of the thoracoacromial artery	Acromion, coracoid process, sternoclavicular joint; tributary veins from the deltoid, subclavius, pectoralis minor and pectoralis major	Cephalic vein or axillary vein or subclavian vein
thymic (two or three in number)	Thymus	Parenchyma of thymus	Left brachiocephalic and inferior thyroid veins or, at times, superior phrenic veins
tracheal (varying in number)	Along the surface of the trachea	Wall of the trachea	Thyroid plexus and brachiocephalic vein or superior vena cava

VEIN	
acromiothoracic	☞ thoracoacromial vein
anterior mediastinal	☞ mediastinal veins
azygos minor inferior	☞ hemiazygos vein
azygos minor superior	☞ accessory hemiazygos vein
greater azygos	☞ azygos vein
inferior coronary	☞ middle cardiac vein or posterior interventricular vein
innominate of Vieussens	☞ anterior veins of right ventricle or anterior cardiac veins
internal mammary	☞ internal thoracic vein
left azygos	☞ hemiazygos vein
left coronary	☞ great cardiac vein
long thoracic	☞ lateral thoracic vein
Marshall's vein	☞ oblique vein of left atrium
right coronary	☞ small cardiac vein
small coronary or **of Galen**	☞ anterior veins of right ventricle or anterior cardiac veins
Thebesian	☞ smallest cardiac veins

The table alongside lists some veins by their name normally used or eponym, with the corresponding reference to the official term.

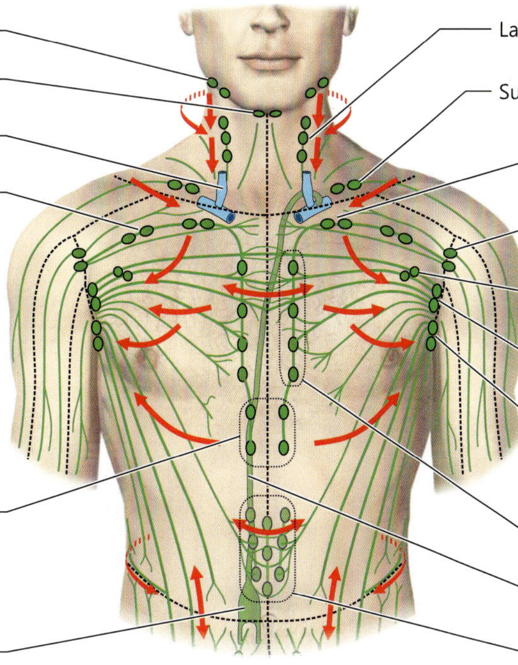

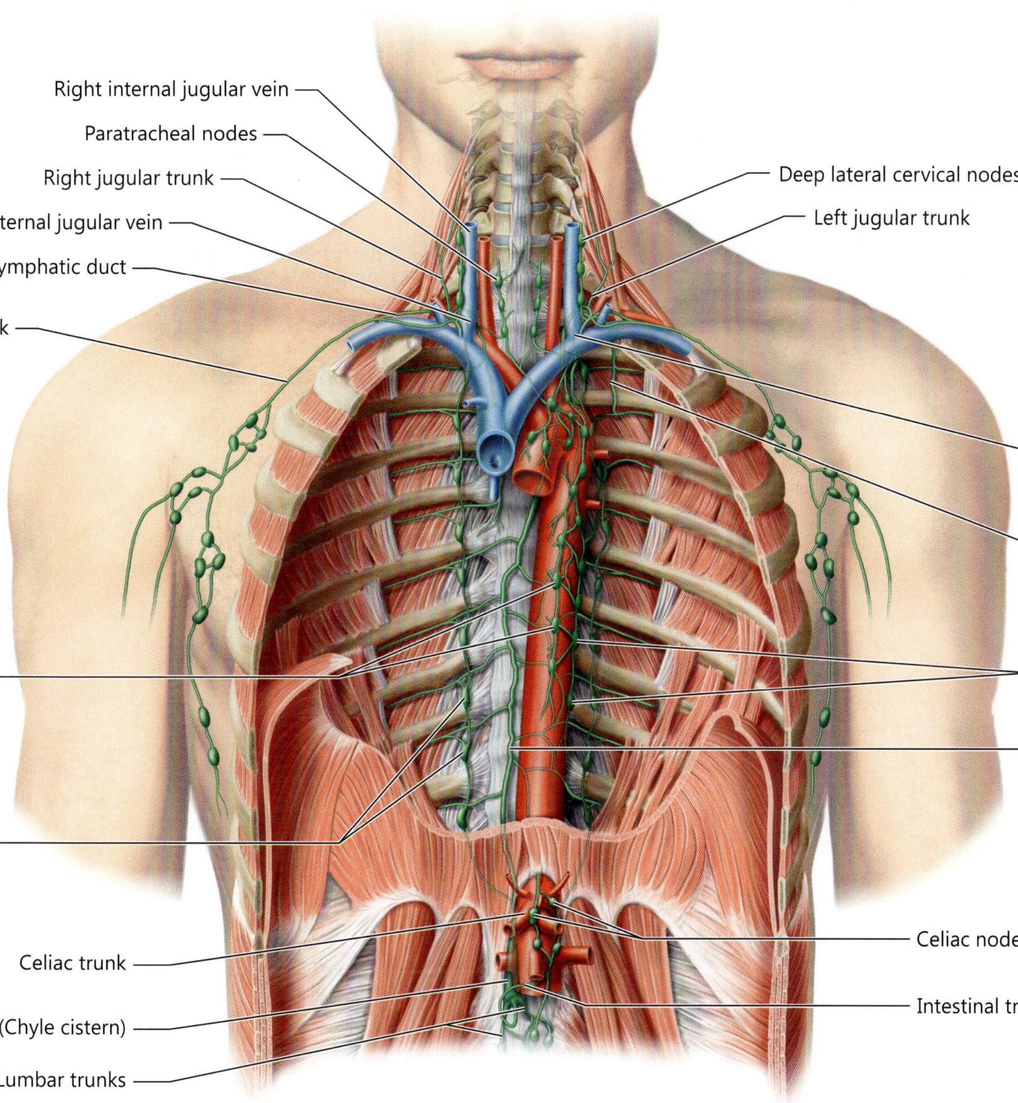

At the top, schematic representation showing the principal **superficial lymphatic vessels** and **lymphatic groups** of the thorax and the flow paths of lymphatic drainage. Below, disposition of the principal deep lymphatic ducts and lymphatic groups of the posterior mediastinum.

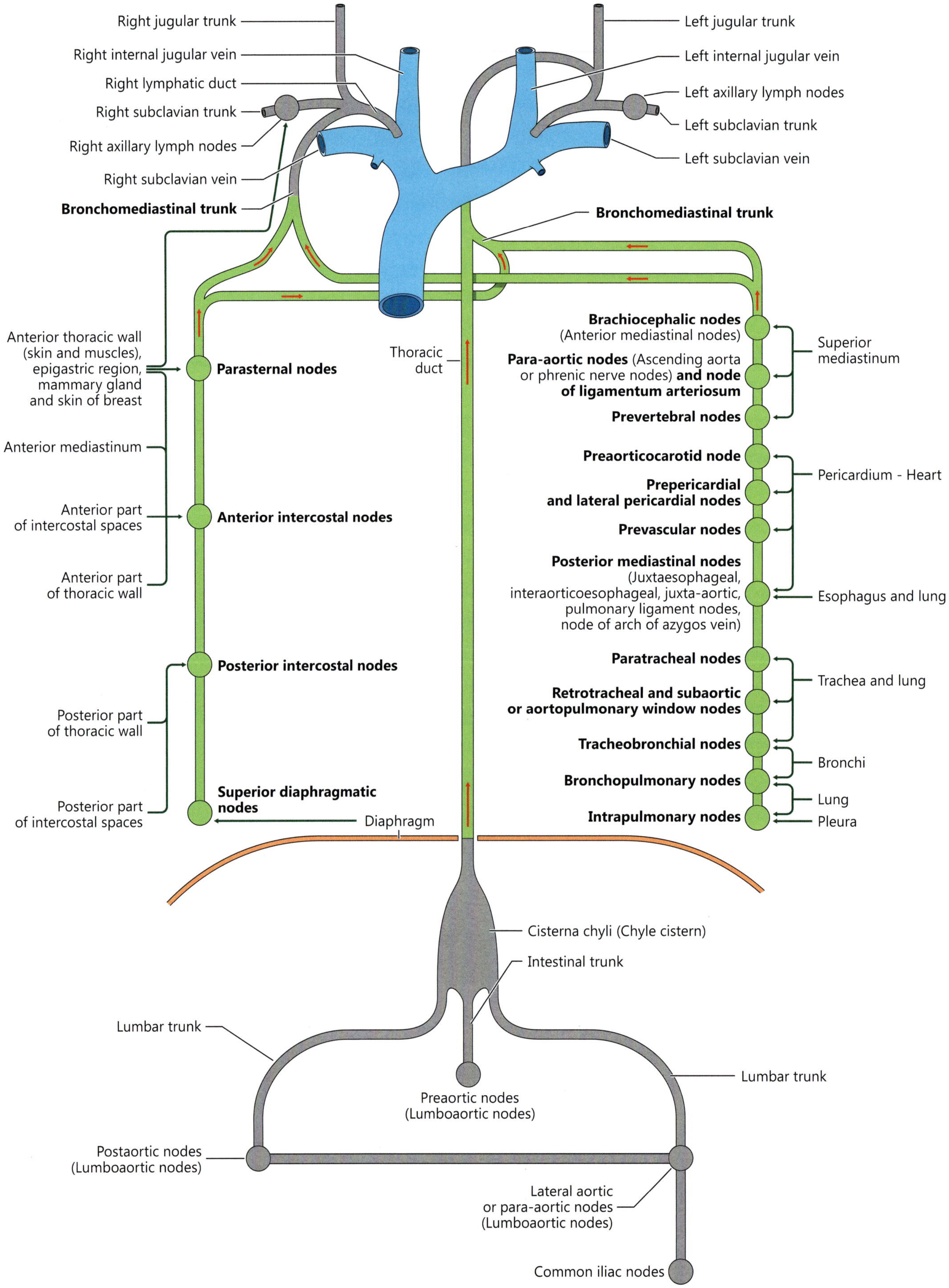

Schematic representation of the principal **lymphatic groups** and **lymphatic ducts**. The lymph nodes and ducts of the thorax and their visceral and parietal territories of drainage are highlighted.

Classification of the lymph nodes of the mediastinum

LYMPH NODE STATION OR GROUP	LYMPH NODES	LOCATION	REGION	AFFERENTS	EFFERENTS
1	**Superior mediastinal** (proper)	Above a horizontal line crossing the left brachiocephalic vein in correspondence to the trachea	Superior mediastinum	Thymus, thyroid gland, heart, pericardium, diaphragmatic pleura and mediastinal pleura, superior diaphragmatic nodes	Right and left bronchomediastinal trunks
2	**Superior paratracheal**	Below the above indicated boundary for the superior mediastinal nodes and above a horizontal line tangential to the superior border of the arch of aorta	Superior mediastinum	Lungs, bronchi, trachea, heart, juxtaesophageal nodes	Inferior paratracheal nodes and inferior cervical nodes
3	**Prevascular and retrotracheal**	Behind the trachea in front of the great vessels	Superior mediastinum	Thymus, thyroid gland, heart, pericardium, diaphragmatic pleura and mediastinal pleura, superior diaphragmatic nodes, superior lobe of left lung (to the prevascular nodes); lungs, bronchi, trachea, heart, juxtaesophageal nodes (to the retrotracheal nodes)	Right and left bronchomediastinal trunks
4	**Inferior paratracheal**	On each side of the median line crossing the trachea between a horizontal line tangential to the superior border of the arch of aorta and a horizontal line passing over the superior borders of the right and left superior lobar bronchi	Superior mediastinum	Lungs, bronchi, trachea, heart, juxtaesophageal nodes	Thoracic duct
5	**Subaortic** (or aortopulmonary window nodes, also known as Aortic)	In the aortopulmonary window laterally to the ligamentum arteriosum or to the aorta or left pulmonary artery	Mediastinum	Lungs, bronchi, trachea, heart, juxtaesophageal nodes	Thoracic duct
6	**Para-aortic** (ascending aorta nodes or phrenic nerve nodes, also known as Aortic)	In front of and laterally to the ascending aorta and arch of aorta or to the brachiocephalic trunk below a line tangential to the superior border of the arch of aorta	Mediastinum	Thymus, thyroid gland, heart, pericardium, diaphragmatic pleura and mediastinal pleura, superior diaphragmatic nodes	Right and left bronchomediastinal trunks
7	**Subcarinal**	Below the carina of trachea not associated to the right and left inferior lobar bronchi	Inferior mediastinum	Lungs, bronchi, trachea, heart, juxtaesophageal nodes	Paratracheal nodes, in particular on the right side
8	**Juxtaesophageal** (paraesophageal)	Adjacent to the wall of the esophagus to the right and left of the median line	Inferior mediastinum	Esophagus, pericardium, diaphragm, inferior diaphragmatic nodes, left lobe of liver	Thoracic duct, tracheobronchial, subcarinal, lateral aortic and celiac nodes
9	**Pulmonary ligament nodes**	Within the pulmonary ligament	Inferior mediastinum	Basal segments of the inferior lobes of lungs, esophagus	Thoracic duct, tracheobronchial, subcarinal, lateral aortic and celiac nodes

SUPERIOR MEDIASTINAL NODES	INFERIOR MEDIASTINAL NODES	ANTERIOR MEDIASTINAL NODES	POSTERIOR MEDIASTINAL NODES
Superior mediastinal nodes (proper) Superior paratracheal nodes Prevascular nodes Prevertebral nodes Inferior paratracheal nodes	Subcarinal nodes Juxtaesophageal nodes Pulmonary ligament nodes	Brachiocephalic nodes (or nodes of the transverse chain) Preaorticocarotid nodes Node of ligamentum arteriosum Prevascular nodes	Juxtaesophageal nodes Interaorticoesophageal nodes Juxta-aortic nodes Node of arch of azygos vein

Summary table of the lymphatic groups of the thorax

LYMPH NODES	GROUP OR STATION	SITE	AFFERENTS	EFFERENTS
			PARIETAL THORACIC LYMPH NODES	
Intercostal	Parietal	Deep	Intercostal collectors	Posterior mediastinal nodes, thoracic duct
Paramammary	Parietal	Superficial	Superficial mammary region	Axillary lymph nodes
Parasternal	Parietal	Deep	Collectors from the skin and muscles of the anterior thoracic wall, from the epigastric region, from the skin of the breast, from the anterior diaphragmatic nodes, and costal part of parietal pleura	Bronchomediastinal trunk
Superior diaphragmatic	Parietal	Deep	Collectors from the diaphragm and deep ascending from the liver	Mediastinal and parasternal nodes
			VISCERAL THORACIC LYMPH NODES	
Brachiocephalic (nodes of the transverse chain or anterosuperior mediastinal)	Anterior mediastinal	Deep	Thyroid gland, thymus, heart, pericardium, lateral diaphragmatic nodes	Bronchomediastinal trunk
Bronchopulmonary (pulmonary) – right – left (hilar or left hilar nodes)	Tracheobronchial	Deep	Lungs, visceral pleura and other thoracic organs	Tracheobronchial nodes (only some directly into the thoracic duct)
Interaorticoesophageal	Posterior mediastinal and Station 8	Deep	Mediastinal pleura and thoracic part of the esophagus, posterior pericardium	Tracheobronchial nodes (only some directly into the thoracic duct)
Intrapulmonary – interlobar – lobar – segmental – subsegmental		Deep	Lungs	Right thoracic duct or lymphatic duct
Juxta-aortic	Posterior mediastinal	Deep	Mediastinal pleura, thoracic part of the esophagus, posterior pericardium	Tracheobronchial nodes (only some directly into the thoracic duct)
Juxtaesophageal (paraesophageal)	Posterior mediastinal or inferior mediastinal and Station 8	Deep	Mediastinal pleura, thoracic part of the esophagus, posterior pericardium	Tracheobronchial nodes (only some directly into the thoracic duct)
Lateral pericardial		Deep	Thoracic organs	Right thoracic duct or lymphatic duct
Mediastinal – anterior (☞ Anterior mediastinal group) – – diaphragmatic – inferior (☞ Inferior mediastinal group) – posterior (☞ Posterior mediastinal group) – – diaphragmatic – superior (☞ Superior mediastinal group)	 Station 1	Deep	 Diaphragm, diaphragmatic pleura, liver Diaphragmatic pleura	 Right thoracic duct or lymphatic duct Right thoracic duct or lymphatic duct
Node of arch of azygos vein	Posterior mediastinal	Deep	Thoracic organs	Right thoracic duct or lymphatic duct
Node of ligamentum arteriosum	Anterior mediastinal	Deep	Thoracic organs	Right thoracic duct or lymphatic duct
Para-aortic (ascending aorta or phrenic nerve nodes)	Station 6	Deep	Thoracic organs	Right thoracic duct or lymphatic duct
Paratracheal – superior – right and left inferior	Superior mediastinal Station 2 Tracheobronchial and Station 4	Deep	Trachea, bronchi, mediastinal pleura, posterior pericardium	Tracheobronchial nodes or thoracic duct
Preaorticocarotid	Anterior mediastinal	Deep	Left lung	Bronchomediastinal trunk

continued

Summary table of the lymphatic groups of the thorax				*(continued)*
LYMPH NODES	***GROUP OR STATION***	***SITE***	***AFFERENTS***	***EFFERENTS***
Prepericardial		Deep	Thoracic organs	Right thoracic duct or lymphatic duct
Prevascular	Anterior mediastinal or superior mediastinal and Station 3	Deep	Right lung	Nodes of the transverse chain
Prevertebral	Superior mediastinal	Deep	Thoracic organs	Right thoracic duct or lymphatic duct
Pulmonary ligament nodes	Inferior mediastinal and Station 9	Deep	Thoracic organs	Right thoracic duct or lymphatic duct
Retrotracheal	Station 3	Deep	Thoracic organs	Right thoracic duct or lymphatic duct
Subaortic (aortopulmonary window nodes)	Station 5	Deep	Thoracic organs	Right thoracic duct or lymphatic duct
Subcarinal	Station 7	Deep	Thoracic organs	Right thoracic duct or lymphatic duct
Tracheobronchial – right superior (hilar or right hilar nodes) and left superior – inferior	Tracheobronchial	Deep	Heart, trachea, bronchi, lungs, posterior mediastinal nodes	Bronchomediastinal trunk

Summary table of the lymphatic ducts involved in the drainage of the thorax			
LYMPH NODES	***ORIGIN***	***TERRITORIES OF DRAINAGE***	***OPENING***
Right and left bronchomediastinal trunks	Brachiocephalic and tracheobronchial lymphatic groups	*Right*: thoracic wall (deep), right lung, right bronchial tree, trachea, esophagus, right part of the heart, liver *Left*: thoracic wall (deep), left lung, left bronchial tree, trachea, most of the esophagus, left part of the heart	*Right*: right jugulosubclavian confluence or right lymphatic duct *Left*: left jugulosubclavian confluence or terminal part of the thoracic duct
Right and left subclavian trunks	Apical group of the axillary lymph nodes	Upper limb, part of the thoracic wall, most of the breast, anterosuperior (supraumbilical) part of the anterior abdominal wall	*Right*: right jugulosubclavian confluence or right lymphatic duct *Left*: left jugulosubclavian confluence or terminal part of the thoracic duct
Right lymphatic duct	Right jugular, subclavian and at times bronchomediastinal trunks	Territories of drainage of the right bronchomediastinal, subclavian and jugular trunks	Right jugulosubclavian confluence
Thoracic duct	Right and left lumbar trunks and intestinal trunk (cisterna chyli)	Territories of drainage of the right and left lumbar trunks, and of the left intestinal, bronchomediastinal, subclavian and jugular trunks	Left jugulosubclavian confluence

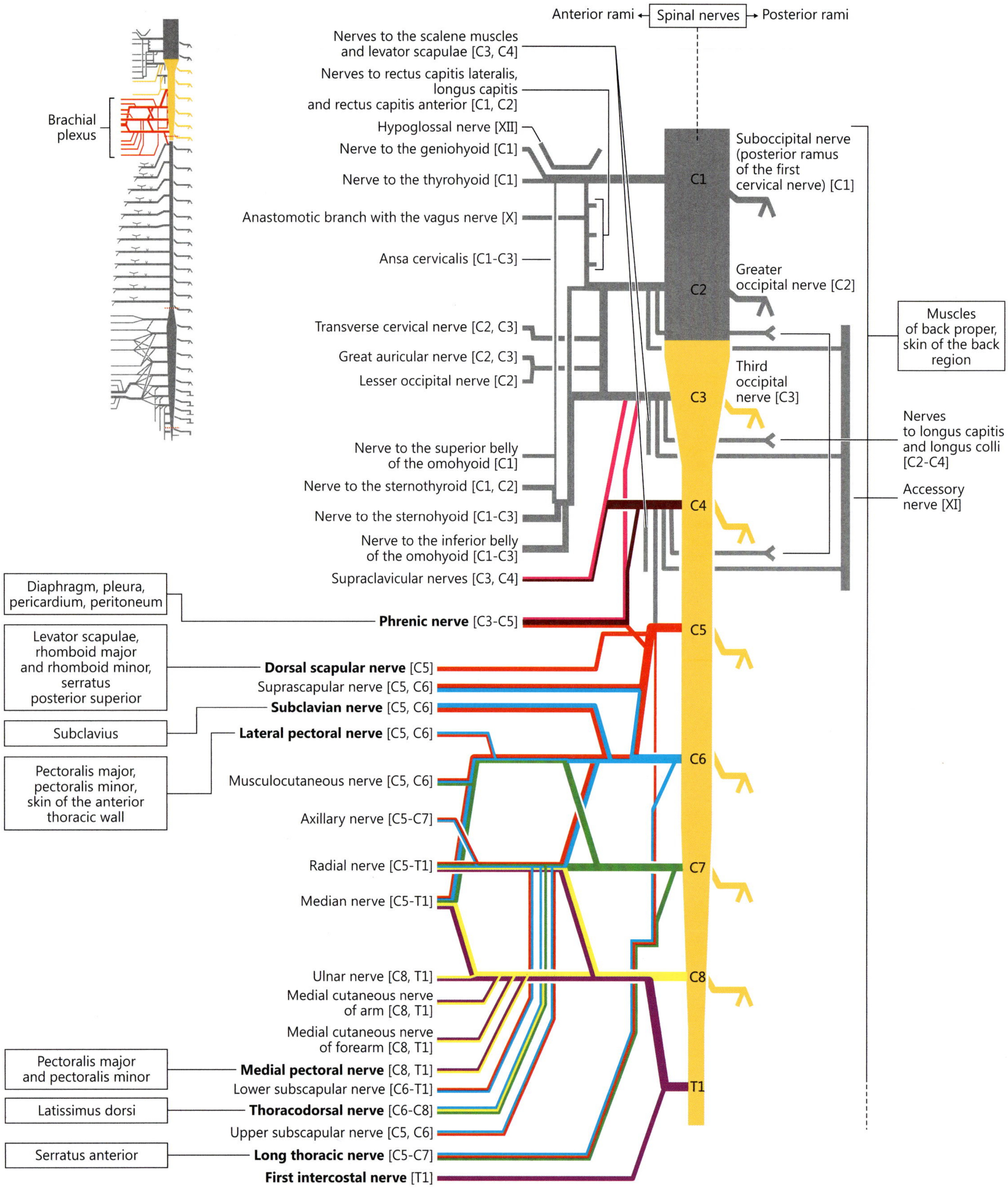

Schematic representation of the **cervical** and **brachial plexuses**. In the left part of the picture, the cervical plexus (a description of which is given in the chapter on the neck) is represented in *gray*. It is formed by the anterior rami of the first four cervical nerves. Note that each anterior ramus, with the exception of the 1st cervical nerve, divides into two branches, an ascending and a descending one, which unite with the corresponding rami of the contiguous nerves to construct the cervical loops; the descending branch of the 4th cervical nerve anastomoses with the anterior ramus of the 5th cervical nerve, which forms part of the brachial plexus. From the cervical plexus arise cutaneous and muscular anastomotic branches. The brachial plexus is represented in different colors. It is composed of the anterior rami of the 5th, 6th, 7th and 8th cervical nerves. From this plexus originate, besides the terminal branches, also collateral branches. In the right part of the picture, the dorsal branches of the cervical nerves are represented.

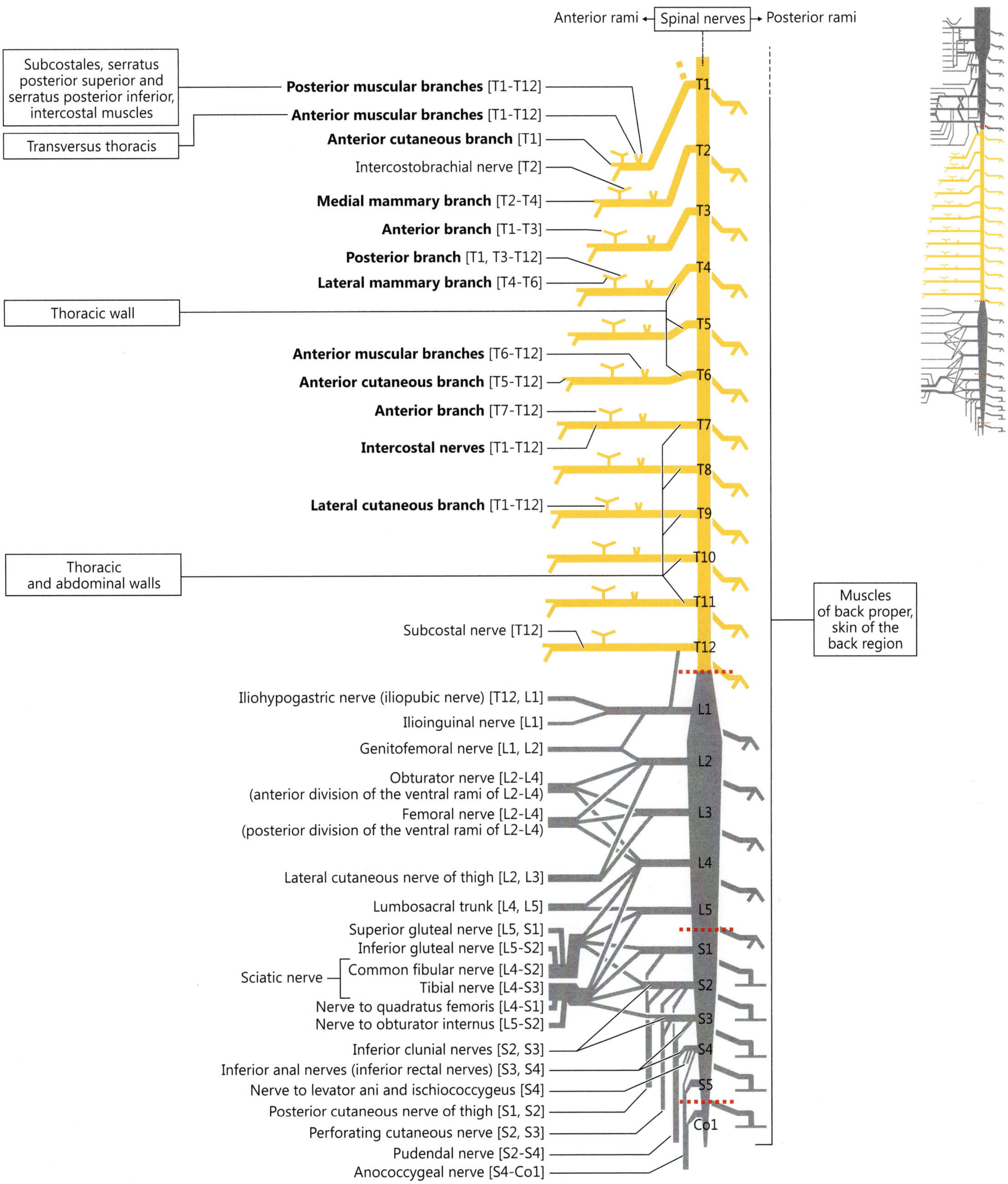

Schematic representation of the **intercostal nerves**, and of the **lumbar**, **sacral** and **coccygeal plexuses**. In the left part of the picture, the intercostal nerves are represented in *yellow*. Composed of the anterior rami of the twelve pairs of thoracic nerves, these are mixed nerves which provide cutaneous innervation to the thoracoabdominal wall and muscles of the thorax. The lumbar, sacral and coccygeal plexuses are represented in *gray*, and will be illustrated in the section on the abdomen. In the right part of the picture, the dorsal branches of the intercostal nerves are represented.

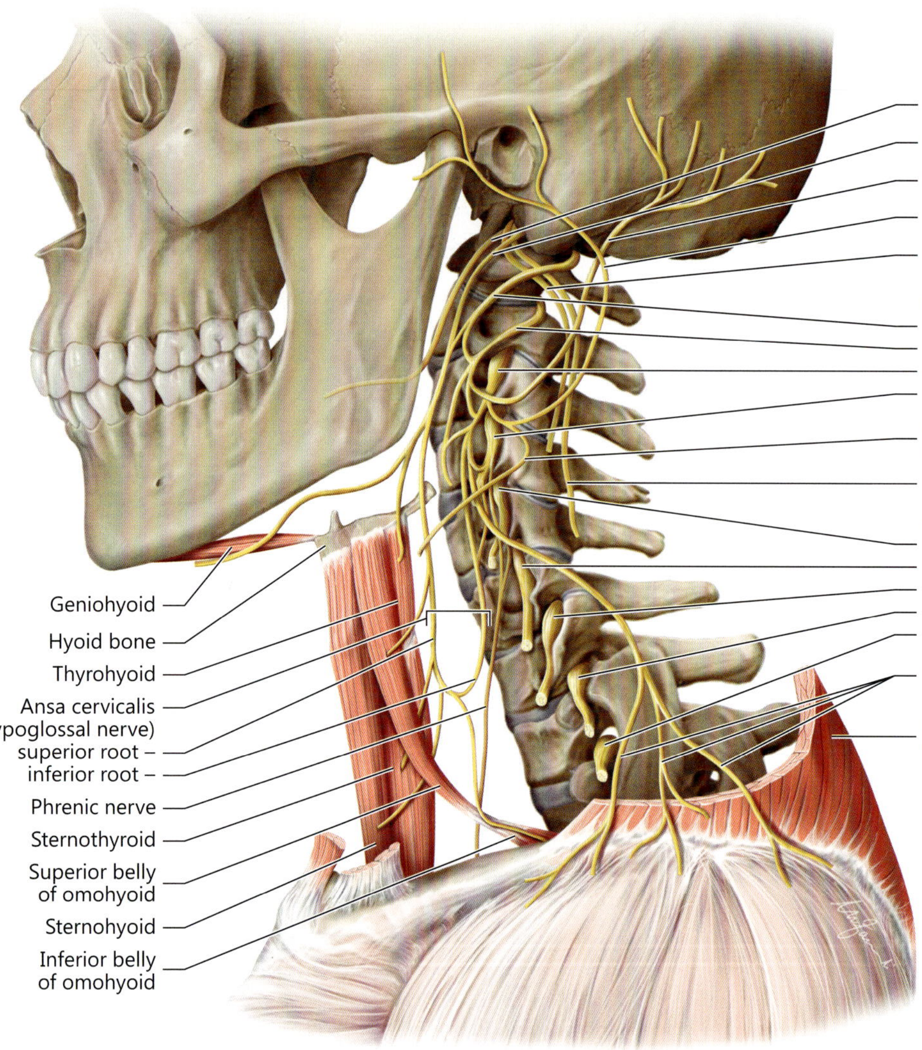

Illustration showing the **cervical plexus** in relation to the skeleton of the vertebral column.

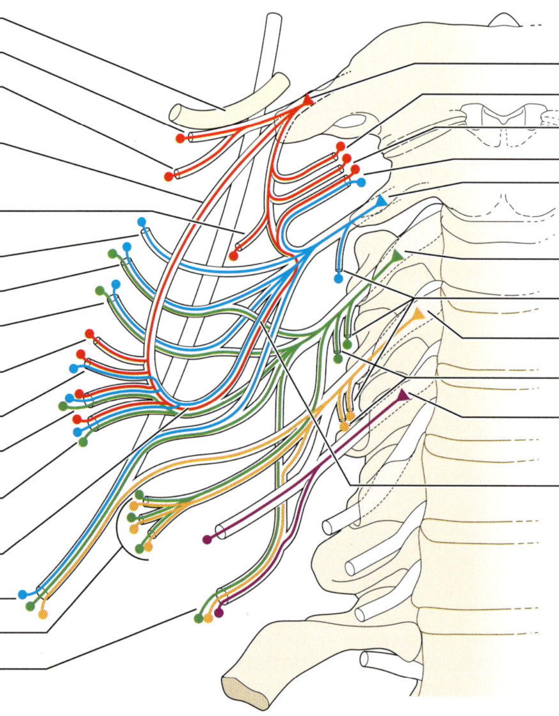

Schematic representation showing the structure of the **cervical plexus**.

Schematic representation showing the **brachial plexus** in relation to the skeleton of the vertebral column.

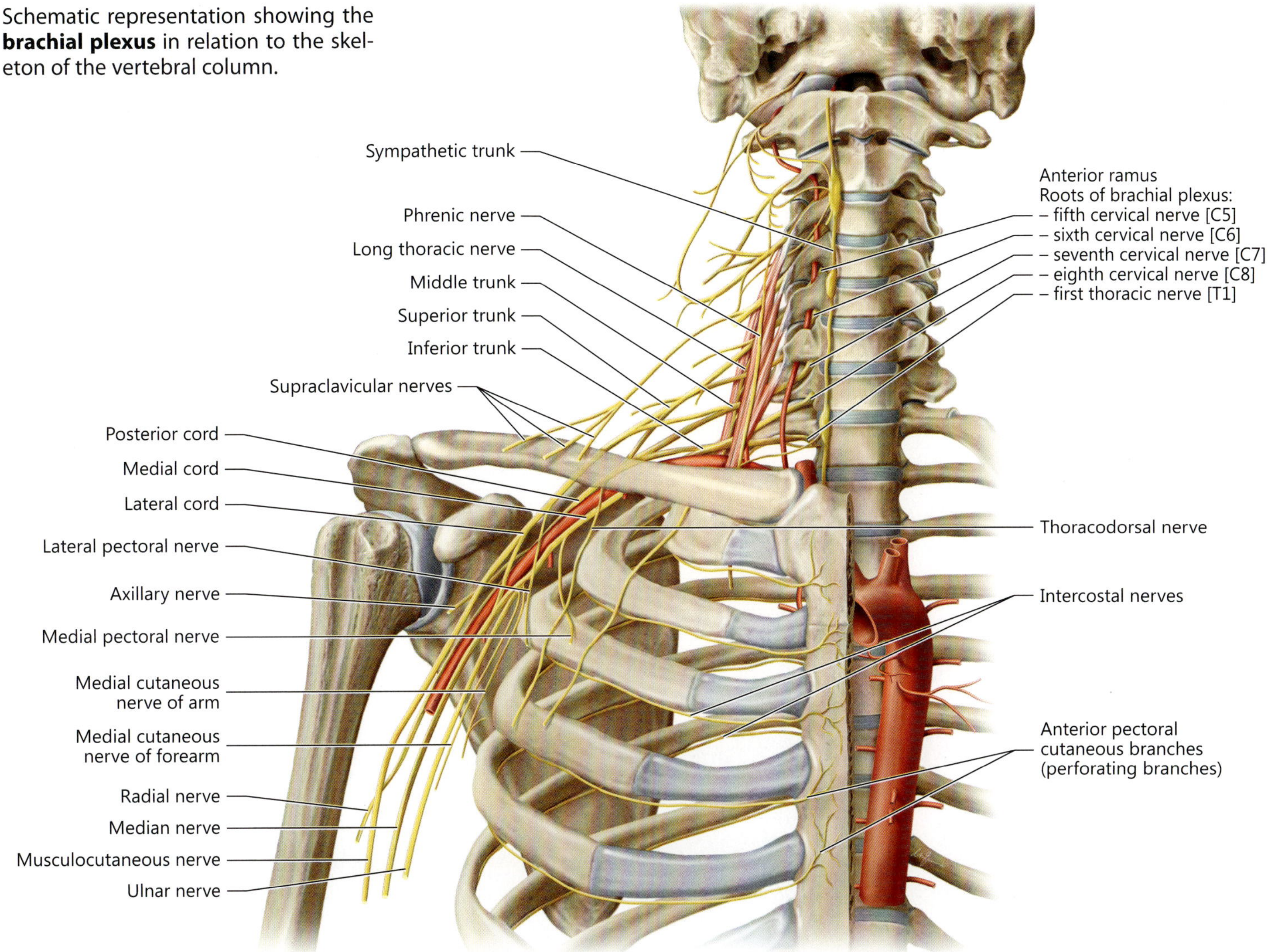

Schematic representation showing the structure of the **brachial plexus**. One can see the position of the anterior branches (ant. b.), with the formation of the trunks (superior, middle and inferior) and cords, and of the posterior (post. b.) and terminal branches (term. b.). The phrenic nerve [C3, C4, C5] belongs to the cervical plexus; the first intercostal nerve to the thoracic nerves (anterior ramus of the first thoracic nerve).

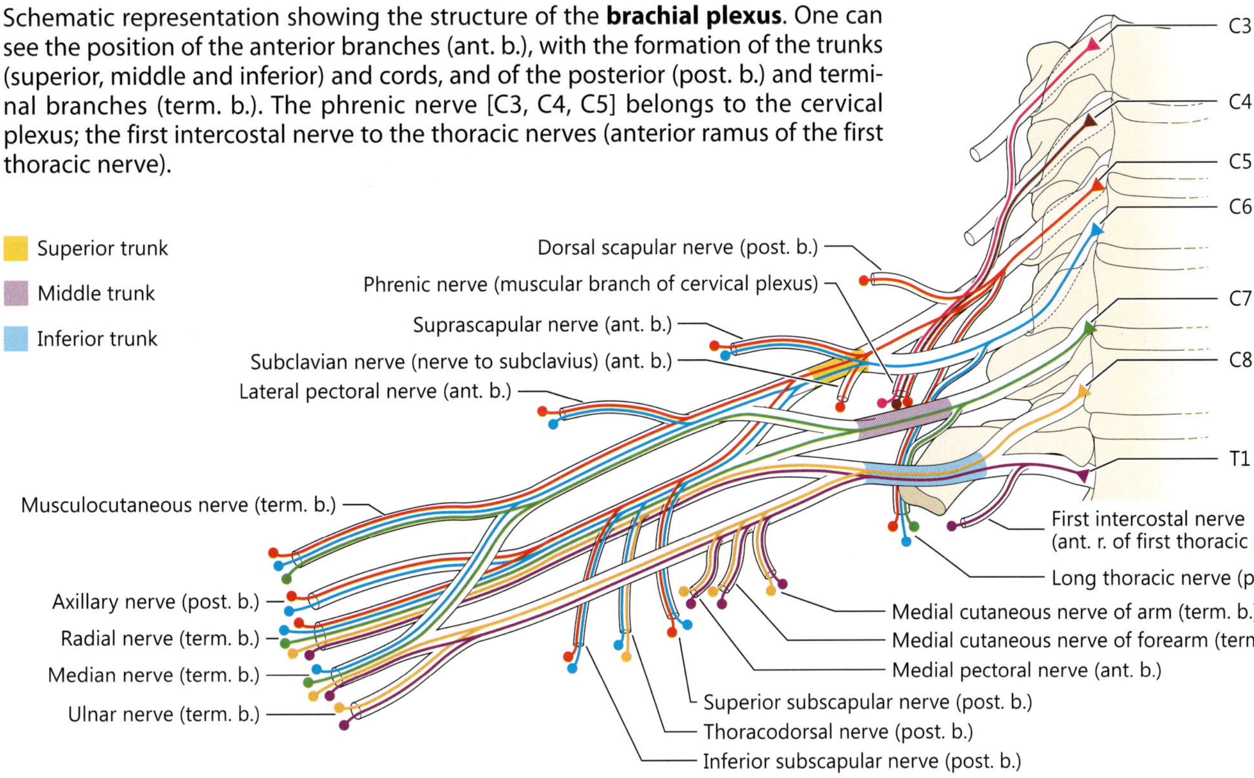

Course of the **posterior rami of the spinal nerves** which, heading dorsally, divide into a lateral branch and a medial branch. Note the particular disposition of the dorsal branches of the first three cervical rami, in particular of the third occipital nerve which ascends in the nuchal region.

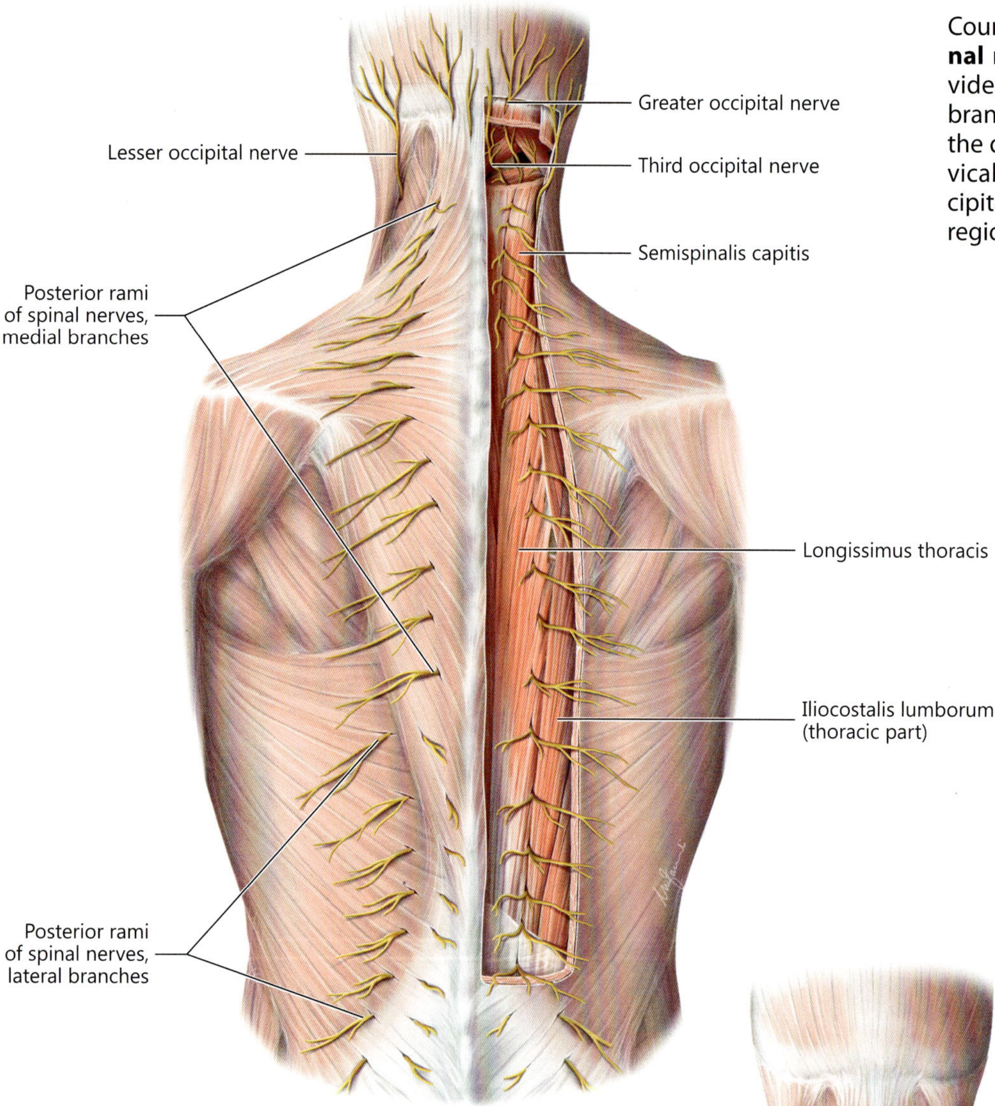

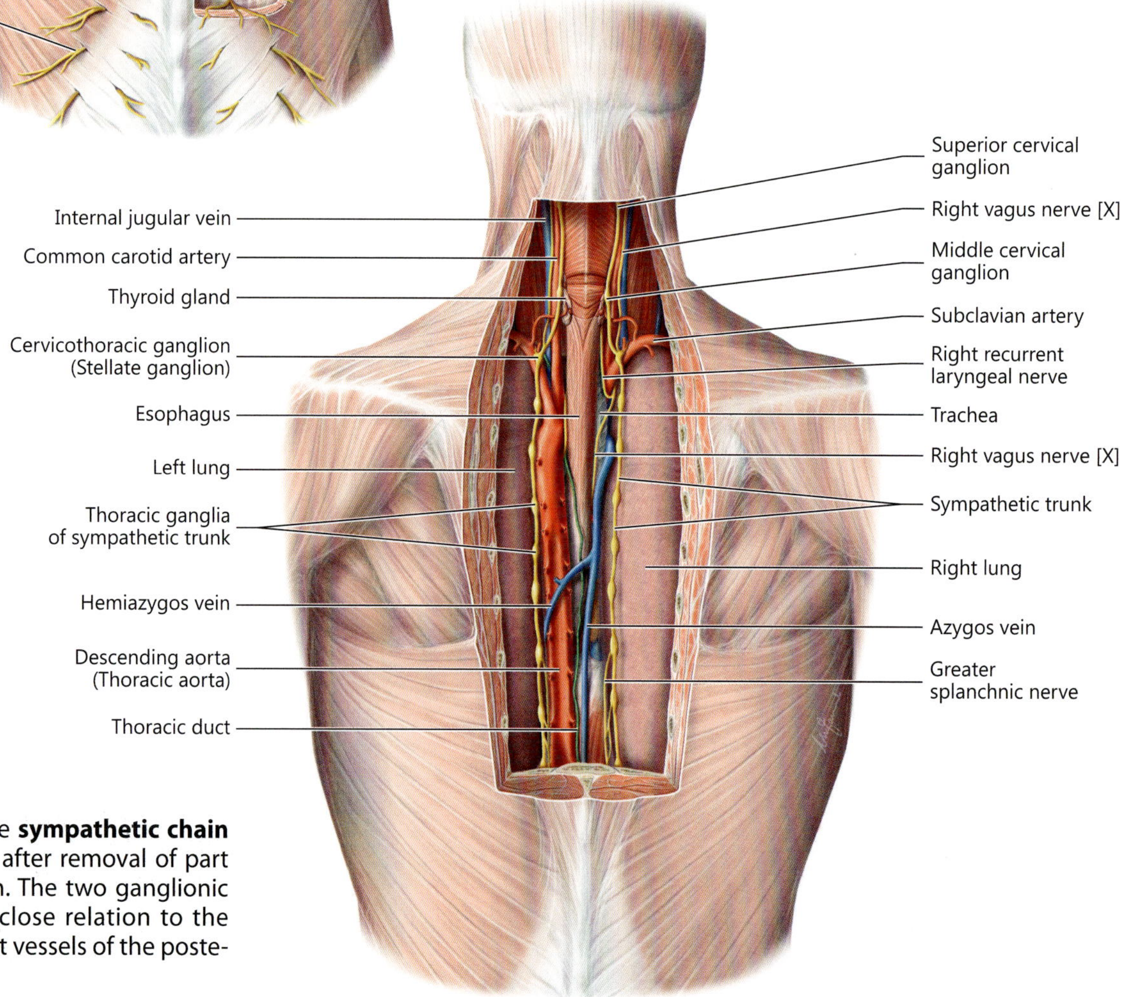

Thoracic segment of the **sympathetic chain** in posterior projection, after removal of part of the vertebral column. The two ganglionic chains are situated in close relation to the parietal pleura and great vessels of the posterior mediastinum.

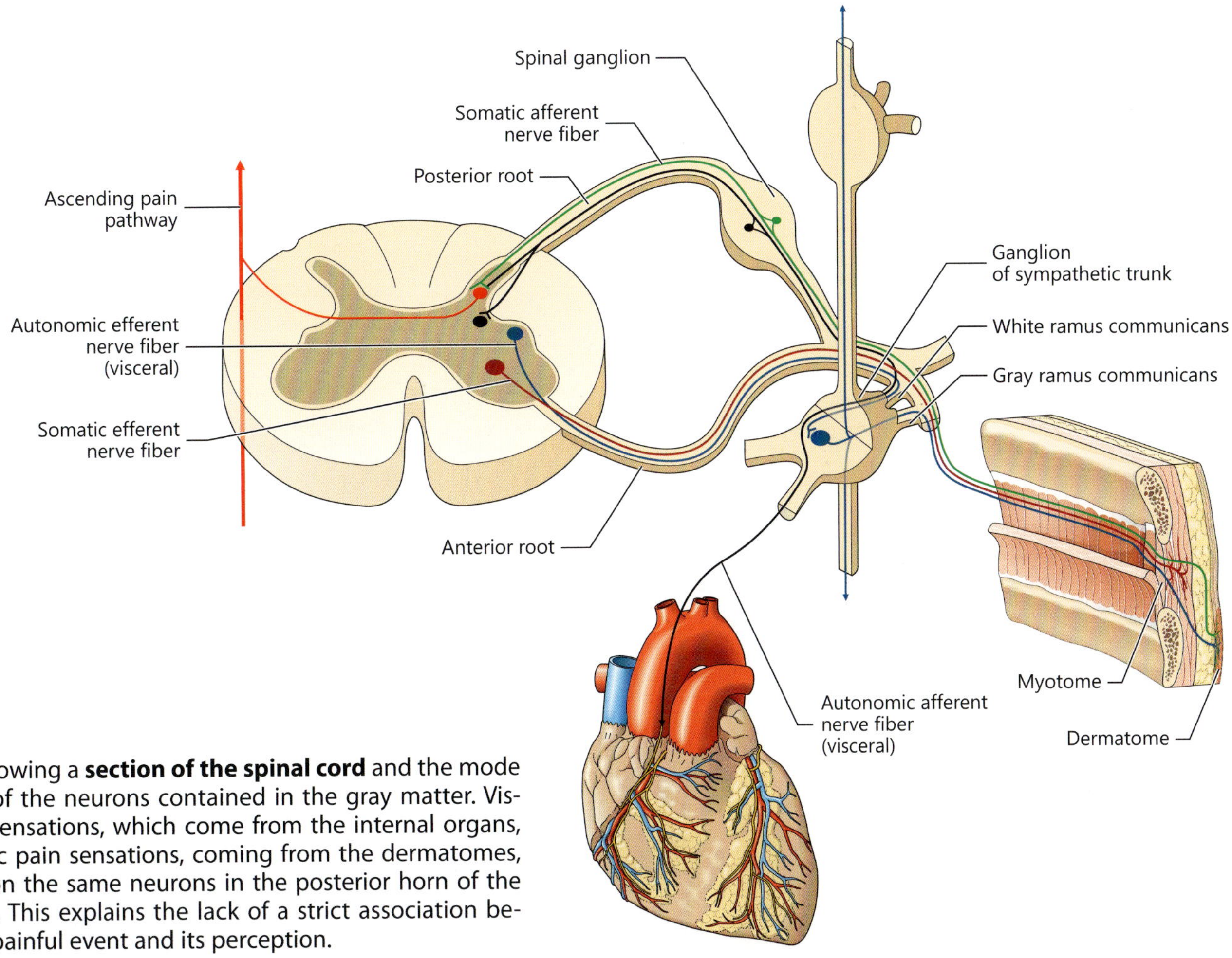

Diagram showing a **section of the spinal cord** and the mode of activity of the neurons contained in the gray matter. Visceral pain sensations, which come from the internal organs, and somatic pain sensations, coming from the dermatomes, terminate on the same neurons in the posterior horn of the spinal cord. This explains the lack of a strict association between the painful event and its perception.

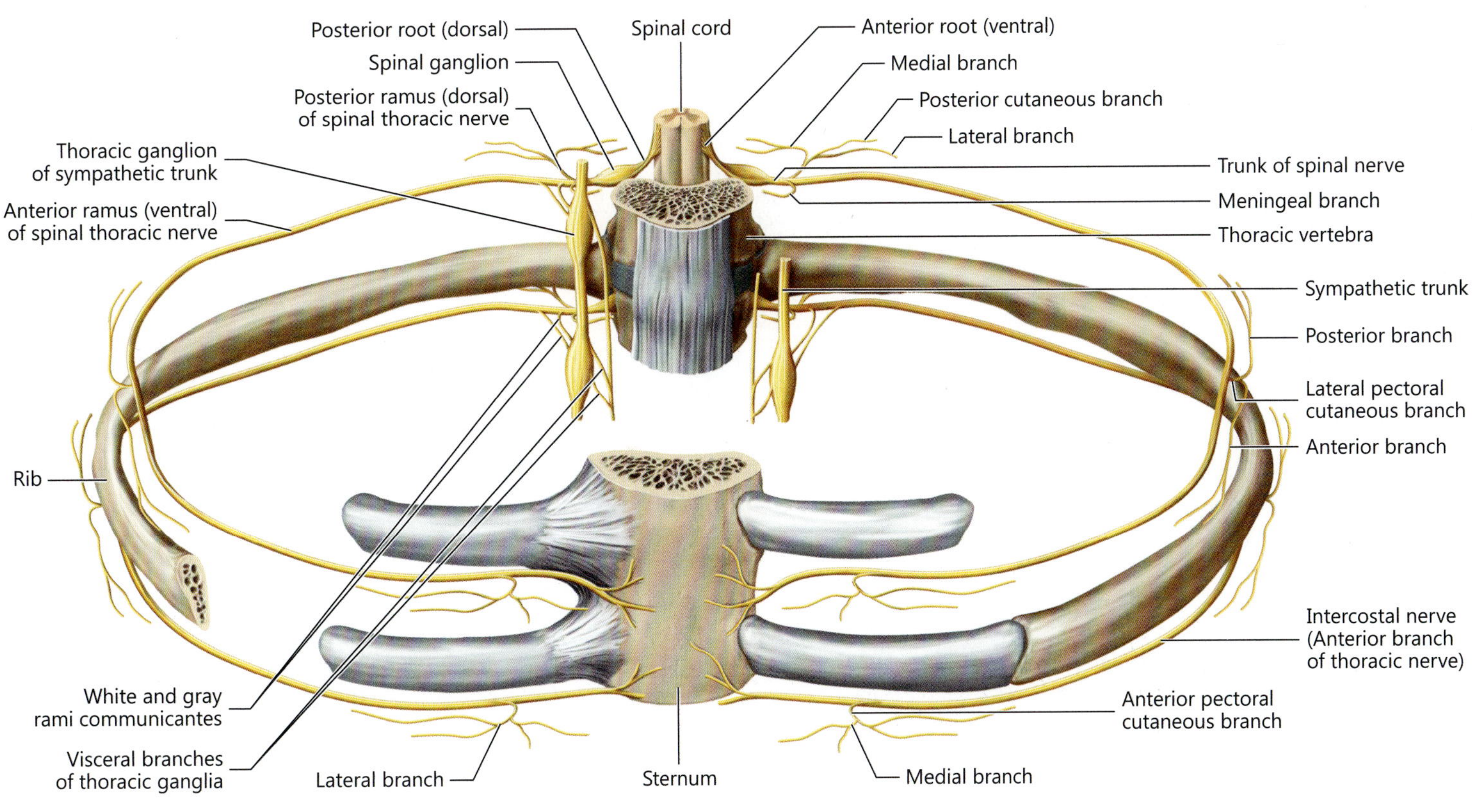

Schematic representation showing the course of the **thoracic nerves** in relation to the ribs and sternum. The anterior rami of the thoracic nerves (intercostal nerves) head forwards following the same course as the ribs and giving off anterior, lateral and medial cutaneous branches.

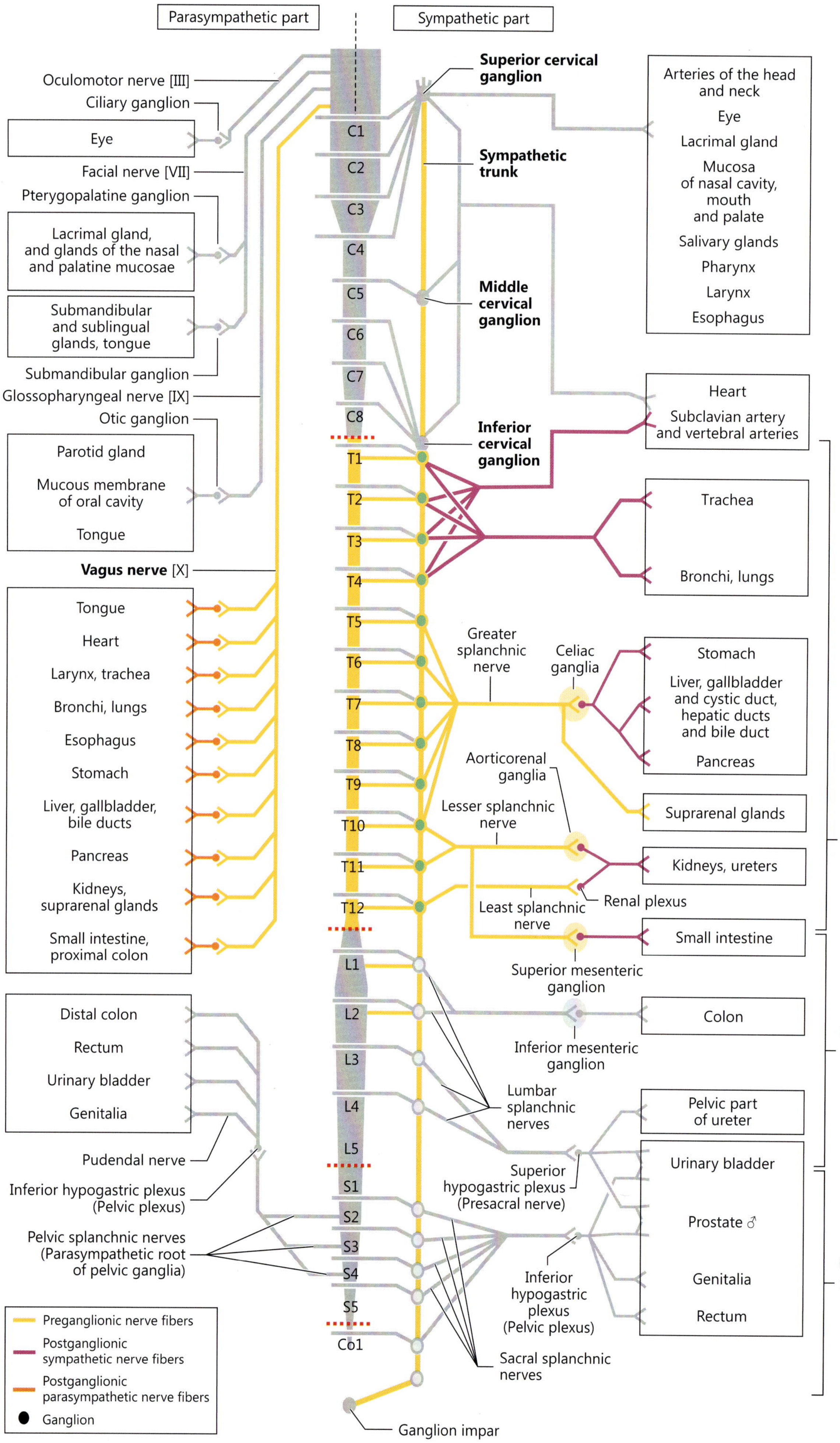

Schematic representation of the **autonomic division** composed of the sympathetic nervous system (on the right) and parasympathetic nervous system (on the left). The autonomic division is the part of the central nervous system that controls the secretory functions of glands and wall motility of internal organs and vessels, thus regulating the vital functions of the organs and all body systems. The organs that are innervated by nerve fibers of the autonomic division are listed, in detail, in the boxes. The preganglionic nerve fibers are represented in *yellow*; in *purple*, the postganglionic fibers of the sympathetic nervous system, and in *orange* those of the parasympathetic nervous system. The parasympathetic (cranial and sacral) nervous system comprises the neuraxial visceral centers situated, respectively, in the brainstem and sacral segment of the spinal cord. Note, in particular, the elevated number of visceral efferent (motor) fibers of the parasympathetic part of the vagus nerve.

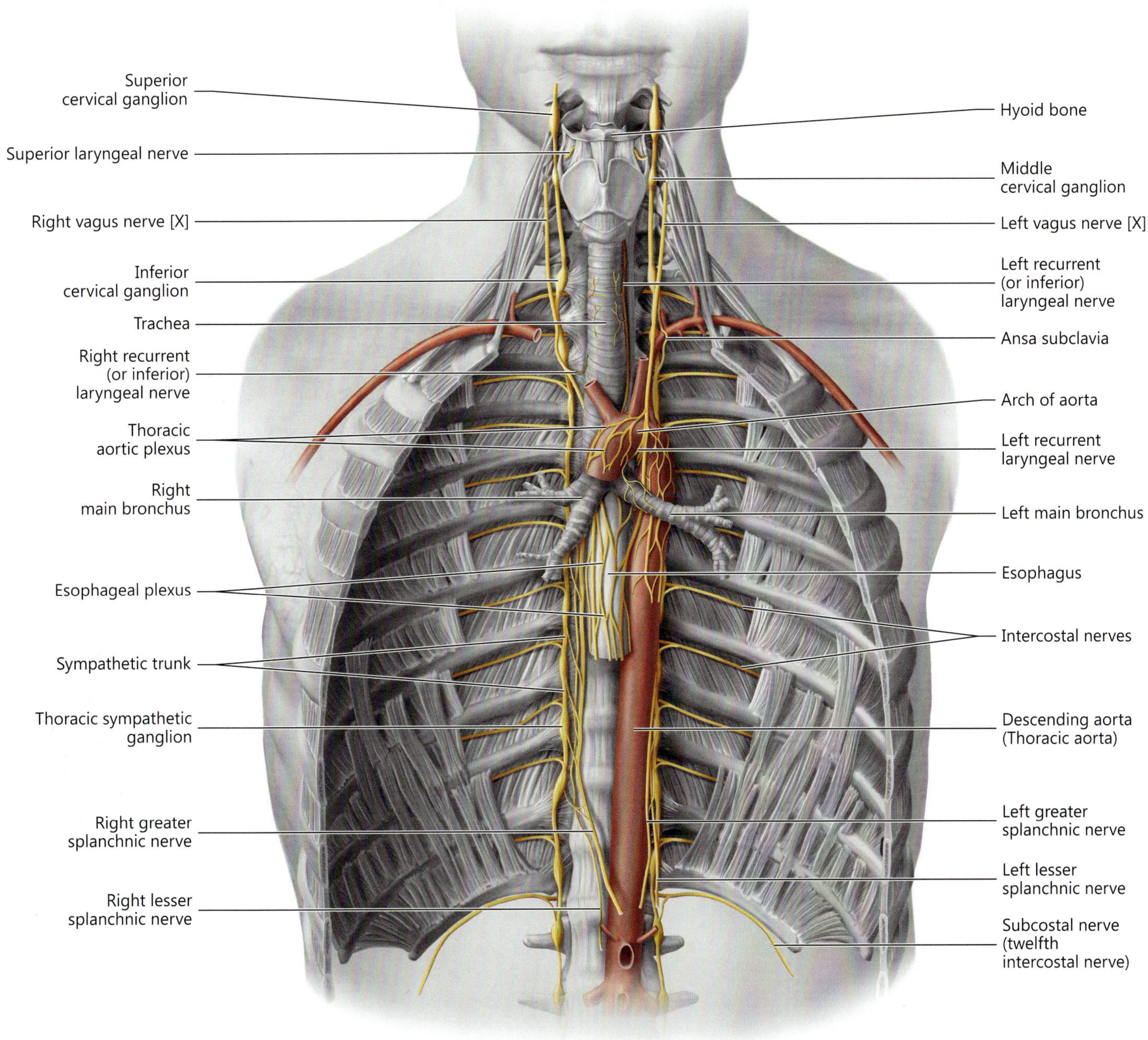

Disposition of the **sympathetic chain** in the cervical and thoracic segments.

Summary table of the nerves of the thorax. In simple bold, the nerves that originate from the spinal nerves; in bold underlined, the nerves of the sympathetic nervous system; in *italics*, the vagus nerve, whose visceral component is an afferent of the parasympathetic nervous system

NERVE(S)	ORIGIN	RAMIFICATIONS	DISTRIBUTION
accessory phrenic	Inconstant branch of the fifth cervical nerve which originates together with the subclavian nerve	Unites with the phrenic nerve	Diaphragm
ansa subclavia	Branch connecting the cervicothoracic ganglion with the middle cervical ganglion forming an ansa around the subclavian artery		
bronchial branches	From the vagus nerve [X], in the thorax	To the pulmonary plexus	Lungs
dorsal scapular (first posterior thoracic nerve)	Supraclavicular part of the brachial plexus, from the superior trunk [C4, C5]	Filaments	Levator scapulae, rhomboid major, rhomboid minor and serratus posterior superior
esophageal branches	From the thoracic segment of the sympathetic trunk		Esophagus
greater splanchnic	From the thoracic segment of the sympathetic trunk with four or five roots; runs in the thorax and abdomen	To the celiac plexus and celiac ganglia	Through the celiac plexus, to the other visceral plexuses of the abdominal part
inferior cervical cardiac	Inferior cervical ganglion and first thoracic ganglion (the two ganglia can fuse together to form the cervicothoracic ganglion or stellate ganglion)	To the cardiac plexus	Heart
intercostal (anterior rami of thoracic nerves from T I to T XI; the anterior ramus of T XII is the subcostal nerve)	Thoracic nerves	White and gray rami communicantes, lateral pectoral cutaneous branch, lateral mammary branch of the fourth, fifth and sixth intercostal nerve, anterior pectoral cutaneous branch, medial mammary branch of the second, third and fourth intercostal nerve, muscular branches, collateral branch, anterior and lateral abdominal cutaneous branches, intercostobrachial nerve	The first 2 nerves supply fibers to the upper limbs and thoracic wall; the 4 successive nerves to the thoracic wall; the 5 inferior nerves to the thoracic and abdominal walls; subcostales, serratus posterior superior, serratus posterior inferior external, internal and innermost intercostal muscles, transversus thoracis, abdominal muscles (rectus abdominis, external oblique, internal oblique, transversus abdominis, pyramidalis)
intercostobrachial (posterior branch of the lateral pectoral cutaneous branch of the second intercostal nerve)	Second intercostal nerve	Anastomoses with the medial and posterior cutaneous nerves of arm	Skin of the superior half of the medial and posterior surfaces of the arm
intermediate supraclavicular	Cervical plexus [C3, C4]	Filaments	Skin over the pectoralis major and deltoid
lateral pectoral (first anterior thoracic nerve)	Infraclavicular part of the brachial plexus, from the lateral cord [C5, C6]	Filaments	Pectoralis major
lateral supraclavicular	Cervical plexus [C3, C4]	Filaments	Skin over the superior and posterior parts of shoulder
lesser splanchnic	From the thoracic segment of the sympathetic trunk, in general with three roots; runs in the thorax and abdomen	To the celiac plexus and renal and suprarenal plexuses	Through the celiac plexus, to the other visceral plexuses of the abdominal part
long thoracic (second posterior thoracic nerve)	Supraclavicular part of the brachial plexus, from the superior and middle trunks [C5, C6, C7]	Filaments	Serratus anterior
medial pectoral (second anterior thoracic nerve)	Infraclavicular part of the brachial plexus, from the medial cord [C8, T I]	Filaments	Pectoralis minor and inferior part of pectoralis major
medial supraclavicular	Cervical plexus [C3, C4]	Filaments	Skin of the medial part of the infraclavicular region until the median line, sternoclavicular joint
middle cervical cardiac	Middle cervical ganglion	To the deep part of the cardiac plexus	Heart
phrenic	Cervical plexus, with a principal root from the fourth cervical nerve and two accessory, inconstant, roots from the third and fifth cervical nerves	Pericardial branch and phrenicoabdominal branches	Diaphragm, pericardium, pleura, great vessels passing through the diaphragm, peritoneum
posterior rami of thoracic nerves	Thoracic nerves	Medial and lateral branches	Skin of the vertebral region and muscles of back proper

continued

Summary table of the nerves of the thorax. In simple bold, the nerves that originate from the spinal nerves; in bold underlined, the nerves of the sympathetic nervous system; in *italics*, the vagus nerve, whose visceral component is an afferent of the parasympathetic nervous system *(continued)*

NERVE(S)	*ORIGIN*	*RAMIFICATIONS*	*DISTRIBUTION*
recurrent laryngeal (inferior laryngeal)	Vagus nerve [X]	Tracheal, esophageal and pharyngeal branches	Intrinsic muscles of the larynx with the exception of the cricothyroid, innervated by the superior laryngeal nerve; mucosa of larynx below the vocal folds, trachea, esophagus, inferior constrictor of pharynx
subclavian	Supraclavicular part of the brachial plexus, from the superior trunk [C5]	Filaments, anastomosis with the phrenic nerve	Subclavius, sternoclavicular joint
subcostal	Anterior ramus of the twelfth thoracic nerve	Lateral pectoral cutaneous branch, anastomotic branch with the lumbar plexus	Abdominal wall and skin of the gluteal region
superior and inferior cervical cardiac branches	From the vagus nerve [X], in the neck	To the cardiac plexus	Heart
superior cervical cardiac	Inferior part of the superior cervical ganglion	To the cardiac plexus	Heart
thoracic cardiac branches	From the second to the fifth thoracic ganglion	To the cardiac plexus	Heart
thoracic cardiac branches	From the vagus nerve [X], in the thorax	To the cardiac plexus	Heart
thoracic nerves [T I-T XII] (12 pairs of spinal nerves)	Thoracic segment of the spinal cord	Anterior and posterior rami	Thoracic and abdominal walls, skin of the buttocks
thoracic pulmonary branches	From the second to the fifth or sixth thoracic ganglion	To the pulmonary plexus	Lungs
thoracic segment of sympathetic trunk	Sympathetic trunk in the thorax; generally eleven thoracic ganglia, the first thoracic ganglion often being fused with the inferior cervical ganglion	White and gray rami communicantes with the thoracic nerves and perivascular and visceral peripheral branches (greater and lesser splanchnic nerves and esophageal branches)	Thoracic aortic, cardiac, pulmonary and celiac plexuses through the greater and lesser splanchnic nerves
thoracodorsal	Infraclavicular part of the brachial plexus, from the posterior cord [C6, C7, C8]	Filaments	Latissimus dorsi
vagus [X]	Myelencephalon (medulla oblongata or bulb)	Meningeal, auricular, communicating branch with glossopharyngeal nerve, pharyngeal, superior and inferior cervical cardiac branches and thoracic cardiac, bronchial, renal branches; anterior and posterior vagal trunks (anterior and posterior gastric branches, hepatic and celiac branches); superior and recurrent laryngeal nerves (tracheal, esophageal and pharyngeal branches)	Organs of the thorax and abdomen: heart, wall of the aorta and of its large branches; glands and smooth muscle of the airways, digestive tract (except for its terminal part) and of part of the urinary system; striated muscle of pharynx, larynx and proximal part of the esophagus; aortic sinus, aortic body, mucosa of the larynx, pharynx, trachea, esophagus and of the other thoracic and abdominal organs; taste buds in the mucosa of the epiglottis and in the oropharynx; skin of the auricle, of the external acoustic meatus and of the lateral surface of the tympanic membrane

NERVE	
anterior supraclavicular	☞ medial supraclavicular nerves
great cardiac	☞ middle cervical cardiac nerve
internal respiratory nerve of Bell	☞ phrenic nerve
long subscapular	☞ thoracodorsal nerve
middle supraclavicular	☞ intermediate supraclavicular nerves
pneumogastric	☞ vagus nerve [X]
posterior scapular	☞ dorsal scapular nerve
to pectoralis major	☞ lateral pectoral nerve
to pectoralis minor	☞ medial pectoral nerve
to serratus anterior	☞ long thoracic nerve

The table alongside lists some nerves by their name normally used or eponym, with the corresponding reference to the official term.

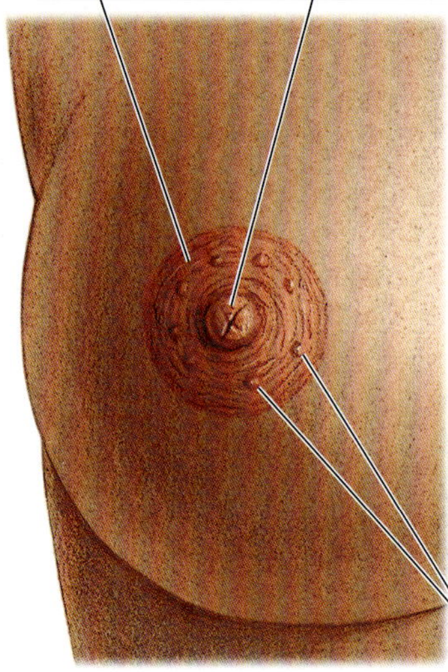

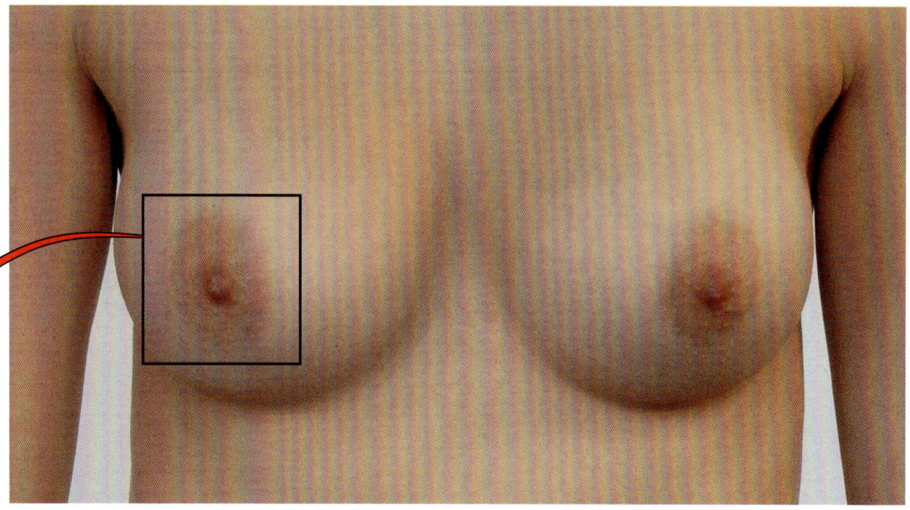

The area occupied by the **breast** of an adult woman extends from the third to the seventh rib on the thoracic cage (inframammary sulcus). The surface of the breast presents a hyperpigmented area (areola) surmounted by a raised zone, the nipple. At its apex open the outlets of the lactiferous ducts. The nipple is generally situated in correspondence to the fourth rib, lateral with respect to the midclavicular line. On the surface of the areola, the areolar tubercles (Montgomery's tubercles) are evident. These are sebaceous glands whose secretion has a lubricating effect and increases during lactation. The breast also contains the mammary gland.

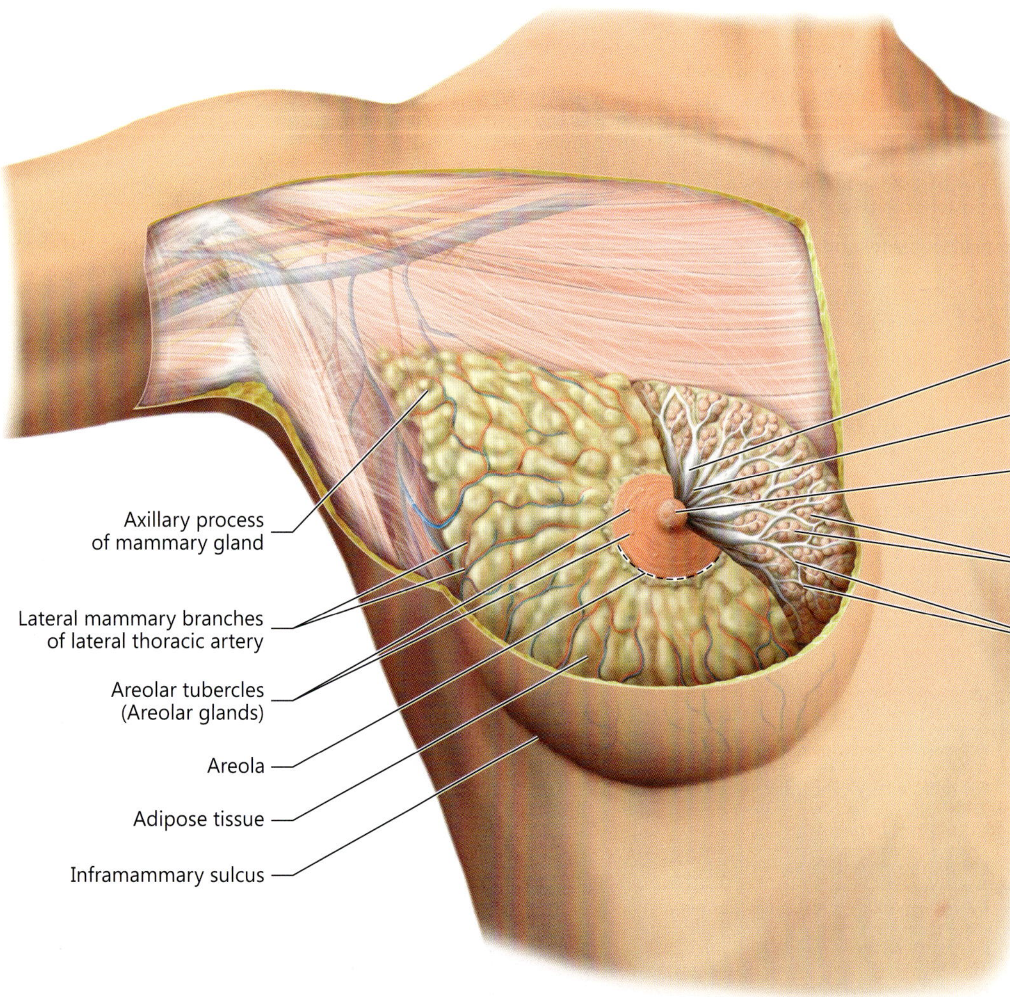

Representation of the **mammary gland** and of the investing layer of the pectoralis major. The medial part of the breast has been transected to show the lobular aspect of the gland, and the lactiferous sinuses and ducts. In the lateral part, one can see the abundant adipose tissue of the subcutaneous layer.

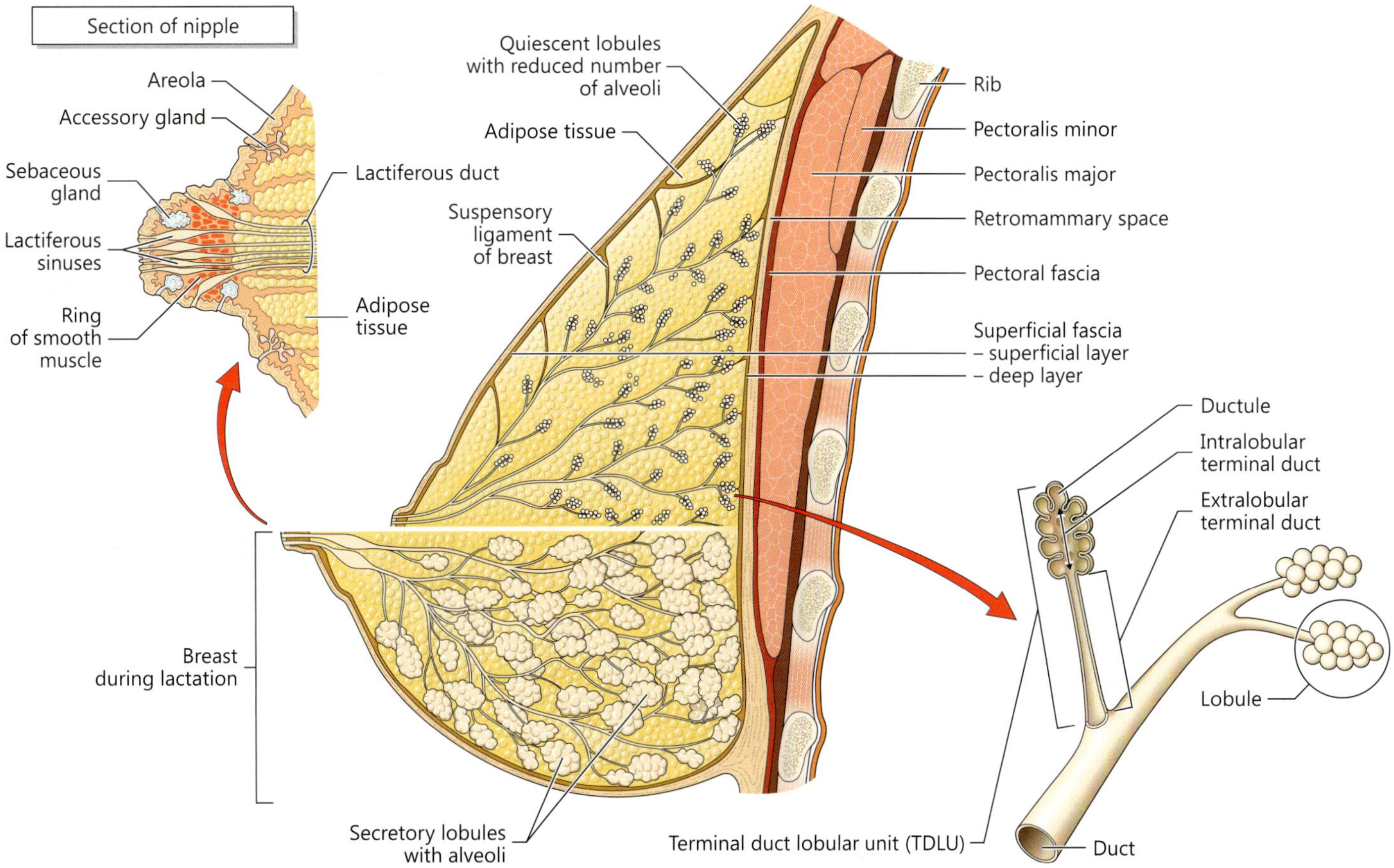

Schematic representation of a **sagittal section of the breast**. The upper part shows a breast in resting phase; the lower part a breast during lactation. The pectoral fascia splits into two layers, between which the mammary gland is located. The deep layer invests the muscle; the superficial layer extends in the subcutaneous layer and sends out fibrous septa which, extending into the thickness of the gland, constitute its stroma (Cooper's ligament or suspensory ligament of the breast). At the top, a close-up detail of a section of the nipple is presented, showing the lactiferous sinuses, the absence of adipose tissue and the presence of smooth muscle tissue. Below is shown the structure of the parenchyma of the gland during lactation: the interlobular ducts ramify into extralobular ducts which, terminating inside lobules, form the intralobular ducts. From these stem numerous ductules which drain the single alveoli of the gland.

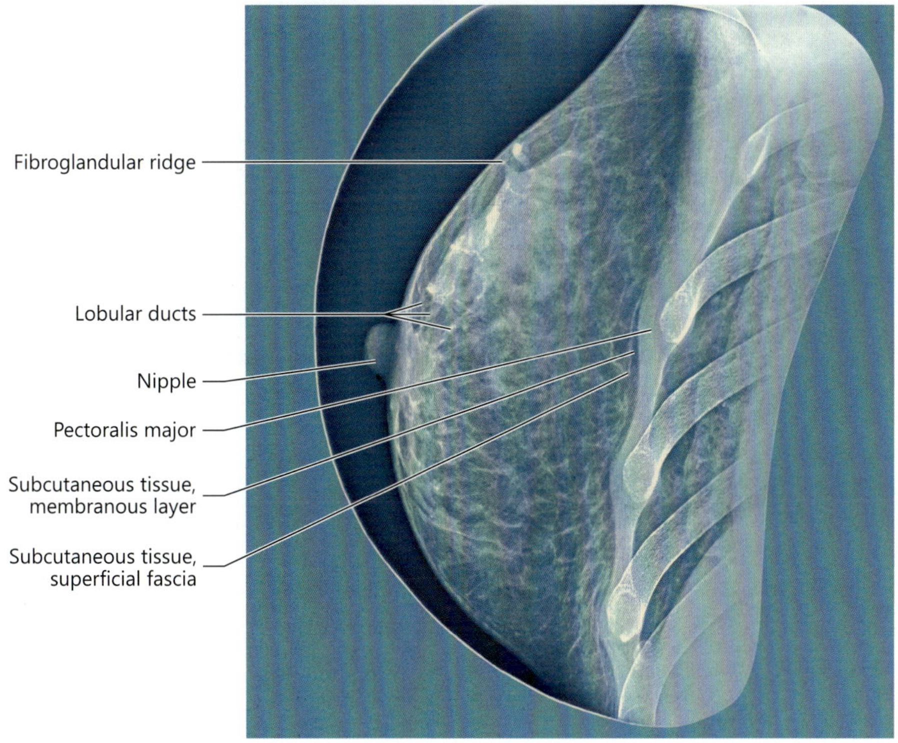

A **mammography** is a radiographic technique at low dosage that consents to visualize the connective tissue of the glandular stroma of the breast and of the lobular ducts. Alterations of this tissue can indicate the presence of neoplasias.

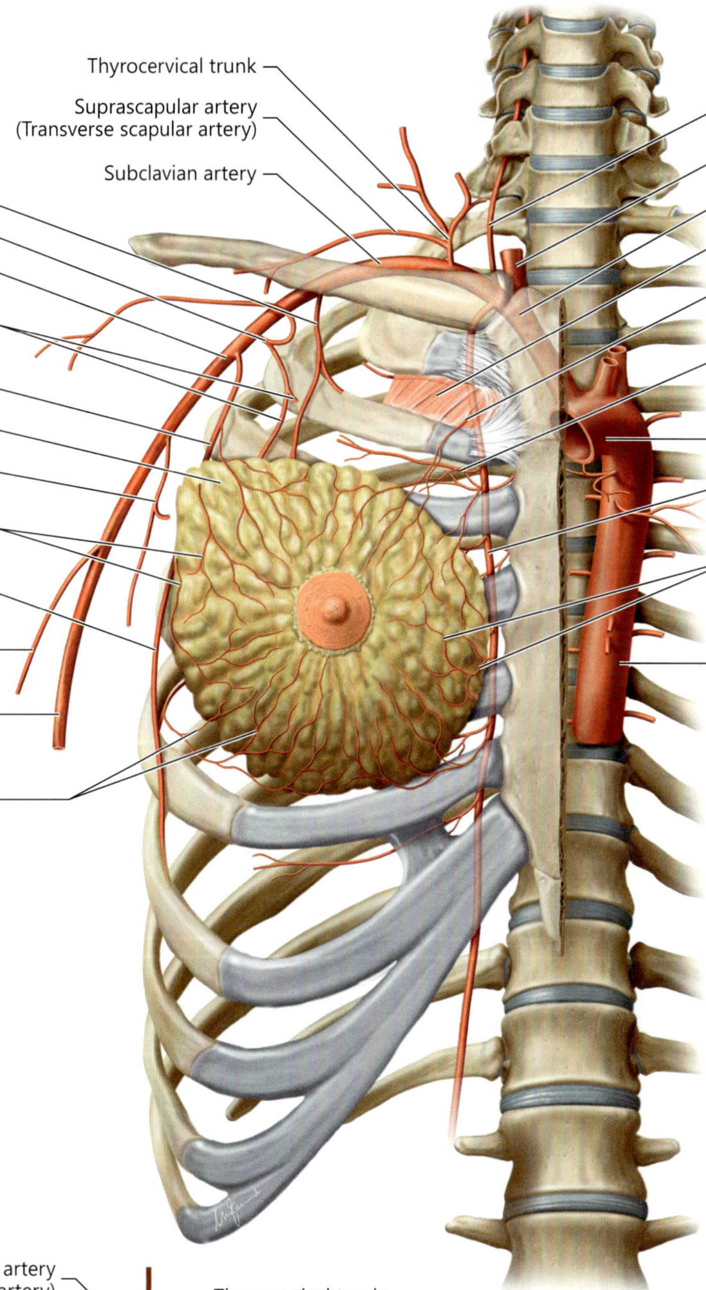

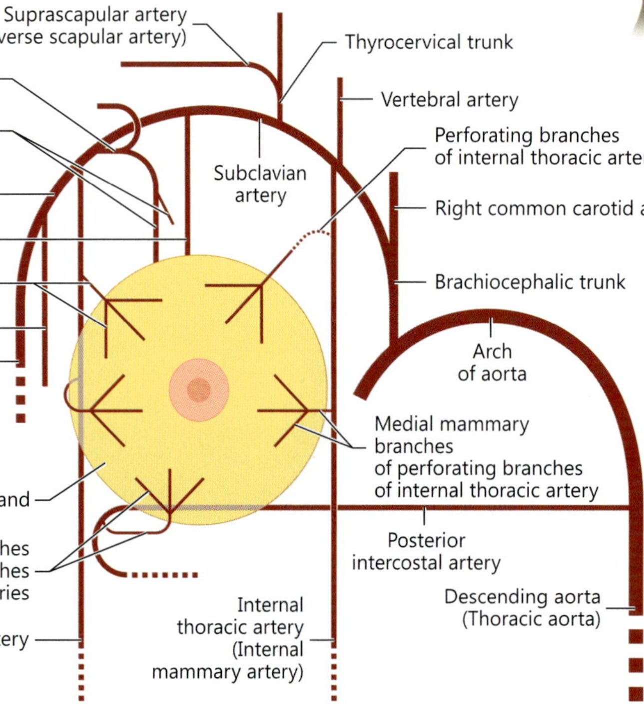

Arterial blood supply of the breast is carried out prevalently by branches of the subclavian artery (internal thoracic artery) and of the axillary artery (lateral thoracic artery). In lesser measure, also the posterior intercostal arteries (branches of the descending thoracic aorta) and the thoracoacromial artery (branch of the axillary artery) are involved.

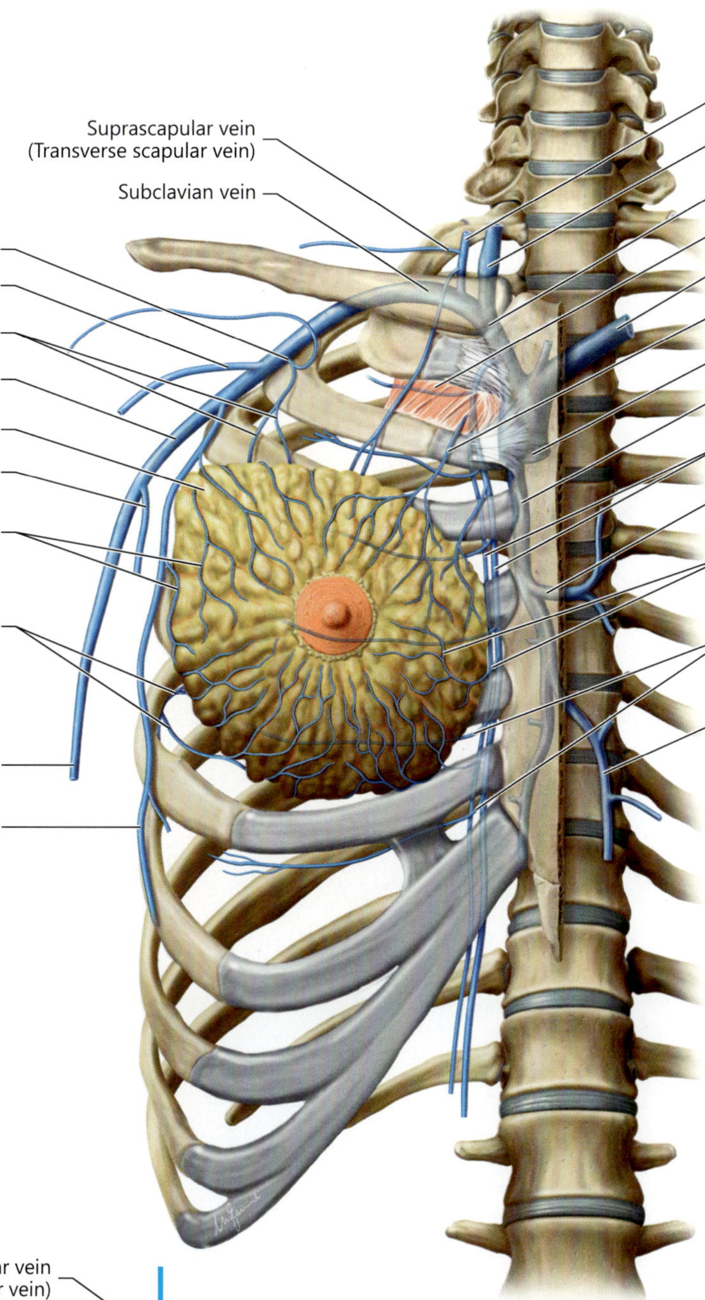

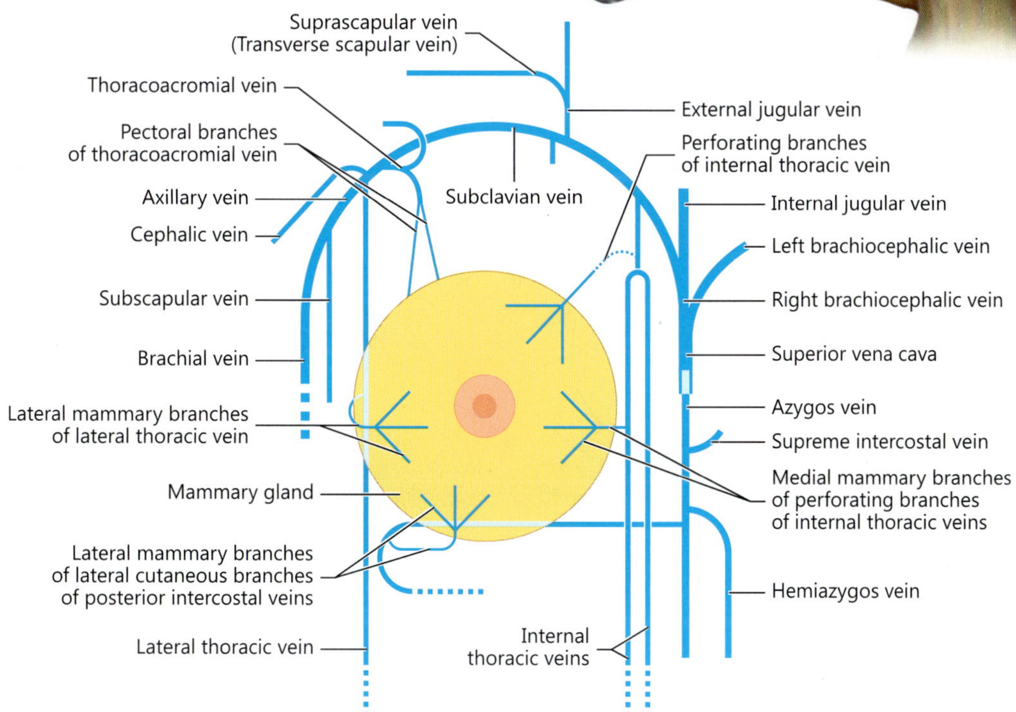

Venous drainage of the breast is carried out prevalently by satellite veins of the arteries involved in the breast.

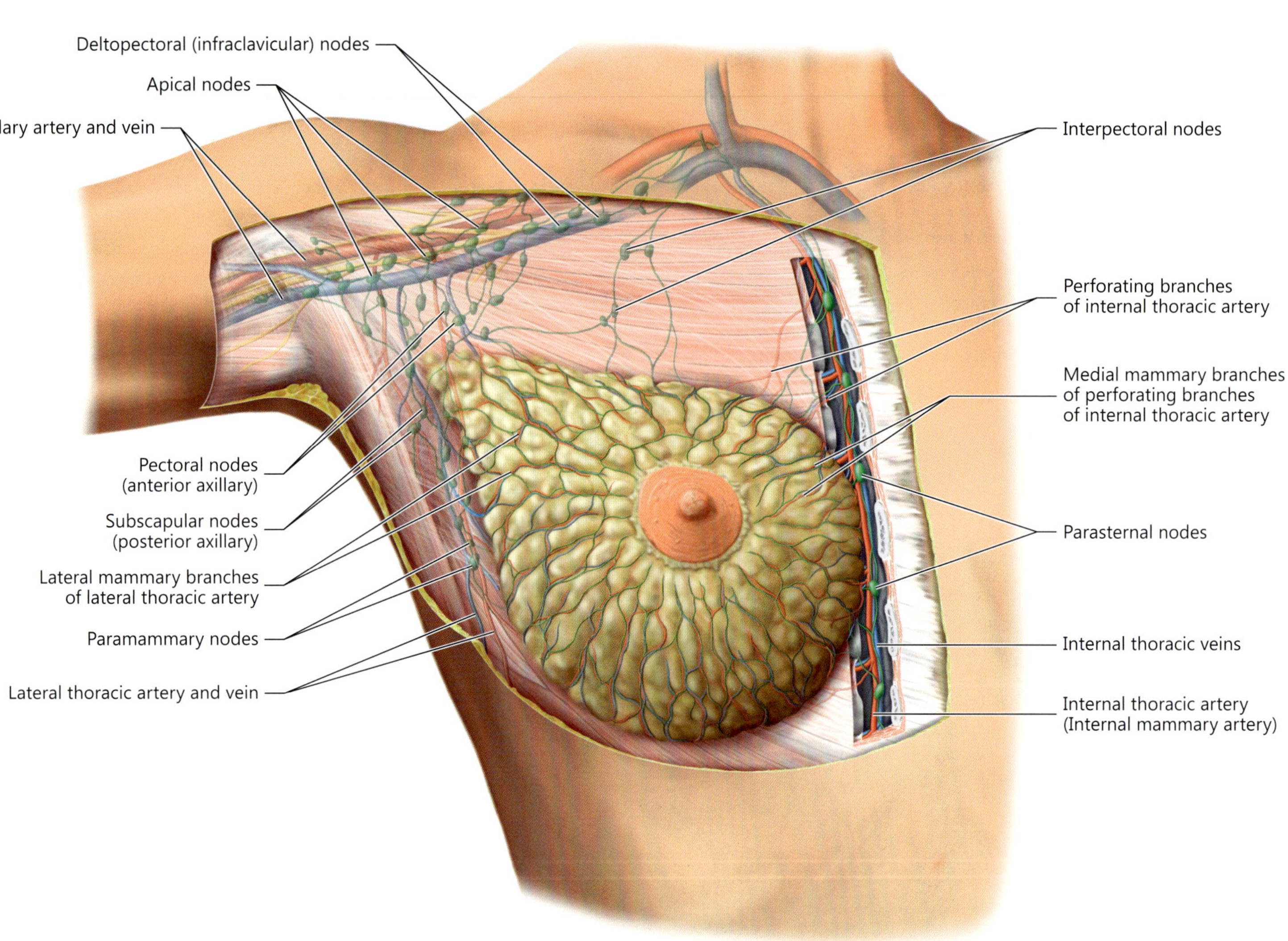

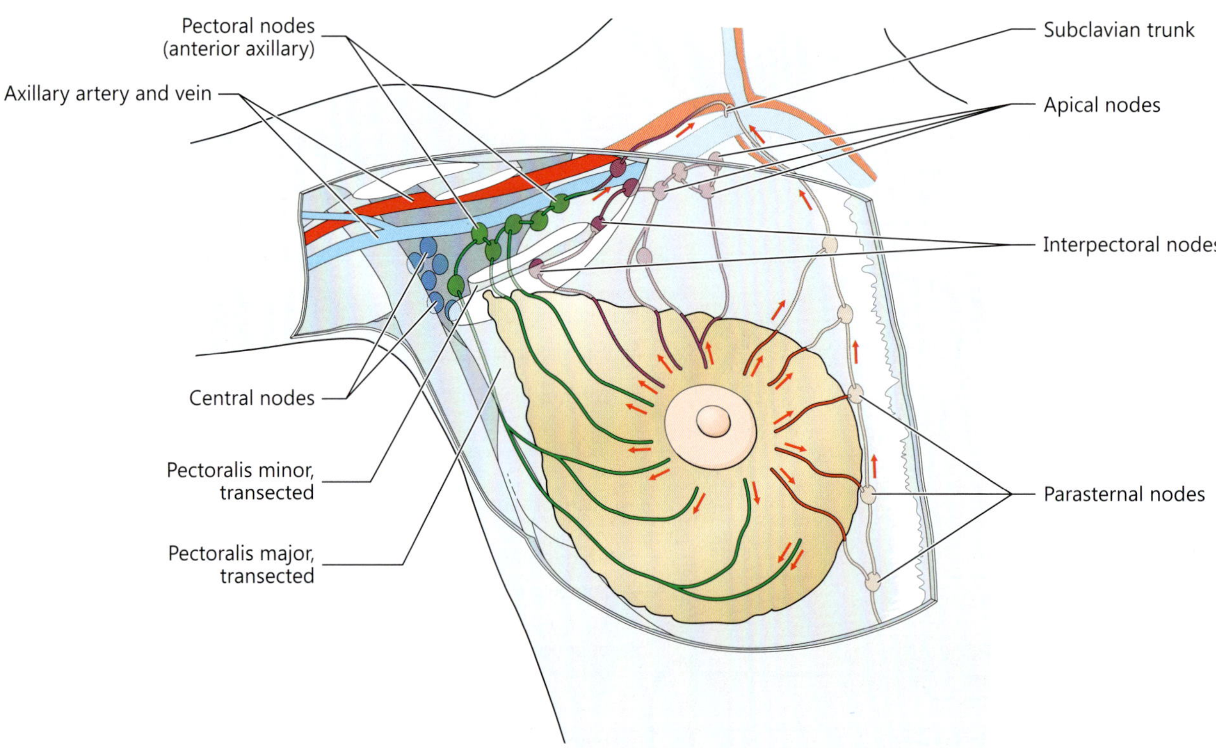

The **lymphatic drainage of the breast** follows the same path as that of the veins. Drainage of the lateral quadrants is carried out prevalently by the axillary lymphatic group. The superomedial quadrant is handled by the deltopectoral (infraclavicular) nodes of the axillary lymphatic group and by the parasternal nodes. The inferomedial quadrant is handled by the parasternal nodes.

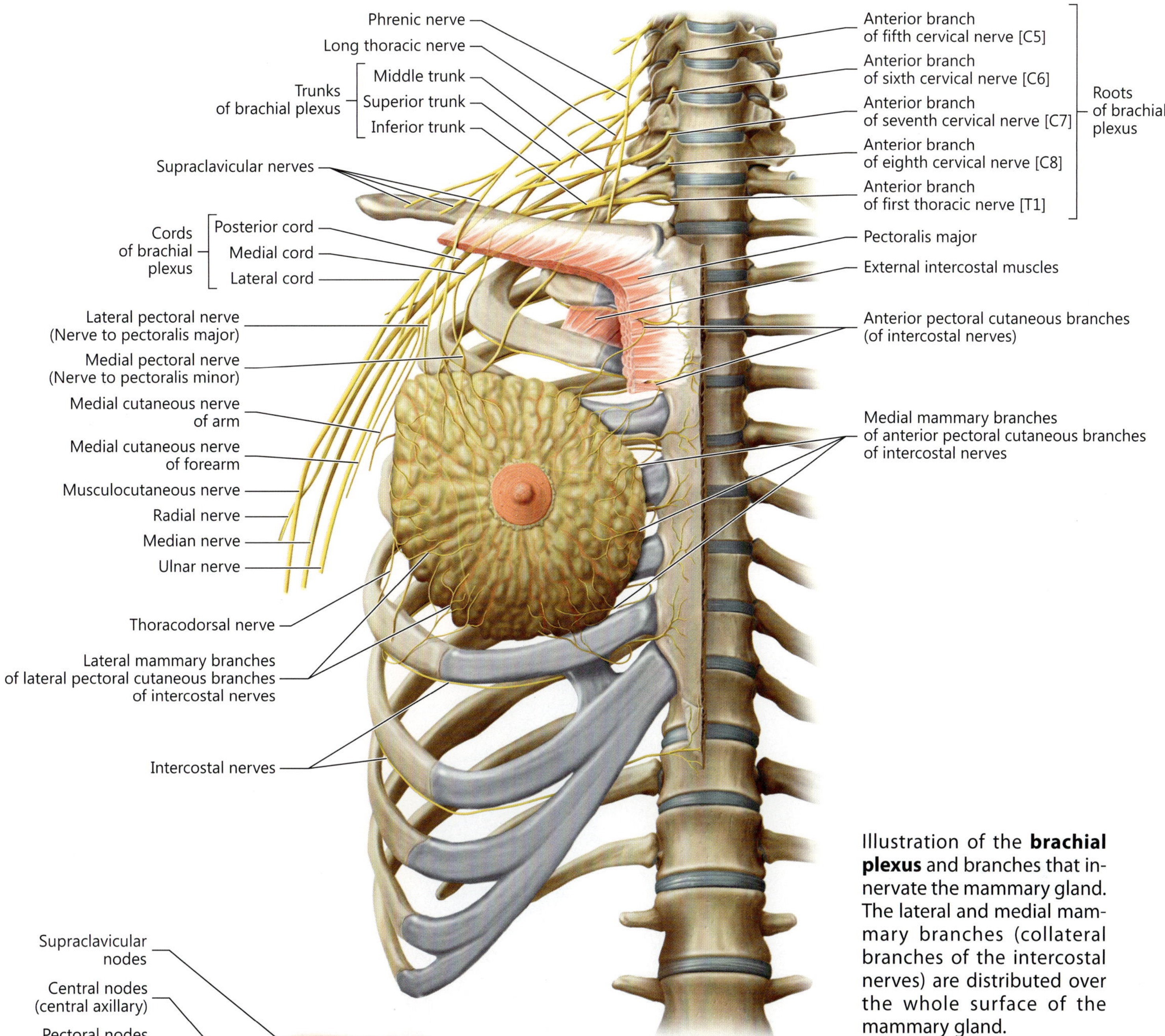

Illustration of the **brachial plexus** and branches that innervate the mammary gland. The lateral and medial mammary branches (collateral branches of the intercostal nerves) are distributed over the whole surface of the mammary gland.

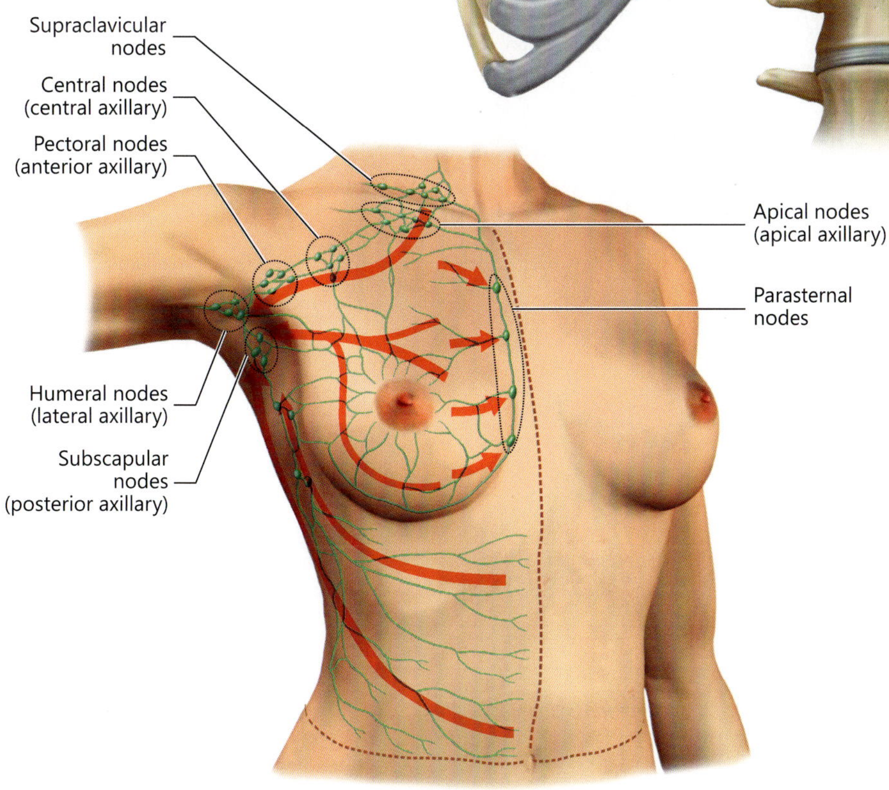

The physiologic **drainage of the breast** is essentially conducted in the direction of the axillary nodes and of the internal mammary lymphatic chain, situated at homolateral parasternal level. As an accessory channel, drainage can also be directed towards the homolateral supraclavicular nodes.

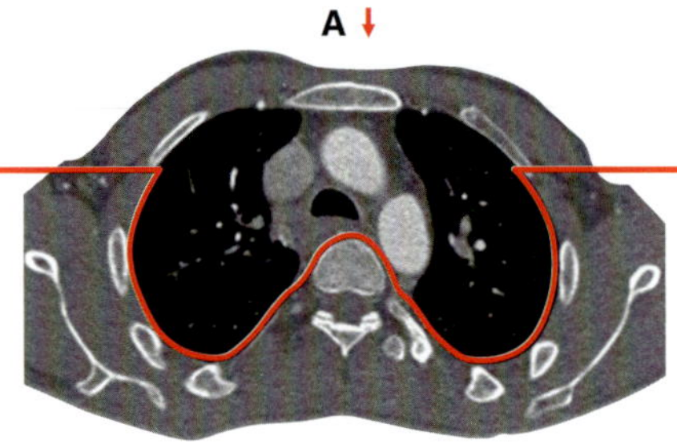

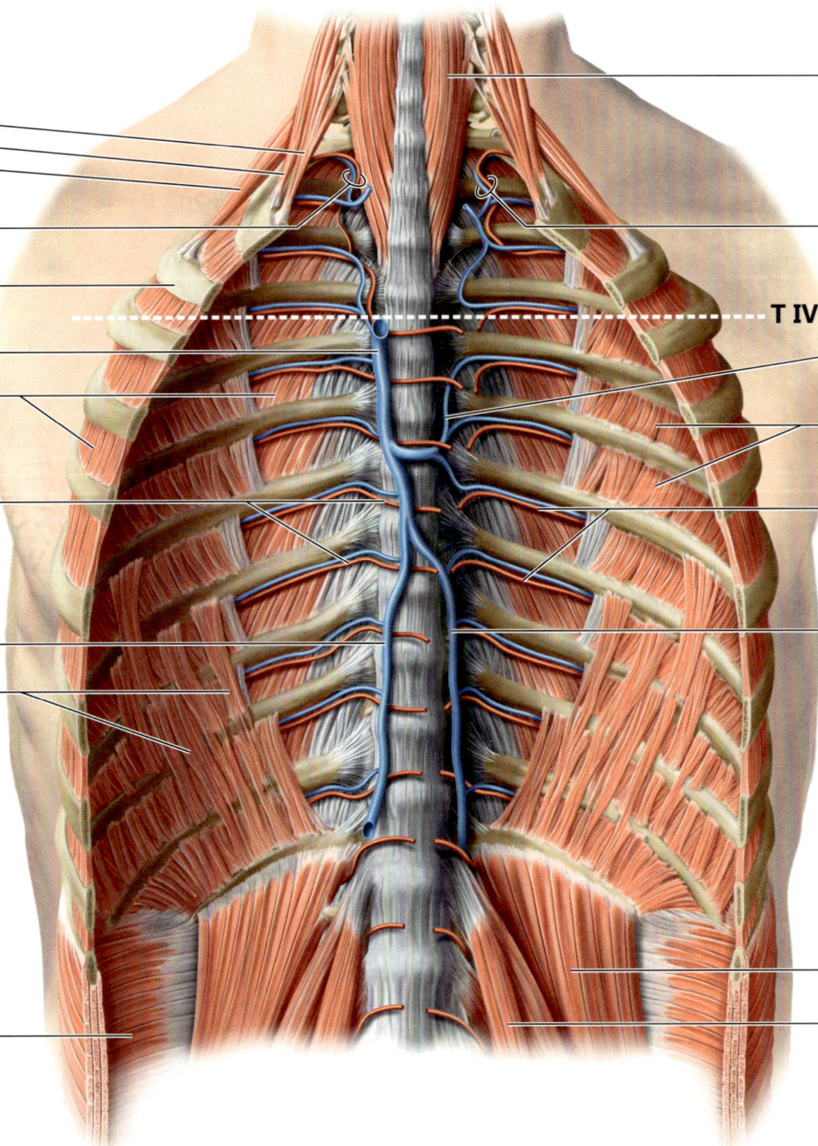

CONTENTS OF THE THORAX (in bold are the structures added to the posterior wall)

- Accessory hemiazygos vein
- Azygos vein, on the right
- Hemiazygos vein
- Insertions of medial and lateral inferior parts of longi colli, T I-T III (right and left)
- Posterior intercostal arteries from 4th to 12th (the right arteries pass in front of the vertebral column)
- Supreme intercostal arteries (right and left) (1st, 2nd and 3rd posterior intercostal arteries)
- Supreme intercostal veins (right and left) (intercostal veins from 1st to 2nd)

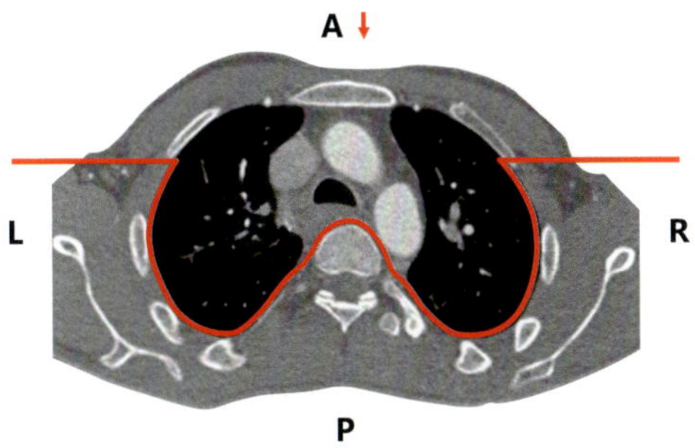

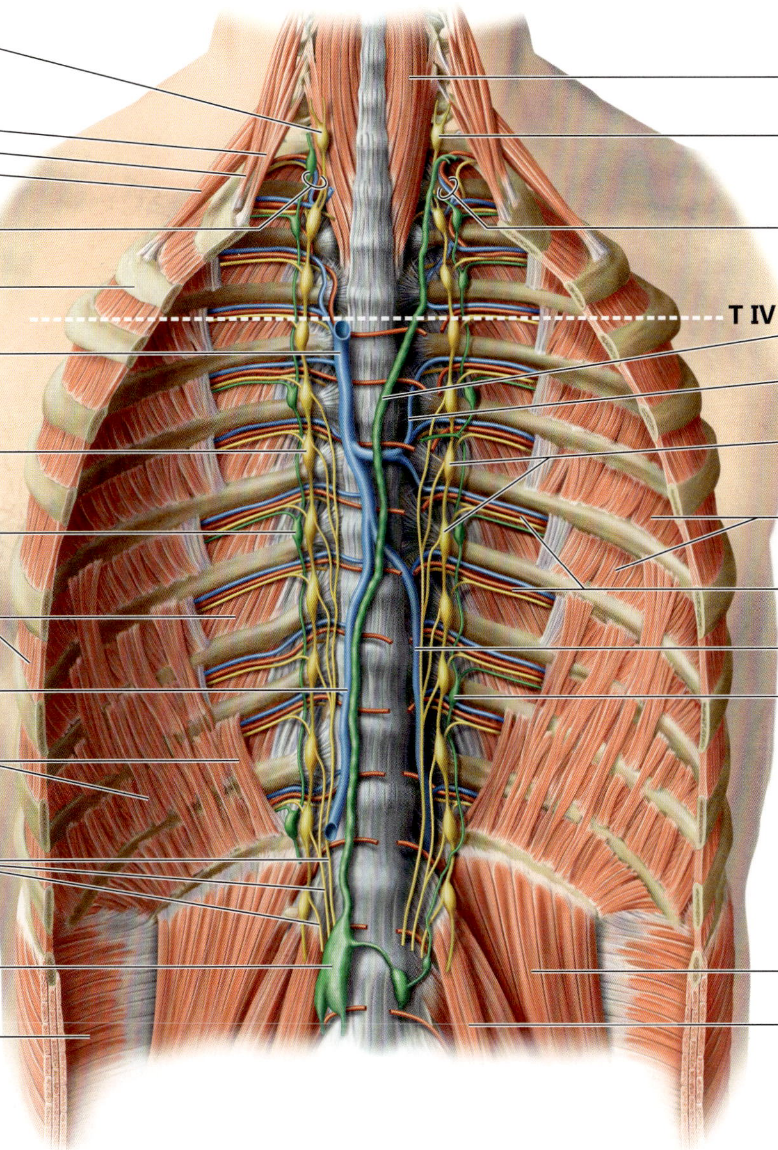

CONTENTS OF THE THORAX (in bold are the structures added with respect to the preceding table)
• Cervicothoracic (stellate) ganglion (right and left) • Greater, lesser and least splanchnic nerves (right and left) • Left intercostal nerves • Posterior intercostal nodes (right and left) • Thoracic duct • Thoracic ganglia of sympathetic trunk (right and left)

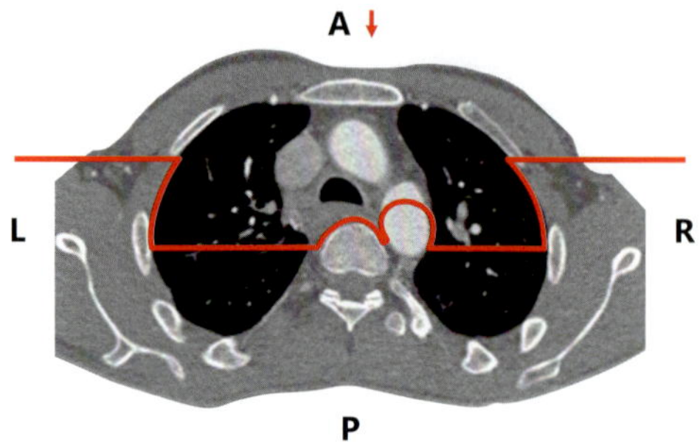

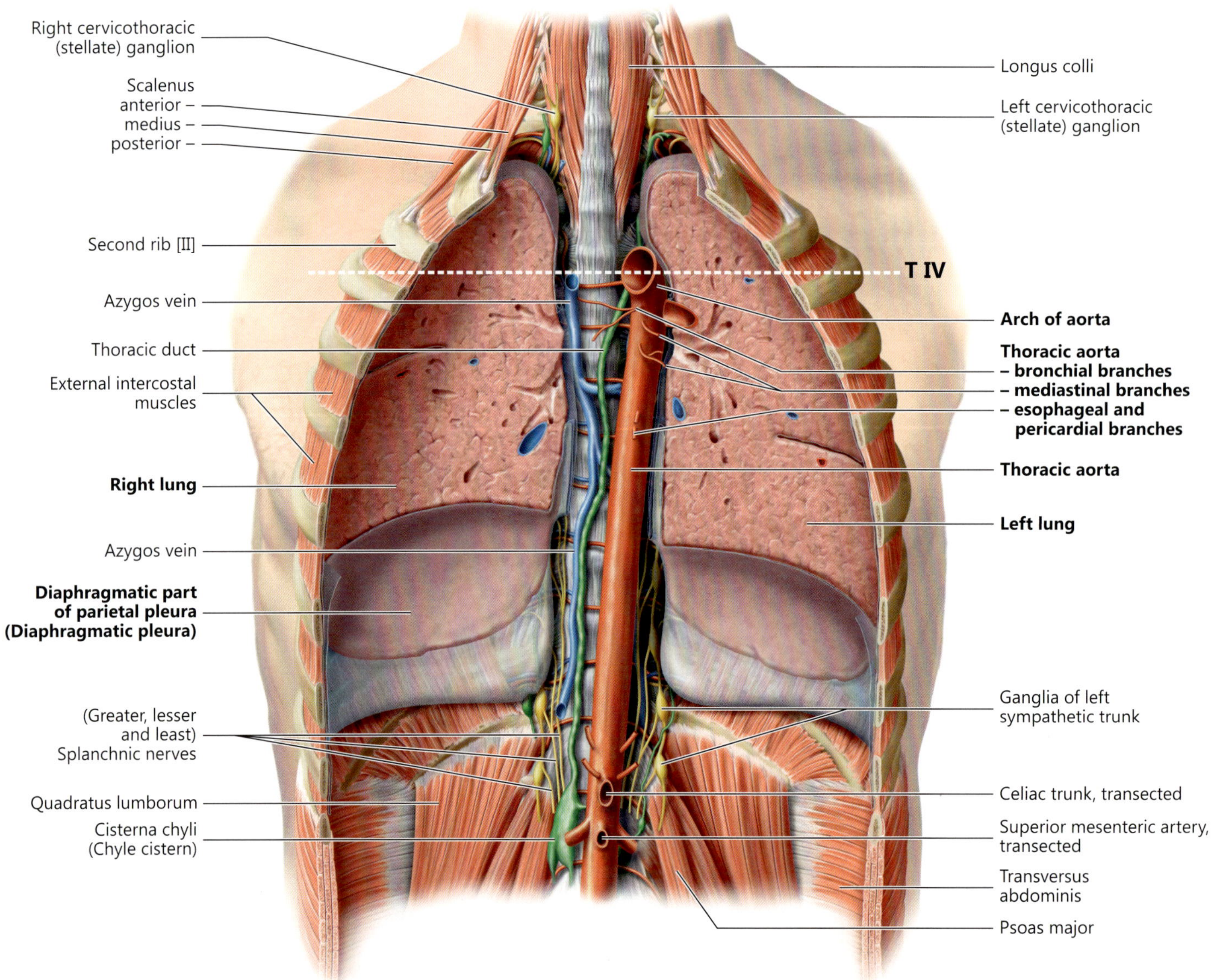

CONTENTS OF THE THORAX (in bold are the structures added with respect to the preceding table)
• Diaphragmatic pleura • Lungs (right and left) • Posterior third of arch of aorta • Thoracic aorta and its collateral branches (bronchial, mediastinal, esophageal and pericardial)

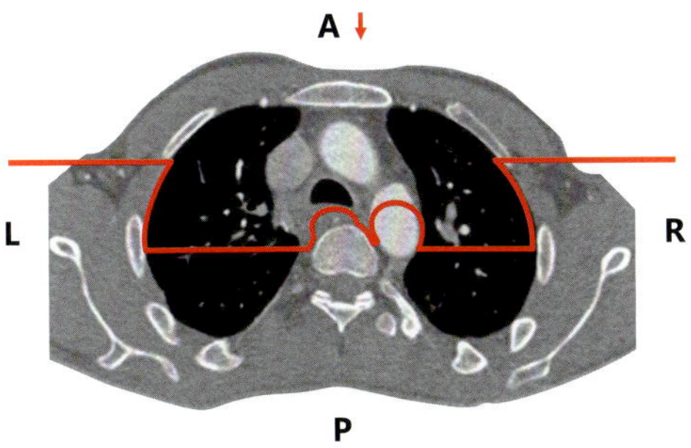

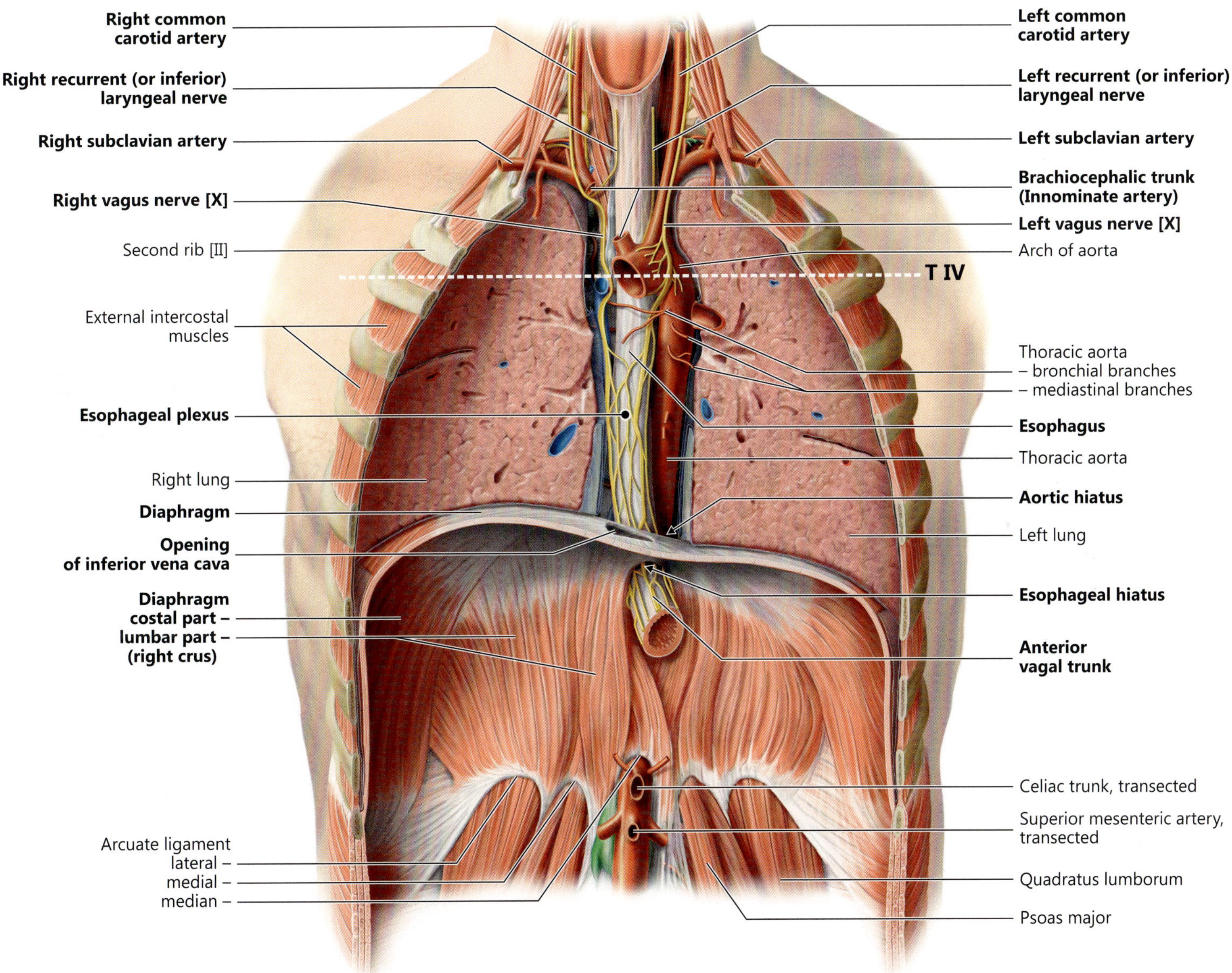

CONTENTS OF THE THORAX (in bold are the structures added with respect to the preceding table)
• Anterior vagal trunk • Branches of arch of aorta (left and right subclavian arteries, left and right common carotid arteries, brachiocephalic trunk) • Central tendon of diaphragm (opening of inferior vena cava, aortic hiatus, esophageal hiatus) • Diaphragm (costal and lumbar parts) • Esophageal plexus • Esophagus • Recurrent laryngeal nerves (inferior laryngeal nerves) (right and left) • Vagus nerves (right and left)

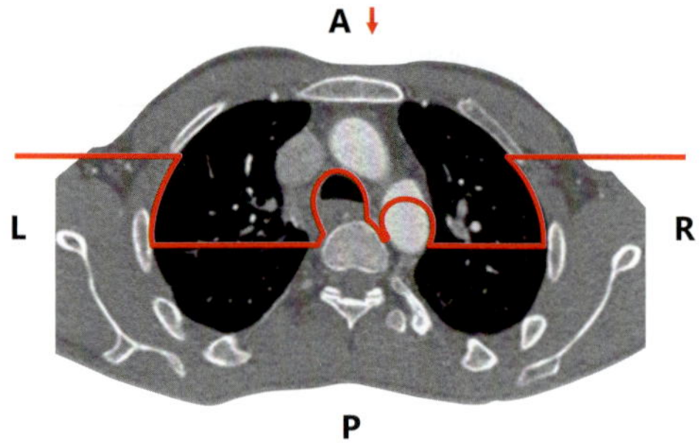

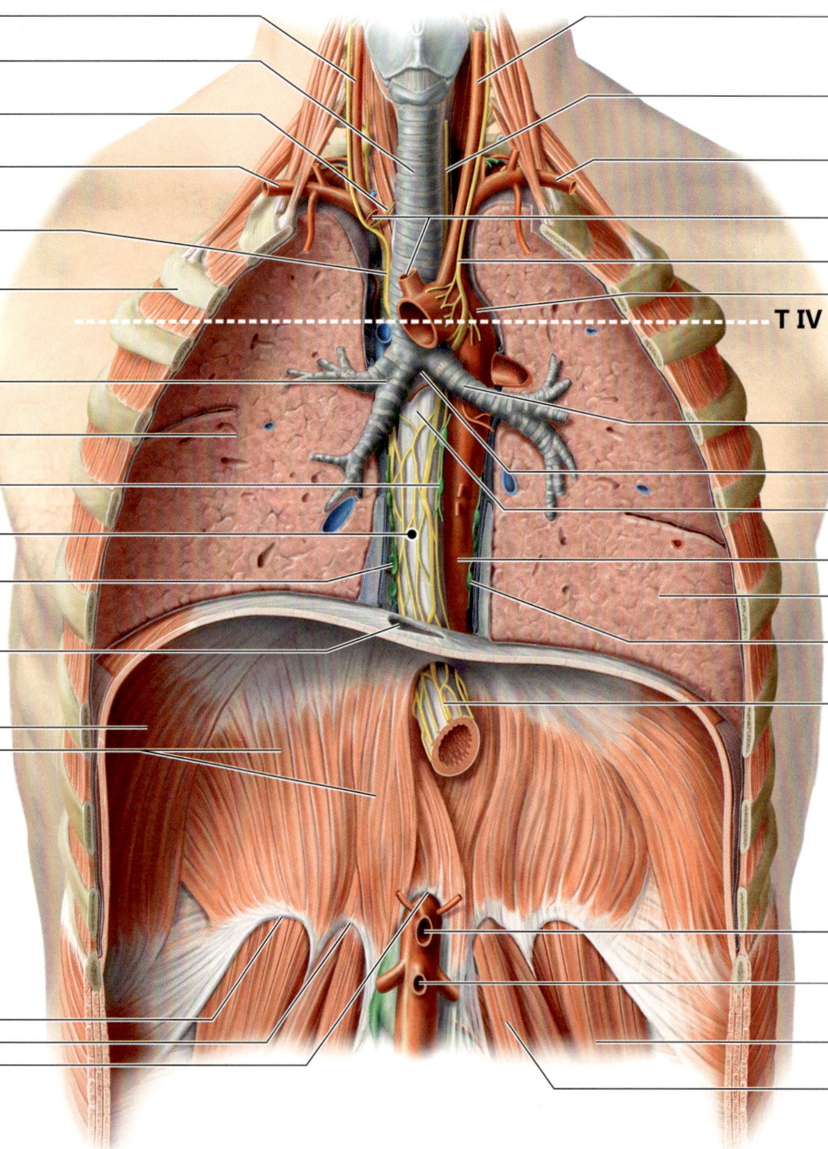

***CONTENTS OF THE THORAX** (in bold are the structures added with respect to the preceding table)*
• Main bronchi (right and left) • Posterior mediastinal nodes (juxtaesophageal, juxta-aortic, interaorticoesophageal) • Trachea • Tracheal bifurcation

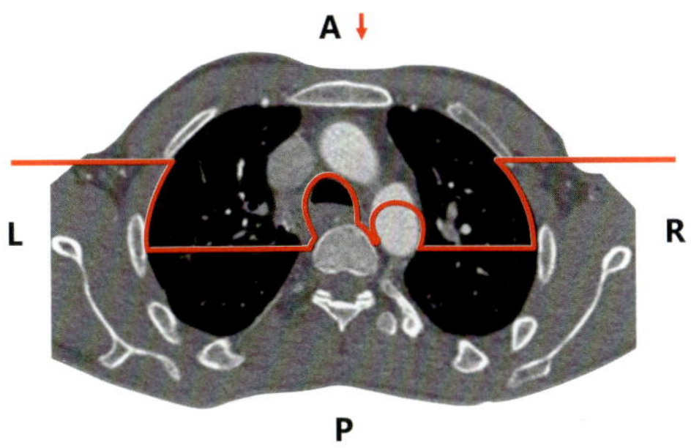

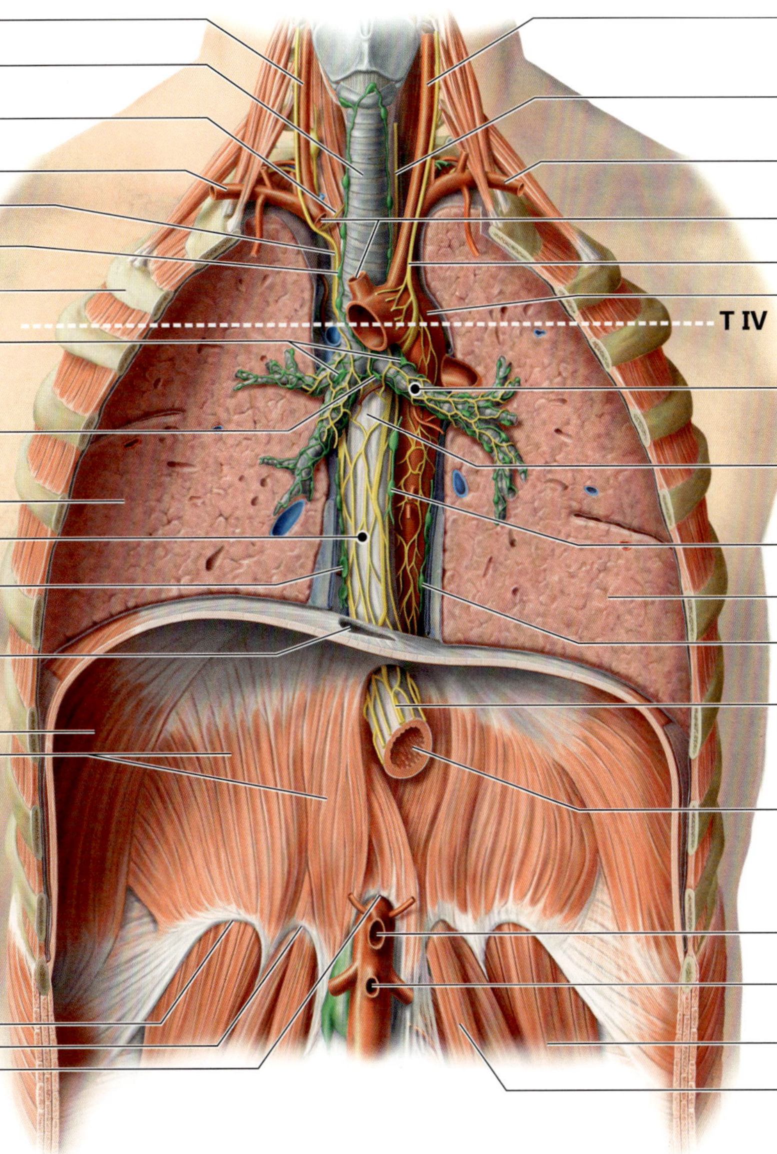

CONTENTS OF THE THORAX (in bold are the structures added with respect to the preceding table)
• Paratracheal nodes (right and left) • Pulmonary plexus • Superior and inferior tracheobronchial nodes

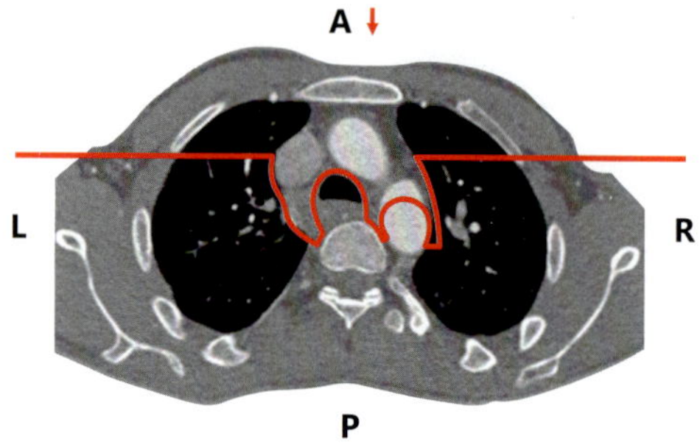

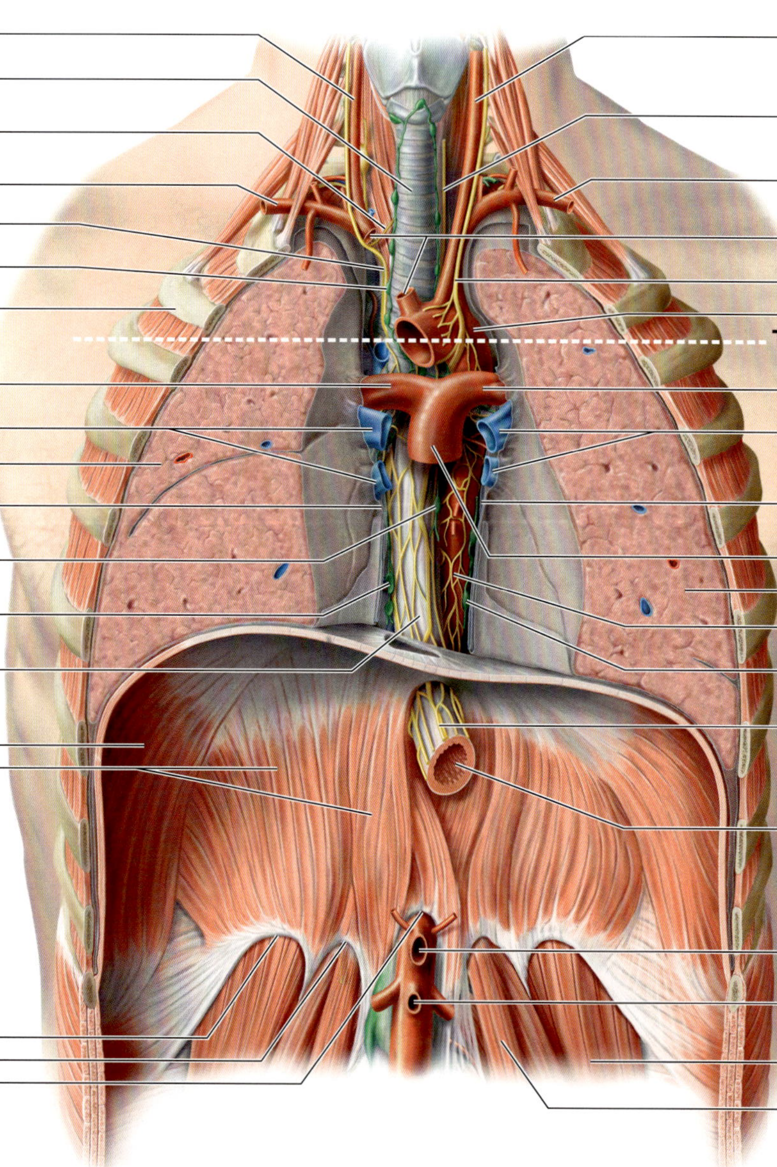

CONTENTS OF THE THORAX (in bold are the structures added with respect to the preceding table)
• Pulmonary arteries (right and left) • Pulmonary (triangular) ligaments (right and left) • Pulmonary trunk • Superior and inferior pulmonary veins (right and left)

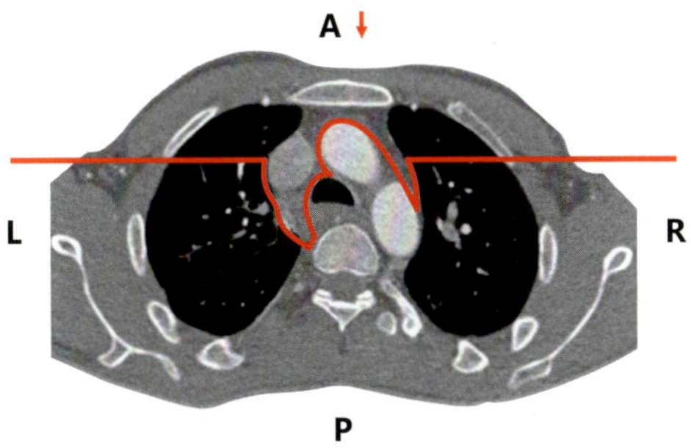

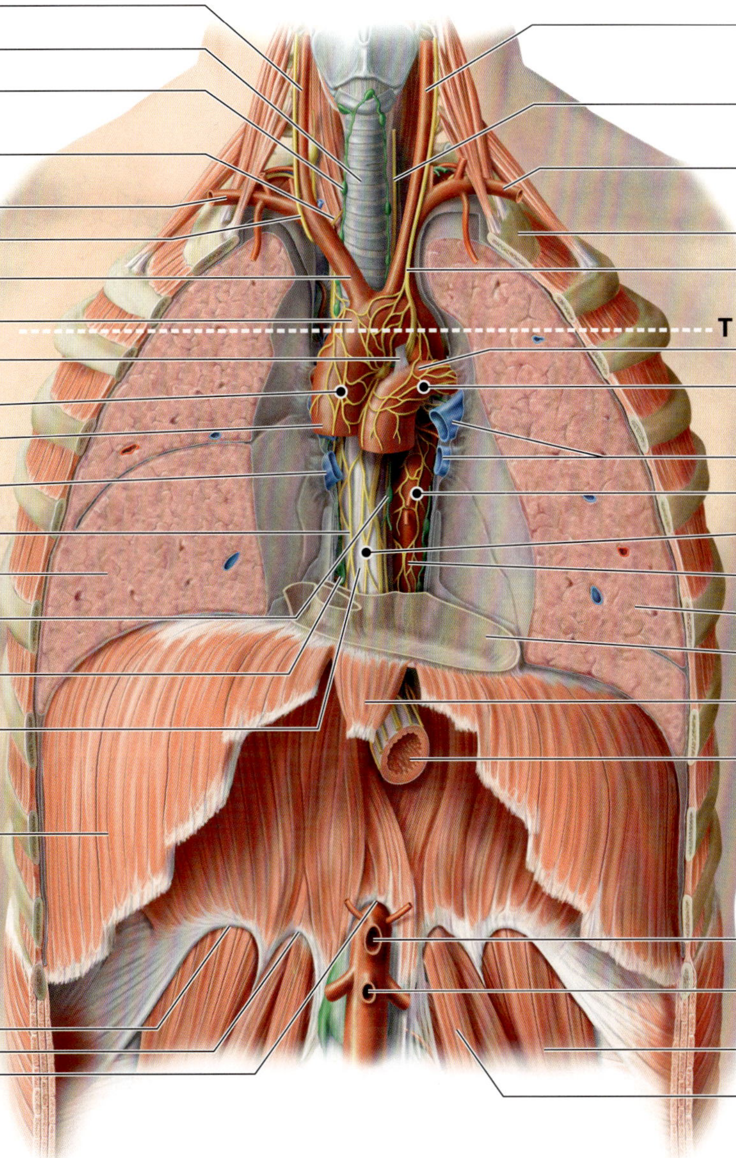

CONTENTS OF THE THORAX (in bold are the structures added with respect to the preceding table)

- Anterior vagal trunk
- Ascending aorta
- Cardiac plexus
- Esophageal plexus
- Ligamentum arteriosum (ligamentum of Botallo)
- Pericardium (diaphragmatic surface)
- Pulmonary plexus
- Thoracic aortic plexus

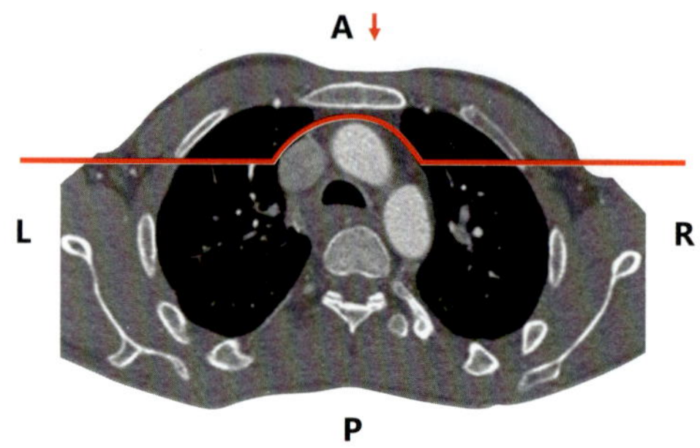

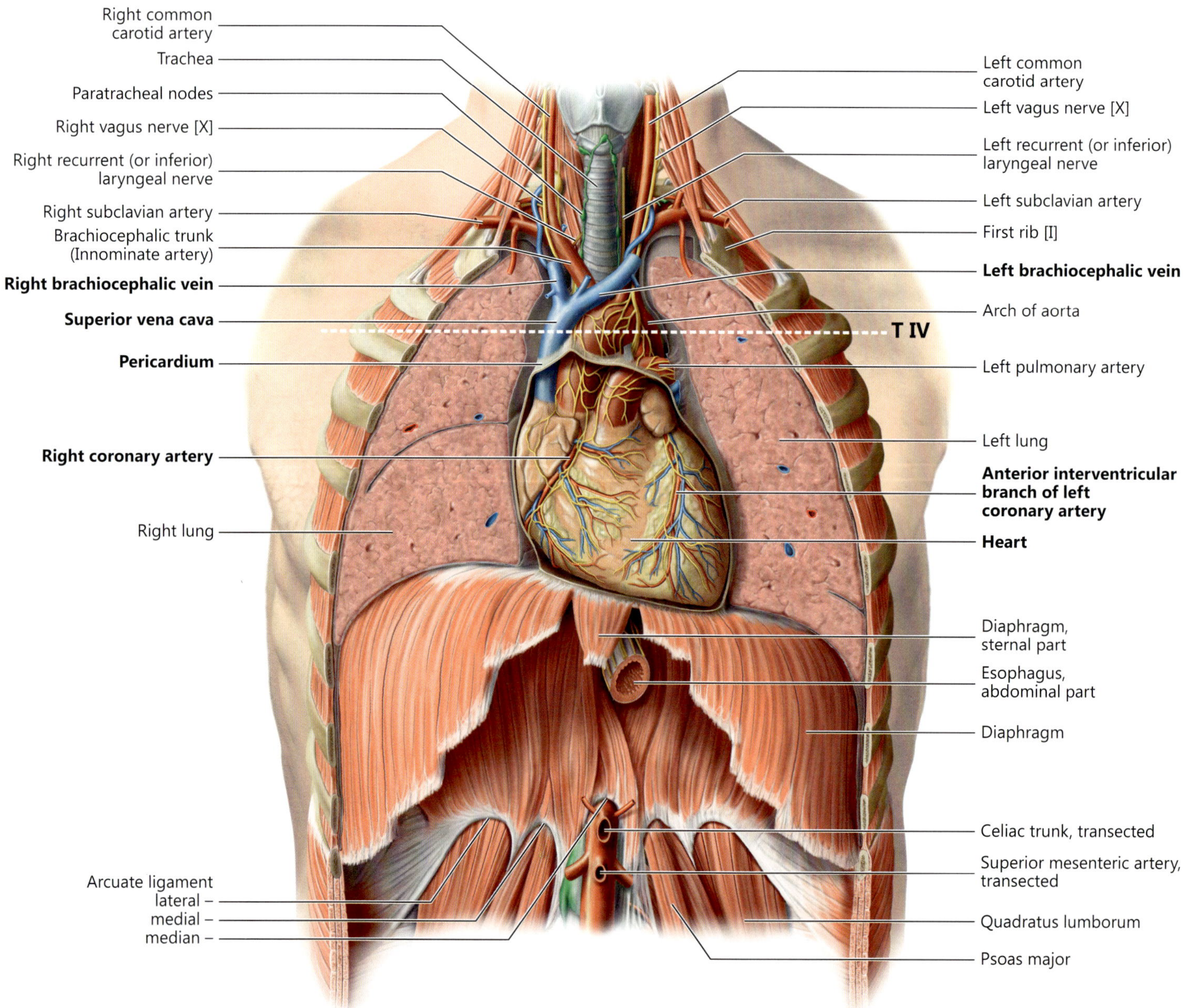

CONTENTS OF THE THORAX (in bold are the structures added with respect to the preceding table)
• Brachiocephalic veins (right and left) • Heart • Left coronary artery, anterior interventricular branch • Pericardium • Right coronary artery • Superior vena cava

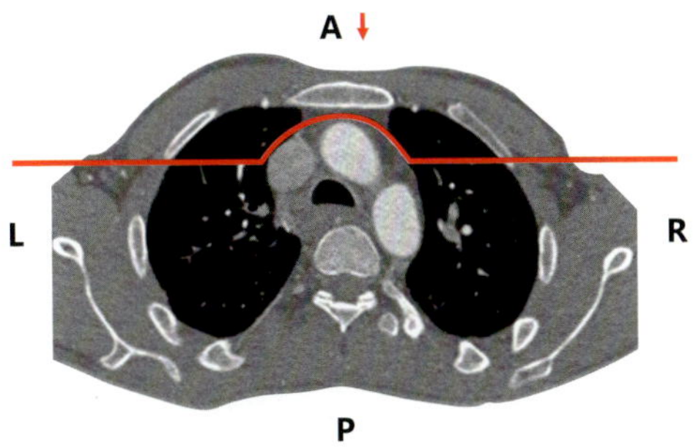

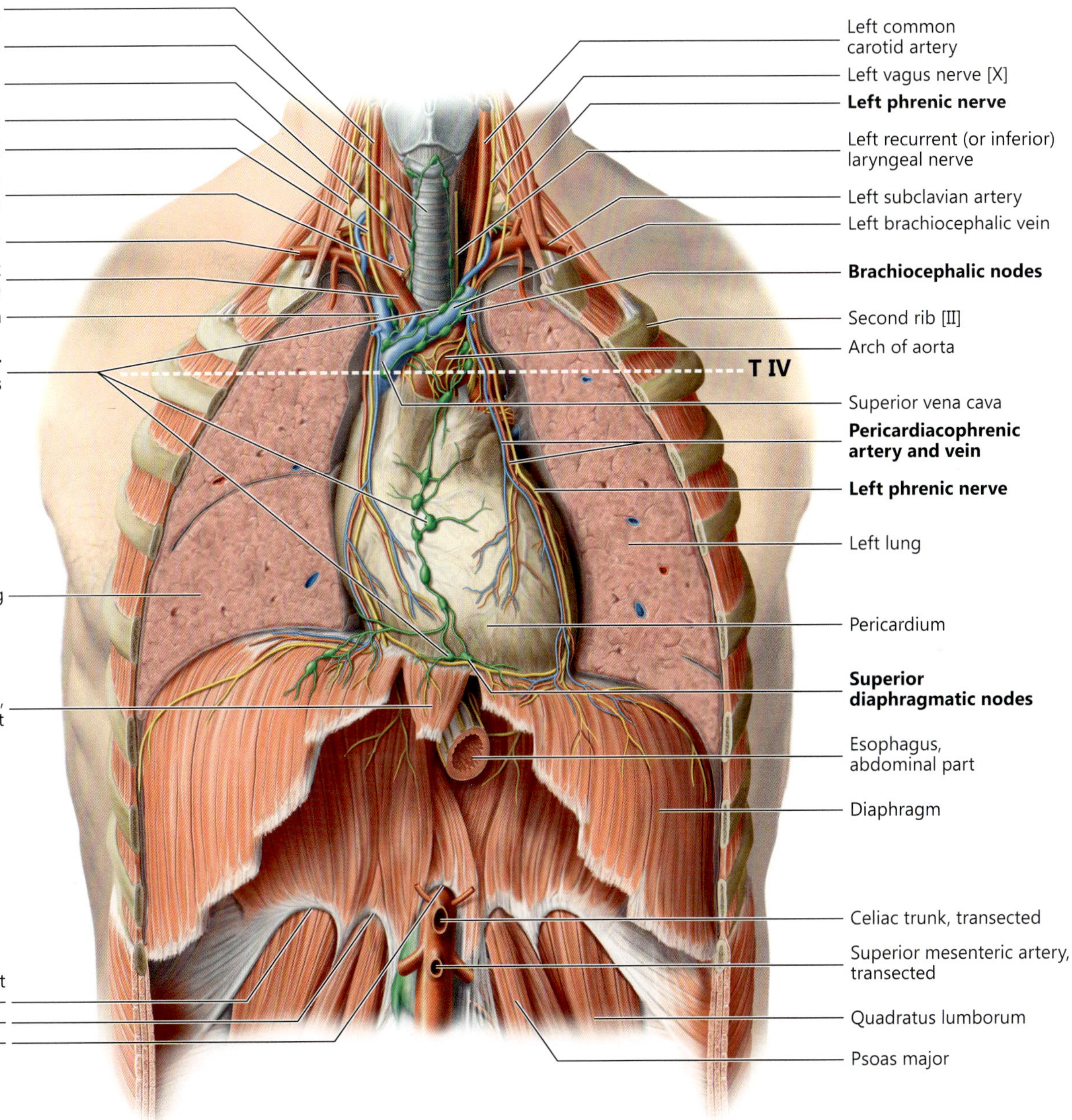

***CONTENTS OF THE THORAX** (in bold are the structures added with respect to the preceding table)*
• Brachiocephalic nodes • Middle and anterior mediastinal nodes • Pericardiacophrenic arteries and veins (right and left) • Phrenic nerves (right and left) • Superior diaphragmatic nodes

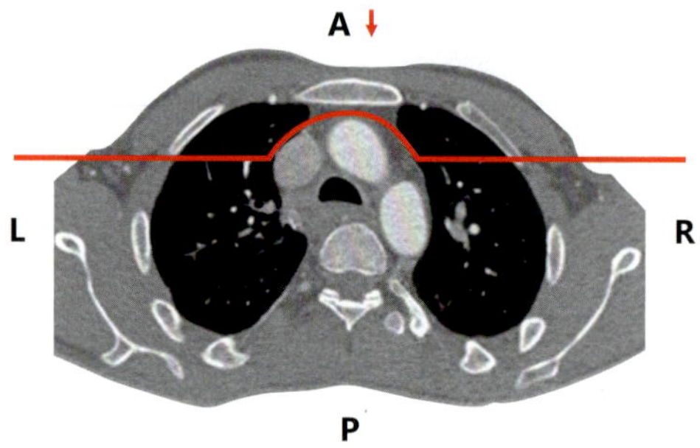

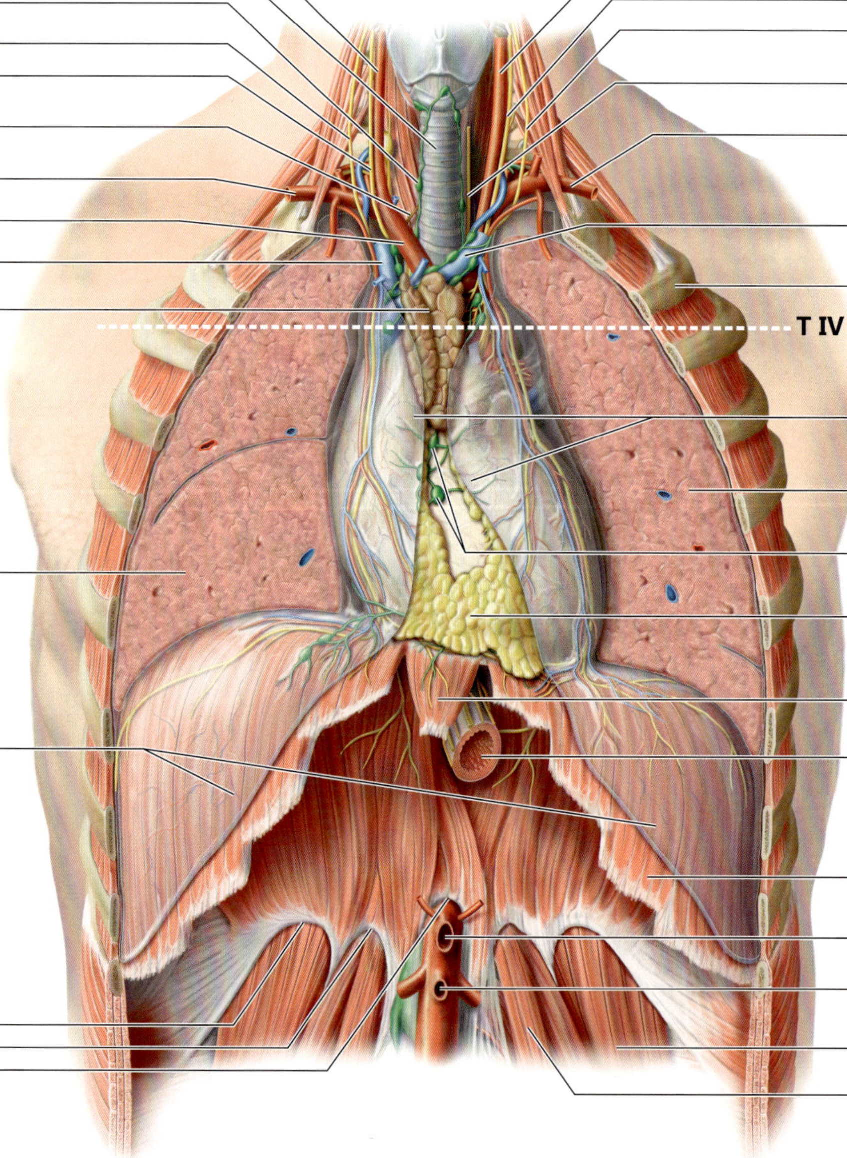

CONTENTS OF THE THORAX (in bold are the structures added with respect to the preceding table)
• Costodiaphragmatic recesses • Costomediastinal recesses • Retrosternal fat pad • Thymus or residual thymic tissue and fibroadipose tissue

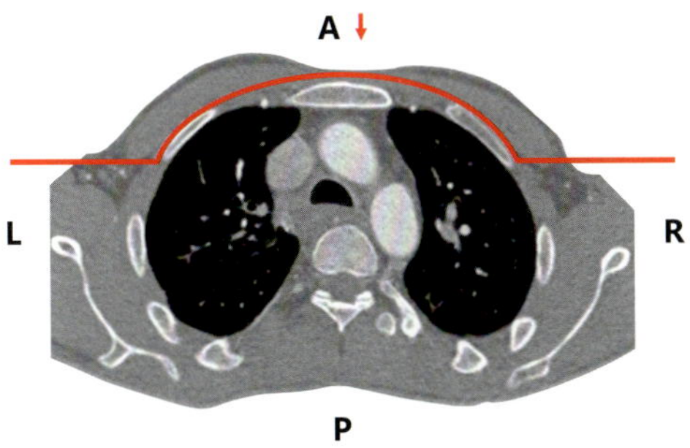

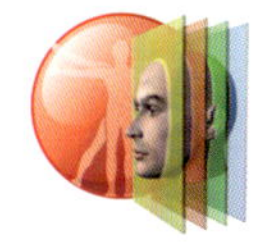

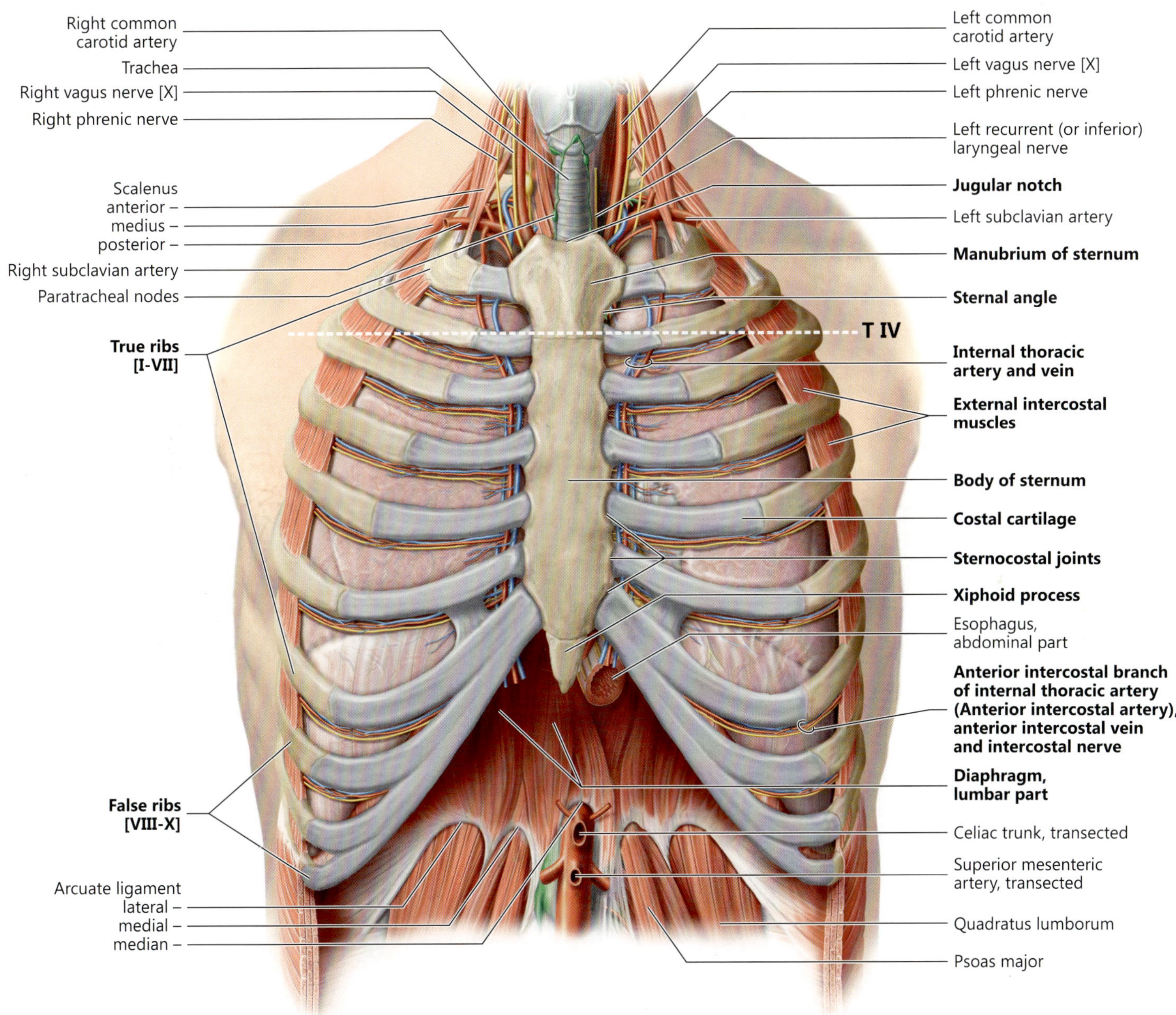

***CONTENTS OF THE THORAX** (in bold are the structures added with respect to the preceding table)*	
• Anterior intercostal arteries	• Intercostal nerves
• Anterior intercostal branches of internal thoracic artery	• Internal thoracic arteries
• Anterior intercostal veins	• Internal thoracic veins
• Costal cartilage	• Ribs
• Diaphragm (lumbar part)	• Sternocostal joints
• External intercostal muscles	• Sternum

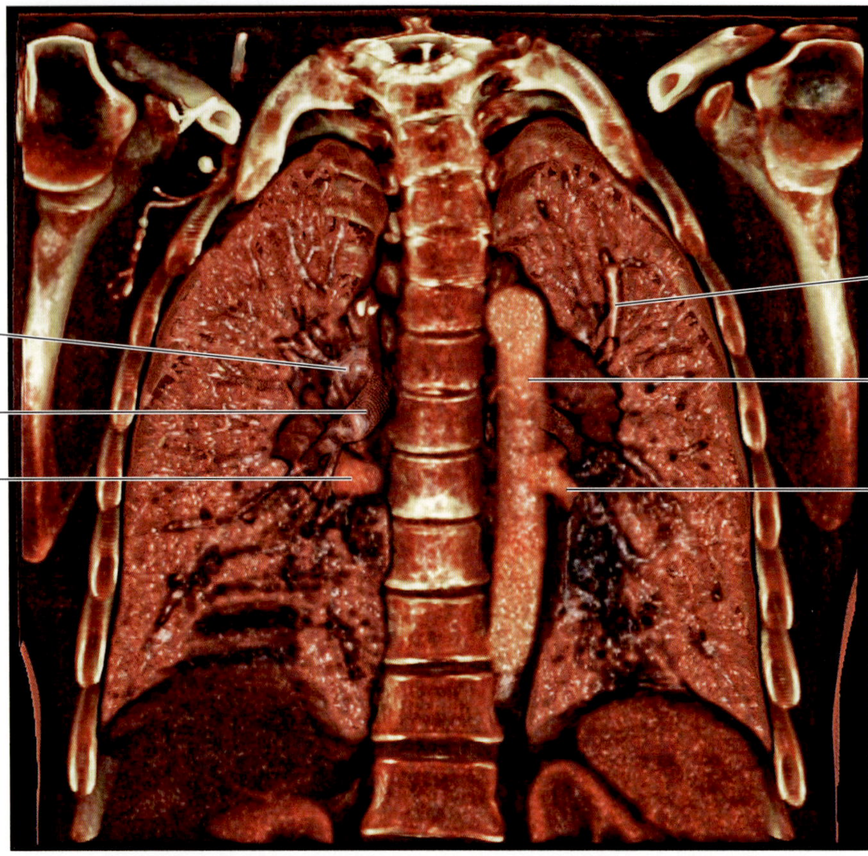

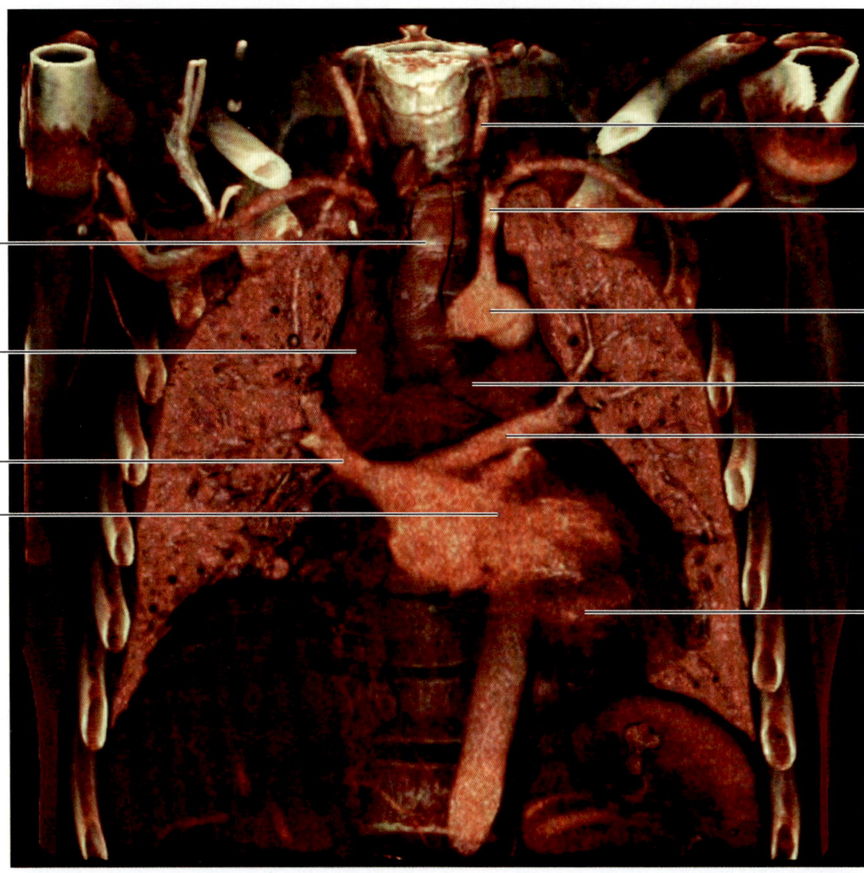

Series of four three-dimensional images of a living human body, obtained from frontal sections in dorso-ventral direction by CT scan using a 3D volume rendering technique. View from in front. The sequence starts with a section at the level of the vertebral bodies. To the left of the vertebral column, one can see the **descending aorta** (**thoracic aorta**) from its origin at T IV level to the point at which it moves in front of the column (transected). Superimposed on the aorta one can see a portion of the left **pulmonary veins**. In the successive image, one can see the left **atrium** and, above it, part of the **arch of the aorta** and its left branches.

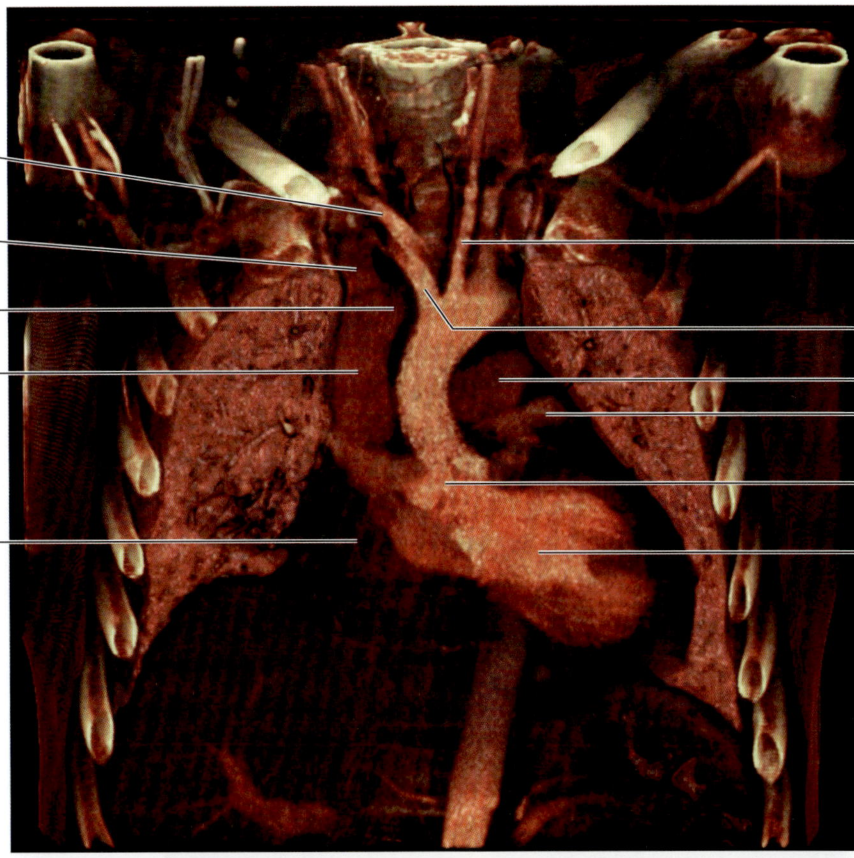

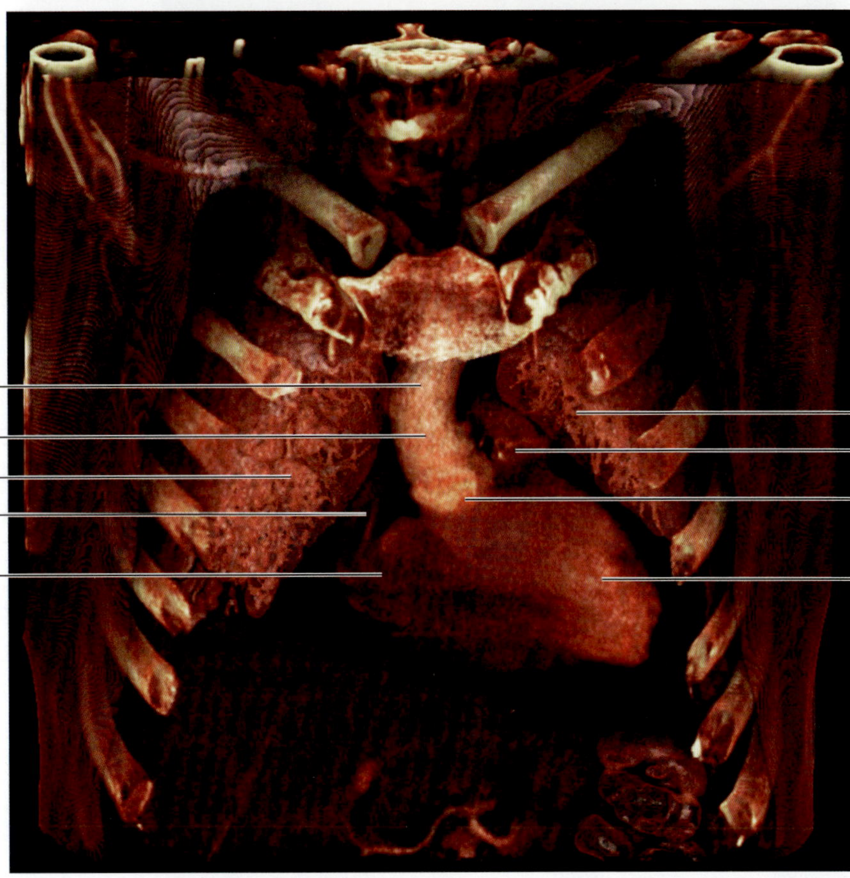

Following in sequence from the previous image, the section at the top shows the left **ventricle**, the **arch of the aorta** and its branches. The arch passes over the left pulmonary veins. To the right of the ascending aorta, one can see the superior vena cava. Note the aortic semilunar cusps.
In the section below, the lungs partially envelop the heart.

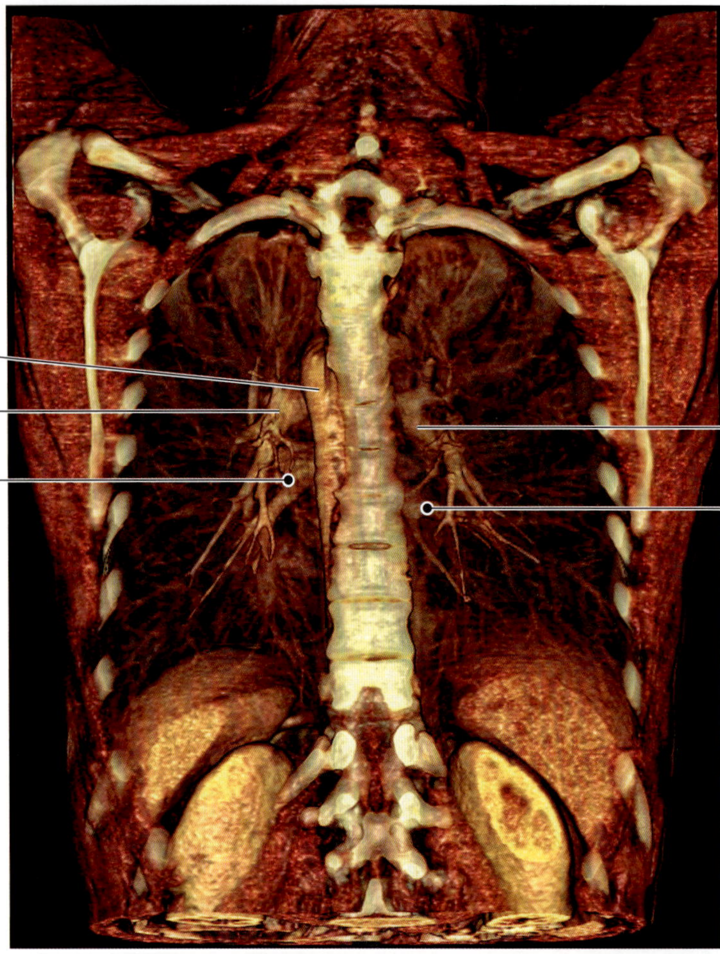

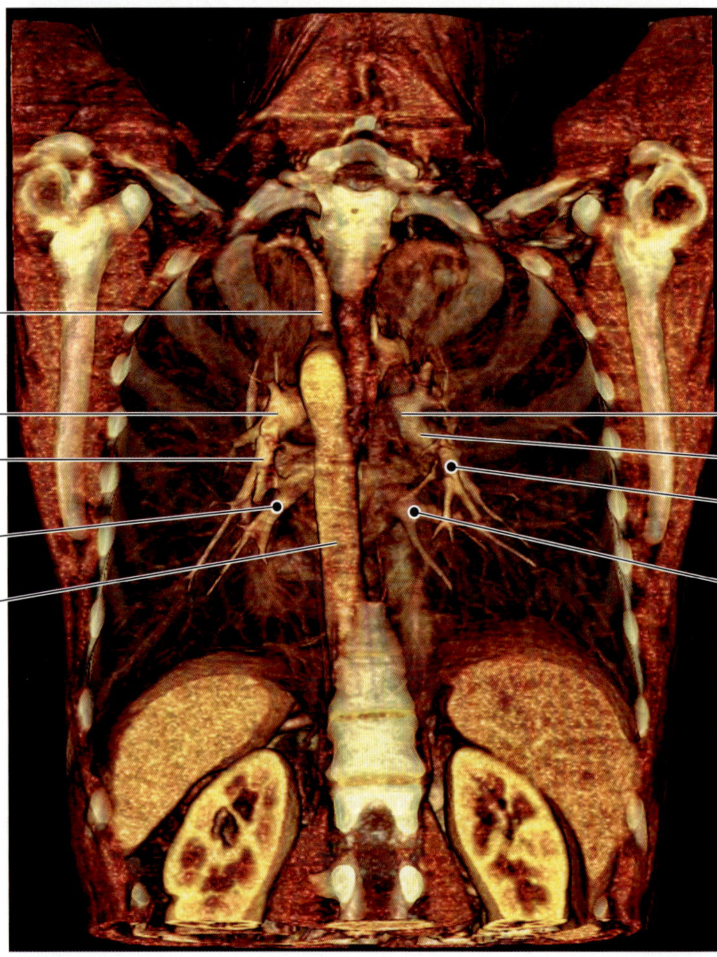

Series of two three-dimensional images of a living human body, obtained from frontal sections in a dorso-ventral direction by CT scan using a 3D volume rendering technique. View from behind. The sequence starts with a section at the level of the vertebral bodies. To the left of the vertebral column, one can see the **descending aorta** (**thoracic aorta**) and laterally, on both sides, the **pulmonary vessels**. The successive section passes in front of the vertebral column.

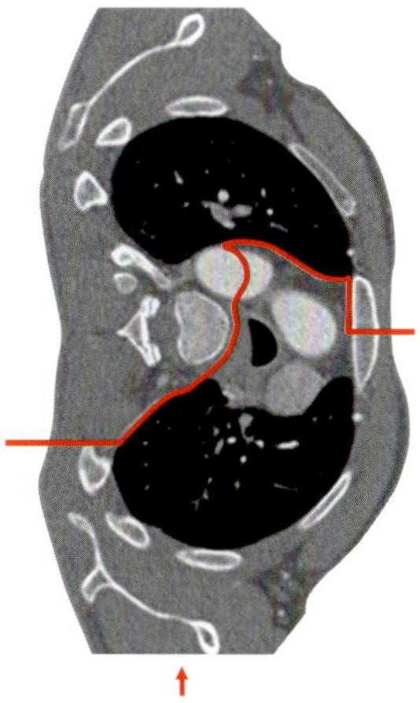

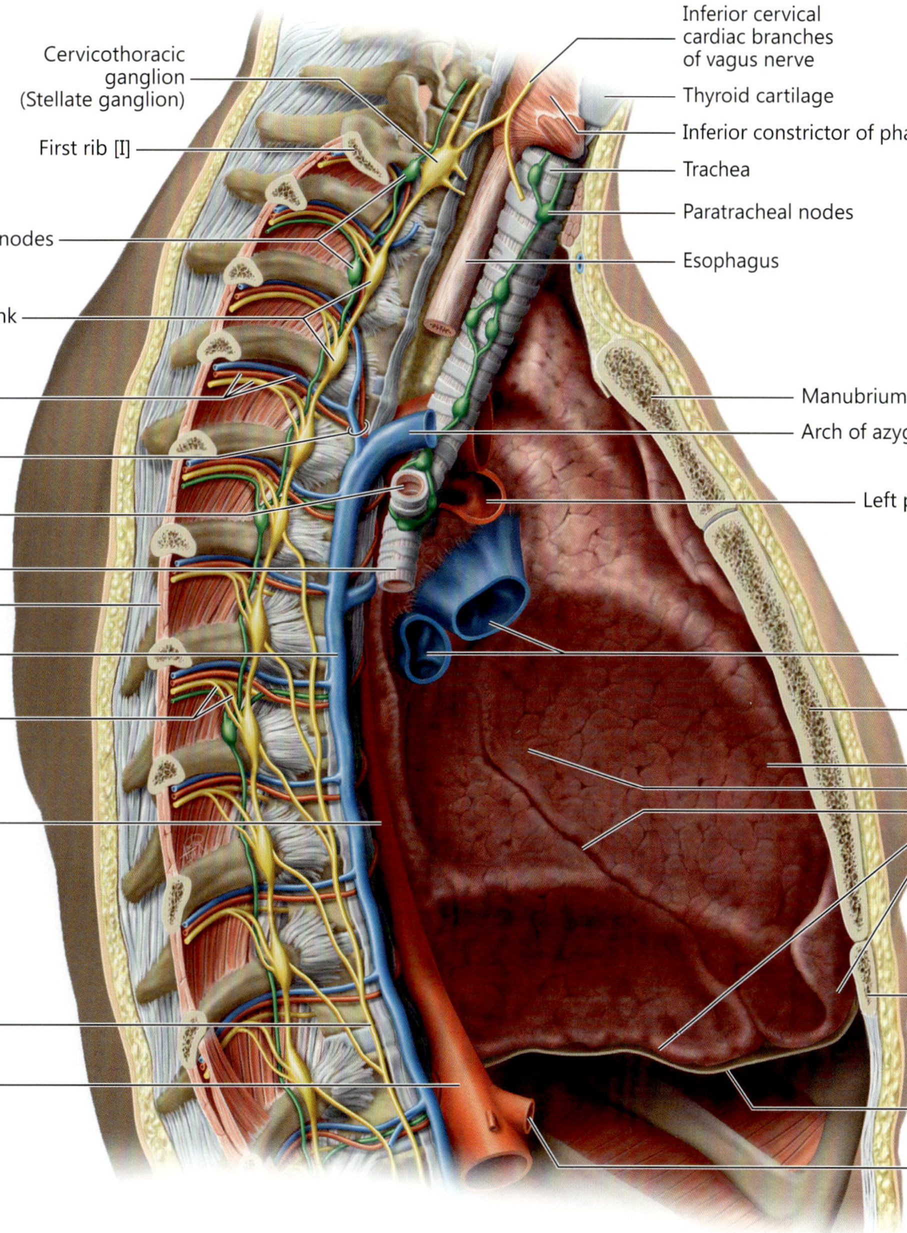

CONTENTS OF THE THORAX

- Arch of azygos vein
- Azygos vein
- Esophagus
- Ganglia of sympathetic trunk
- Greater splanchnic nerve
- Intercostal nodes
- Left lung, cardiac impression
- Left lung, inferior border

- Left lung, lingula
- Left lung, oblique fissure
- Left pulmonary artery
- Left pulmonary veins
- Paratracheal nodes
- Posterior intercostal vein and artery and intercostal nerve
- Right main bronchus

- Right superior intercostal vein
- Right superior lobar bronchus (epiarterial bronchus)
- Right supreme intercostal artery
- Thoracic aorta
- Trachea
- White and gray rami communicantes

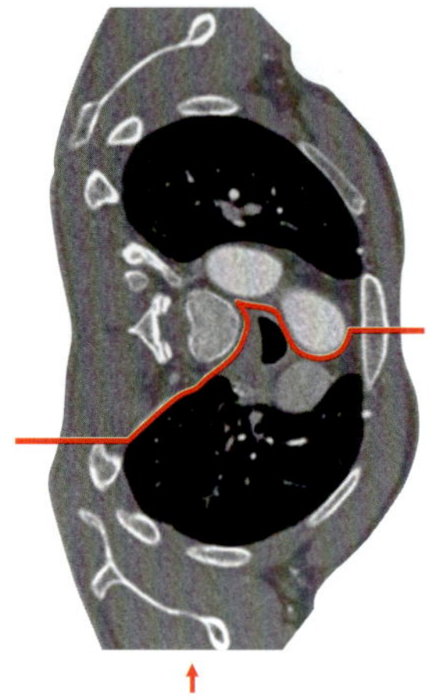

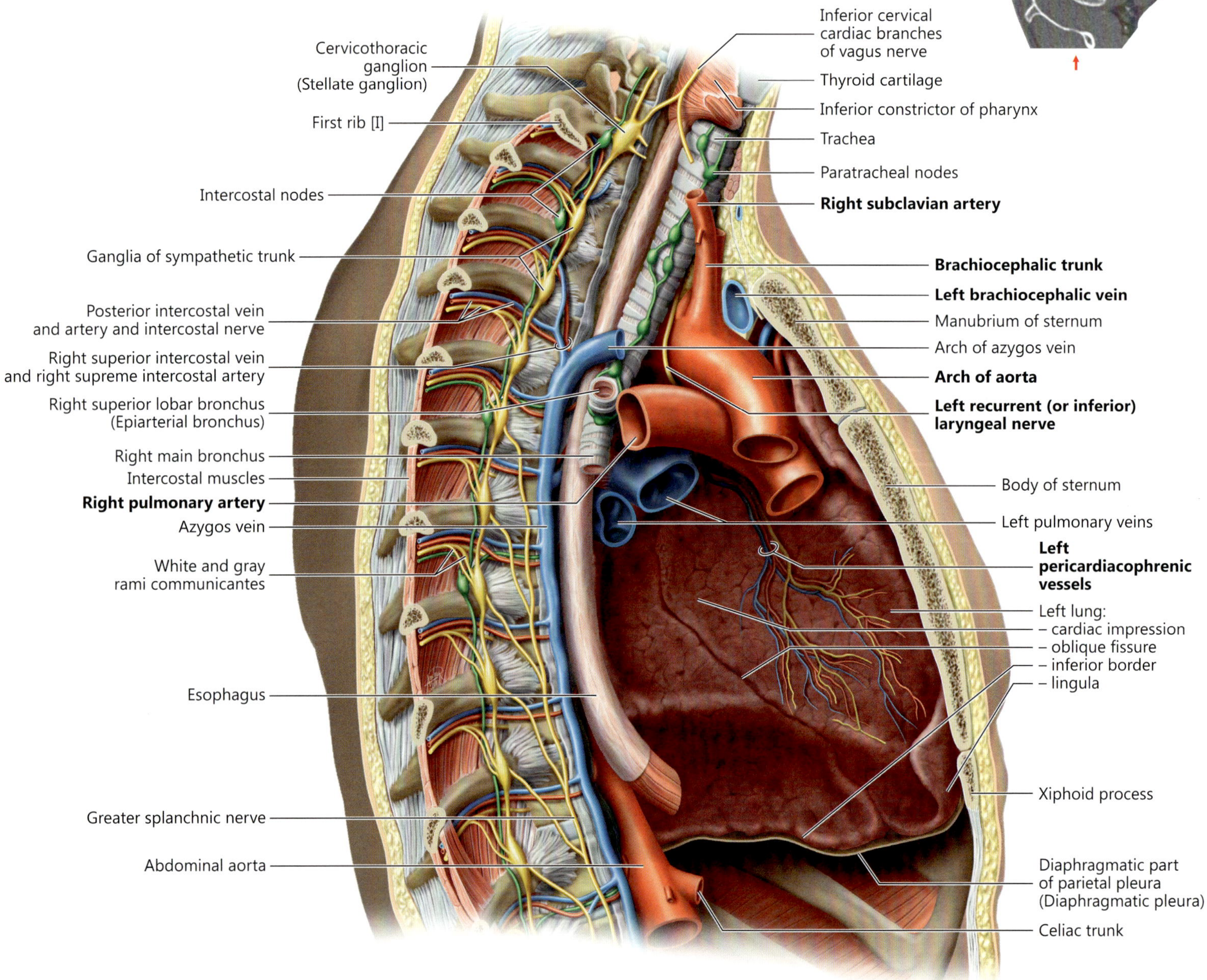

CONTENTS OF THE THORAX (in bold are the structures added with respect to the preceding table)
• Arch of aorta • Brachiocephalic trunk • Left brachiocephalic vein • Left pericardiacophrenic vessels • Left recurrent (or inferior) laryngeal nerve • Right pulmonary artery • Right subclavian artery

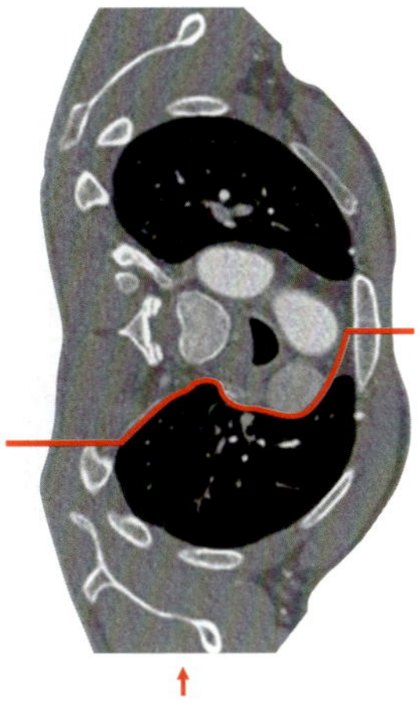

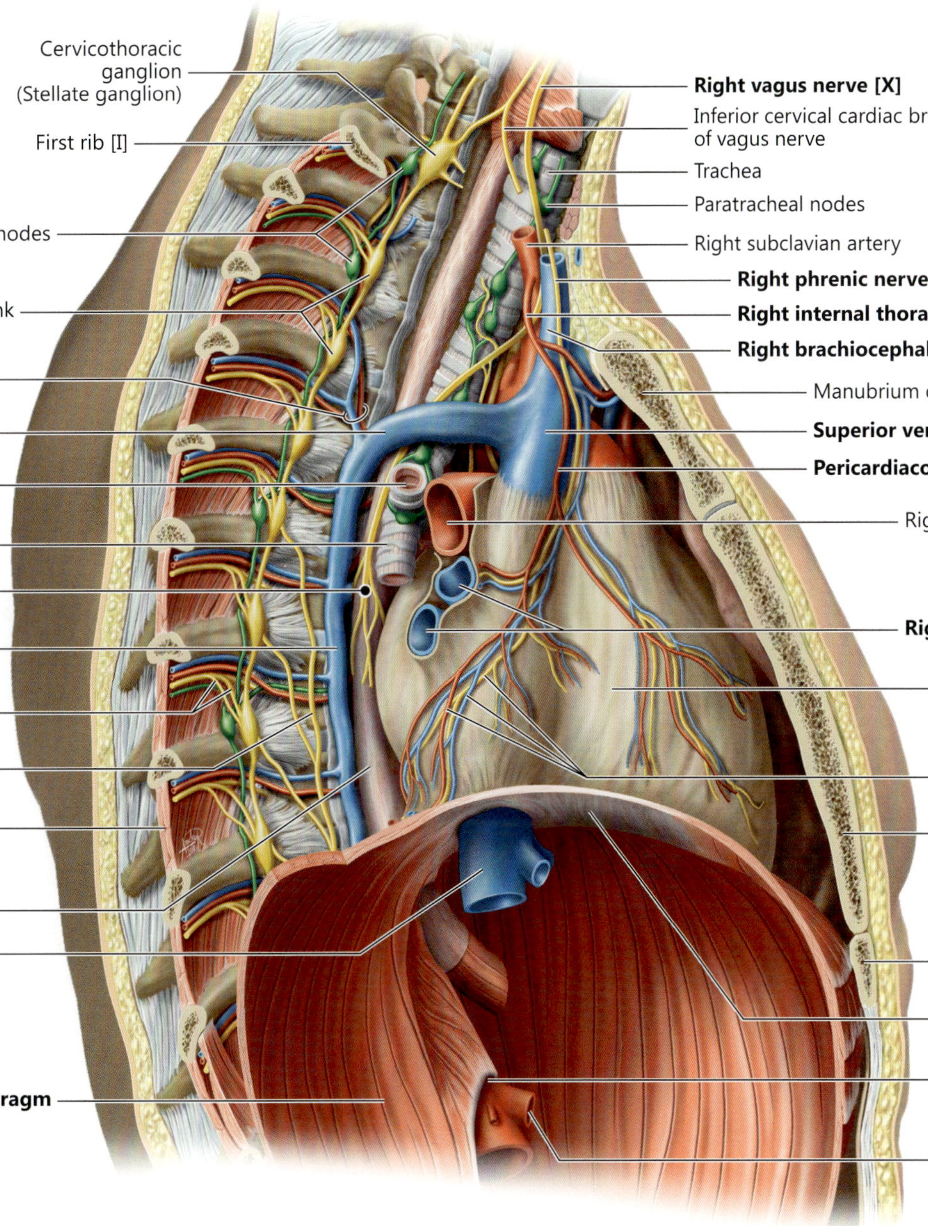

CONTENTS OF THE THORAX (in bold are the structures added with respect to the preceding table)	
• Aortic hiatus • Diaphragm • Esophageal plexus • Fibrous pericardium • Inferior vena cava • Pericardiacophrenic artery • Pericardiacophrenic veins	• Right brachiocephalic vein • Right internal thoracic artery • Right phrenic nerve • Right pulmonary veins • Right vagus nerve [X] • Superior vena cava

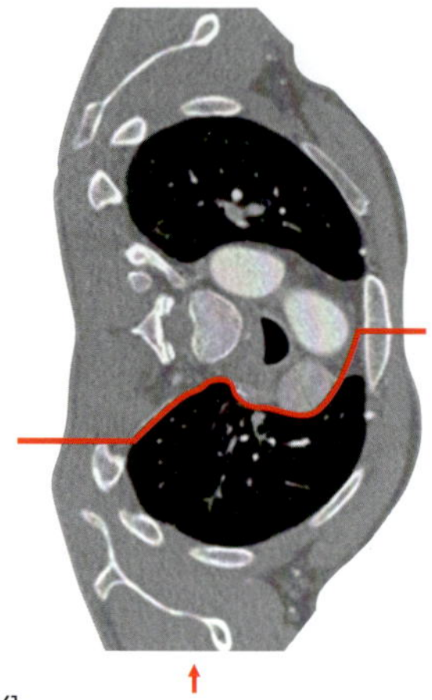

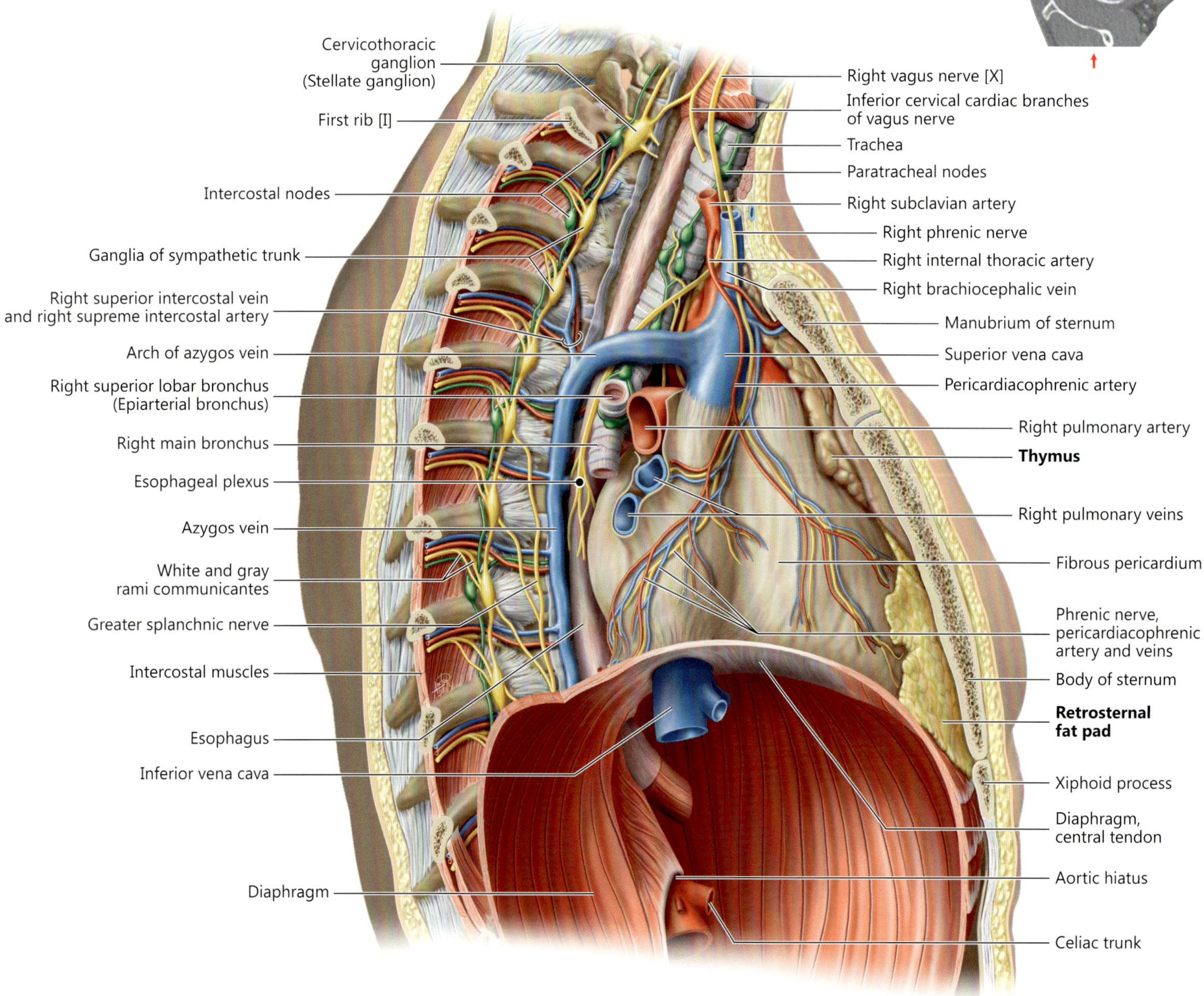

CONTENTS OF THE THORAX (in bold are the structures added with respect to the preceding table)
• Retrosternal fat pad • Thymus

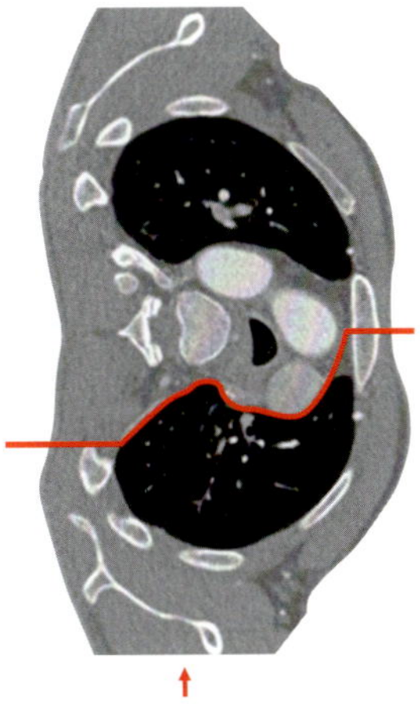

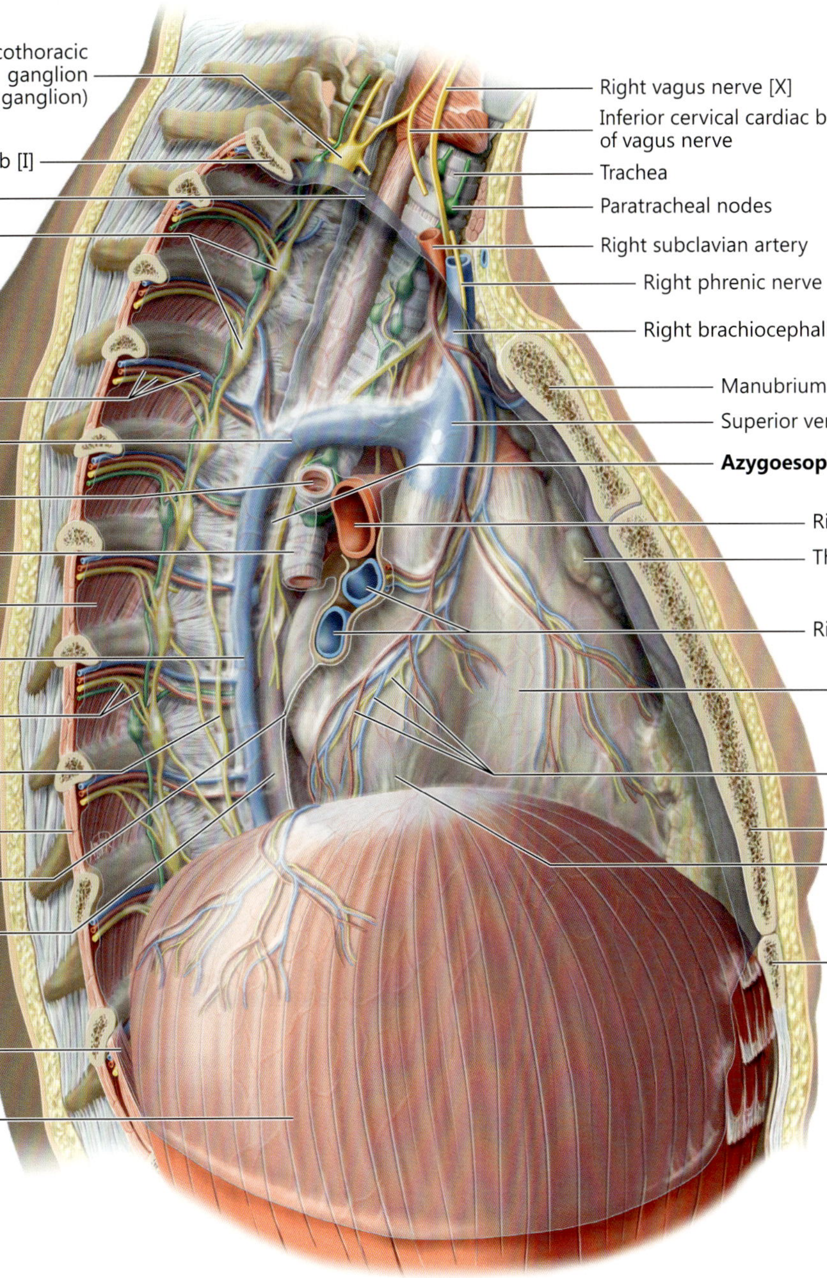

CONTENTS OF THE THORAX (in bold are the structures added with respect to the preceding table)
• Azygoesophageal recess • Costal part of parietal pleura (costal pleura) • Inferior vena cava • Pleura • Pulmonary (triangular) ligament • Right costodiaphragmatic recess

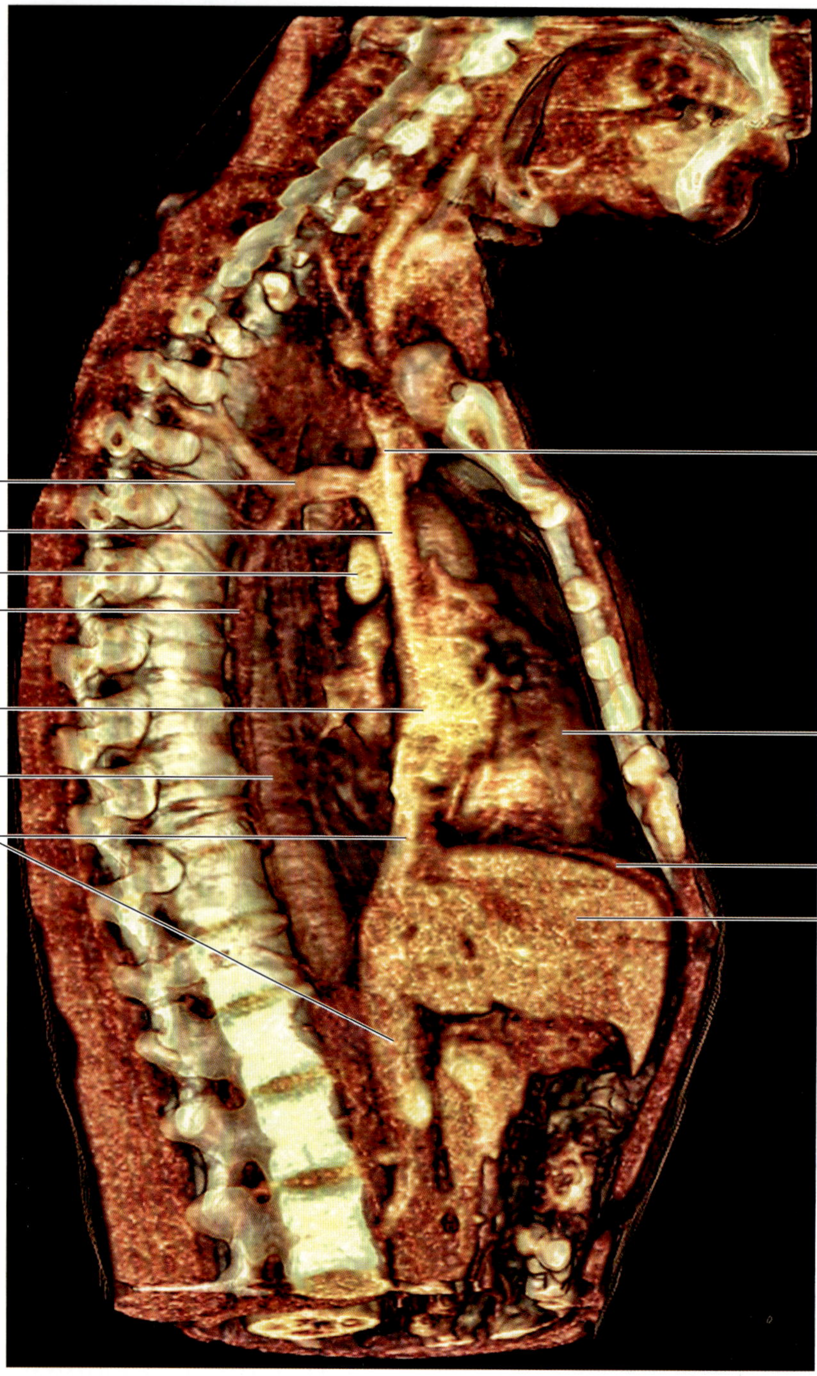

Three-dimensional image of a living human body, obtained by CT scan using a 3D volume rendering technique, in sagittal section. The **mediastinum** is observed from the right. The reconstruction enables one to see the right atrium and opening of the venae cavae. Clearly visible is the arch of the azygos vein on the root of the right lung.

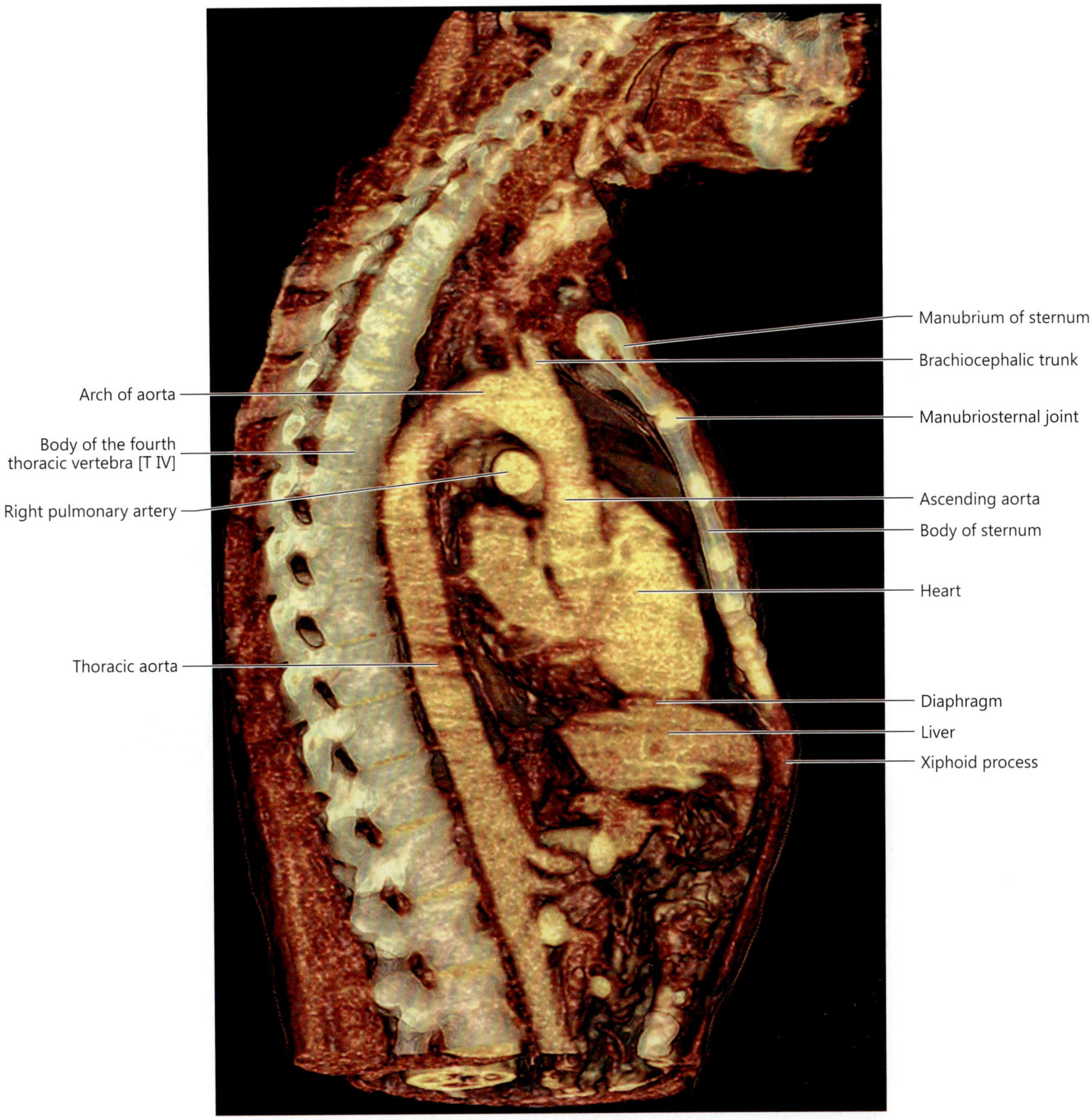

Three-dimensional image of a living human body, obtained by CT scan using a 3D volume, in sagittal section. The **mediastinum** is observed from the right. The reconstruction enables one to see the heart as well as the course of the ascending aorta, of the arch of the aorta, which passes over the root of the right lung, and of the thoracic aorta.

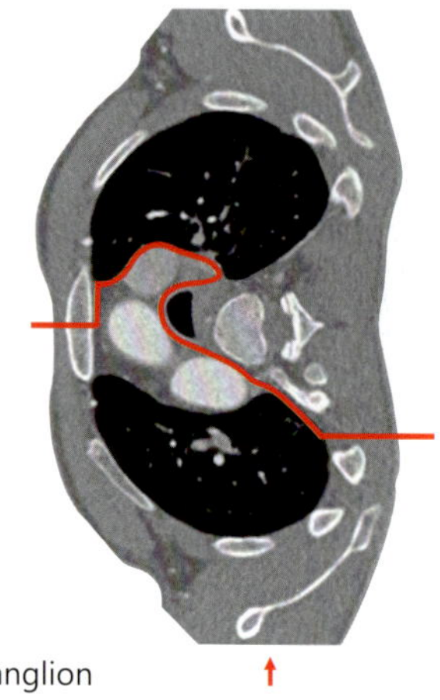

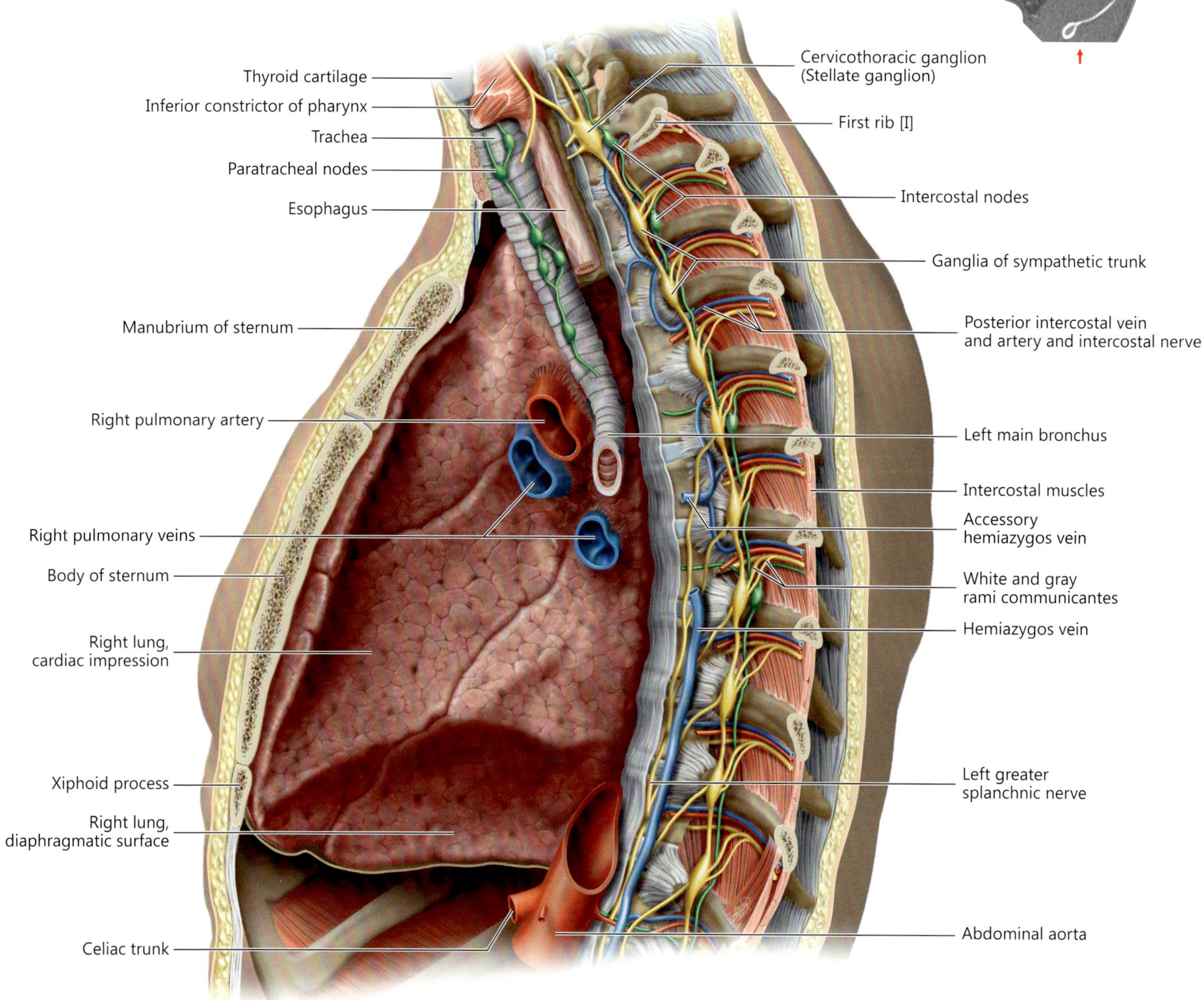

CONTENTS OF THE THORAX	
• Accessory hemiazygos vein • Esophagus • Ganglia of sympathetic trunk • Hemiazygos vein • Intercostal nodes • Left greater splanchnic nerve • Left main bronchus	• Paratracheal nodes • Posterior intercostal vein and artery and intercostal nerve • Right lung, cardiac impression • Right lung, diaphragmatic surface • Right pulmonary artery • Right pulmonary veins • Trachea

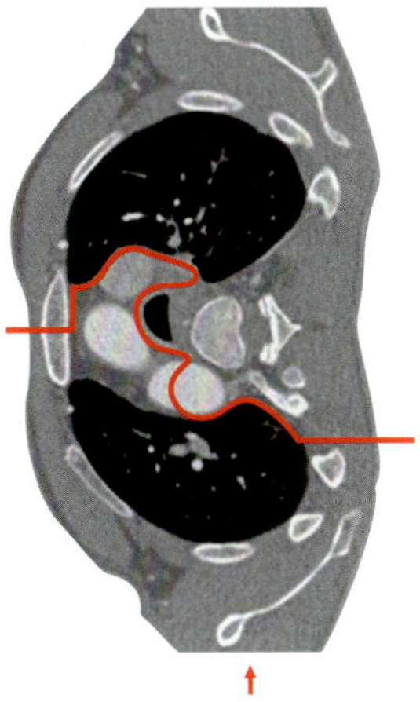

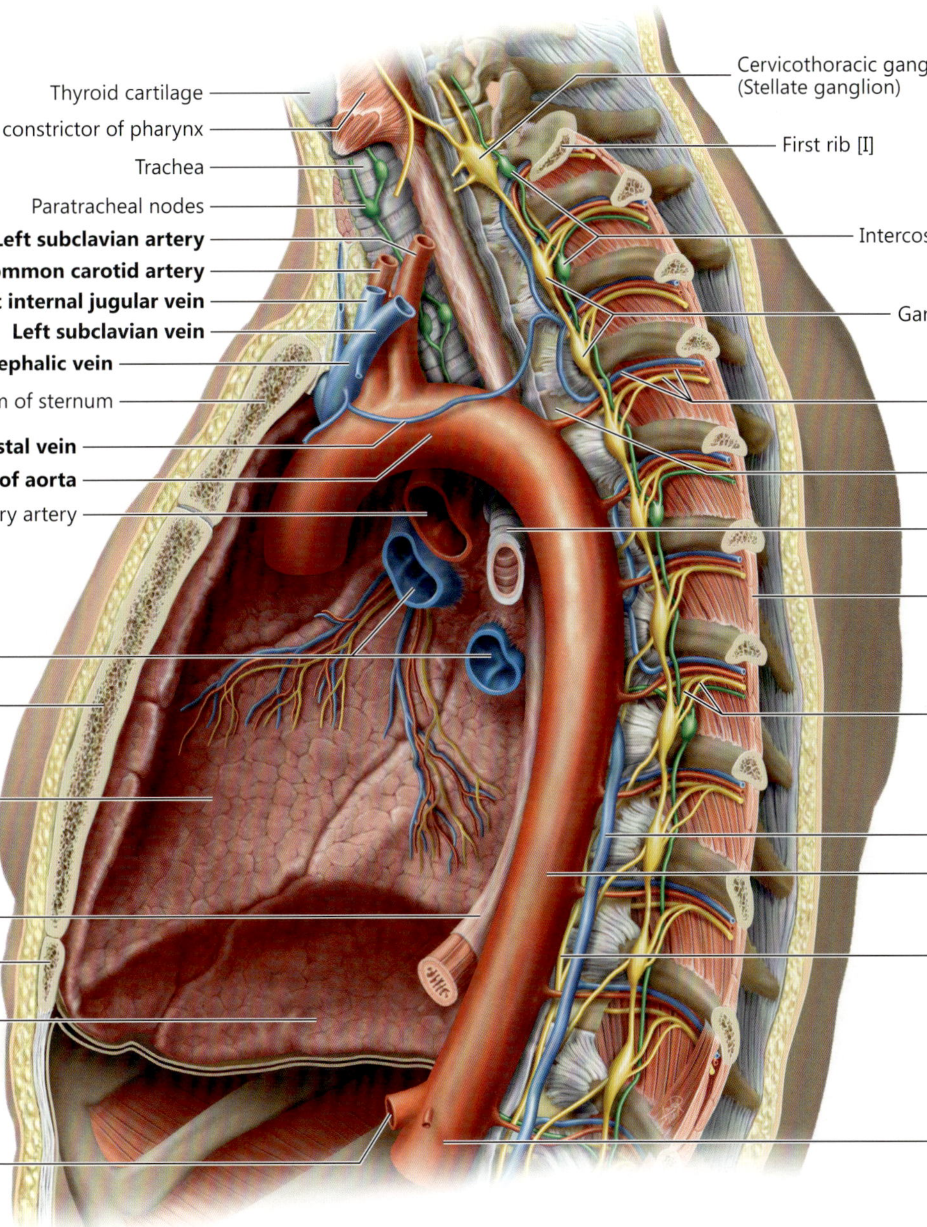

***CONTENTS OF THE THORAX** (in bold are the structures added with respect to the preceding table)*
• Arch of aorta • Left brachiocephalic vein • Left common carotid artery • Left internal jugular vein • Left subclavian artery • Left subclavian vein • Left superior intercostal vein • Thoracic aorta

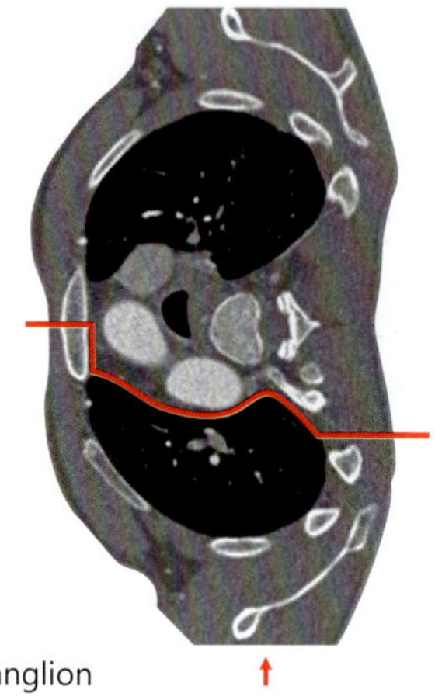

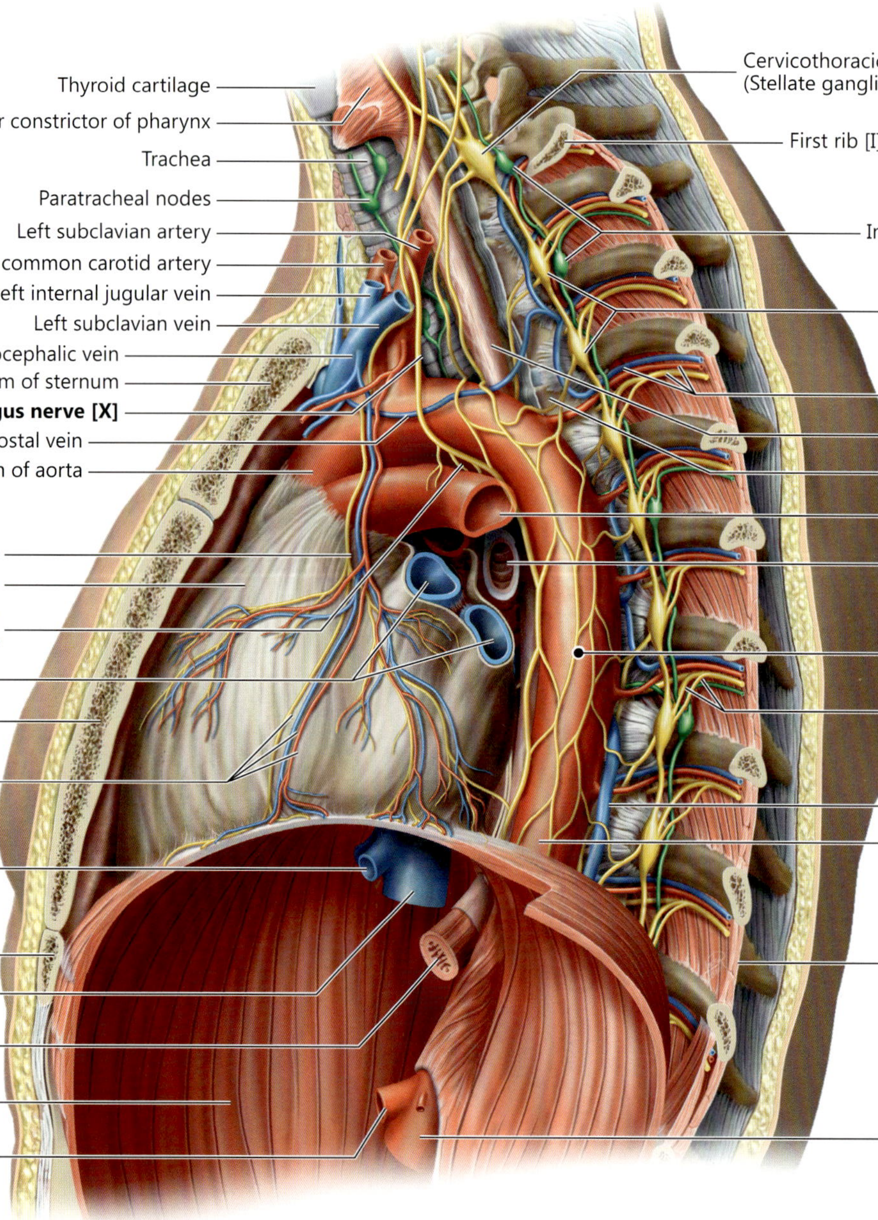

CONTENTS OF THE THORAX (in bold are the structures added with respect to the preceding table)	
• Diaphragm • Fibrous pericardium • Inferior vena cava • Left phrenic nerve • Left pulmonary artery • Left pulmonary veins	• Left recurrent (or inferior) laryngeal nerve • Left vagus nerve [X] • Pericardiacophrenic artery • Pericardiacophrenic veins • Thoracic aortic plexus

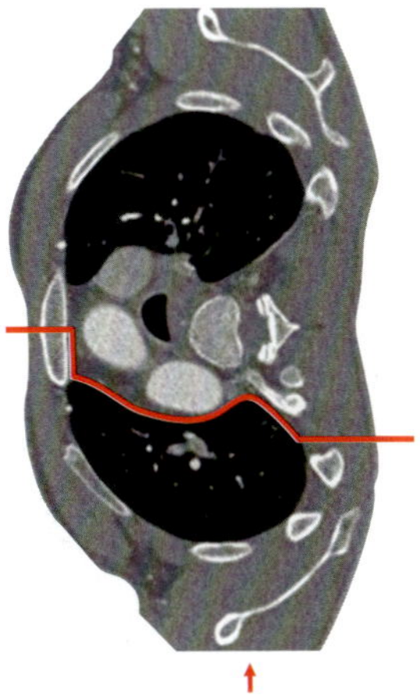

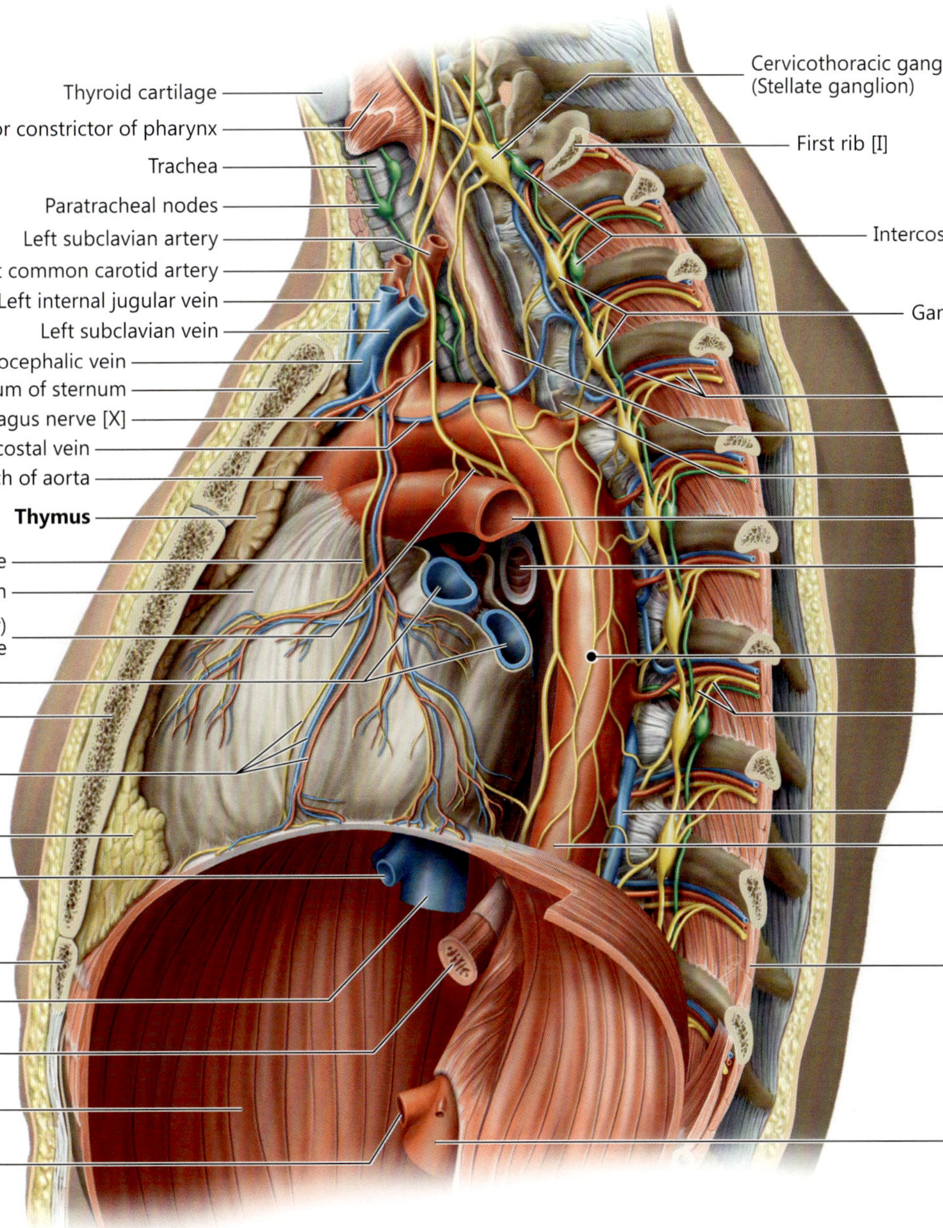

CONTENTS OF THE THORAX (in bold are the structures added with respect to the preceding table)
• Retrosternal fat pad • Thymus

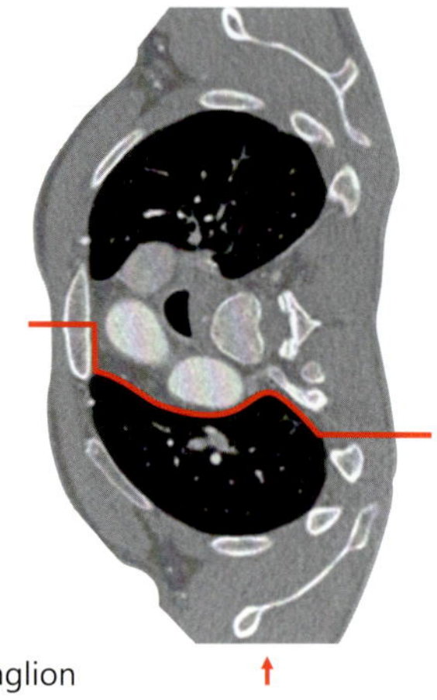

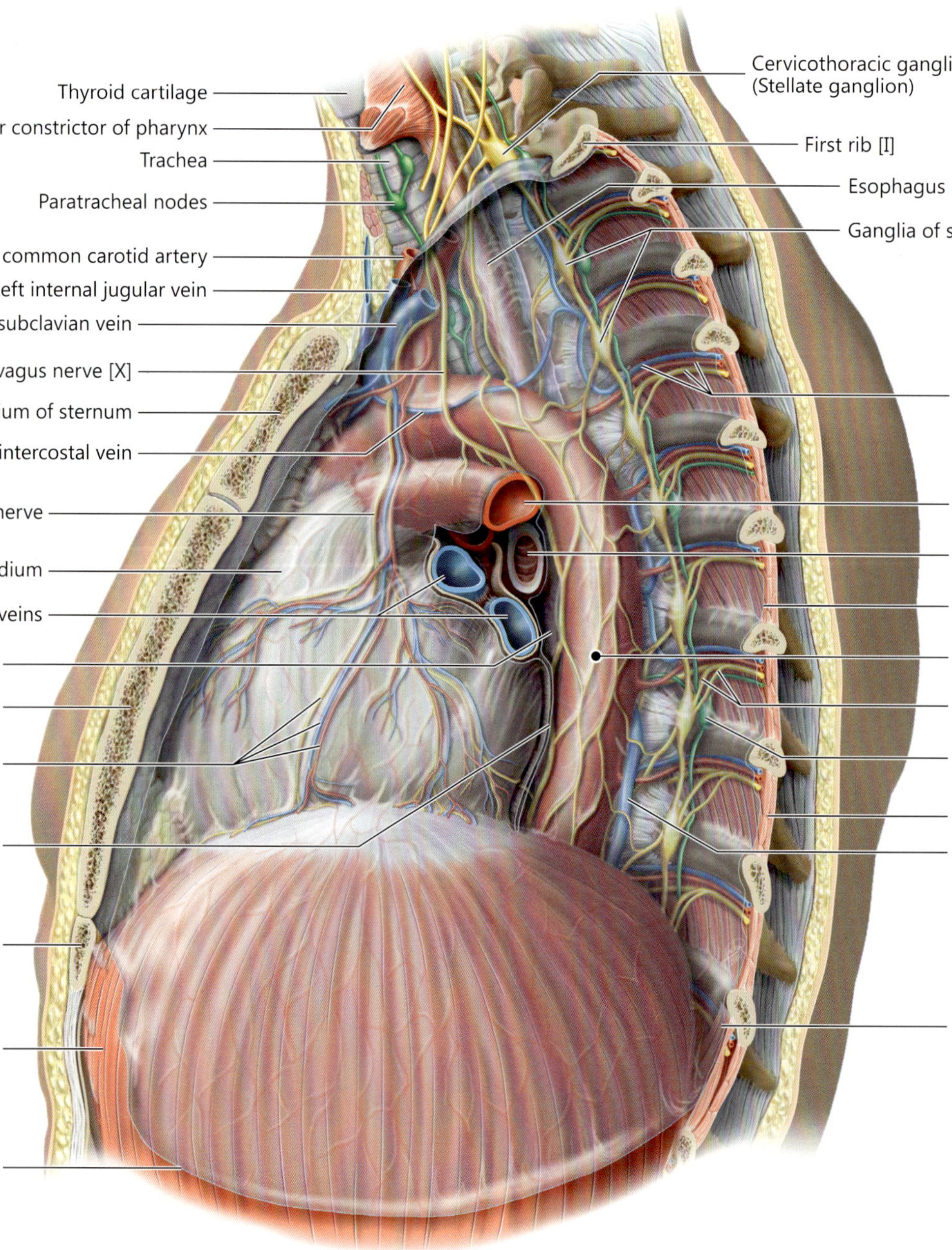

CONTENTS OF THE THORAX (in bold are the structures added with respect to the preceding table)
• Costal part of parietal pleura (costal pleura) • Diaphragmatic part of parietal pleura (diaphragmatic pleura) • Interaortoesophageal recess • Left costodiaphragmatic recess • Left pulmonary (triangular) ligament

The **esophagus** extends for approximately 25 cm, from C VI to T XI. It originates in the neck from the pharynx, at the level of the cricoid cartilage of the larynx (cervical part), and proceeds into the thorax, running in the posterior mediastinum and constituting the thoracic part, which divides in turn into an epibronchial part and a hypobronchial part. It terminates, after passing through the esophageal hiatus of the diaphragm, in the abdominal cavity at the level of the cardias (abdominal part).

The upper third of the esophagus presents also numerous striated muscle fibers, as a continuation of the inferior constrictor of the pharynx, participating in the swallowing process. In the inferior two-thirds, the muscular coat is composed exclusively of two layers of smooth muscle: an inner circular layer and an outer longitudinal layer (transected in the figure). The anterior surface of the esophagus adheres to the posterior surface of the trachea by means of bands of smooth muscle interspersed with loose connective tissue (tracheoesophageal muscle).

The esophagus does not have a sphincter at the level of the esophagogastric junction. This function is delegated to the diaphragmatic musculature at the level of the esophageal hiatus. At this site, some muscle layers of the diaphragm insert on the wall of the esophagus (phrenoesophageal muscle).

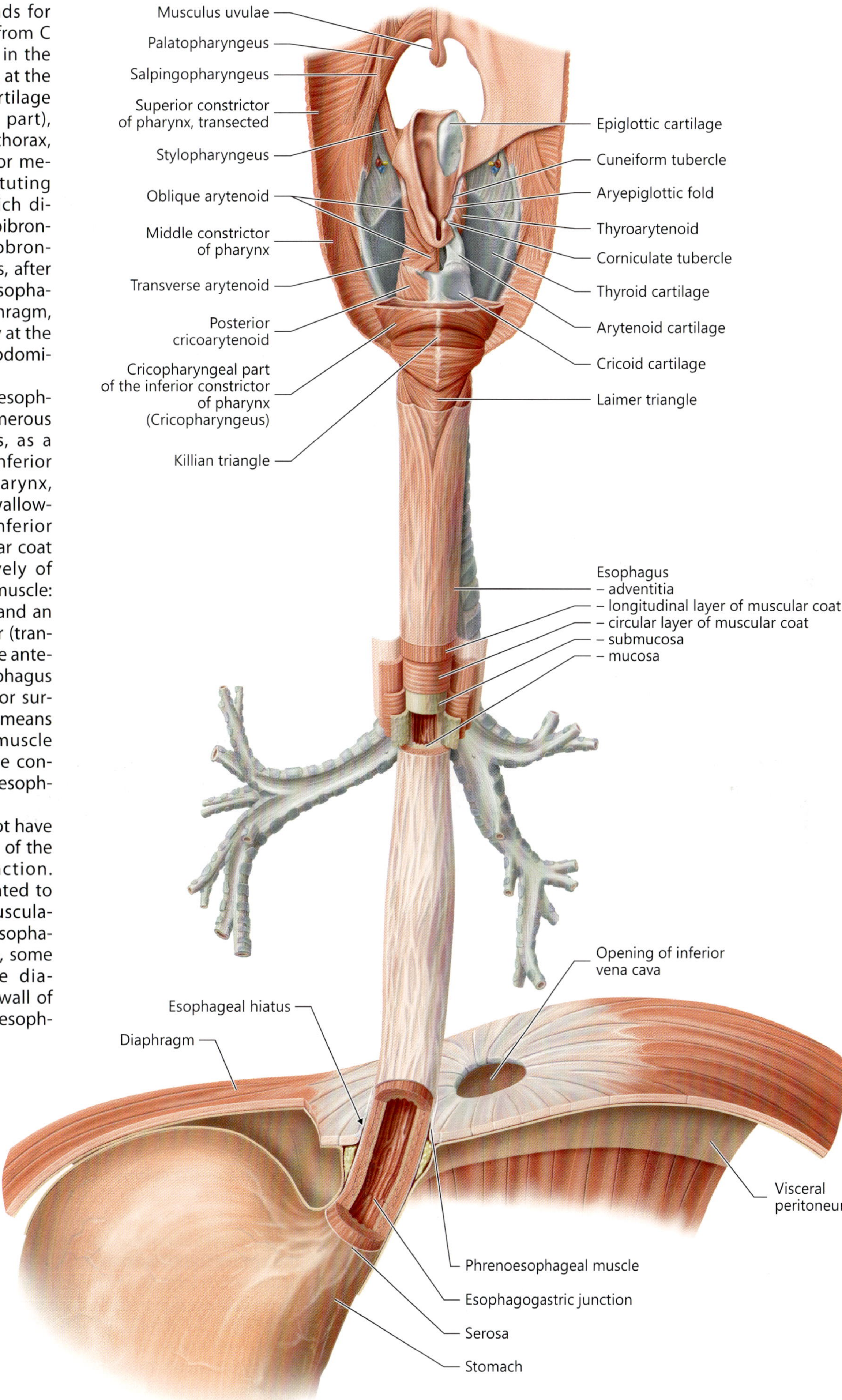

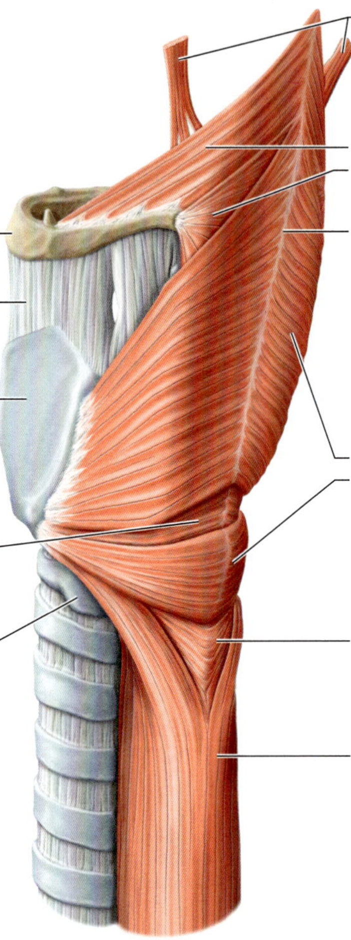

At the level of the pharyngoesophageal junction, there are two regions of minor wall resistance: the **Laimer triangle**, between the cricopharyngeal part of the inferior constrictor, above, and two layers of longitudinal muscle of the esophagus that insert on the sides of the cricoid cartilage of the larynx, below; and the **Killian triangle**, situated between the thyropharyngeal and cricopharyngeal parts of the inferior constrictor.

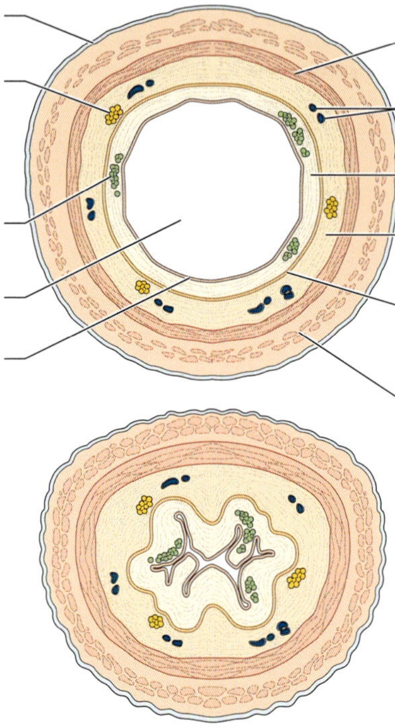

Schematic description of the **wall of the esophagus** in conditions of distension (above) and rest (below).

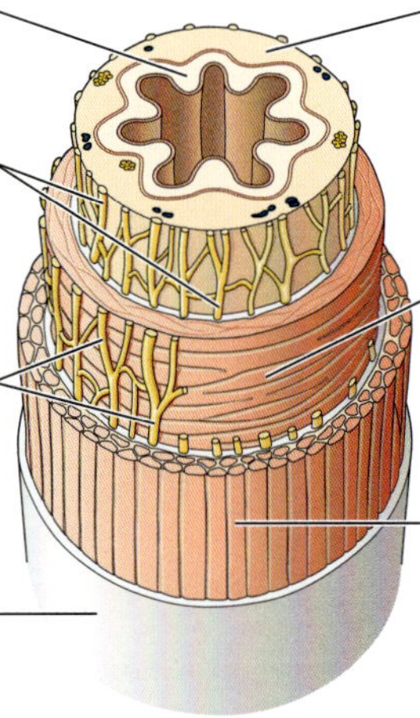

Two nerve plexuses regulate the motility of the gastrointestinal tract from the esophagus down to the rectum: the **submucous plexus** (**plexus of Meissner**), situated between the submucosa and the muscular coat, and the **myenteric plexus** (**plexus of Auerbach**) situated between the longitudinal and circular layers of muscular coat.

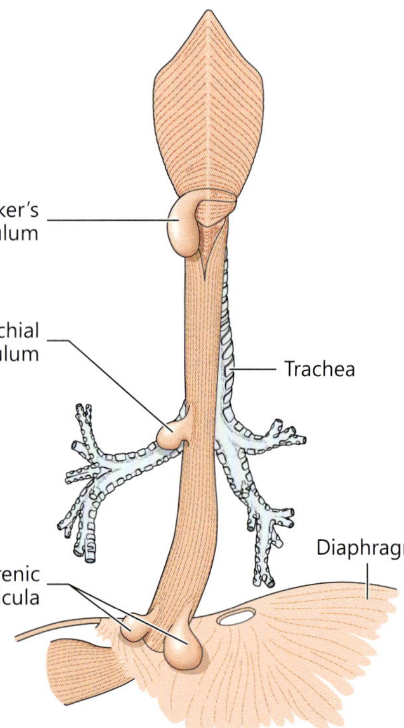

Prolapse of the submucosa and mucosa of the esophageal wall creates diverticula. The diverticula that form in the esophagus can be through pulsion or traction. To the first type belong Zenker's diverticula (pharyngoesophageal diverticula), at the level of the Killian or Laimer triangles, and epiphrenic diverticula, which form due to dyskinesia such as achalasia. Traction diverticula are due to the evaginations of the entire wall of the esophagus on account of adherences to surrounding tissues (e.g. lymph nodes). These adherences can be linked to inflammatory processes. The subsequent post-inflammatory sclerotic retraction exerts traction forming the diverticulum. A preferential site for these diverticula is at the epibronchial level.

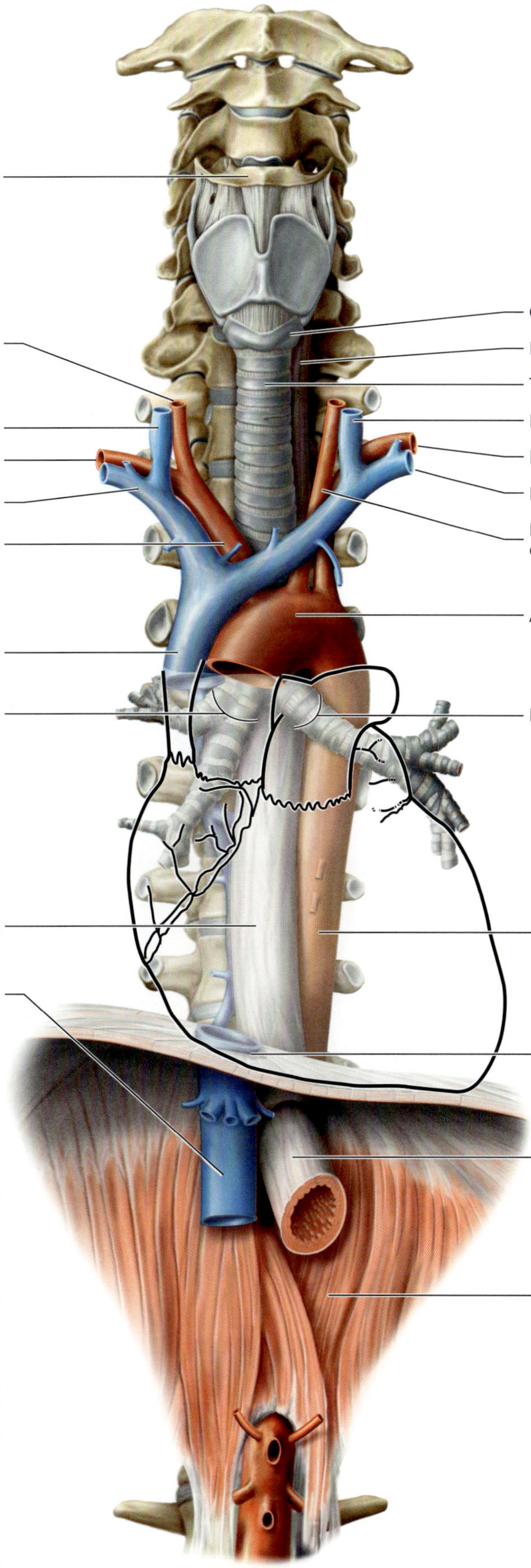

Relationship of the esophagus with contiguous structures, anterior view. At the origin of the esophagus, there is a point of constriction in proximity to the cricoid cartilage (the pharyngoesophageal constriction). In the epibronchial tract, the esophagus runs against the vertebral column in a slightly left paramedian position. The arch of the aorta, running on the left surface of the esophagus, induces a narrowing (aortic constriction) and a curvature on the frontal plane, with concavity to the right. Below the point where it crosses the arch of the aorta, the esophagus regains its paramedian position and is crossed anteriorly by the left bronchus, which induces another narrowing (bronchial constriction) adjacent to the preceding aortic constriction (clinically speaking, these are referred to as the thoracic or bronchoaortic constriction). A final esophageal constriction is found in the passage into the esophageal hiatus of the diaphragm.

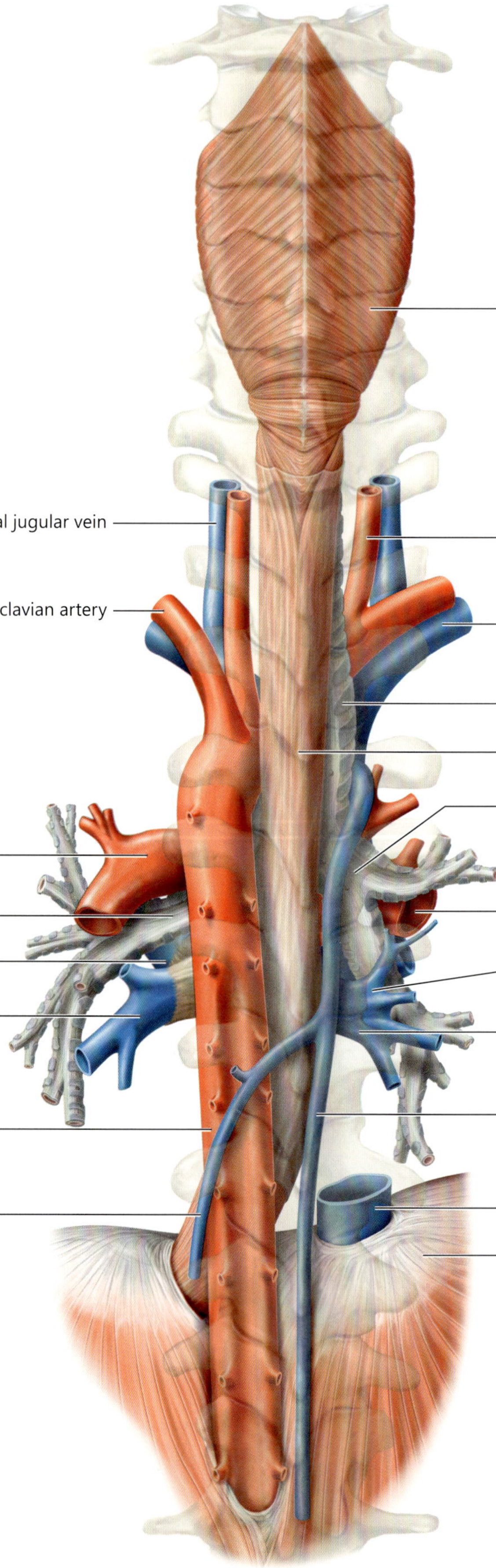

Relationships of the esophagus in the thorax, posterior view. Below the point where the esophagus is crossed by the arch of the aorta, the thoracic aorta shifts behind the esophagus and interposes itself between this and the opening of the hemiazygos vein into the azygos vein at the level of T VII-T VIII.

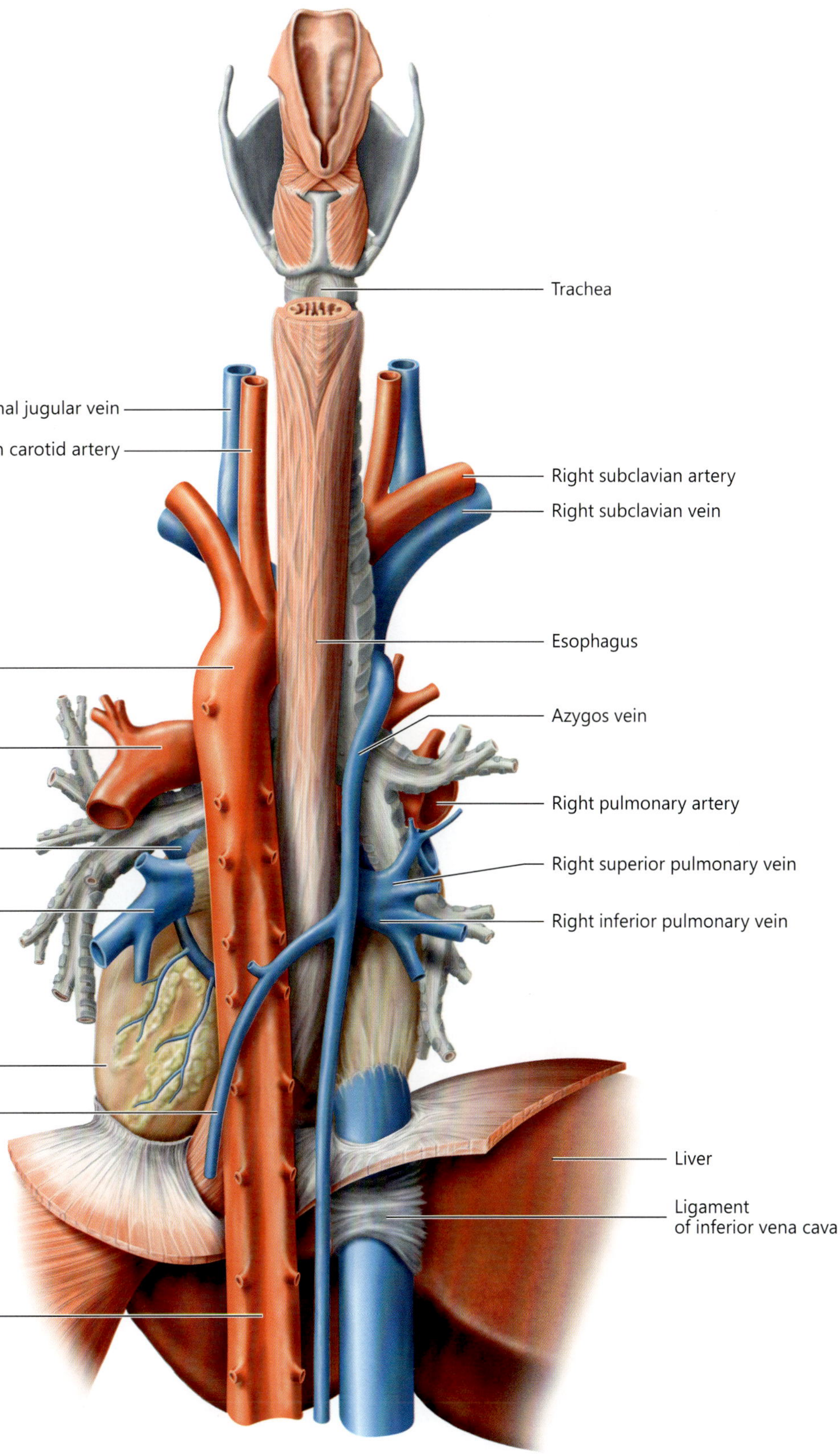

Relationship of the esophagus with the left atrium of the heart, posterior view. Resection of part of the diaphragm allows one to see the ligament of the inferior vena cava.

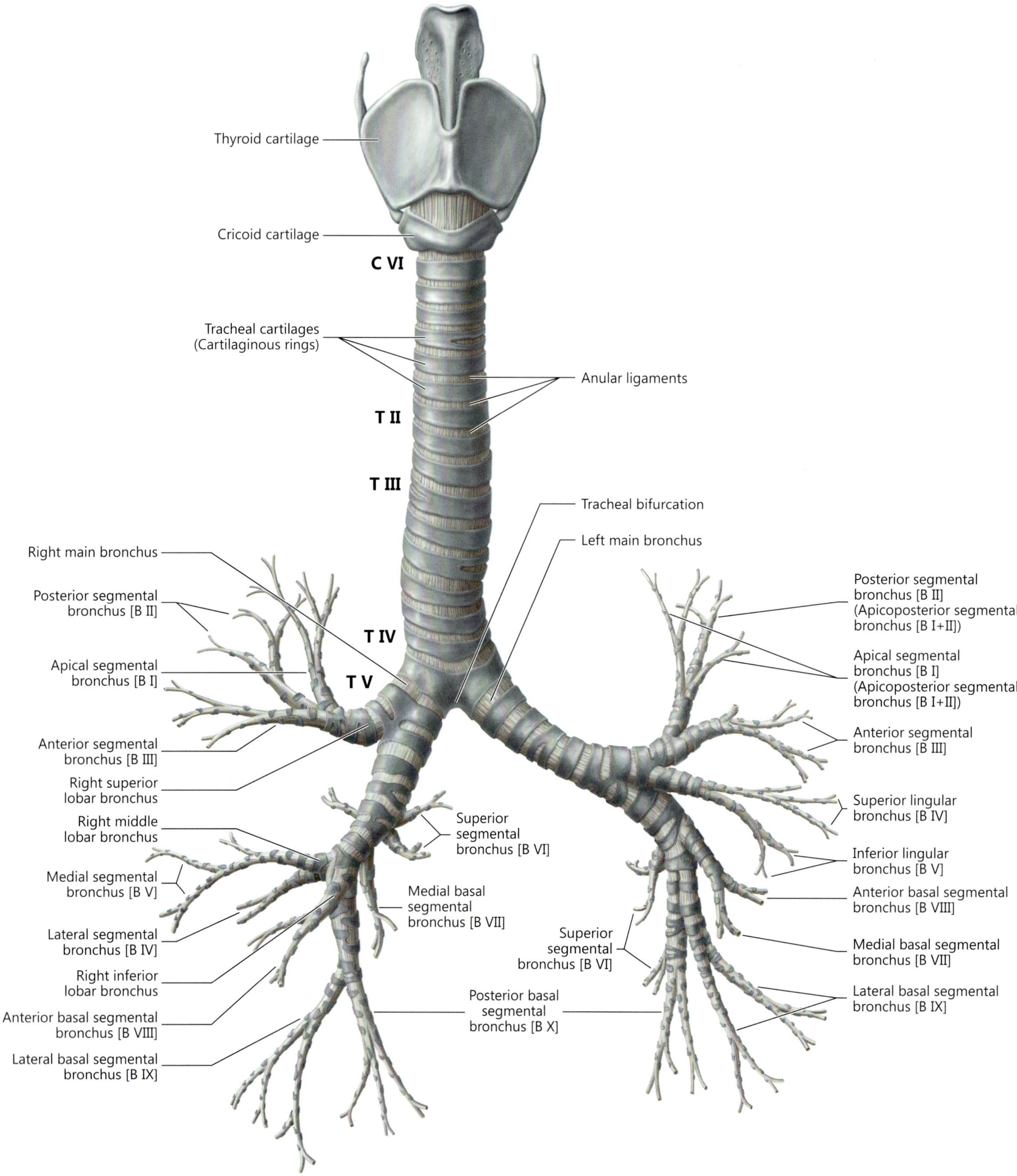

Anterior projection of the **trachea** and the bronchial subdivisions. The trachea extends from the cricoid cartilage of the larynx, at the level of C VI, to the superior border of T V. At this level it divides into the two main bronchi. The right main bronchus has a more vertical path than the left.

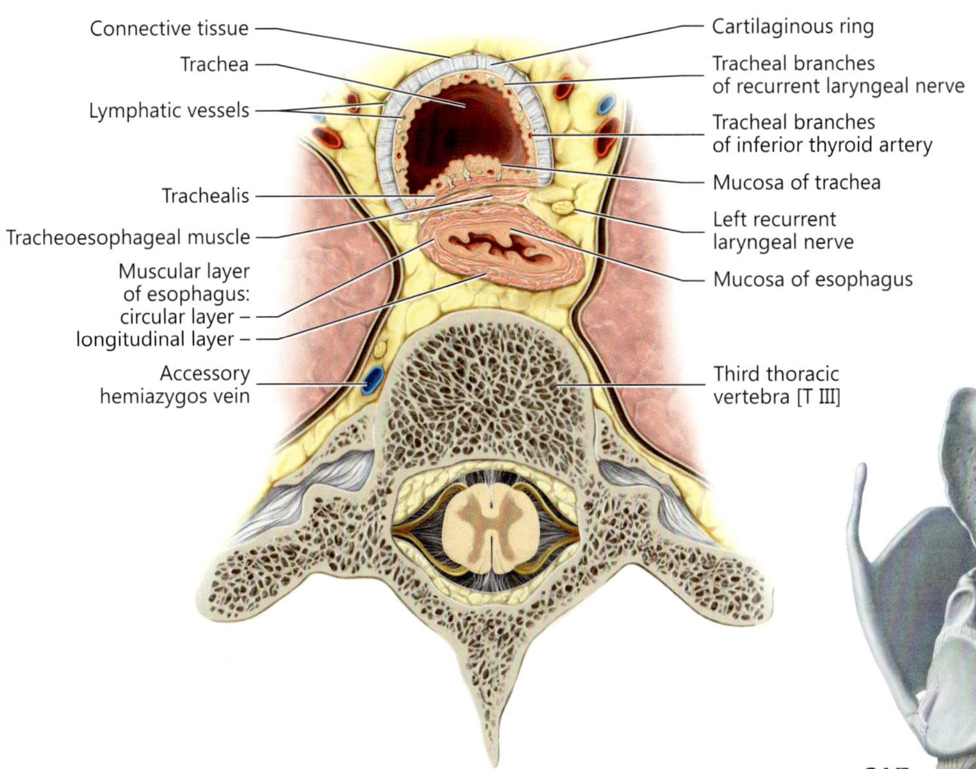

Transverse section of the posterior mediastinum at the level of T III, highlighting the **relationship between trachea and esophagus** (tracheoesophageal muscle).

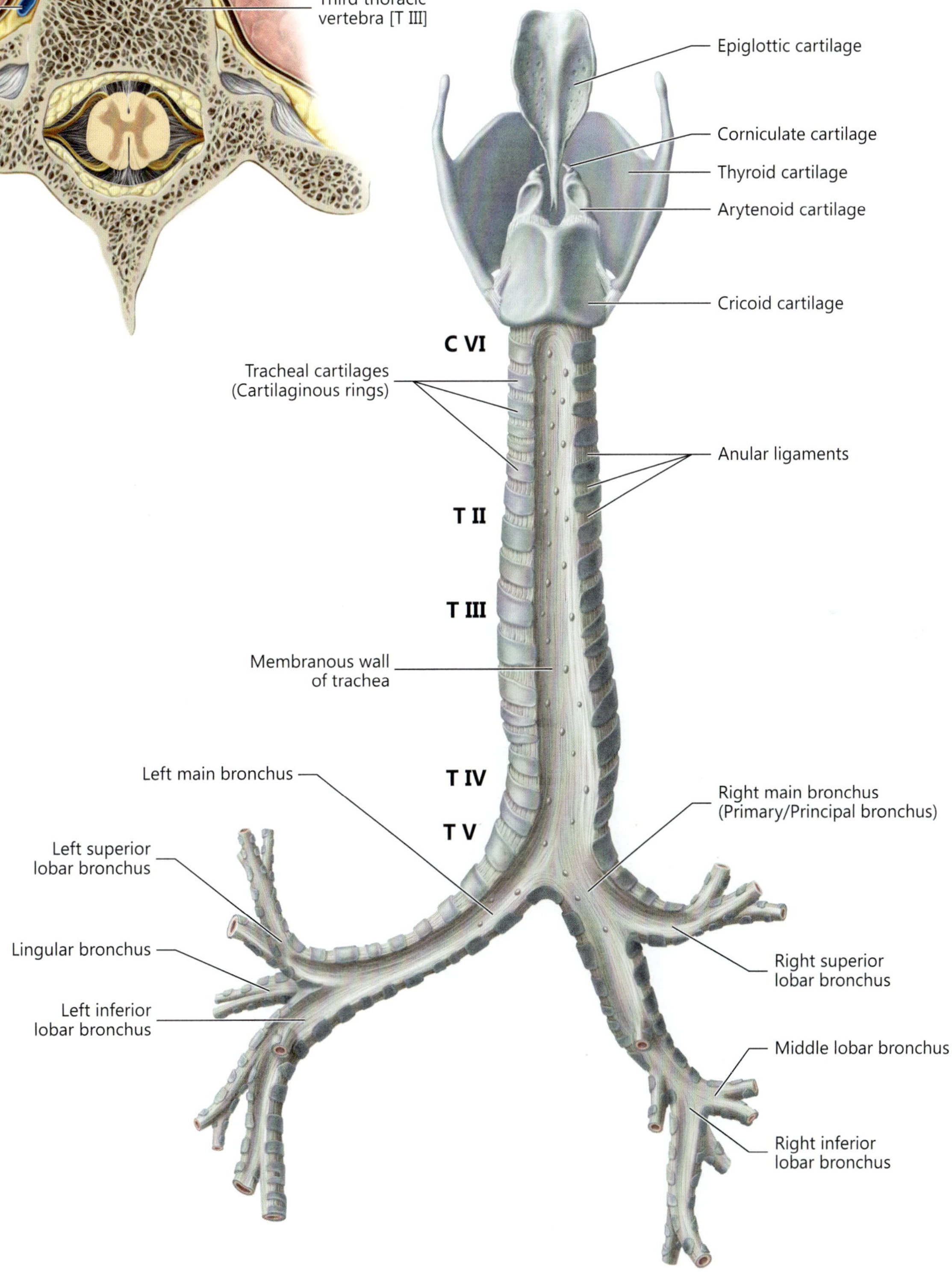

Posterior projection of the **trachea**. The tracheal rings are incomplete posteriorly and the continuity of the wall is ensured by the membranous part of the trachea.

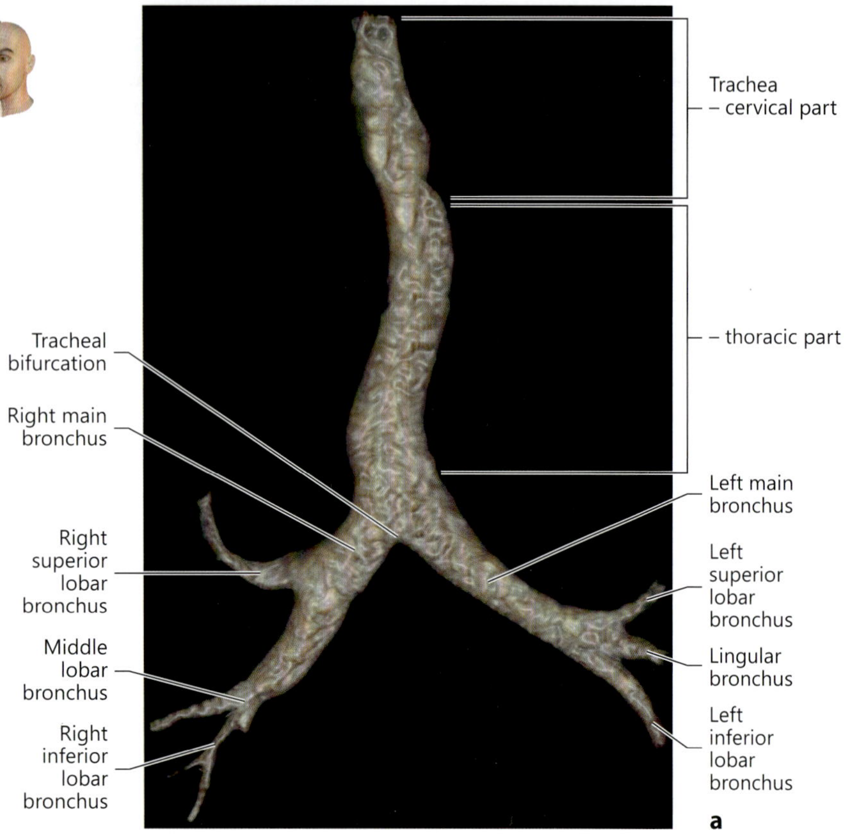

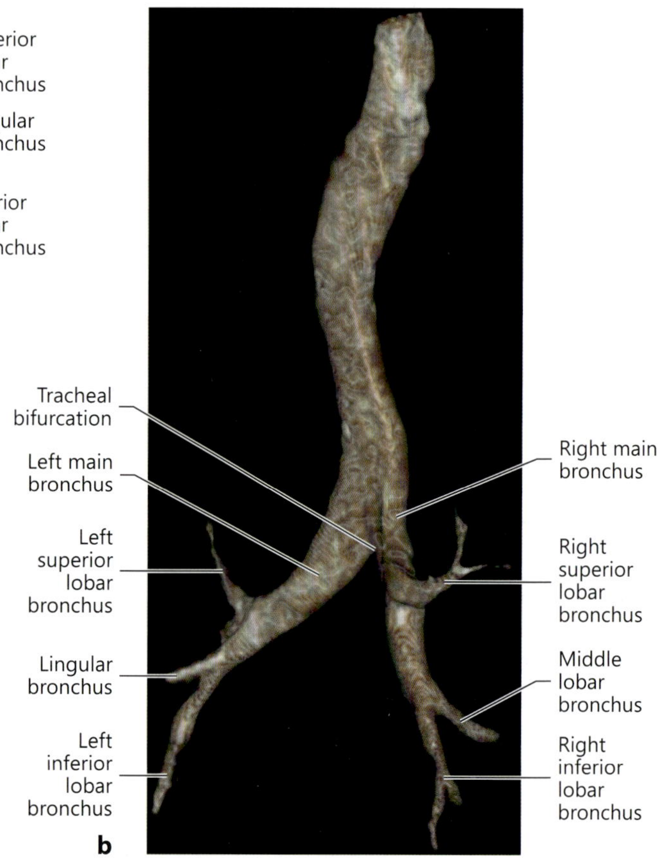

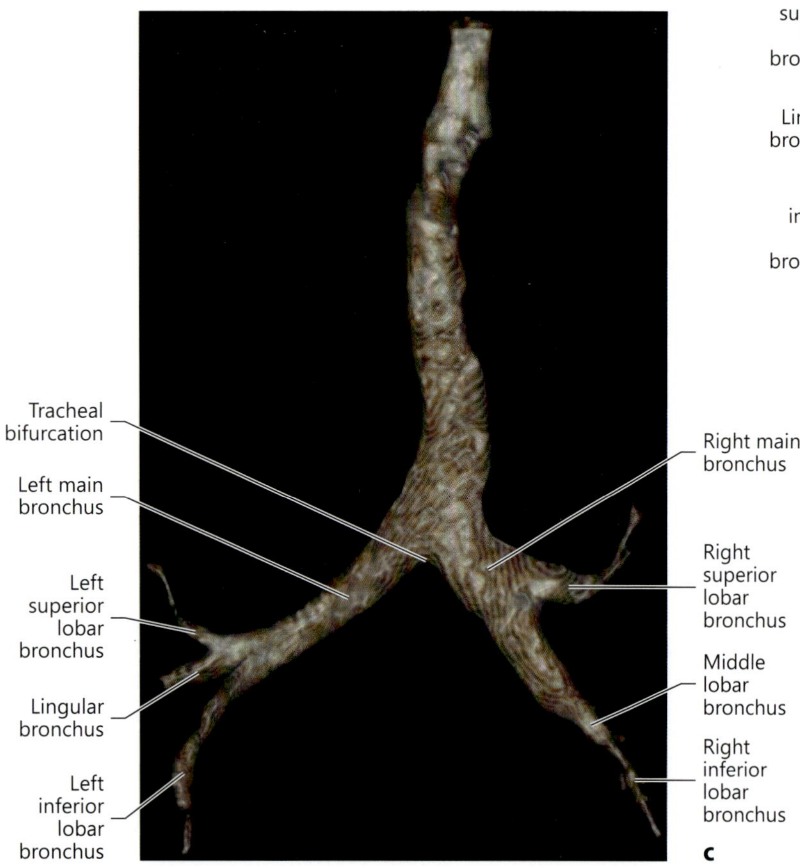

Three-dimensional image of a living human body, obtained by CT scan using a 3D volume rendering technique, showing the **trachea** and first bronchial branches. **a**, Anterior view. **b**, Right lateral view. **c**, Posterior view.

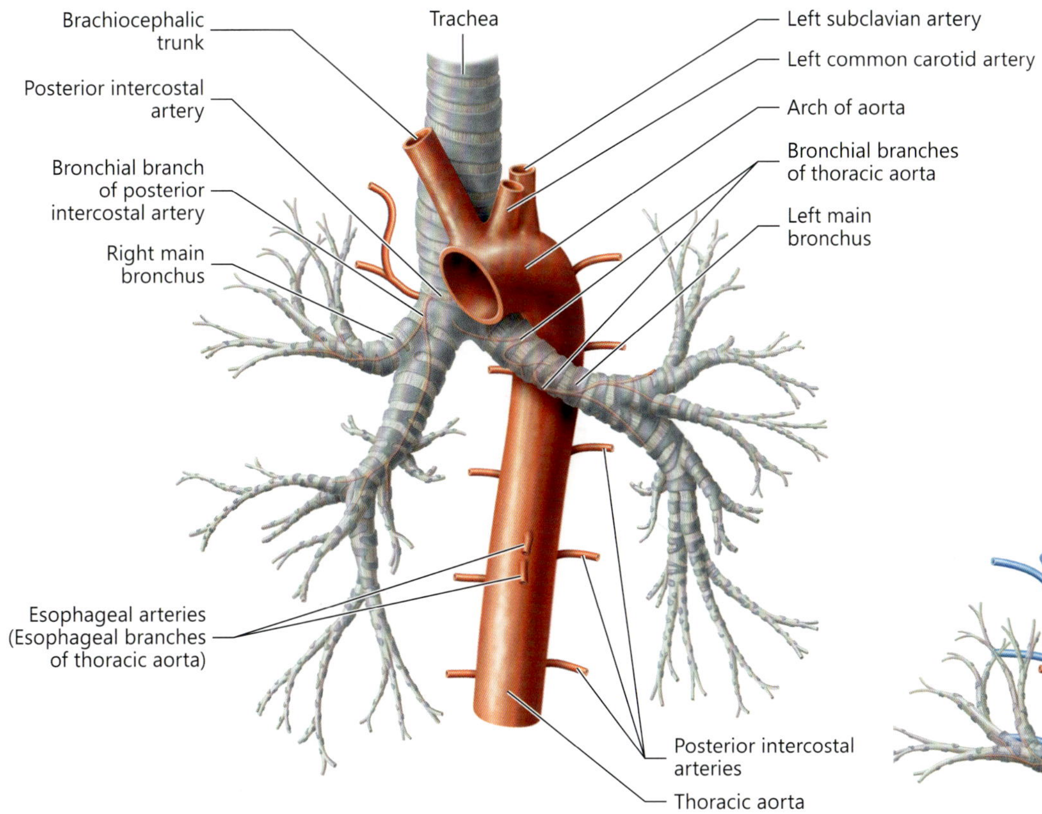

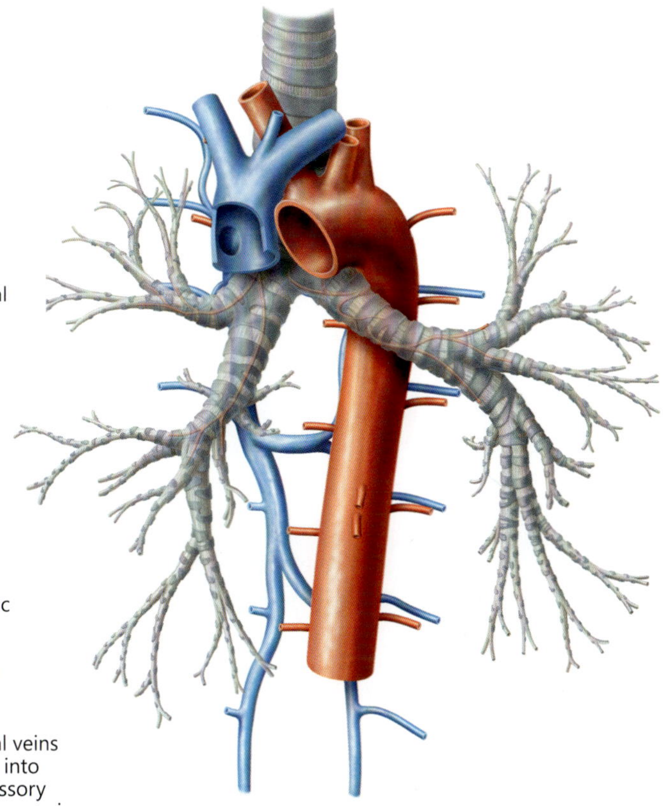

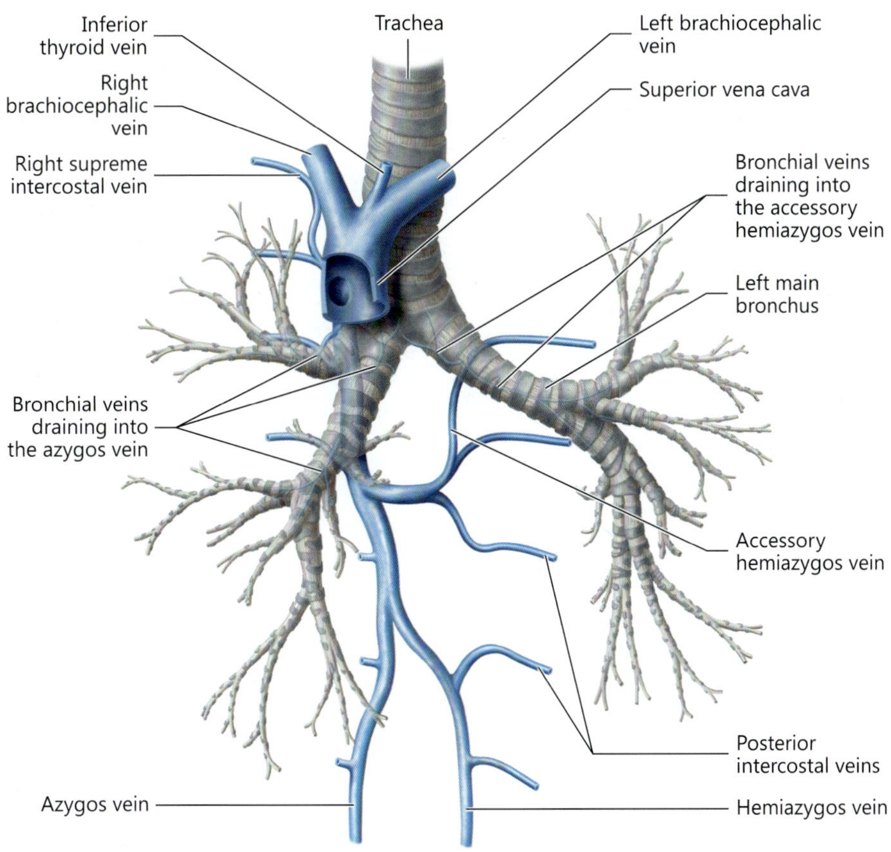

Frontal schematic view showing the relations between the principal **vessels of the large systemic circulation** and the **trachea**.

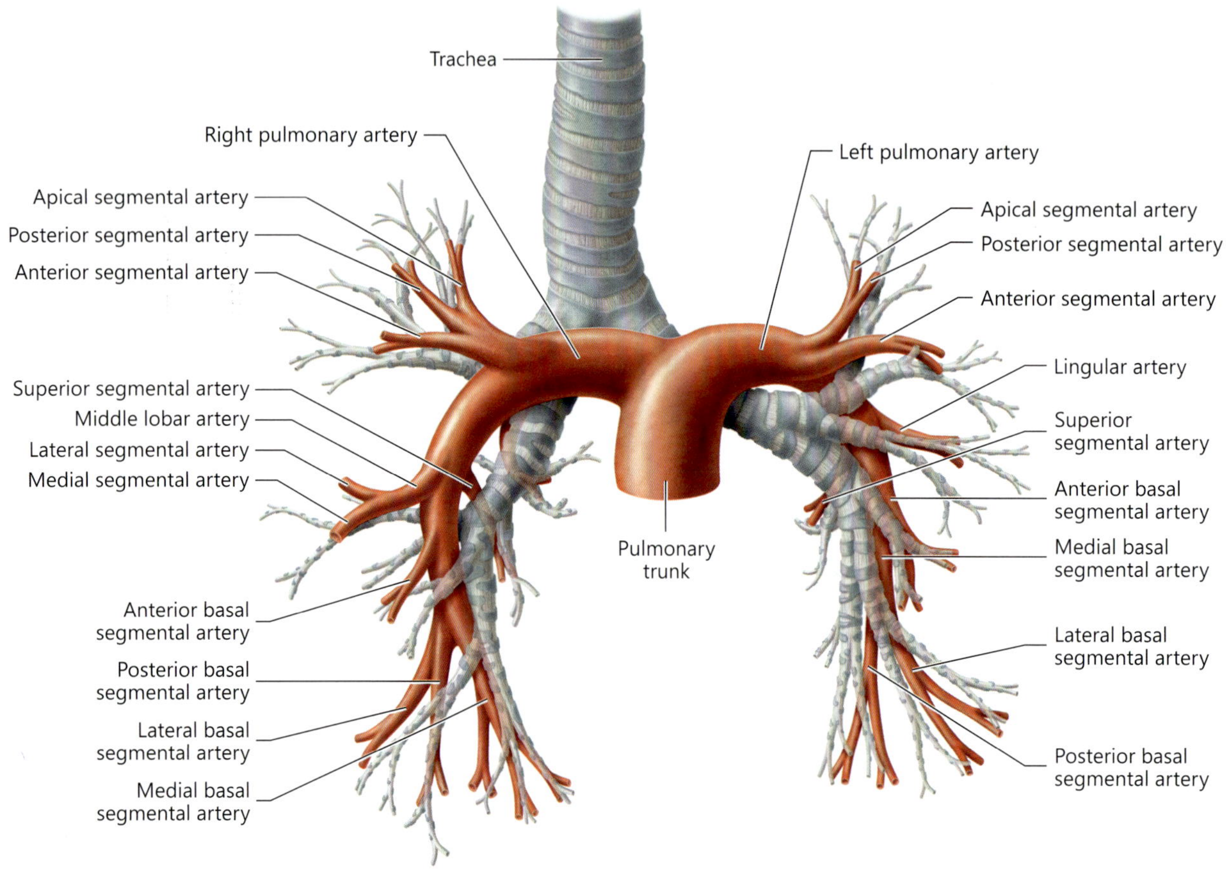

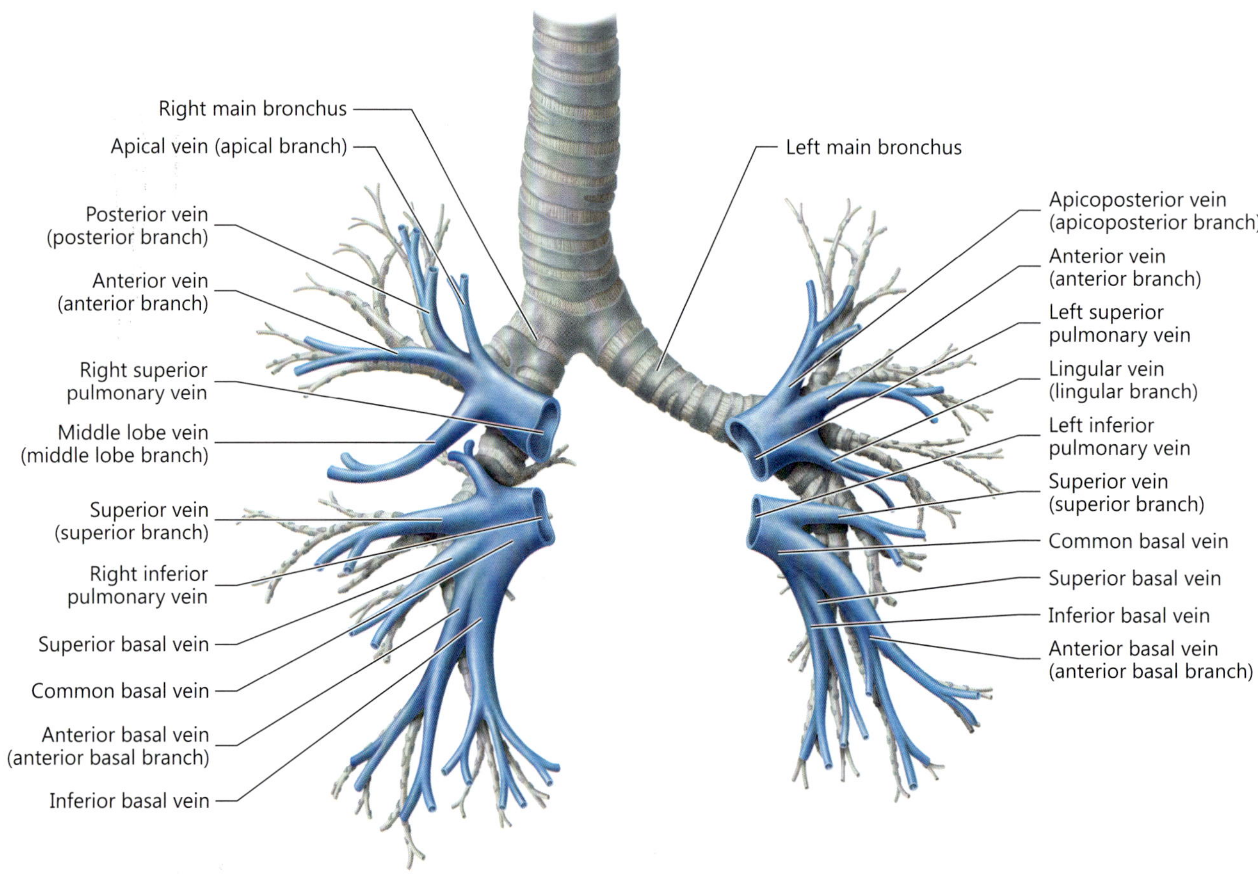

Frontal schematic view showing the relations between the principal vessels of the **pulmonary circulation** and the **trachea**. Above, pulmonary trunk and arteries. Below, pulmonary veins.

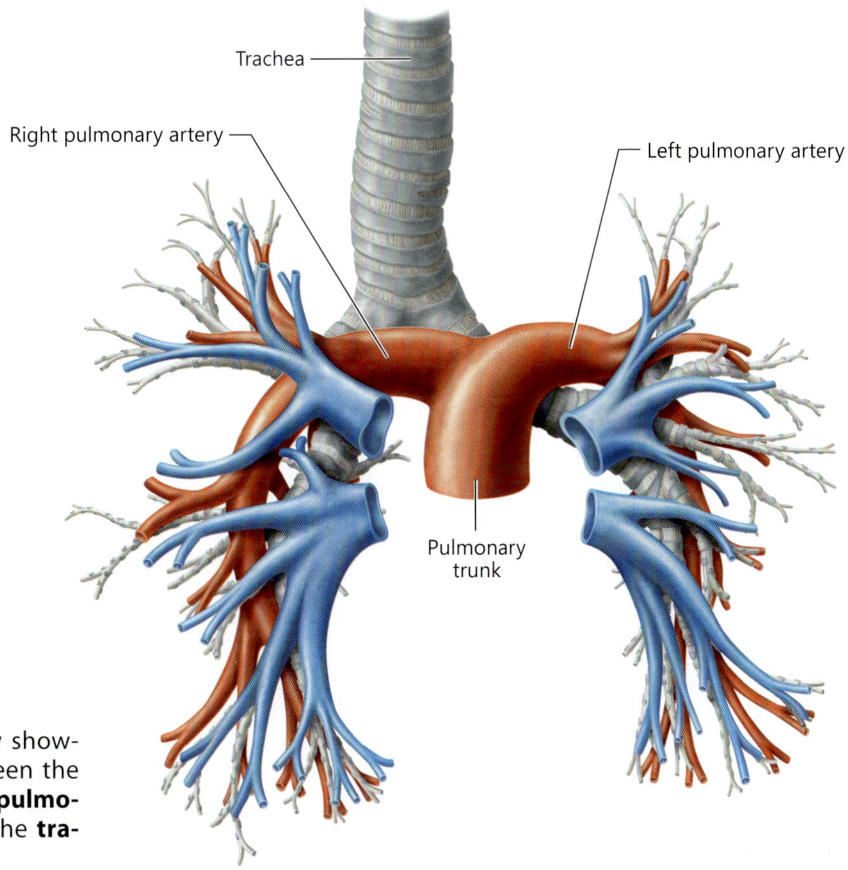

Frontal schematic view showing the relations between the principal vessels of the **pulmonary circulation** and the **trachea**.

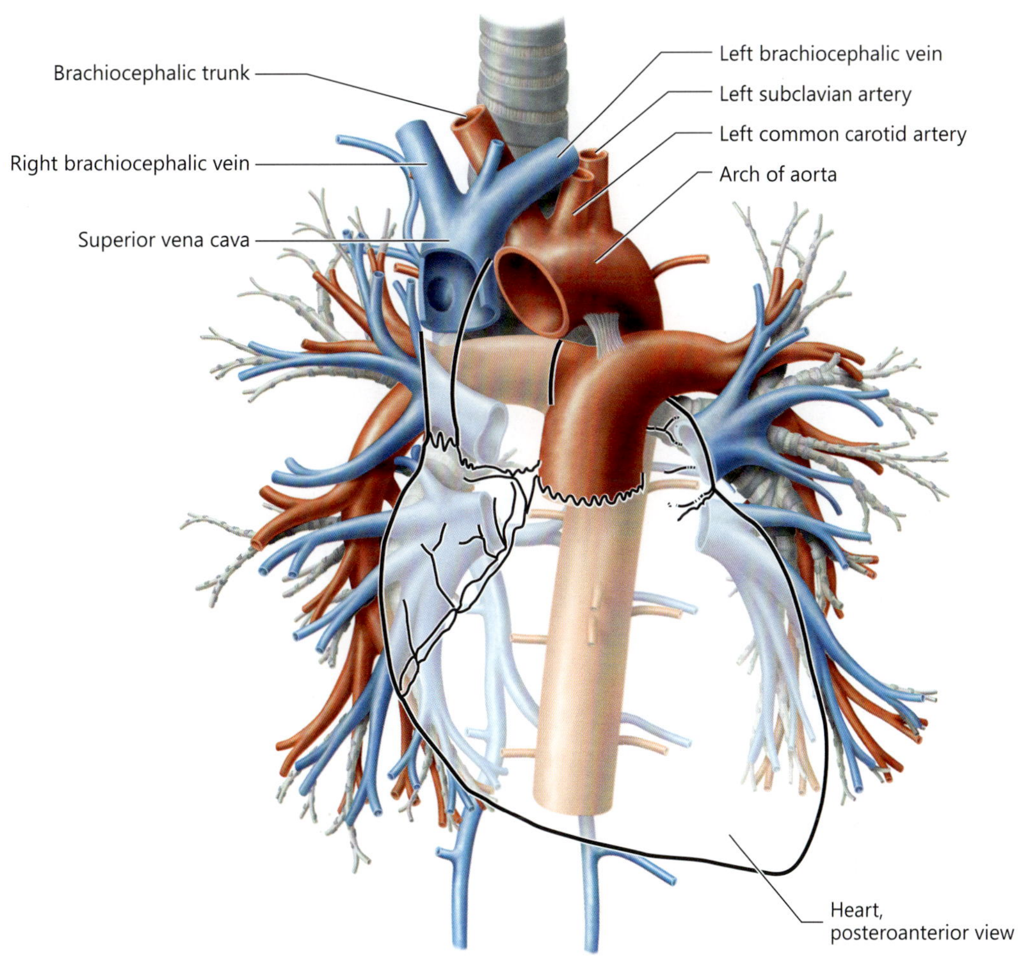

Frontal schematic view showing the relations between the principal vessels of the **large systemic circulation** and **pulmonary circulation**, and the **trachea**. The heart is drawn in transparency to highlight its relationship with the great vessels.

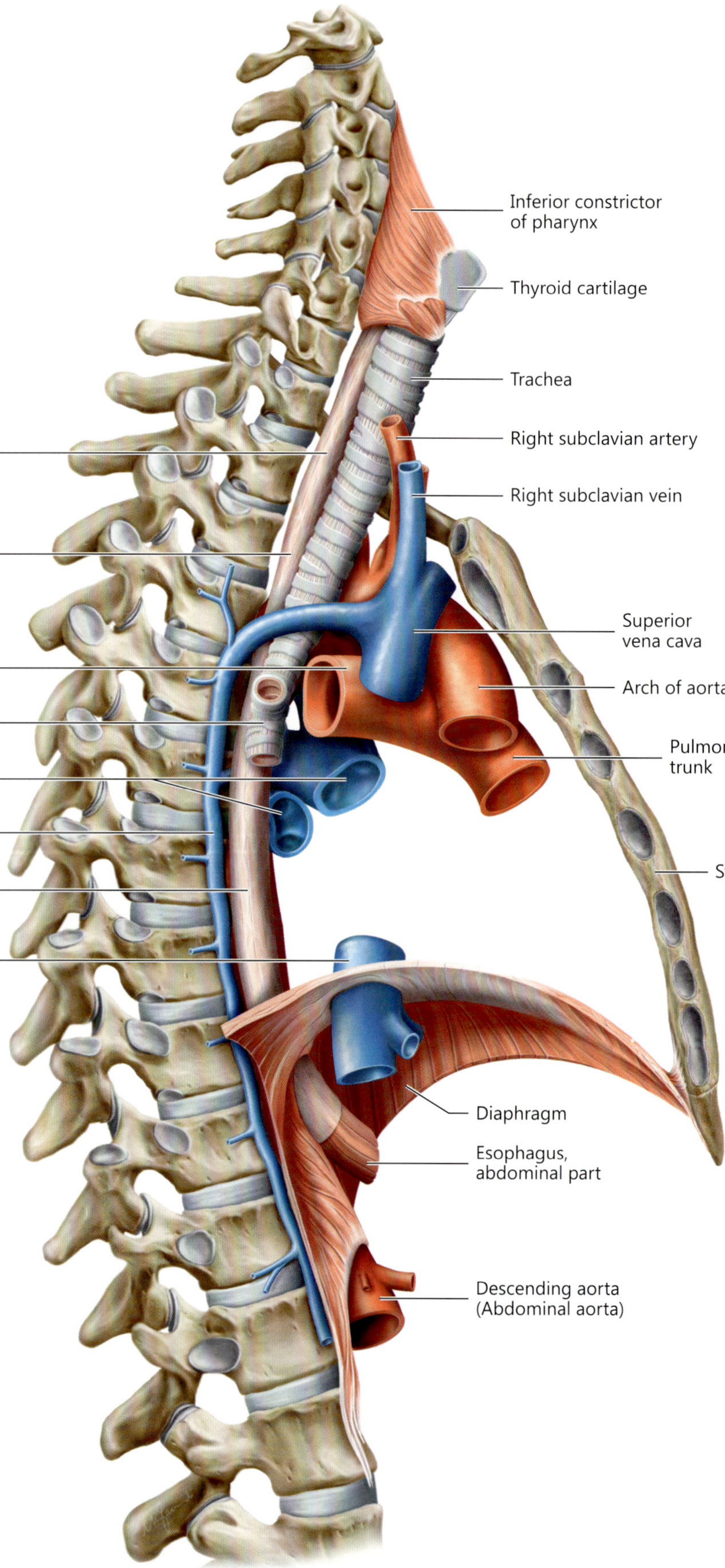

Schematic view showing the great vessels of the **large systemic circulation** and **pulmonary circulation** in relation to the **trachea** and **esophagus**. Right lateral projection.

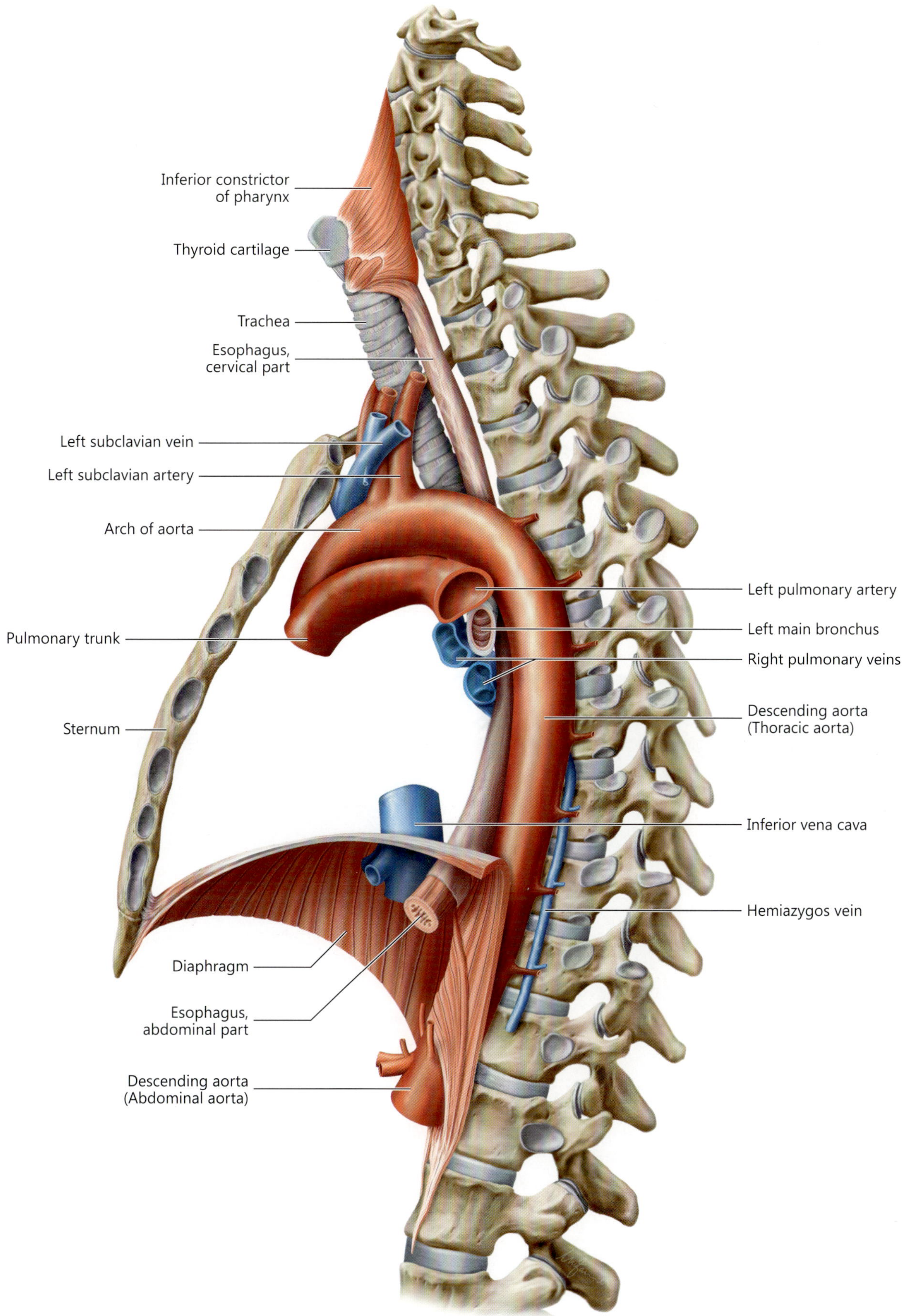

Schematic view showing the great vessels of the **large systemic circulation** and **pulmonary circulation** in relation to the **trachea** and **esophagus**. Left lateral projection.

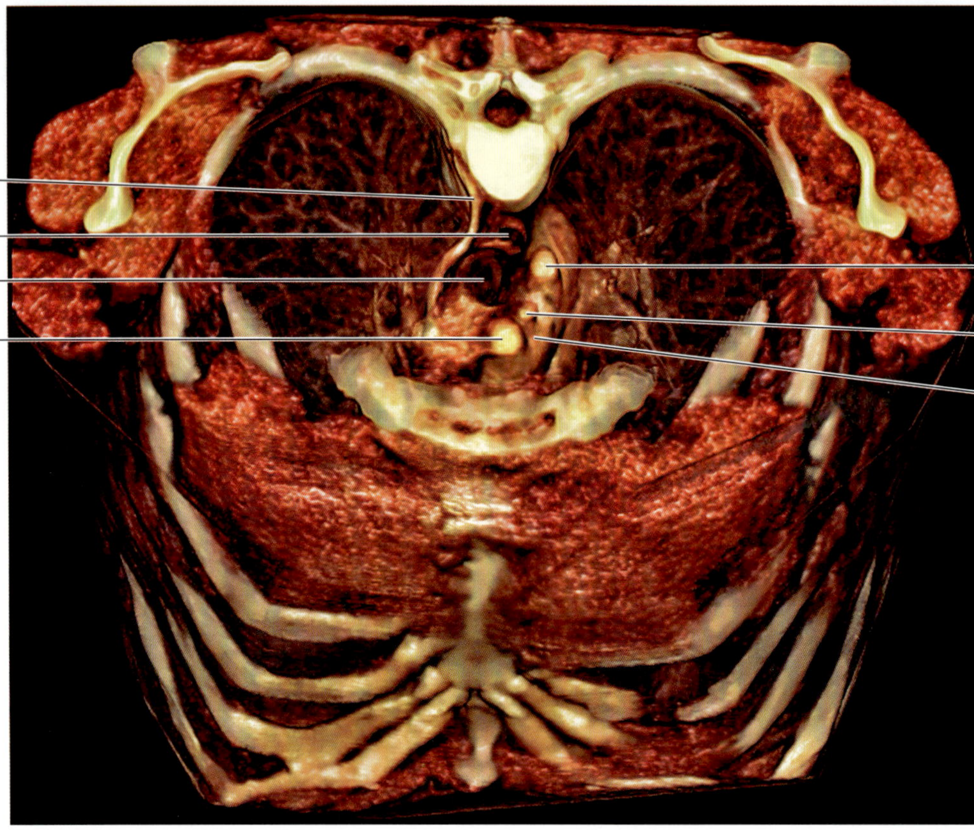

a

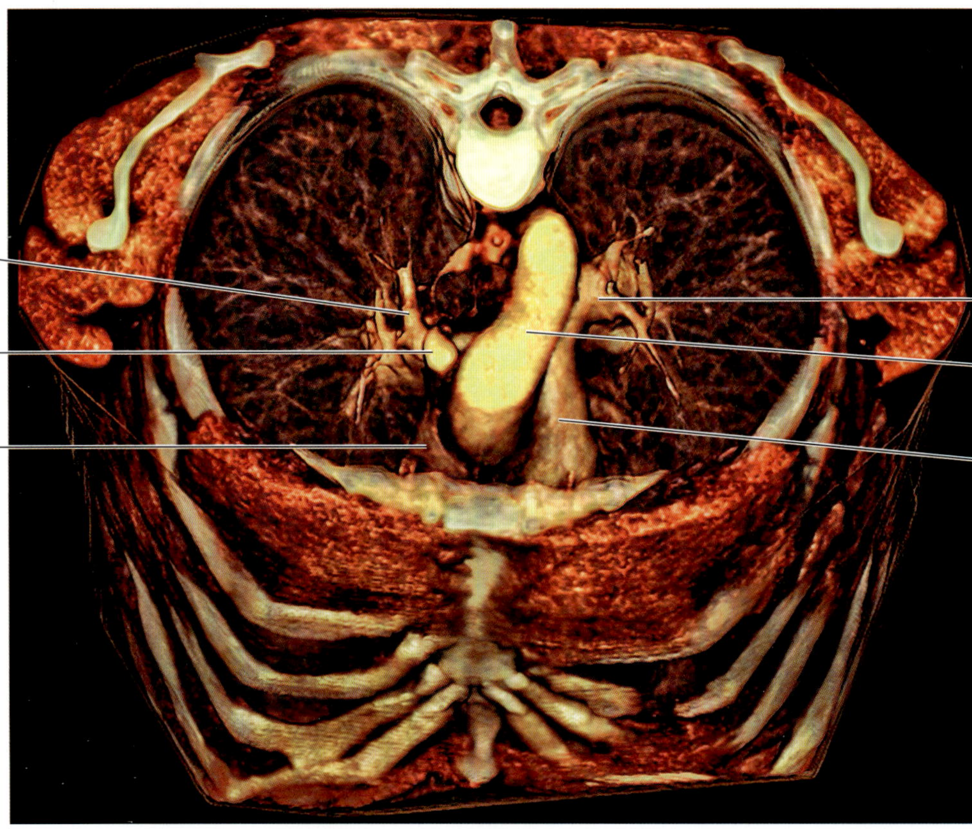

b

Series of four three-dimensional images of a living human body, obtained by CT scan using a 3D volume rendering technique, taken from transverse sections, in craniocaudal direction.

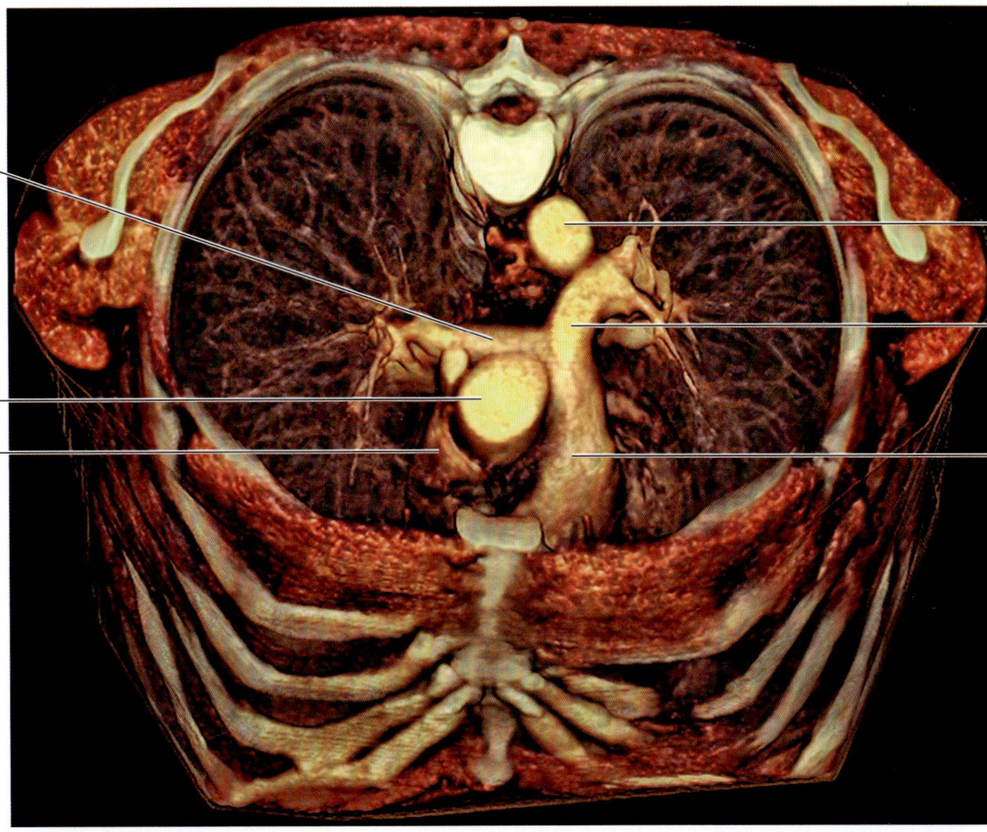

c

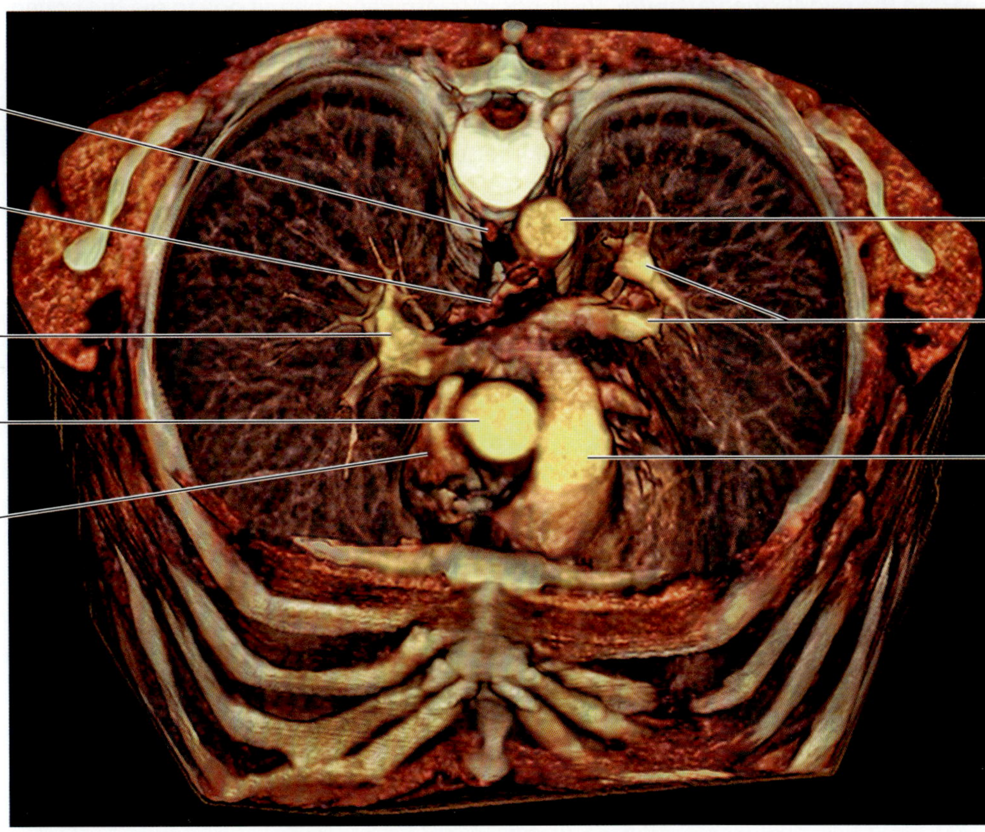

d

The sequence starts from the origin of the **collateral branches of the arch of the aorta** (**a**) and terminates at the origin of the **ascending aorta** from the aortic valve, in front, and the origin of the descending aorta (thoracic aorta), behind (**d**). The sequence shows the oblique orientation from front to back and from right to left of the arch (**b**), from its origin (right of the anterior median, or midsternal, line at the level of the 2nd sternocostal joint), to its termination on the left surface of T IV/T V (**c**). The arch of the aorta passes over the right pulmonary artery (**c**, **d**).

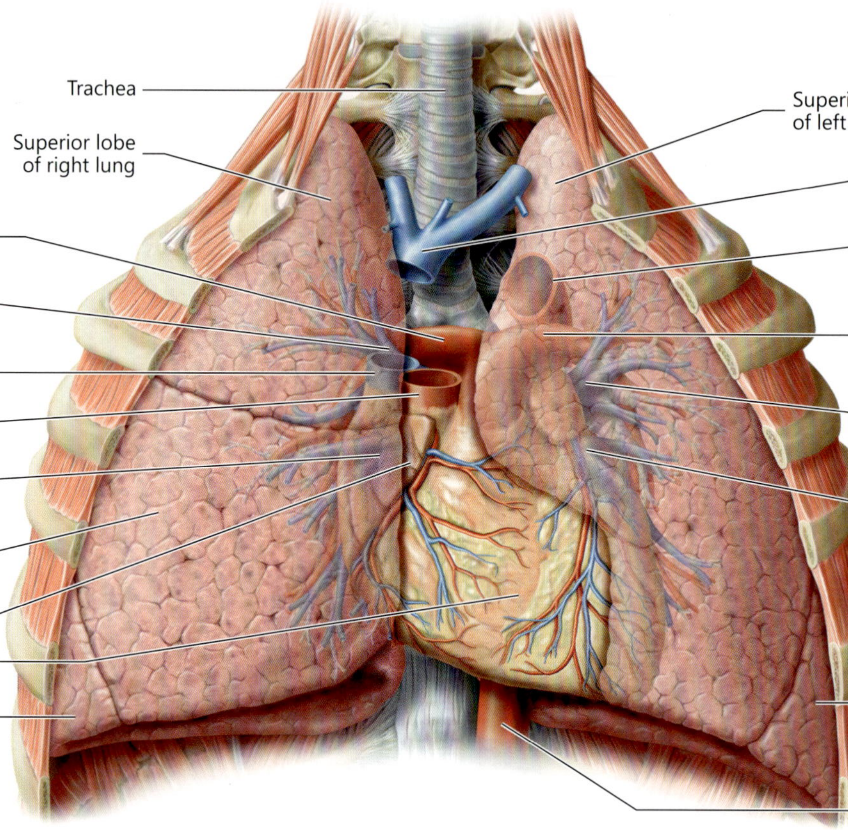

Position of the **heart in the middle mediastinum**. The lungs in transparency permit one to see the boundaries of the anterior surface of the heart (sternocostal surface). The apex is facing down and to the left. The heart, supported on the central tendon of the diaphragm, occupies most of the middle mediastinum, enveloped by the pericardial sac (not shown). The heart is situated between the 3rd and 6th costal cartilages, in front, and T V-T VIII, behind. Two-thirds of it extend to the left of the anterior median (midsternal) line, and one-third to its right. The anterior surface is partially covered by the anterior borders of the lungs and by the costomediastinal pleural recesses (not shown). The superior mediastinum contains the great vessels of the root of the heart.

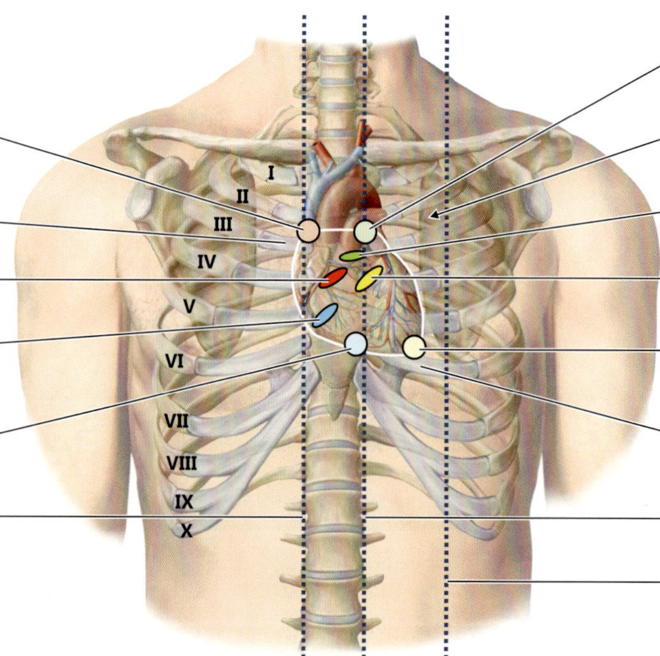

Boundaries of the projection of the heart on the thoracic cage (**surface projection of the heart**), with the projection of the heart valves and relative auscultation sites.

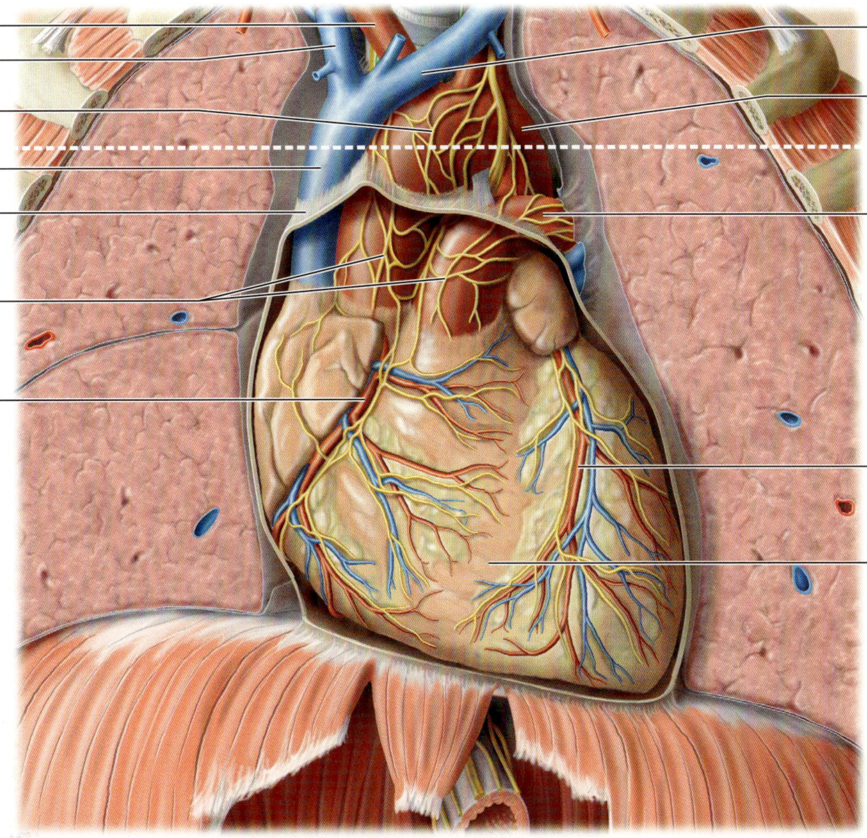

Position of the heart in the **middle mediastinum**. A close-up of the image on the page alongside.

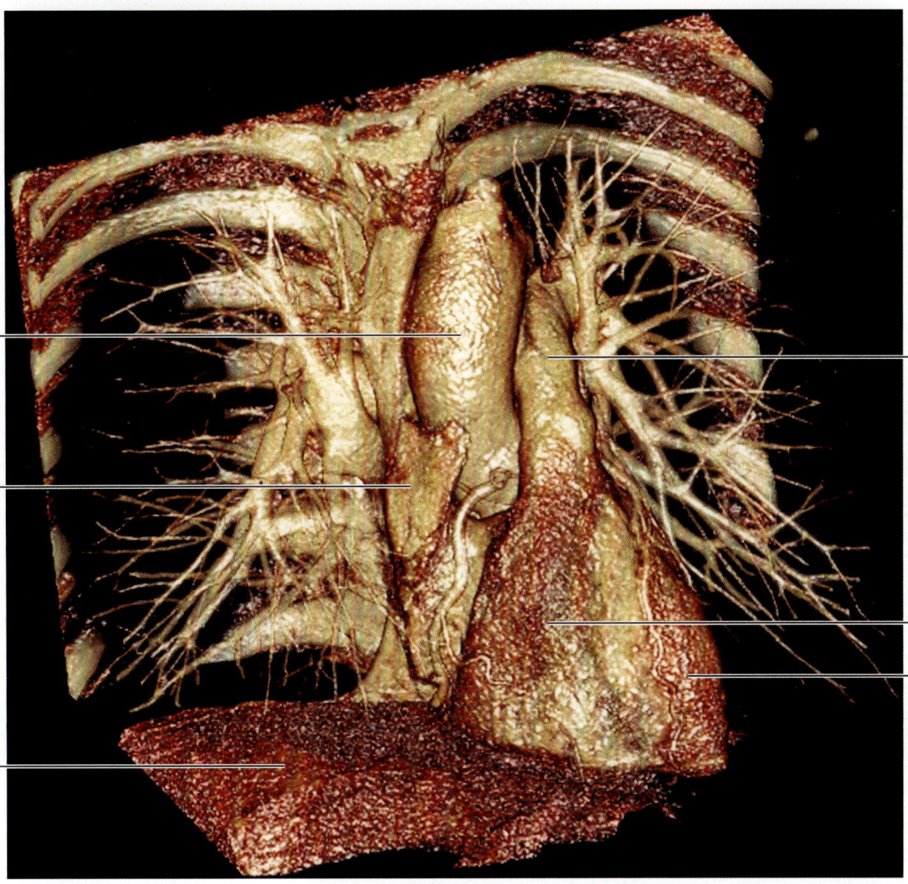

Three-dimensional image of a living human body, obtained by CT scan using a 3D volume rendering technique, showing the **heart**. One can see the ascending aorta, pulmonary trunk, bronchial tree and costal margin.

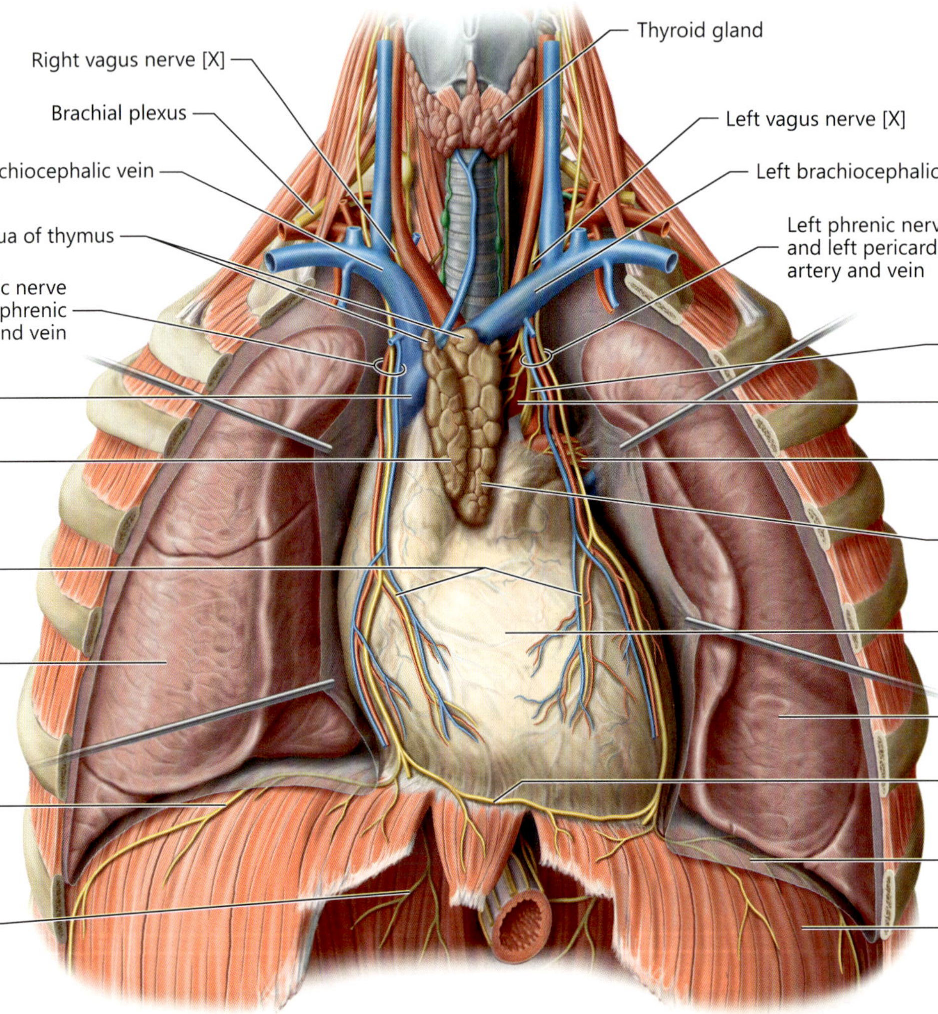

Position of the heart in the **middle mediastinum**. Pinning back the anterior borders of the lung and resecting the costomediastinal pleural recesses, one can see the pericardial sac and, between this and the mediastinal pleura on both sides, the pericardiacophrenic vessels and phrenic nerve. Situated in front are the middle and anterior mediastinal node chains. Before adult age, the point where the great vessels of the heart originate is in contact, in front, with the thymus. Successively, the thymus is replaced by fibroadipose tissue.

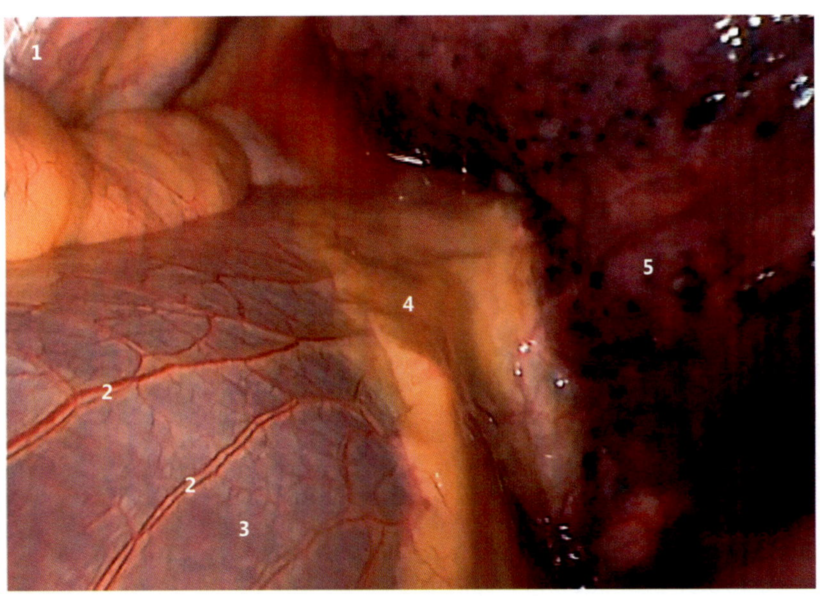

Image of the internal wall of the **thoracic cavity** obtained in the course of a diagnostic thoracoscopy. The endoscope is placed between the parietal and the visceral layers of the pleura. The view is from above. In the image, the lung has been moved aside and one can see the pericardium with the pericardial vessels.

1 Diaphragm
2 Pericardial branches of thoracic aorta
3 Pericardium
4 Pericardial fat
5 Lung

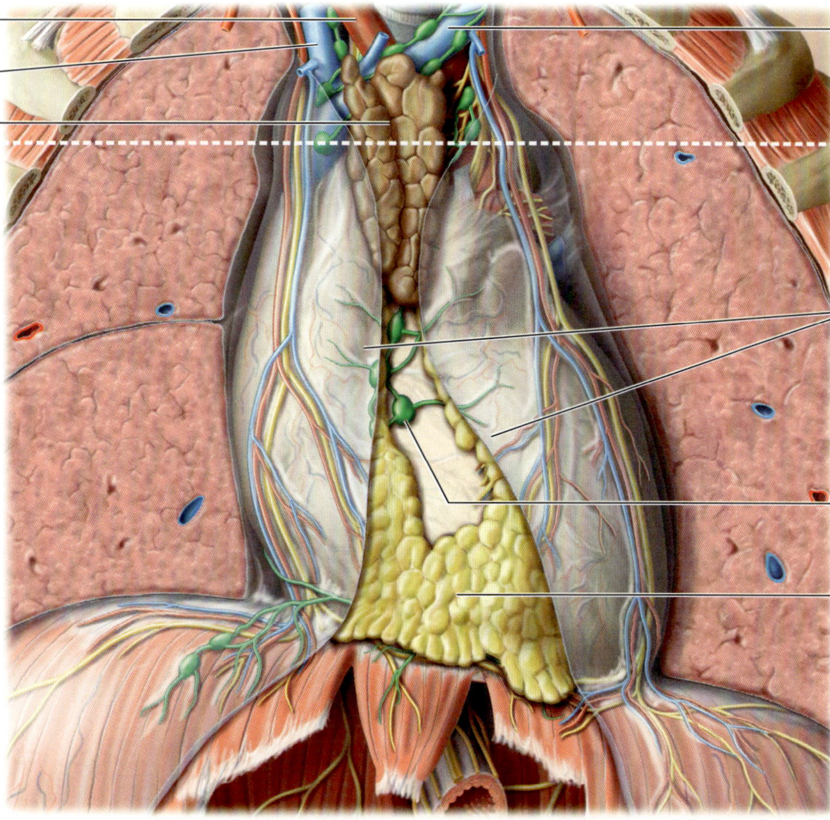

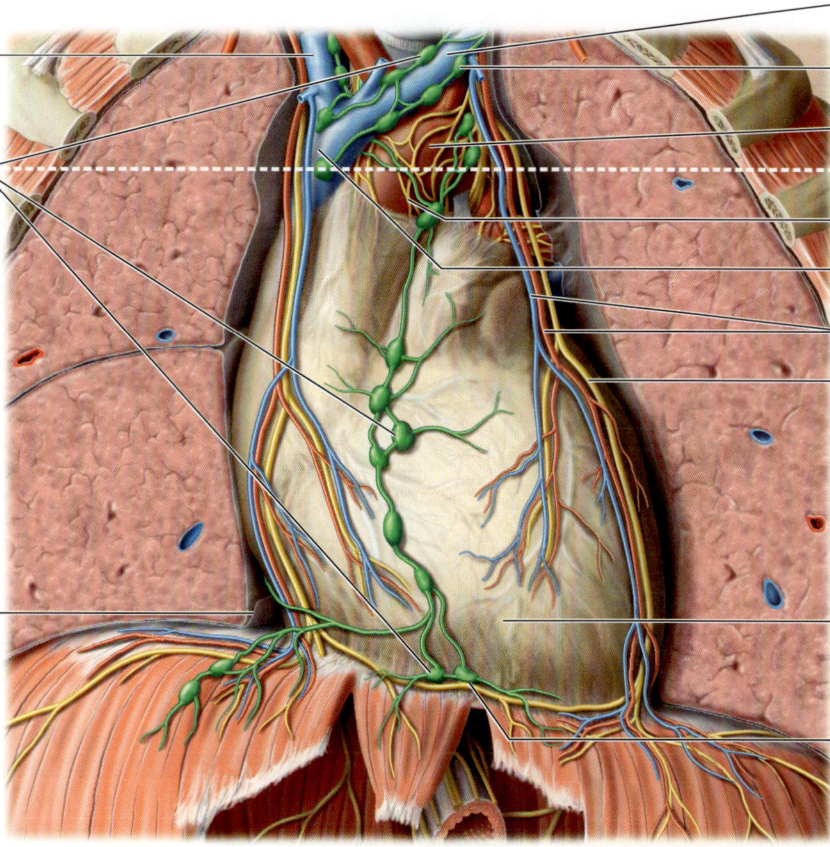

Representation of the **heart in situ**, in relation to the thymus gland and the mediastinal nodes.

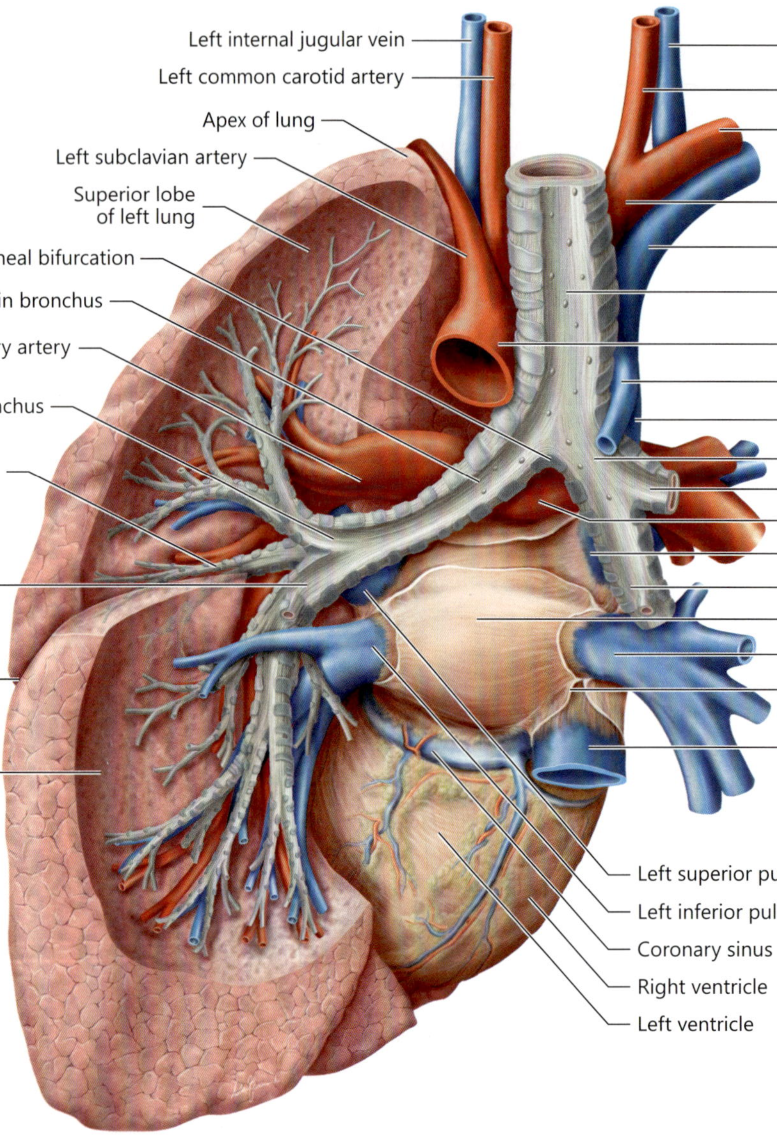

Position of the **heart in the middle mediastinum**, posterior view. The base of the heart faces upwards and to the right; the diaphragmatic or inferior surface, downwards and towards the back. The principal veins of the large and small circulation (the four pulmonary veins and the two venae cavae) arrive at the base of the heart. The vestibule (roof) of the left atrium represents the most posterior surface of the heart, in contact with the organs of the posterior mediastinum (esophagus and, further behind and to the left, the thoracic aorta, not shown).

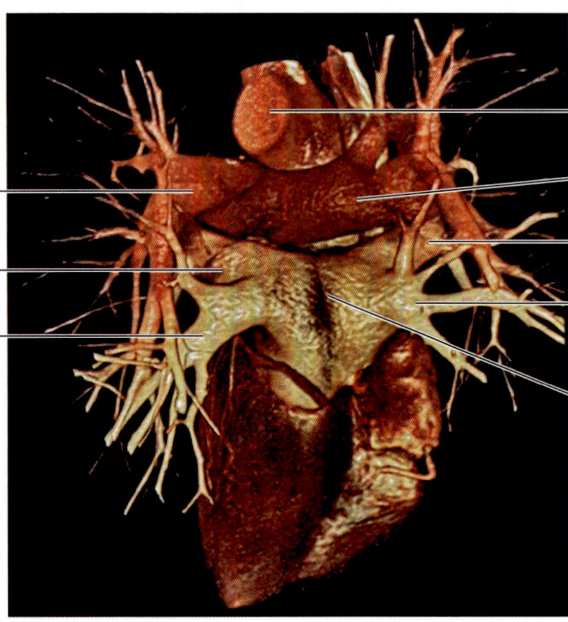

Three-dimensional image of a living human body, obtained by CT scan using a 3D volume rendering technique, taken from transverse sections, in craniocaudal direction, of the **heart**, posterior view. The projection is the same as that shown in the illustration above.

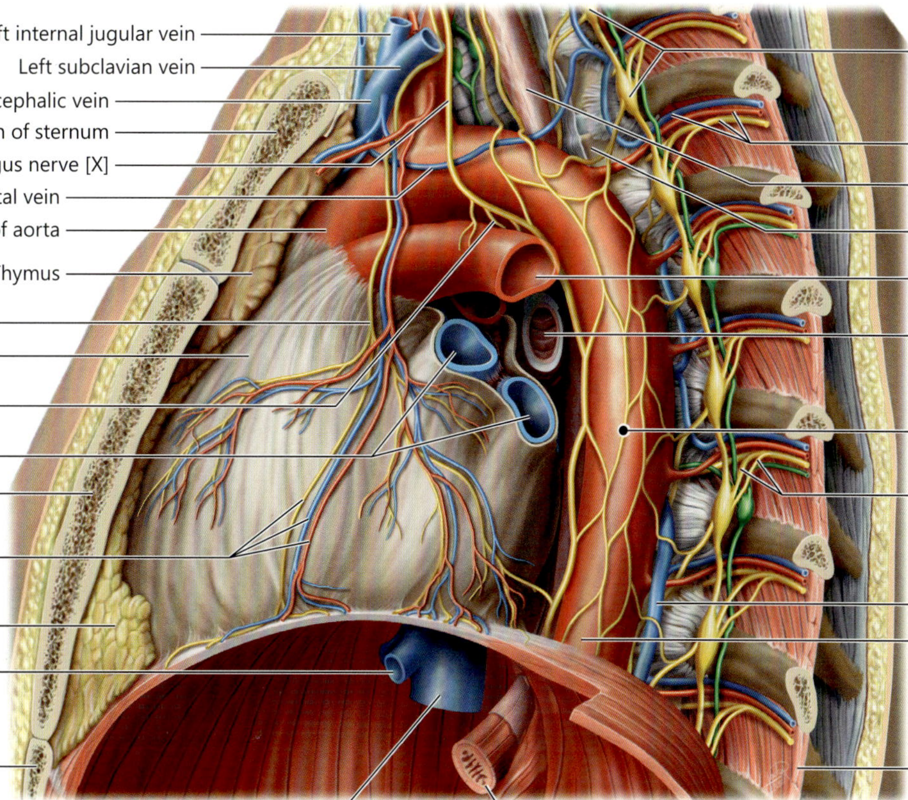

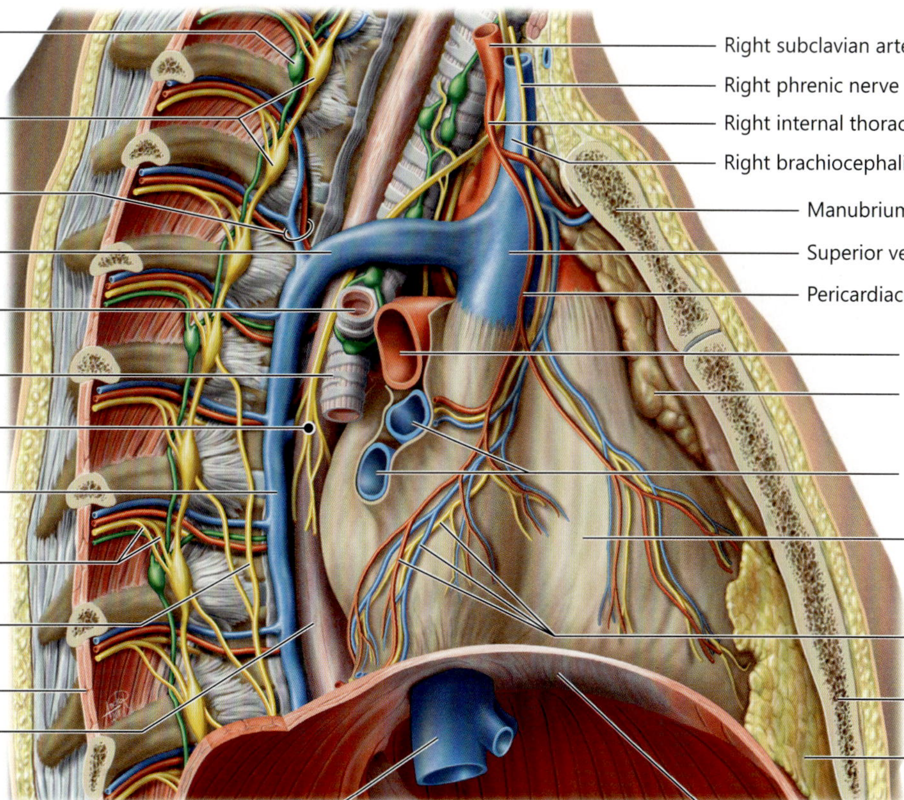

Left (above) and right (below) lateral view of the heart within the **pericardial sac**.

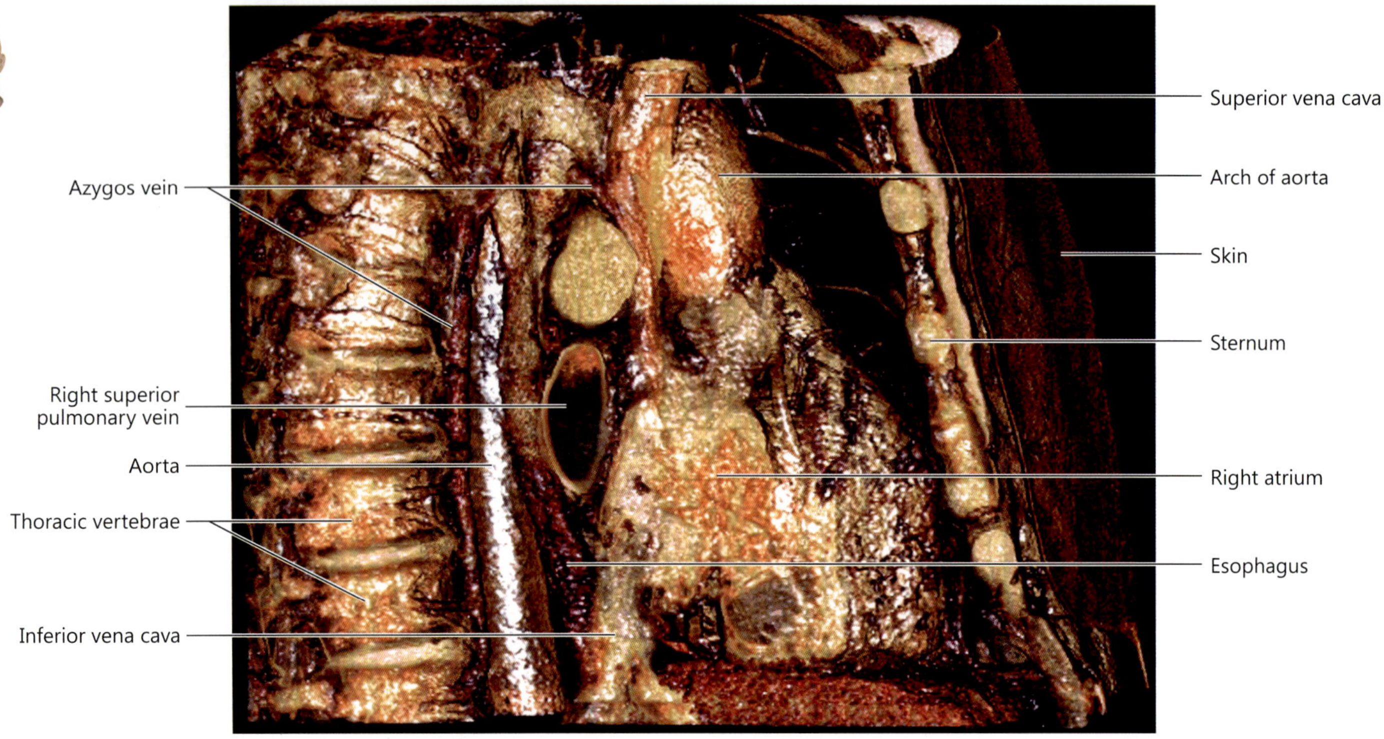

Three-dimensional image of a living human body, obtained by CT scan using a 3D volume rendering technique, taken from transverse sections, in craniocaudal direction, of the **mediastinum** observed from the right.

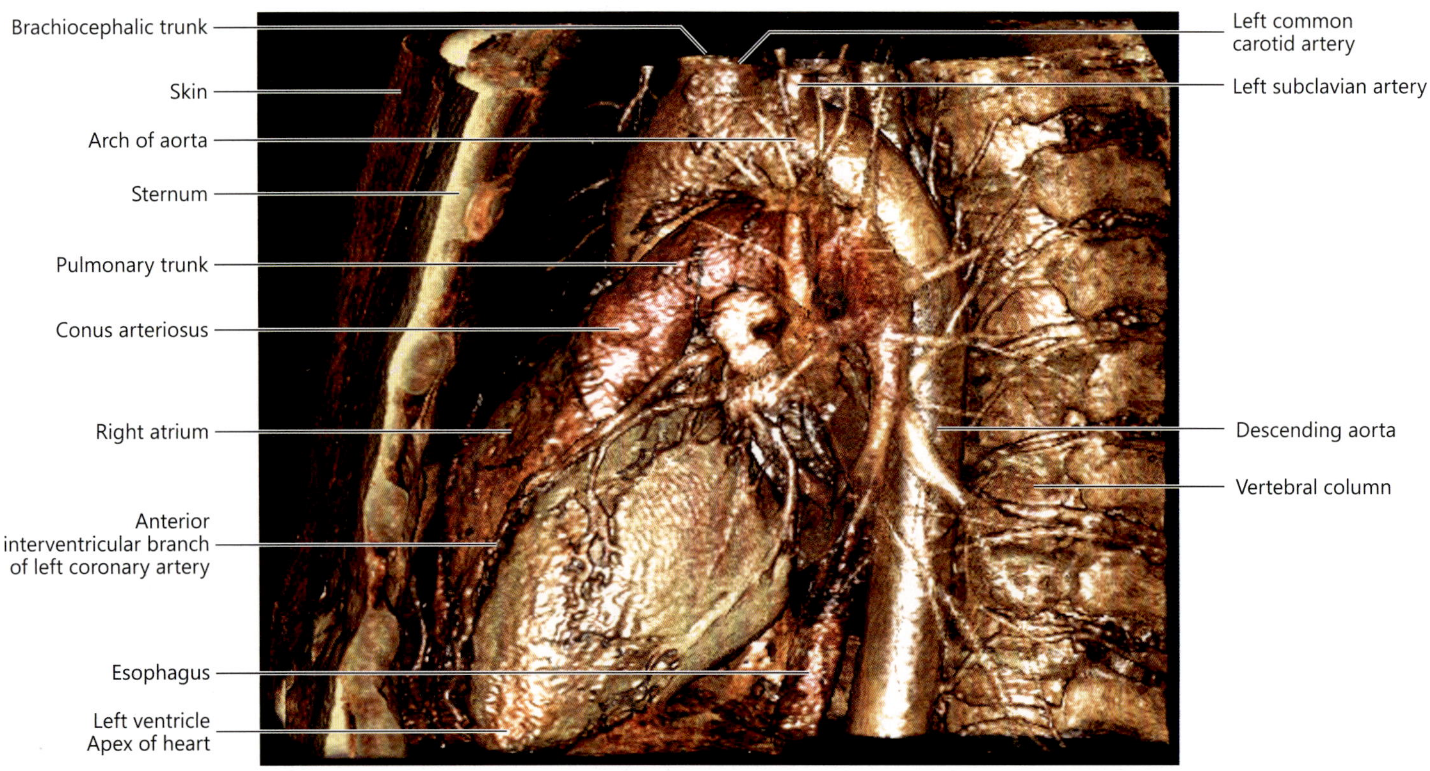

Three-dimensional image of a living human body, obtained by CT scan using a 3D volume rendering technique, taken from transverse sections, in craniocaudal direction, of the **mediastinum** observed from the left.

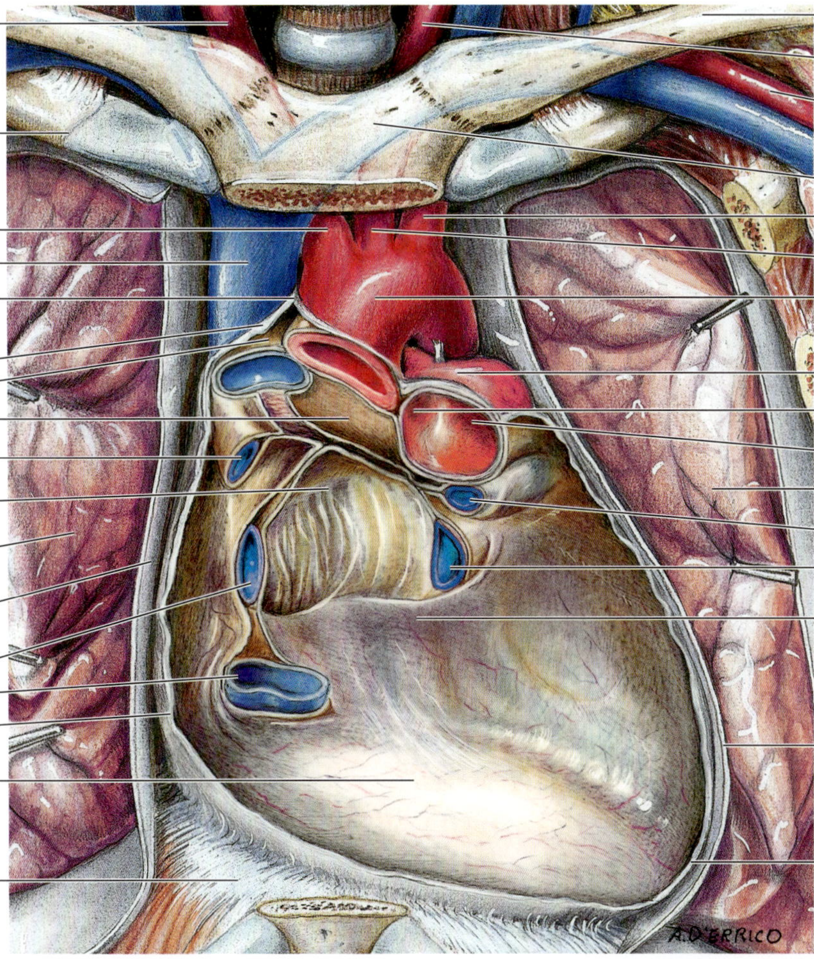

Pericardial sac after removal of the heart, anterior view. One can see the transverse pericardial sinus and oblique pericardial sinus.

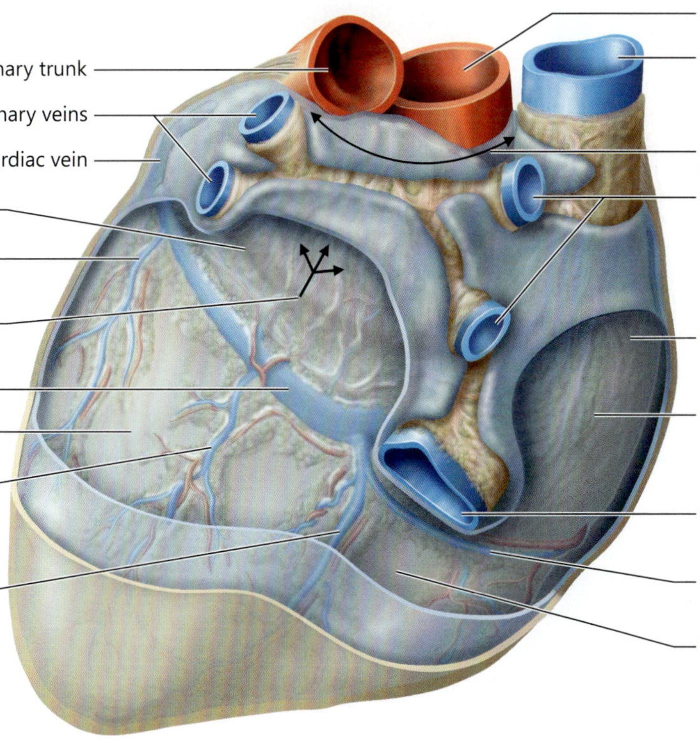

Reflection of the **visceral layer of serous pericardium** (epicardium) onto the parietal layer on the posterior wall of the heart. Arrows indicate the transverse pericardial sinus and oblique pericardial sinus.

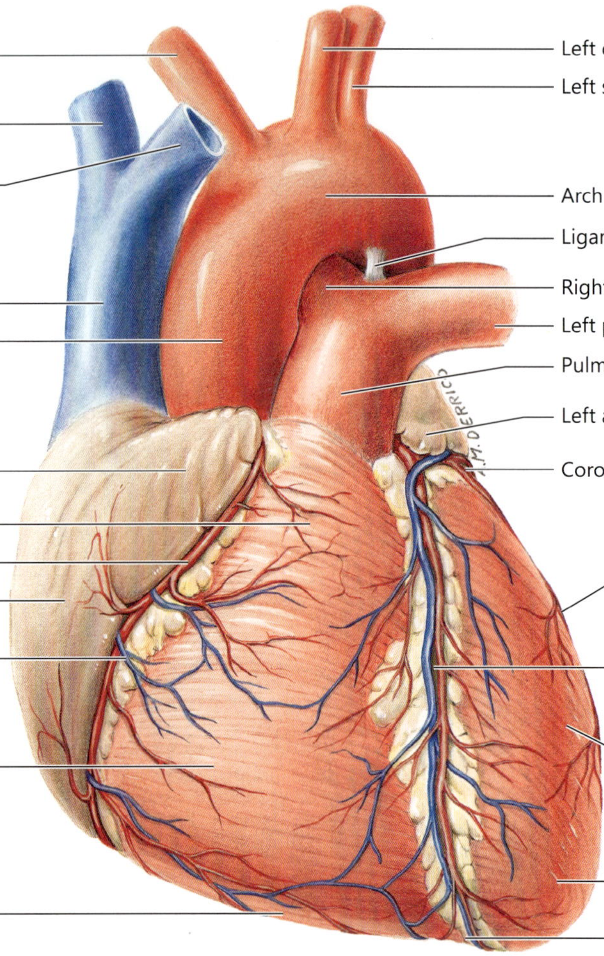

Anterior (sternocostal) surface of the heart.

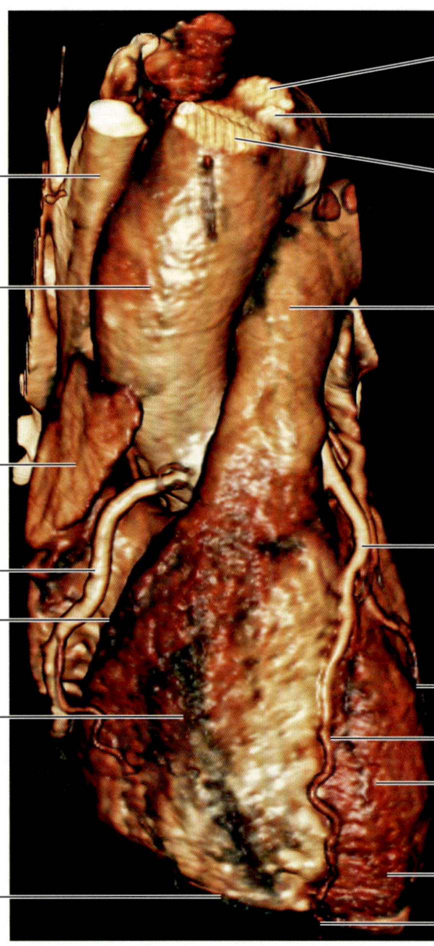

Three-dimensional image of a living human body, obtained by CT scan using a 3D volume rendering technique. **Anterior (sternocostal) surface** of the heart.

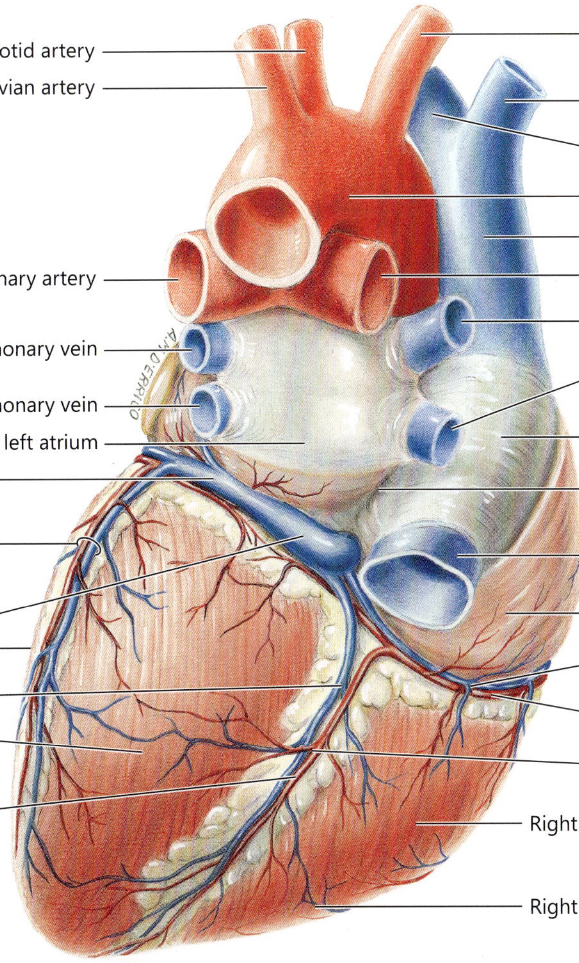

Diaphragmatic (inferior) surface of the heart.

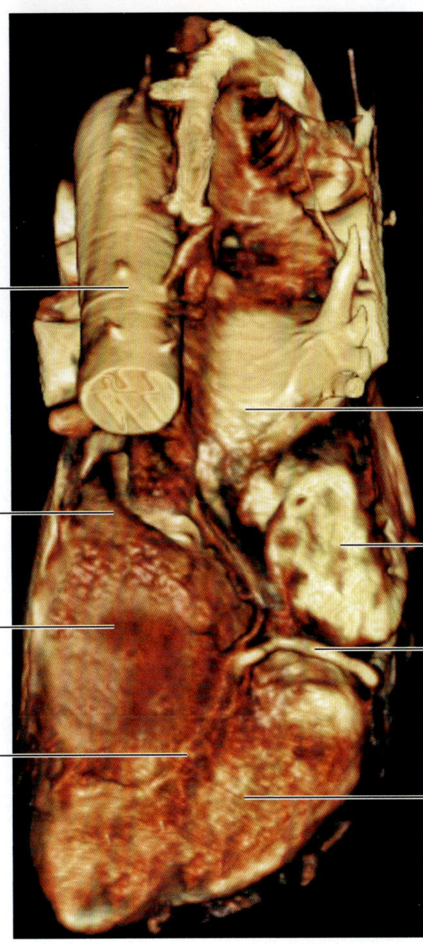

Three-dimensional image of a living human body, obtained by CT scan using a 3D volume rendering technique. **Diaphragmatic (inferior) surface** of the heart.

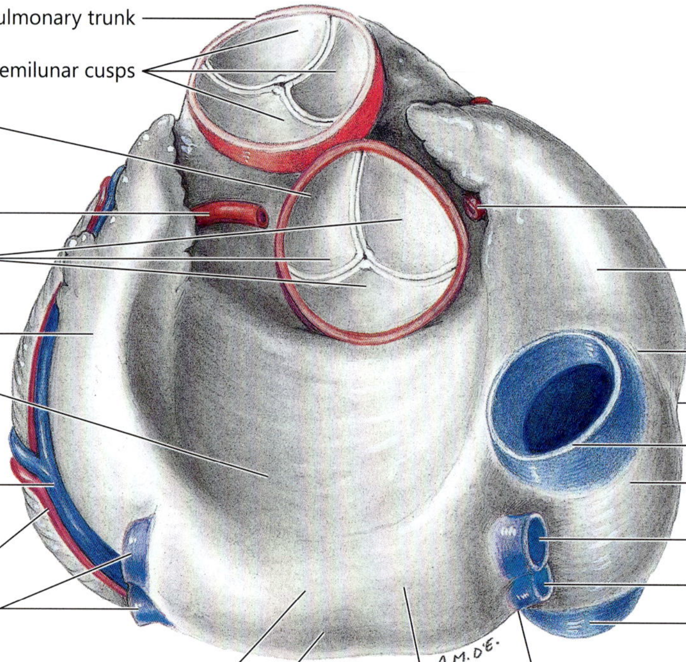

Base of the heart, viewed from above, after resection of the pulmonary trunk and aorta.

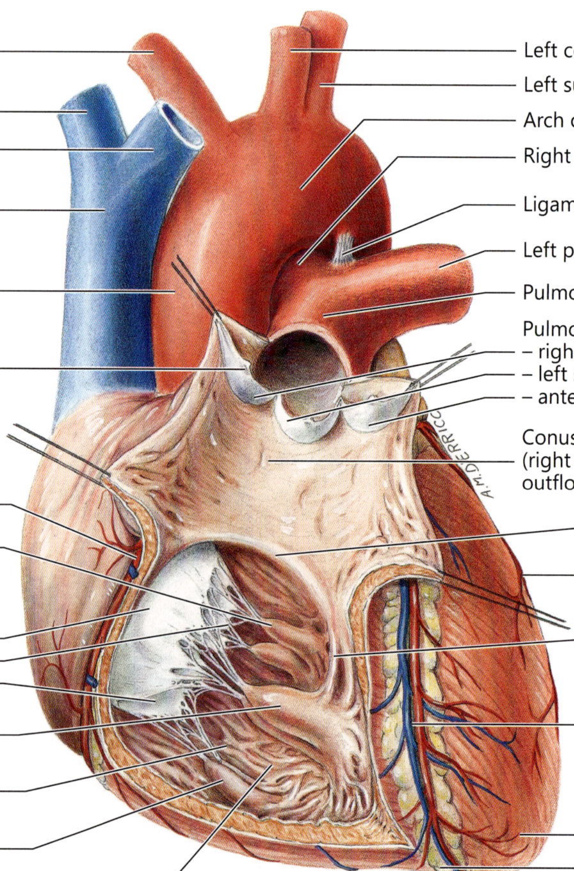

Cavity of the right ventricle, viewed from the front, after partial removal of the anterior wall. The conus arteriosus, open, highlights the valve.

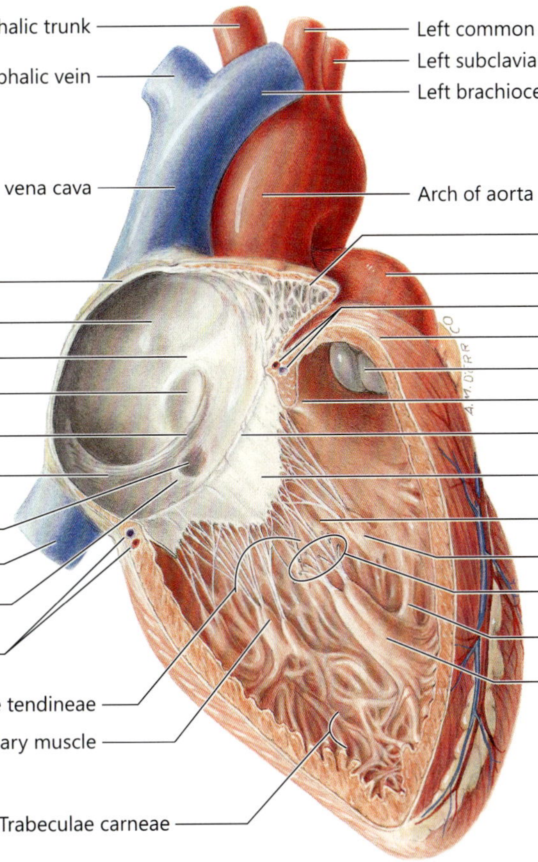

Cavities of the right ventricle and atrium, viewed from the right, after removal of the lateral wall of the sinus of the venae cavae, of the right auricle, and of the right (acute) margin of the heart.

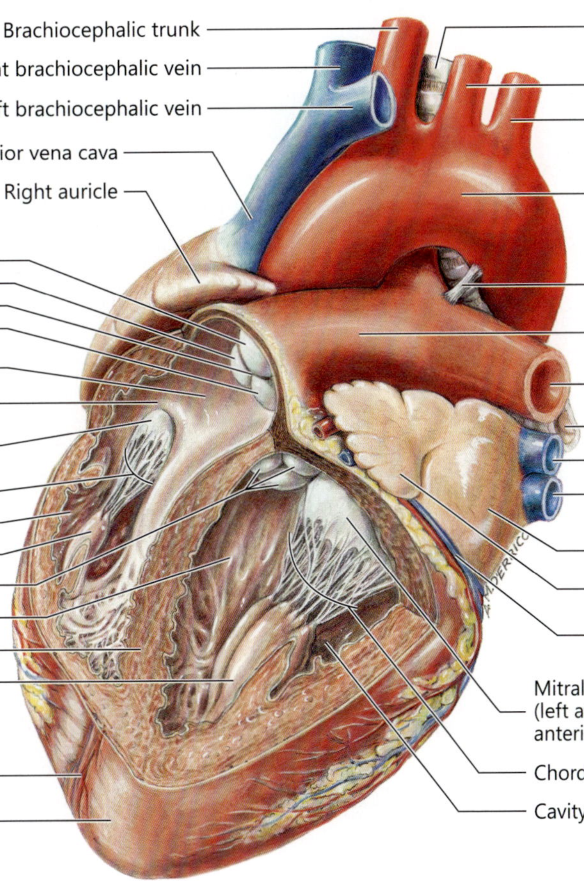

Cavities of the ventricles, viewed from the front and left, after partial removal of the anterior wall.

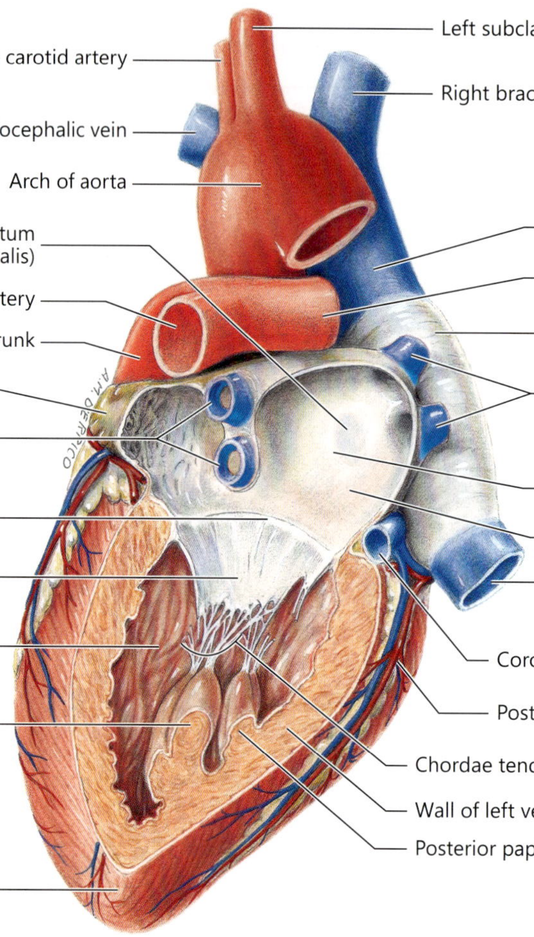

Left atrium and ventricle, viewed from the left, after removal of part of the auricle and of the left (obtuse) margin.

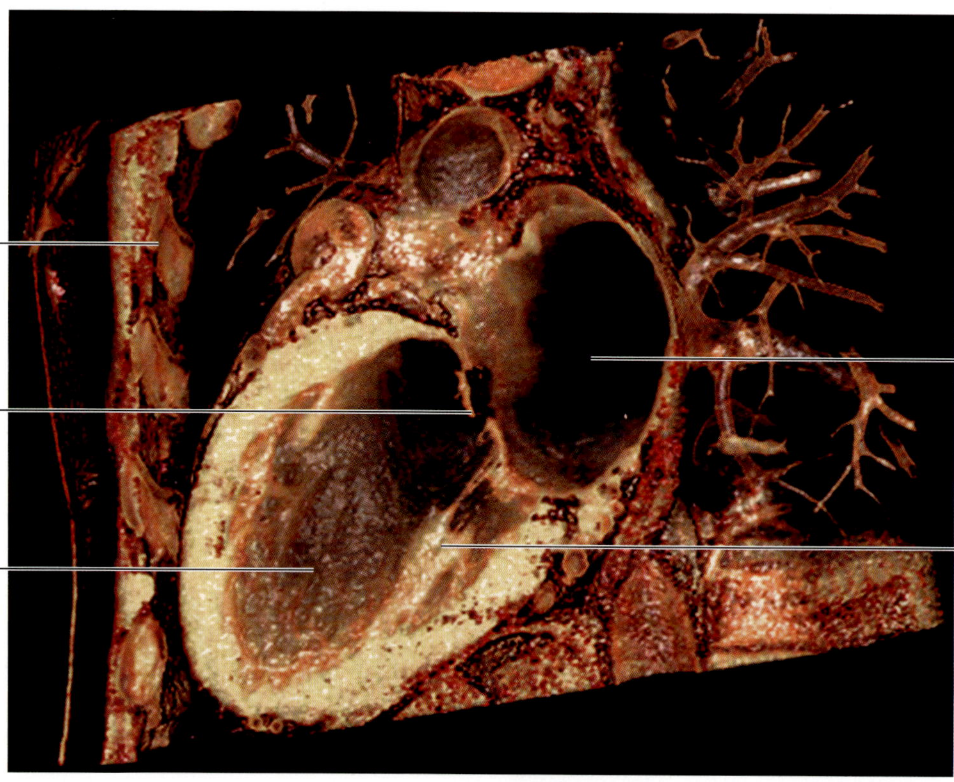

Three-dimensional image of a living human body, obtained by CT scan using a 3D volume rendering technique. **Cavities of the left atrium and ventricle**.

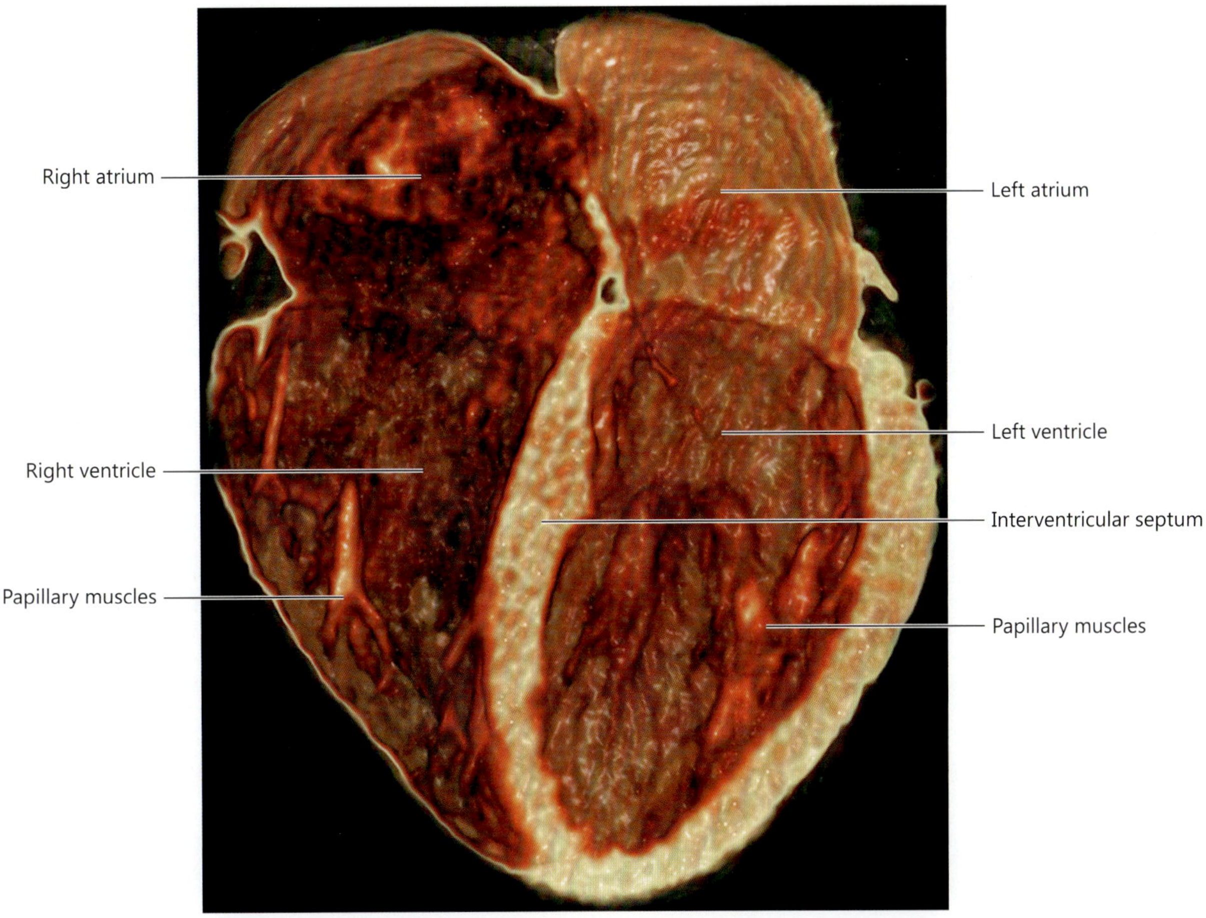

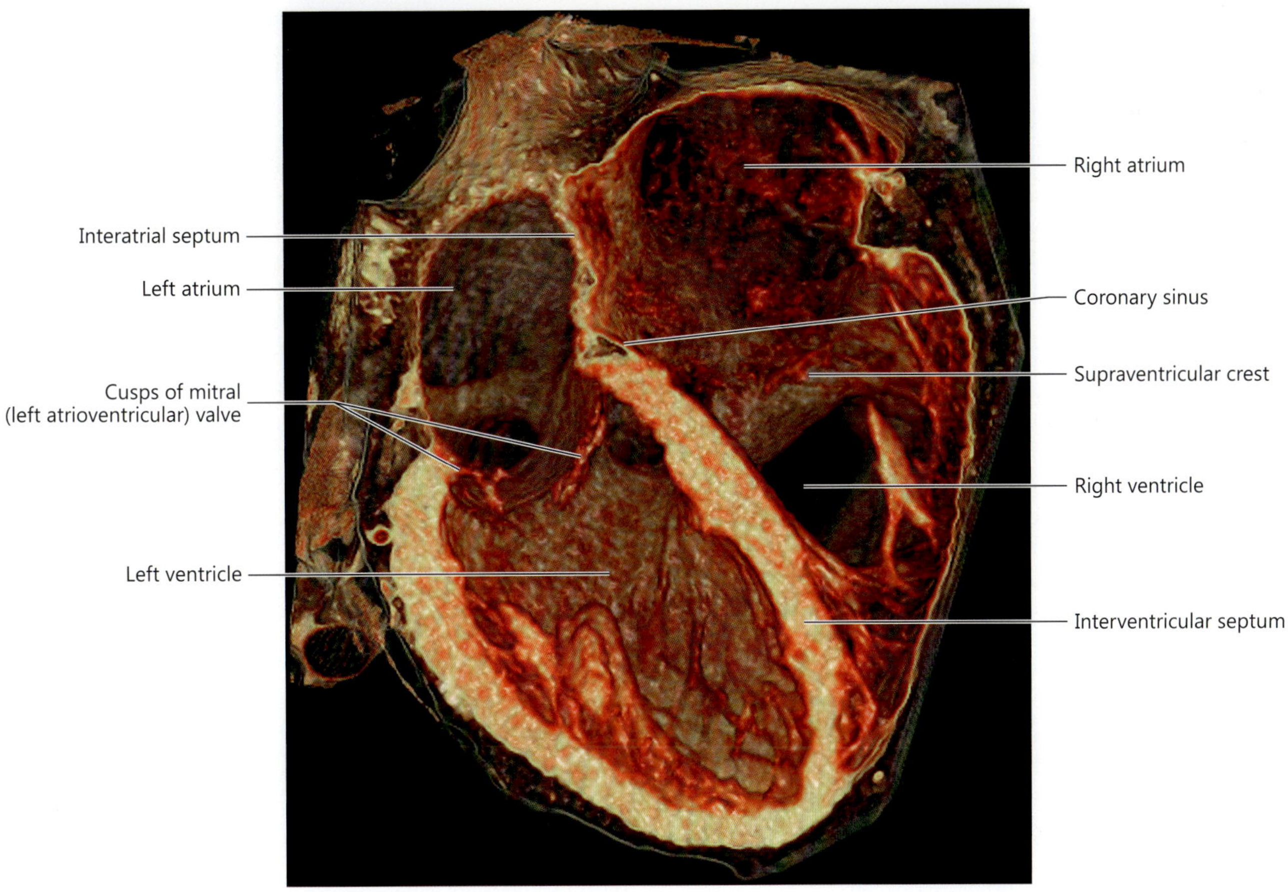

Three-dimensional image of a living human body, obtained by CT scan using a 3D volume rendering technique. **Atrial and ventricular cavities**. Above, view from the anterior (sternocostal) surface. Below, view from the diaphragmatic (inferior) surface.

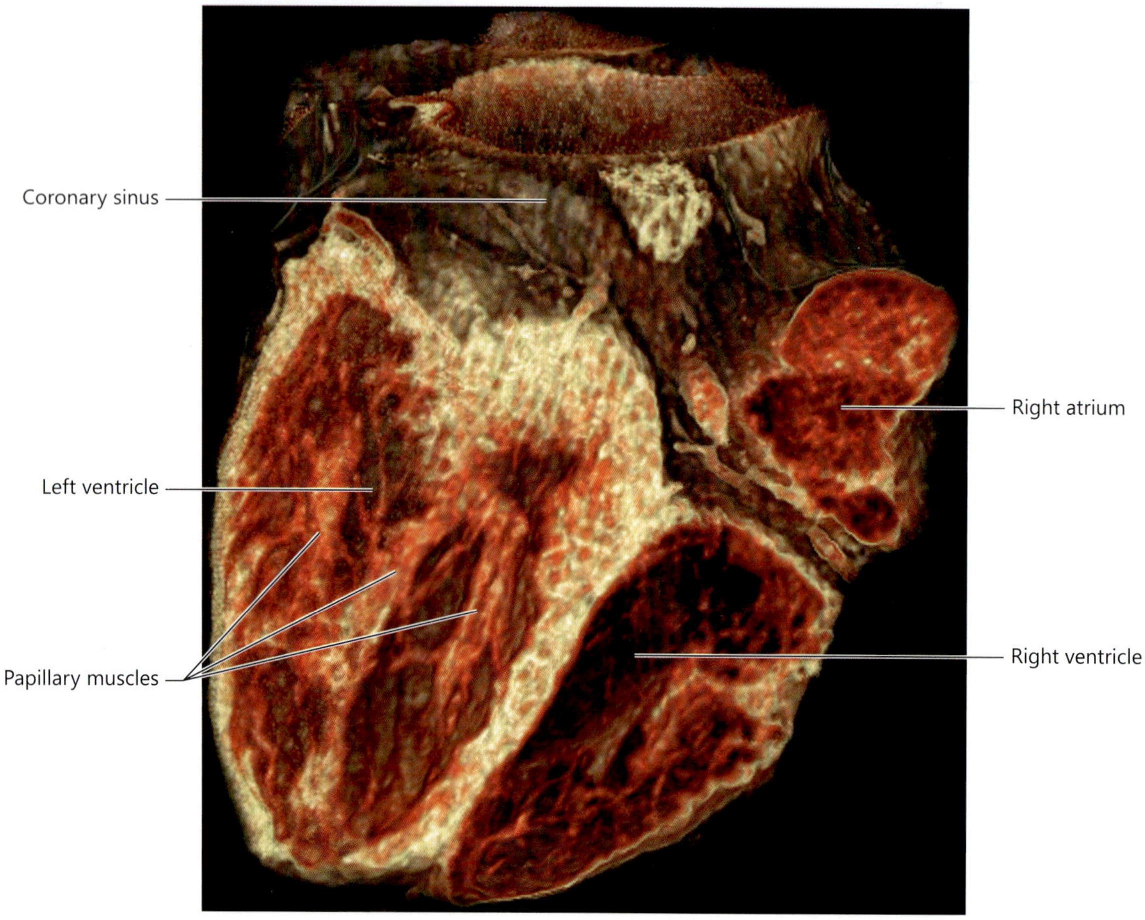

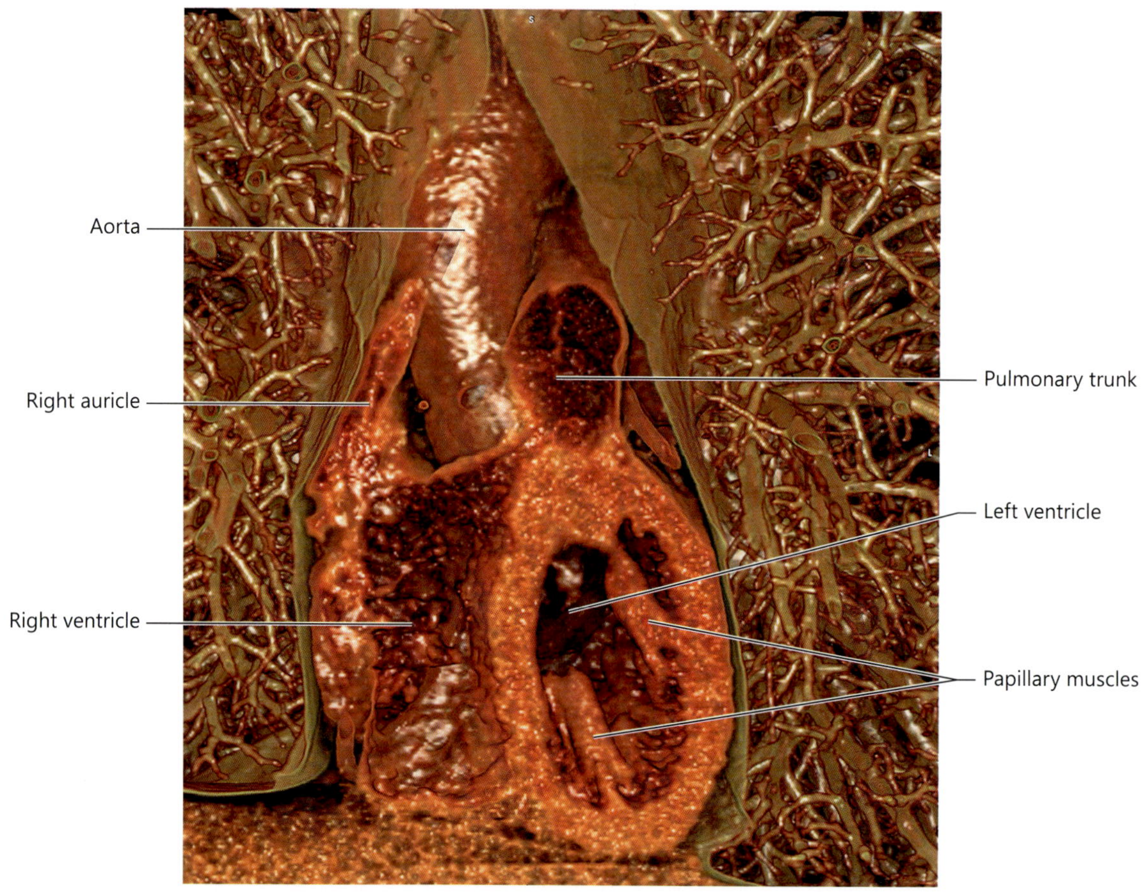

Three-dimensional image of a living human body, obtained by CT scan using a 3D volume rendering technique. **Atrial and ventricular cavities**. Above, view from the diaphragmatic (inferior) surface. Below, anterior view.

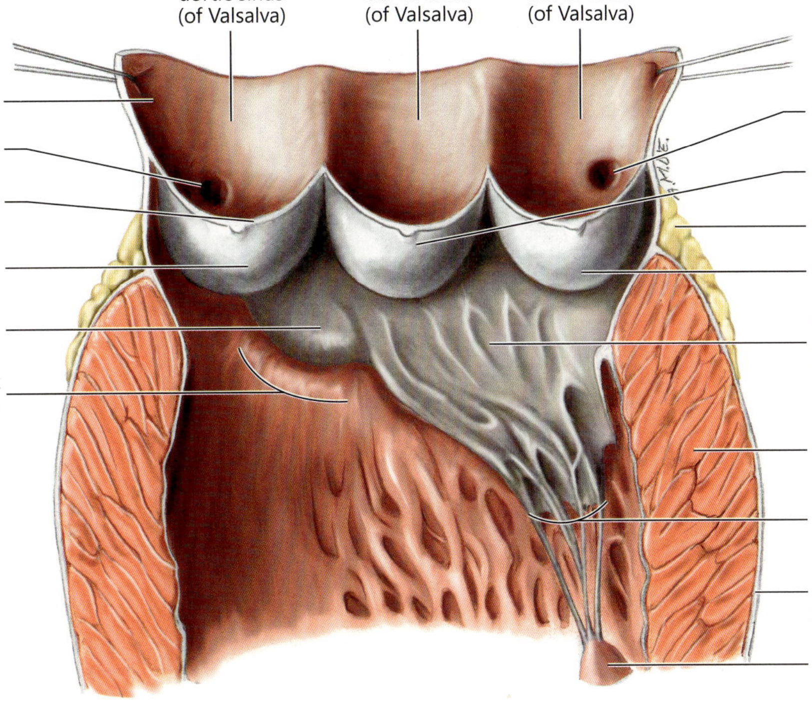

Section of the left ventricle, at the level of the aortic valve, corresponding to the areas inside the box in the figures on the following page. The aortic orifice has been resected and opened. One can see the **cusps of the aortic valve**. At the level of the right and left cusps, the orifices of the coronary arteries open. The membranous part of the interventricular septum extends in between the right and posterior cusps.

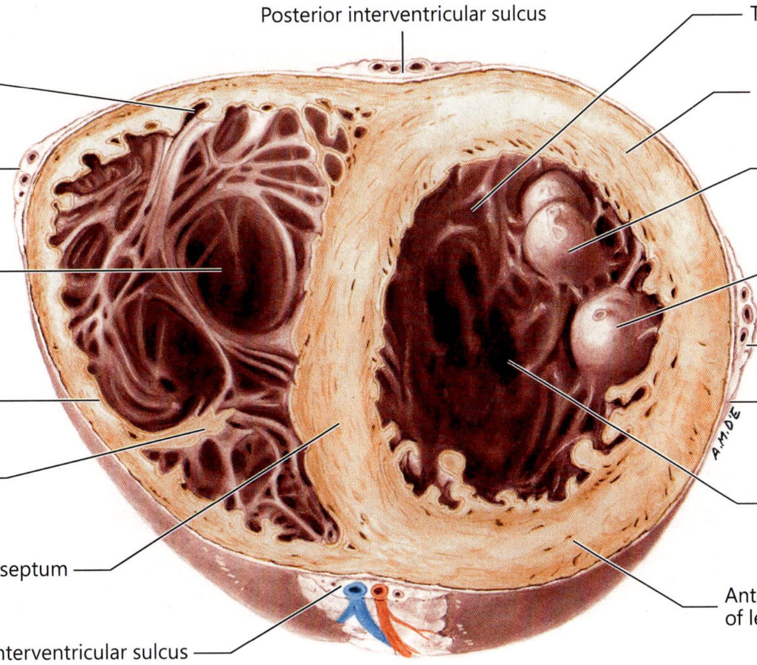

Transverse section of the ventricular part of the heart. Note the different thickness of the **ventricular walls**.

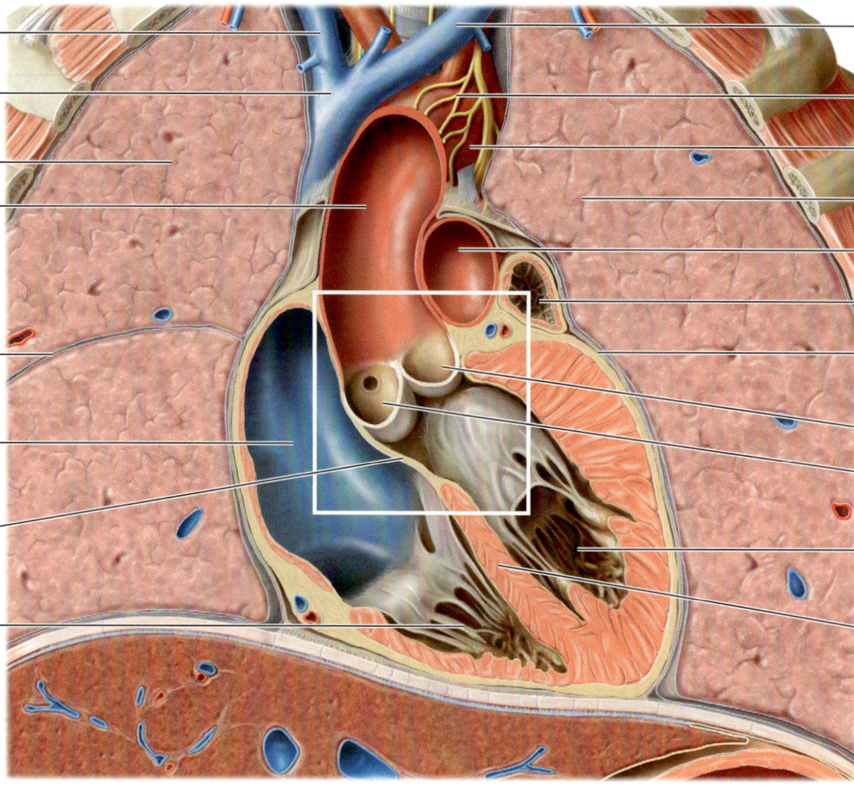

Heart in situ. Frontal section passing through the **aortic valve**. The region in the box corresponds to the area highlighted in the figure below.

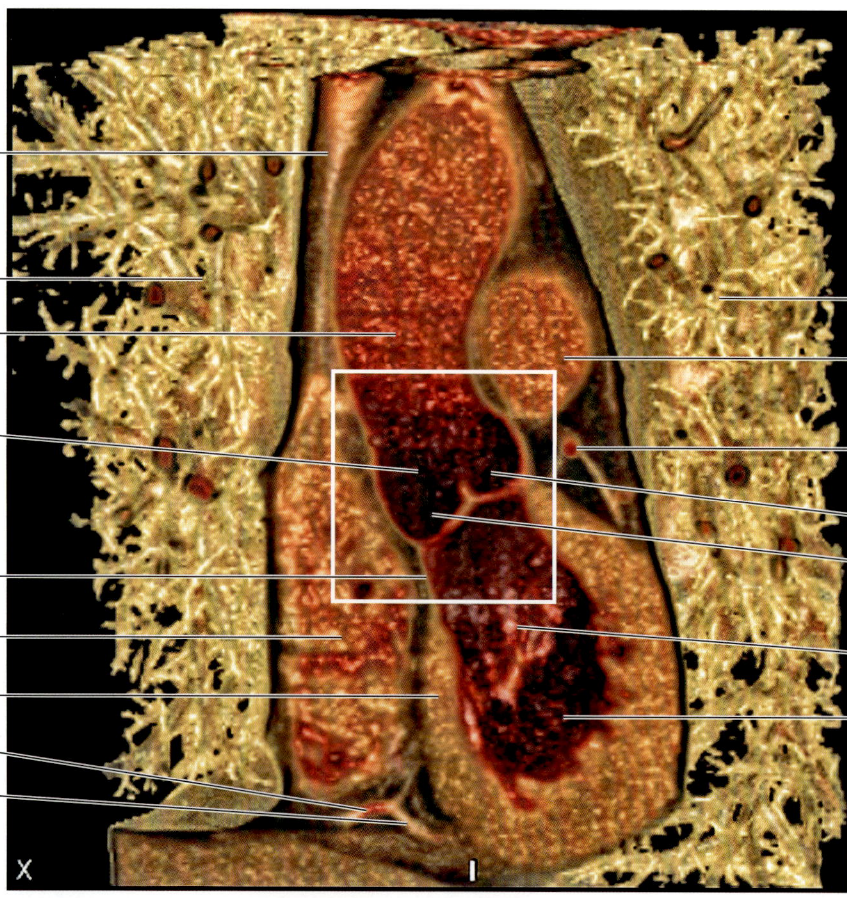

Three-dimensional image of a living human body, obtained by CT scan using a 3D volume rendering technique, showing the atrial and ventricular cavities, ascending aorta, pulmonary trunk and bronchial tree. Inside the box, the **aortic valve** is visible.

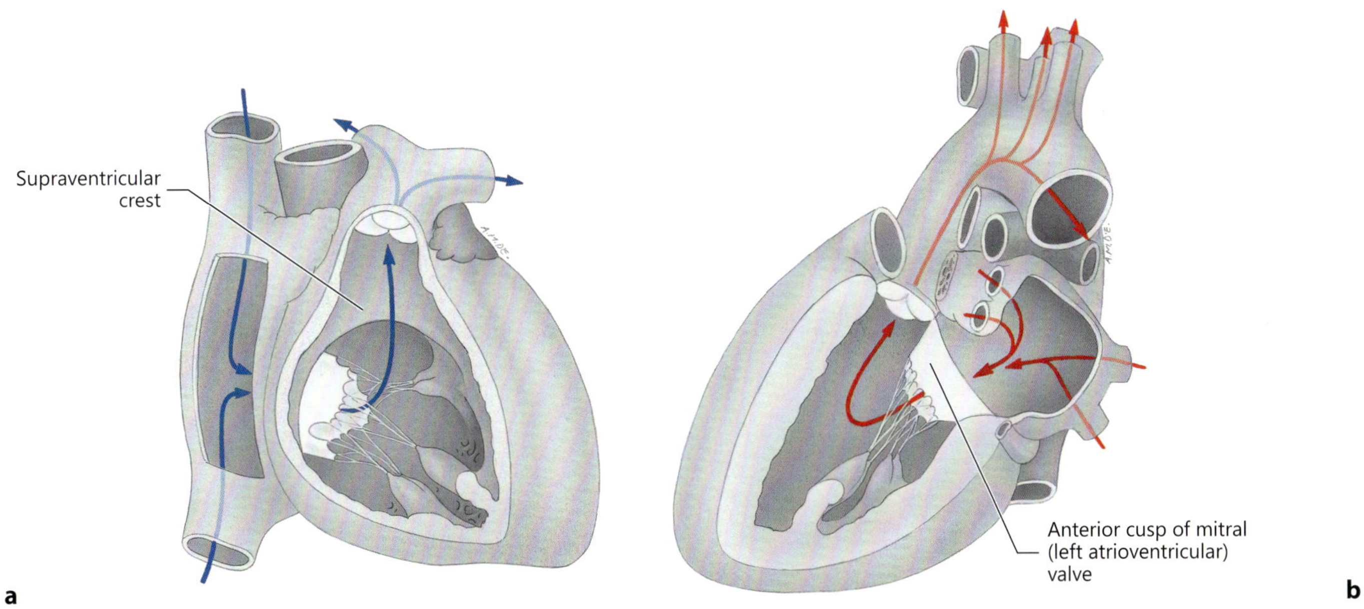

Schematic representation of the direction of **blood flow within the cardiac cavities**. The two pathways of flow into and out of the right ventricular cavity are separated by the supraventricular crest. In the left ventricular cavity, the two pathways are separated by the anterior cusp of the mitral valve.

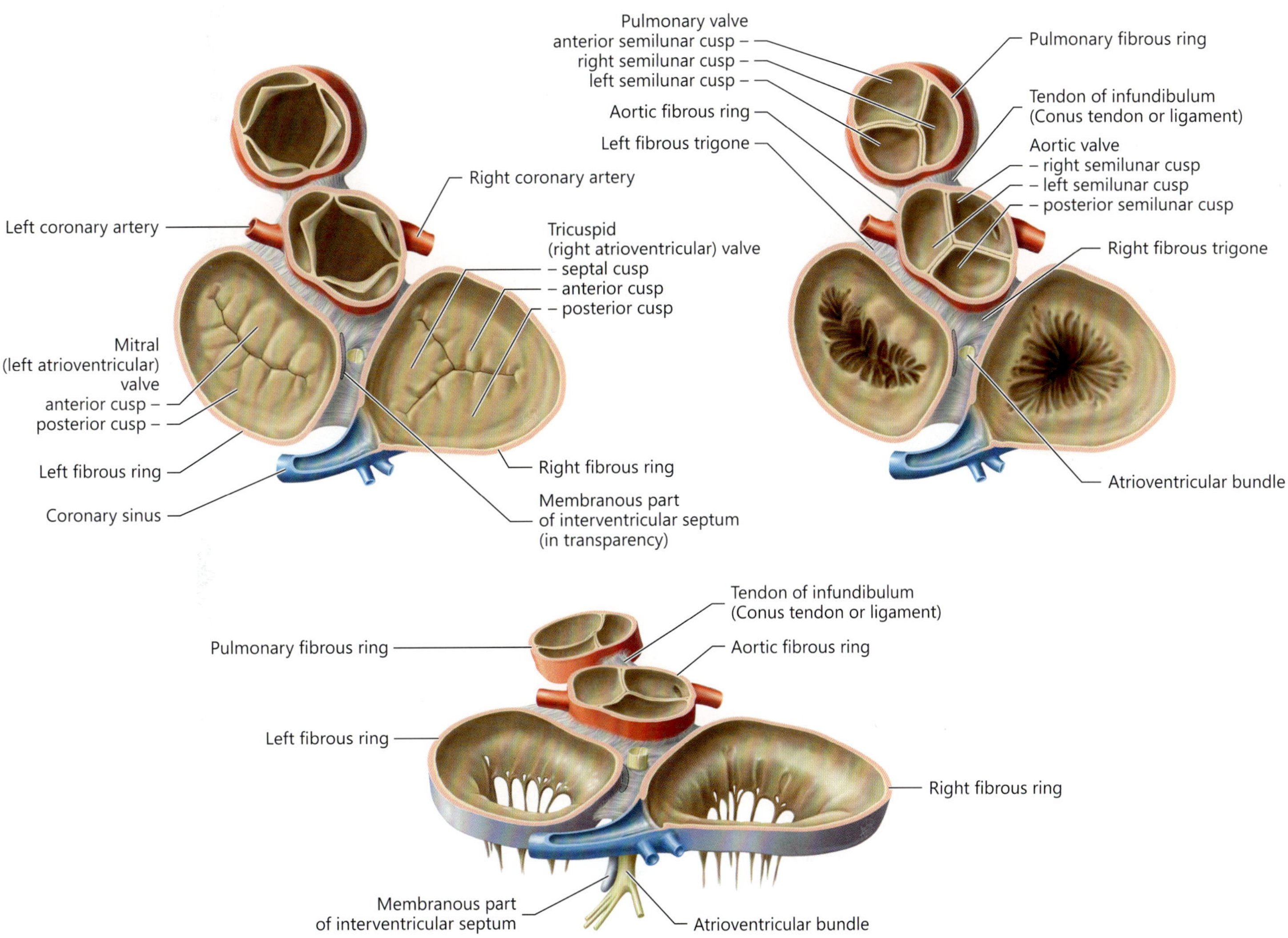

Fibrous skeleton of the heart. Above, the valves are shown in the phases of ventricular systole (on the left) and diastole (on the right). Below, projection viewed from behind. Note the oblique orientation of the pulmonary fibrous ring with respect to the fibrous rings of the atrioventricular and aortic valves. The atrioventricular bundle (of His) of the conduction system passes through the right fibrous trigone.

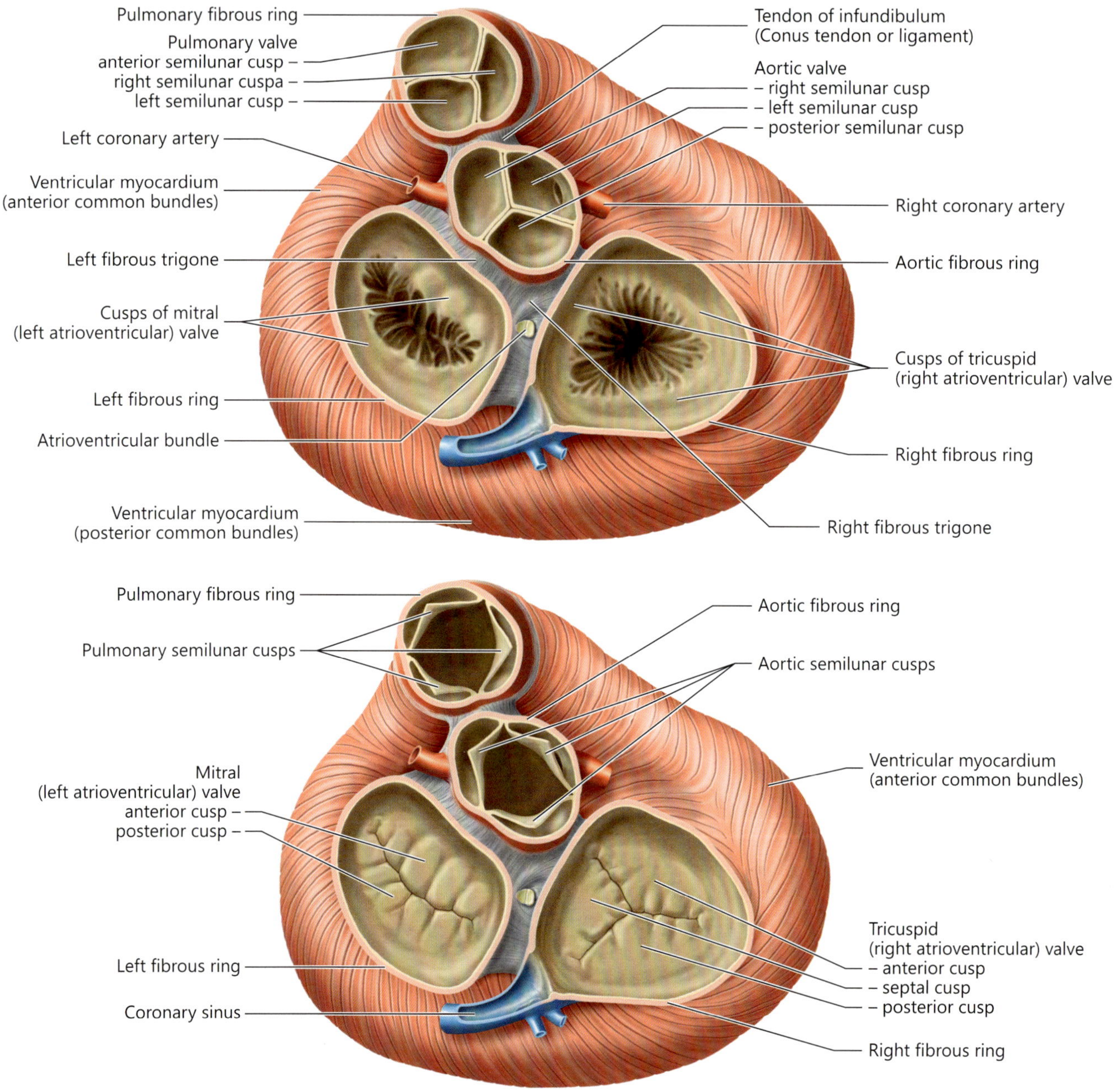

Base of the ventricles, viewed from above, after removal of the atria. Above, phase of ventricular diastole; below, phase of ventricular systole.

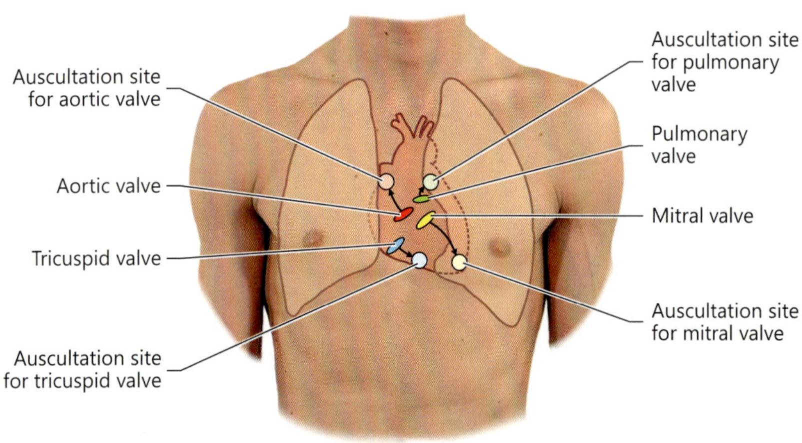

Projection onto the thoracic cage of the cardiac valves and relative **auscultation sites**.

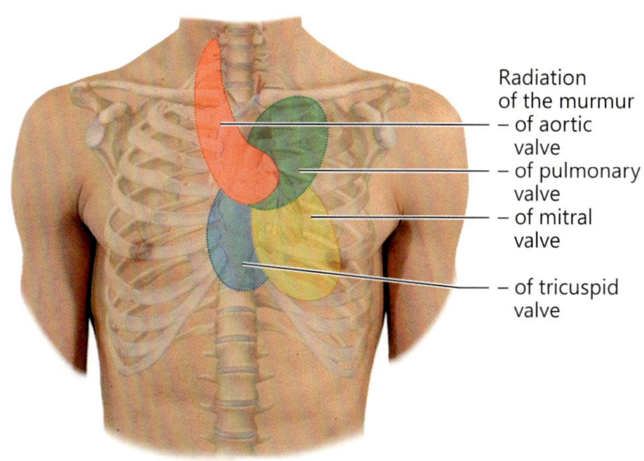

Sites of auscultation of pathological murmurs of the cardiac valves.

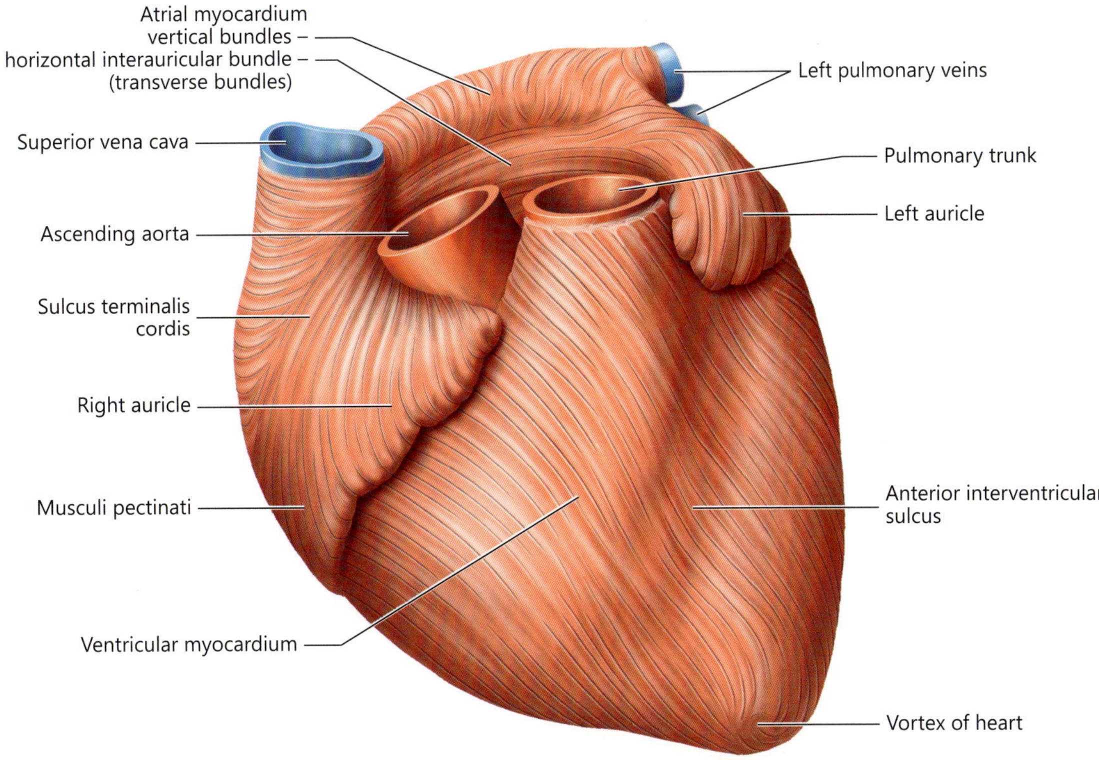

a

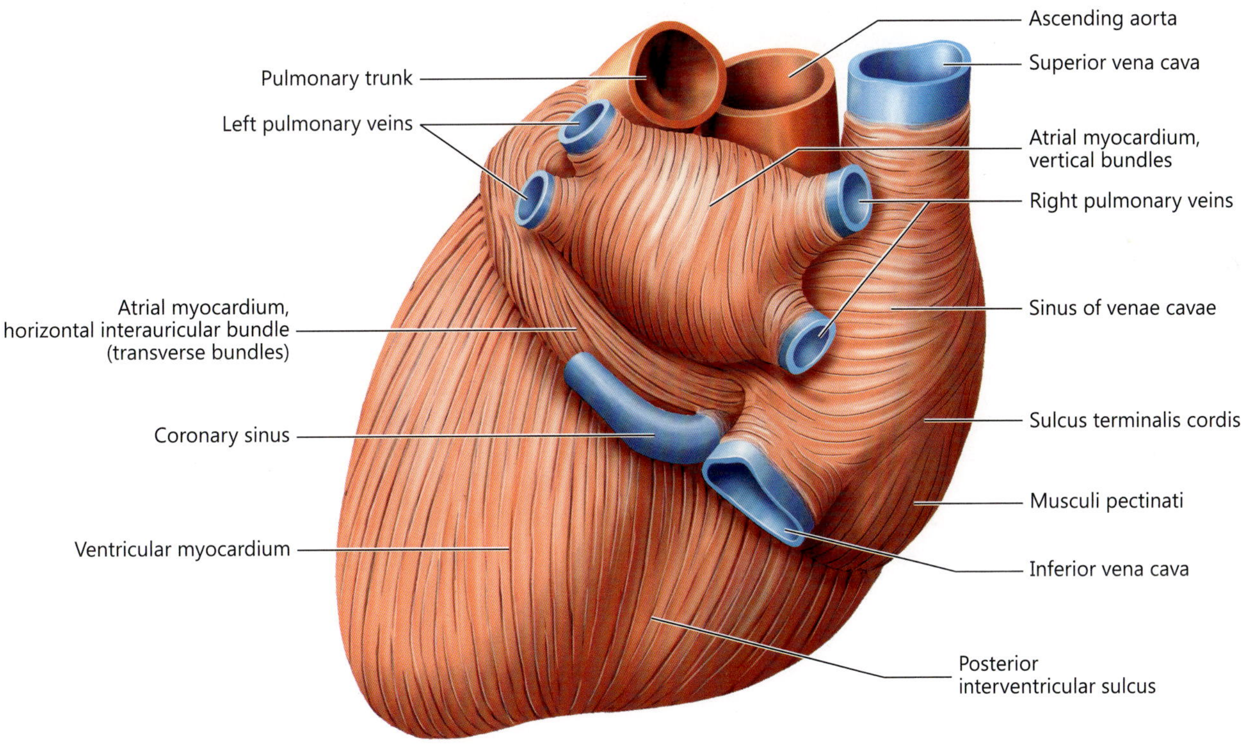

b

a, Disposition of the **atrial and ventricular muscles** on the anterior (sternocostal) surface of the heart; **b**, Disposition of the atrial and ventricular muscles on the diaphragmatic (inferior) surface and base of the heart.

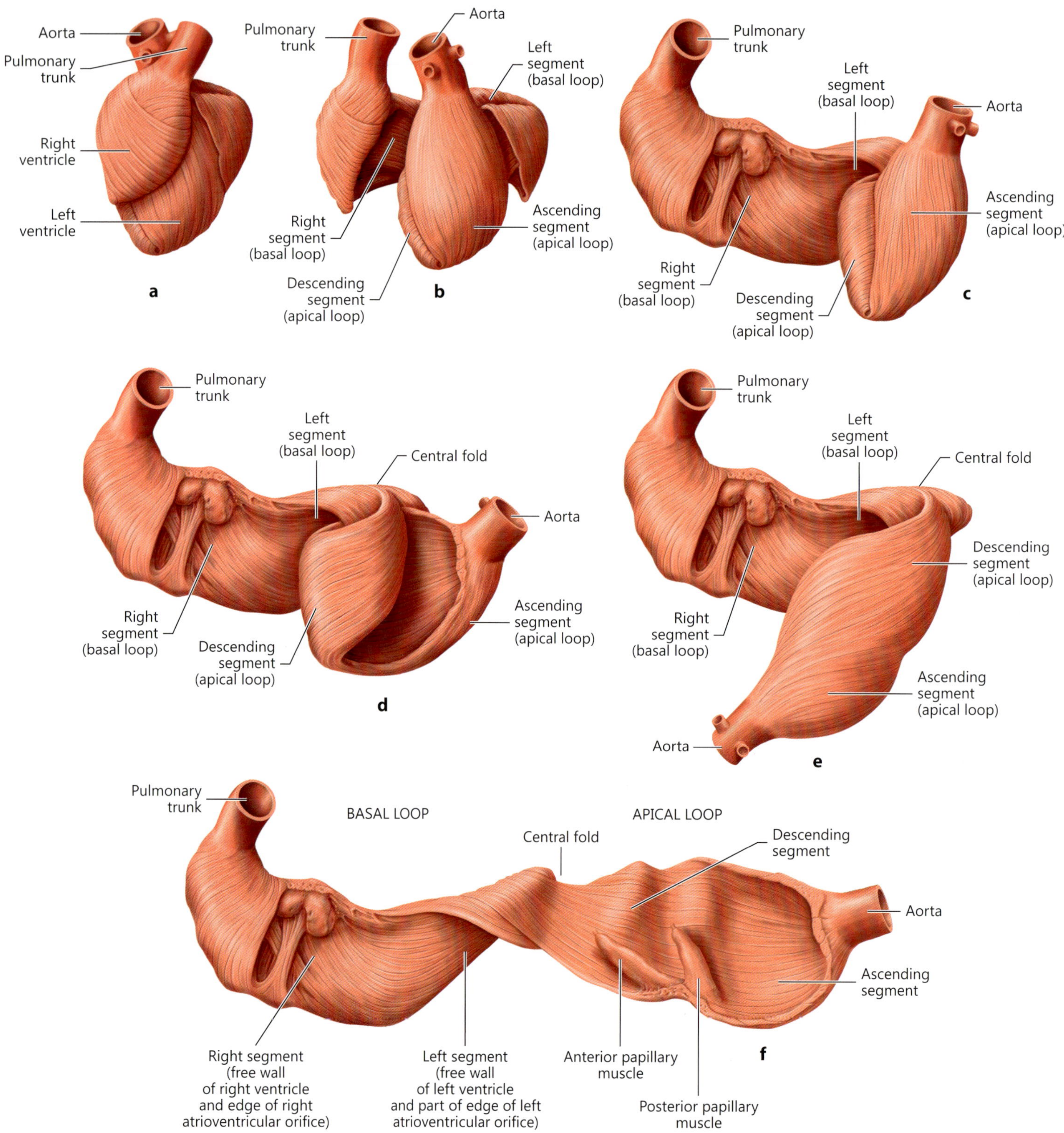

Schematic representation of the succession of unfolding phases of the heart according to Torrent-Guasp, so as to obtain the **ventricular myocardial band**, or helical ventricular myocardial band of Torrent-Guasp. In **a**, the initial arrangement of the myocardial fibers is represented in posterior view; in **b**, **c** and **d**, the successive phases of separation of the pulmonary trunk and right ventricular wall from the aorta are illustrated; note how it is possible to identify and separate, already in this phase, an ascending segment and a descending segment. With the successive pulling apart of the root of the pulmonary trunk from the aortic root, the two segments, ascending and descending, become separated from each other (**e**); in this phase one can identify, furthermore, a right segment and a left segment, corresponding to the basal portion of the heart, and separated from the ascending and descending segments by a zone known as the central fold, corresponding to the apex of the heart. With the complete unfolding of the myocardial structure, one obtains a continuous band of fibers extending from the pulmonary trunk to the aorta; in this band, it is possible to identify a zone corresponding to the basal portion of the heart, extending from the pulmonary trunk to the central fold and known as the basal loop, and an apical part of the heart, extending from the central fold to the aorta, which takes the name of apical loop. In the zone of the basal loop, the right and the left segments can be distinguished; the apical loop, instead, is composed of the descending and the ascending segments.

Schematic representation showing the direction of fibers of the **Torrent-Guasp band** in the initial position of the heart. One can see that this structure is composed of a single band of myocardial fibers that follow a winding helical path from the pulmonary trunk to the root of the aorta; one can easily distinguish the initial position of the descending and ascending segments separated by the central fold; these zones constitute the apical loop. Above the apical loop, one can detect the right and left segments that together constitute the basal loop.

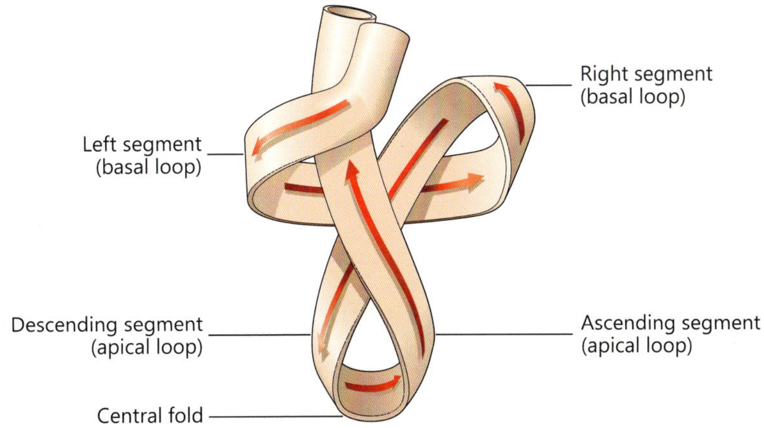

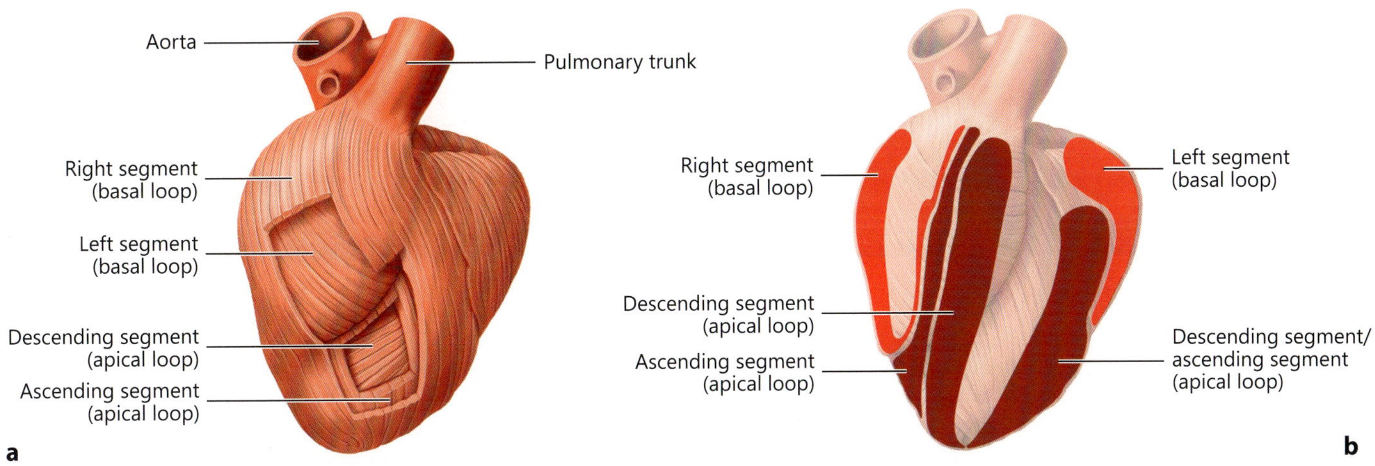

a, Schematic representation of the **Torrent-Guasp band** in which it is possible to distinguish the direction of the **myocardial band** both in correspondence to the apical loop, with the ascending and descending segments, as well as in correspondence to the basal loop, with the right and left segments. **b**, Schematic representation showing the position of the right and left segments with respect to the ascending and descending segments.

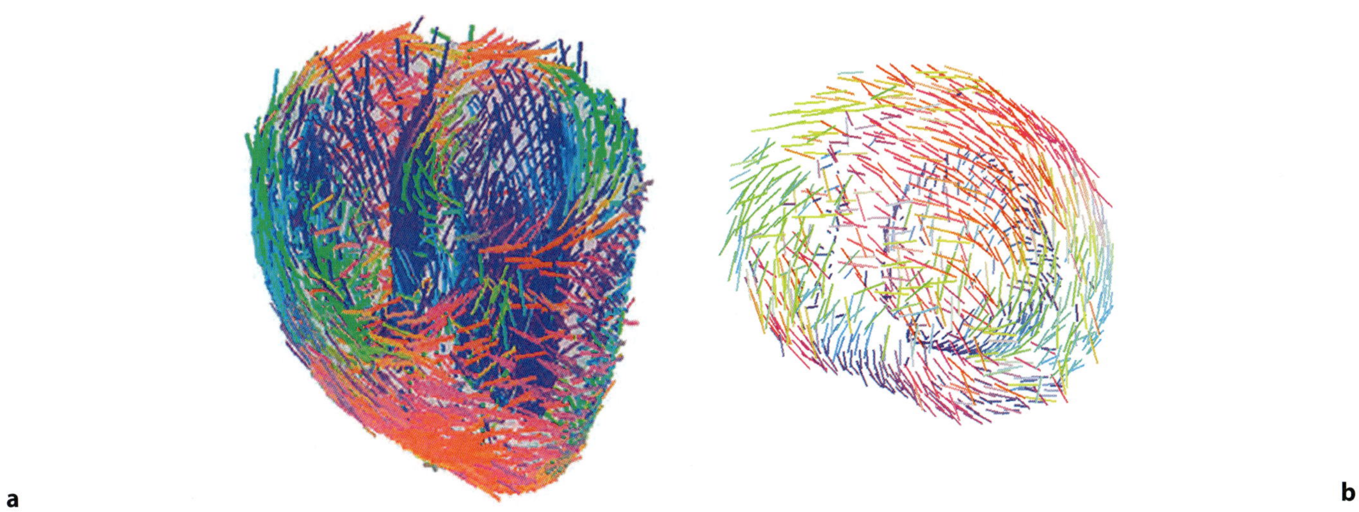

Organization of the **myocardial bands**, visualized by means of Diffusion Tensor Magnetic Resonance Imaging (DT-MRI). The fibers of the myocardium are organized into bundles. Bundles of myofibers of diverse orientation intersect generating a "mesh" (myocardial mesh). The myocardium is formed of three layers of fibers: subendocardial, intermediate and subepicardial. In the subendocardial layer, the fibers are oriented obliquely from the base towards the apex; in the intermediate layer they are oriented in a circular sense. The subepicardial layer is formed by the fibers of the subendocardial layer that re-emerge in correspondence to the apex and ascend in a longitudinal-oblique sense towards the base. The subepicardial fibers form an anticlockwise spiral, while the subendocardial ones form a clockwise spiral (**a**). In **b**, one can distinguish, looking down from above, the typical helical orientation that the myocardial fibers assume in correspondence to the apex of the heart.

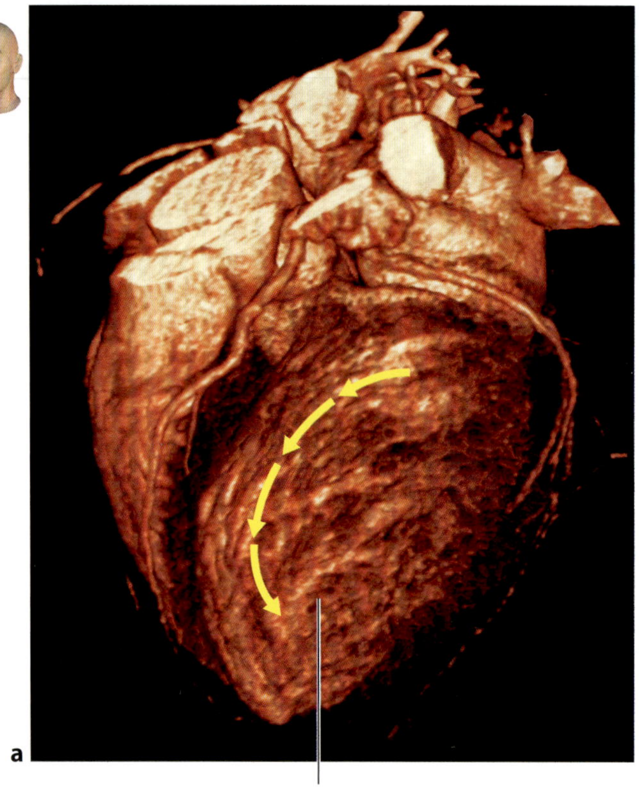

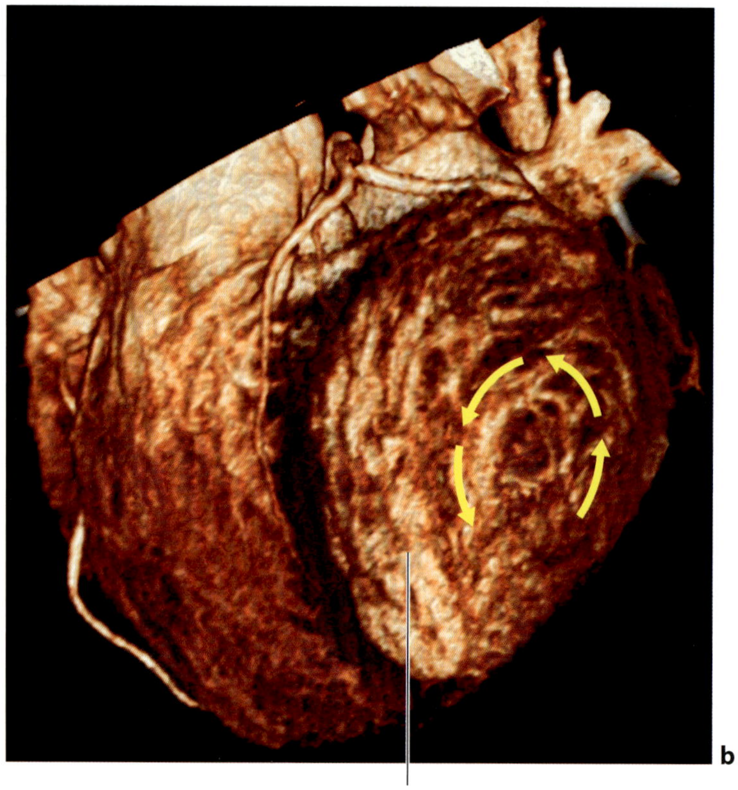

Three-dimensional image of the heart of a live subject, obtained using a 3D volume rendering technique. In **a**, one can see the oblique course of the **myocardial fibers of the left ventricle**. This course becomes helicoidal in correspondence to the ventricular cone (**b**). Thus is formed the helicoidal loop characteristic of the myocardial fibers of this zone.

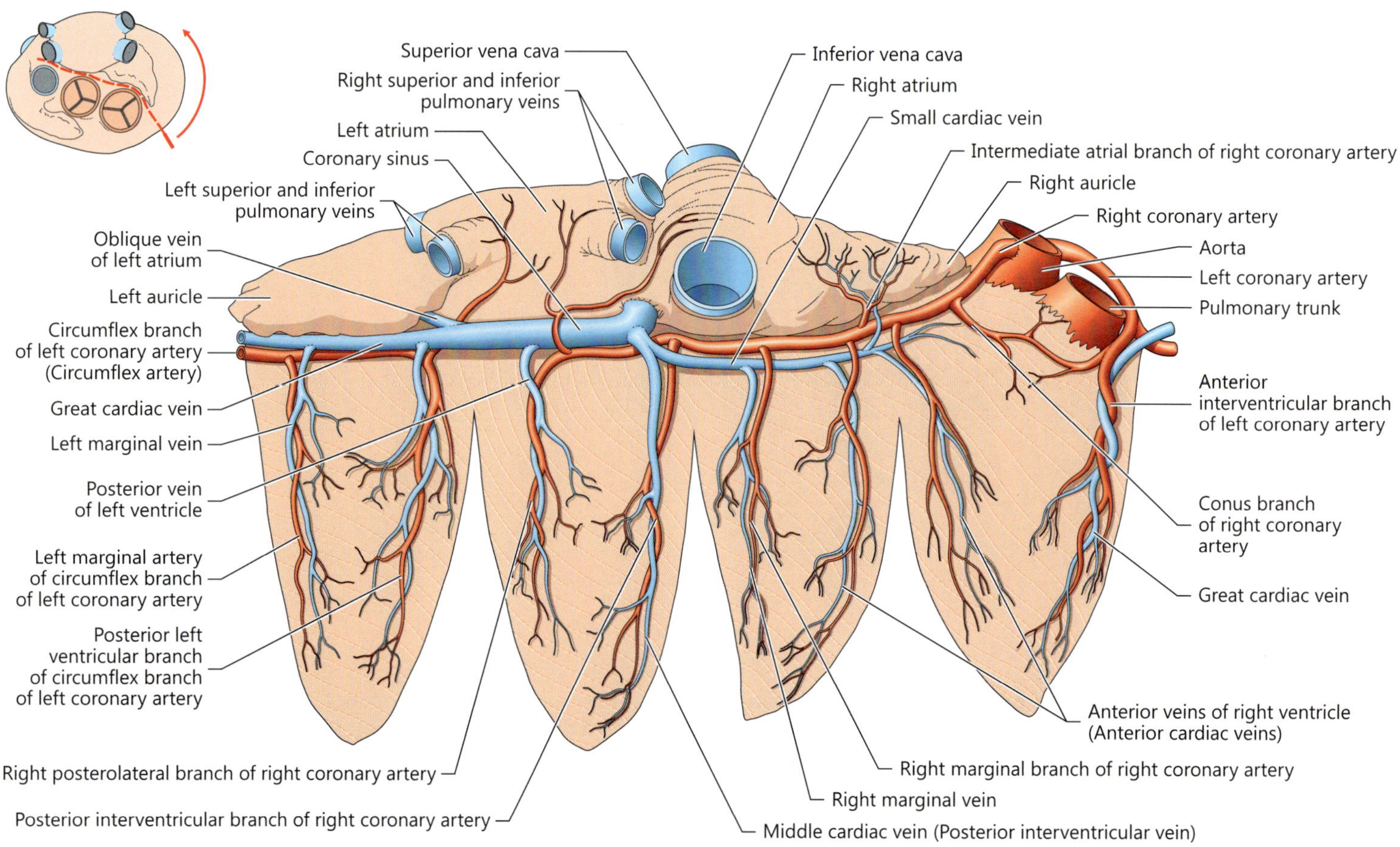

Aphylactic projection of the **cardiac vessels**. The reference relative to the cut surface is illustrated, viewed from above.

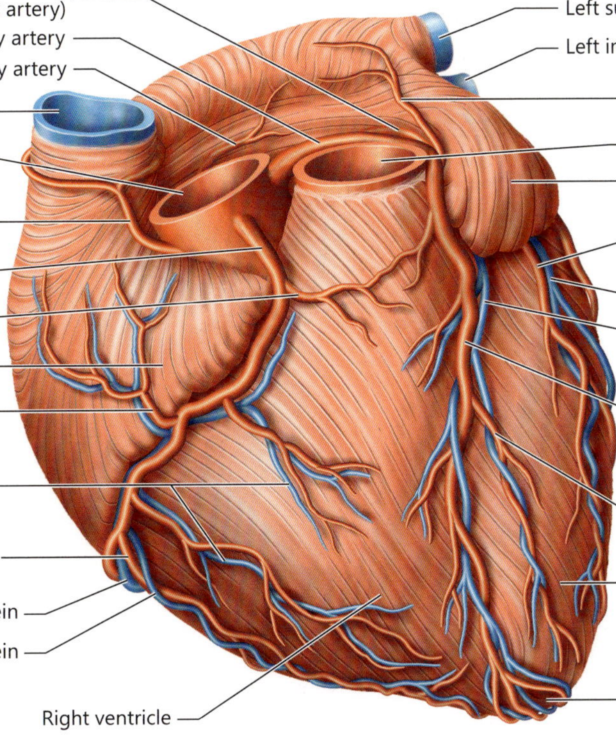

a

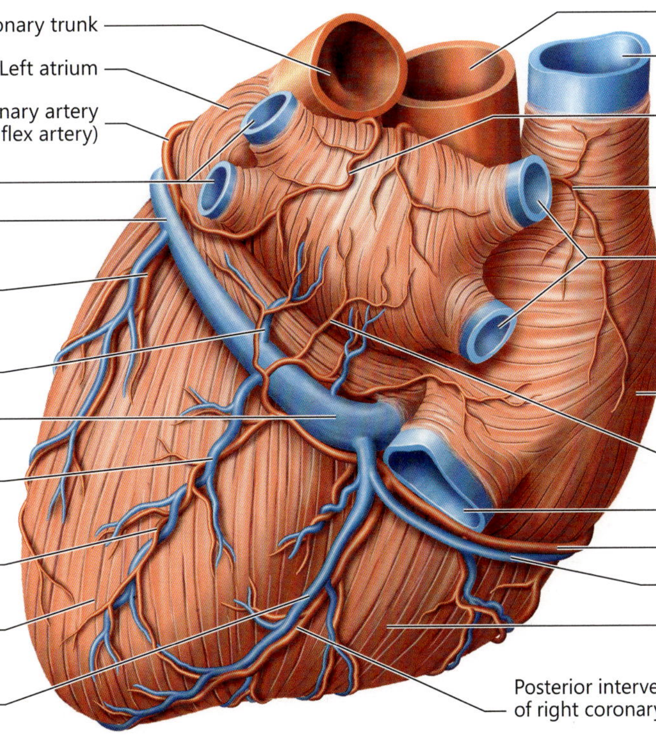

b

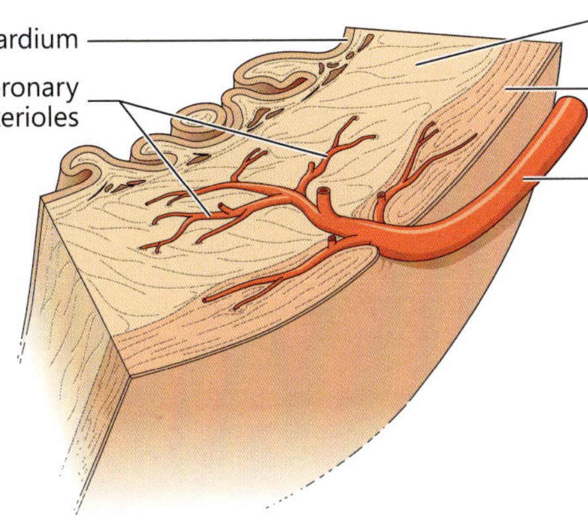

c

a, Distribution of the **arteries and veins of the heart** on the anterior (sternocostal) surface of the heart. **b**, Distribution of the arteries and veins of the heart on the diaphragmatic (inferior) surface and base of the heart. **c**, **Epicardial coronary artery**, with characteristics of a capacitance vessel opposing little resistance to the flow, and its ramification into intramural coronary artery and arterioles, with characteristics of resistance vessels that determine important variations of flow by dilating or contracting.

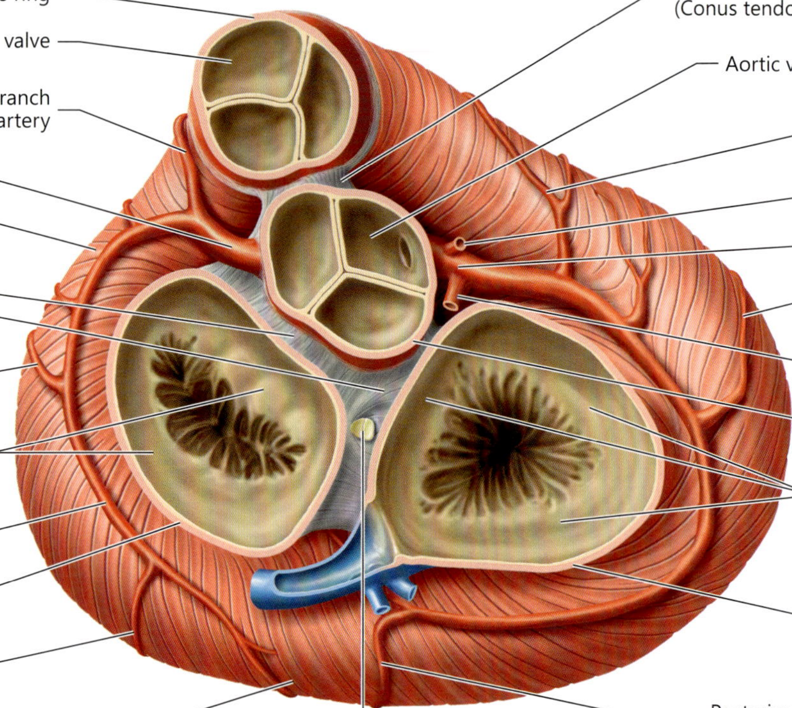

Course of the **coronary arteries** in the coronary sulcus visualized after removal of the atria.

ANATOMIC VARIANTS OF THE ARTERIES OF THE HEART
Conus branch (originates prevalently from the proximal tract of the right coronary artery) can also originate: – from the opening of the right coronary artery – from the aorta
Sinuatrial nodal branch (originates prevalently from the right coronary artery) can also originate: – from the circumflex branch of the left coronary artery – from the right coronary artery and from the circumflex branch of the left coronary artery – from the circumflex branch of the left coronary artery and from the pulmonary trunk – from the aorta
Length of the left coronary artery (prevalent length is 1-2 cm): – <1 cm – >2 cm
Intermediate branch of the left coronary artery (additional branch of the left coronary artery, which prevalently gives off only two branches: the circumflex branch and anterior interventricular branch)
Lateral (diagonal) branches arising from the anterior interventricular branch of the left coronary artery (prevalently two): – 1 – >2
Absence of interventricular septal branches arising from the anterior interventricular branch of the left coronary artery (prevalently present)
Marginal branches originating from the circumflex branch of the left coronary artery (prevalently two): – 1 – >2

ARTERIAL VASCULARIZATION OF THE CONDUCTION SYSTEM	
Sinuatrial node	Sinuatrial nodal branch of the right coronary artery (in approximately 65% of hearts) Sinuatrial nodal branch originating from the circumflex branch of the left coronary artery (in approximately 35% of hearts)
Atrioventricular node	Atrioventricular nodal branch or interventricular septal branch originating from the posterior interventricular branch of the right coronary artery (in approximately 80% of hearts) Atrioventricular nodal branch originating from the circumflex branch of the left coronary artery (in approximately 20% of hearts)
Atrioventricular bundle	Atrioventricular branches of the right coronary artery (in approximately 90% of hearts) Interventricular septal branches originating from the anterior interventricular branch of the left coronary artery (in approximately 10% of hearts)

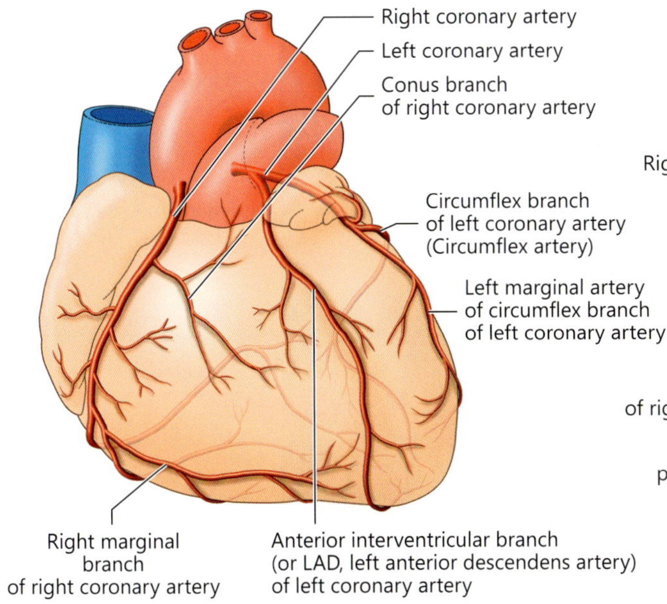

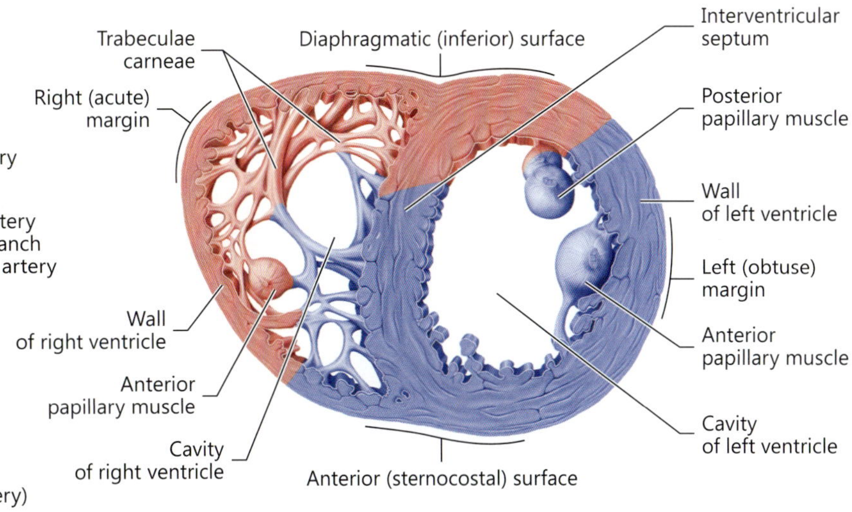

Common disposition: the right coronary artery supplies the posterior wall of the right ventricle and the posterior third of the interventricular septum.

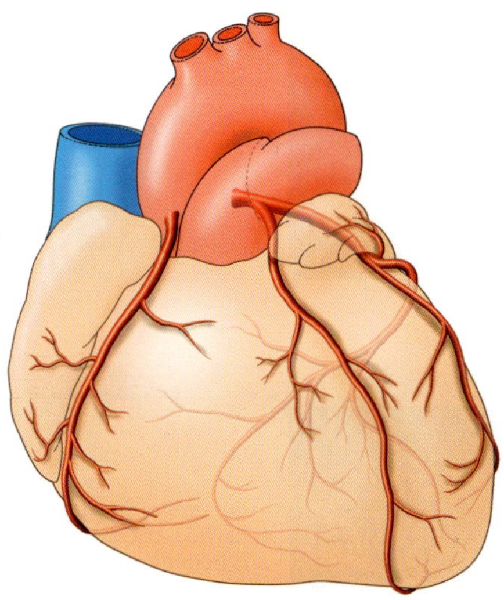

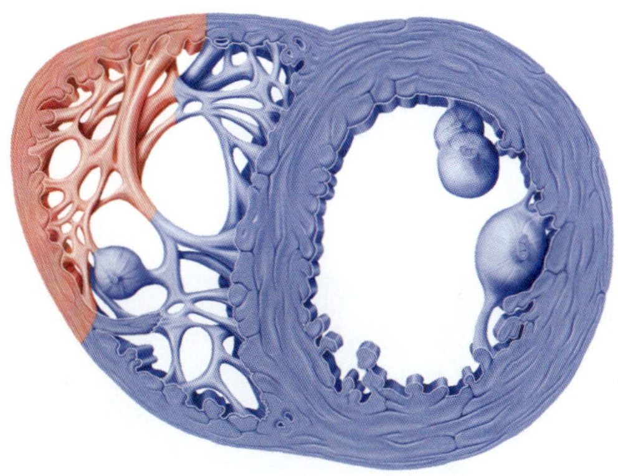

Left dominance: the left coronary artery supplies the posterior wall of the right and left ventricles and the interventricular septum.

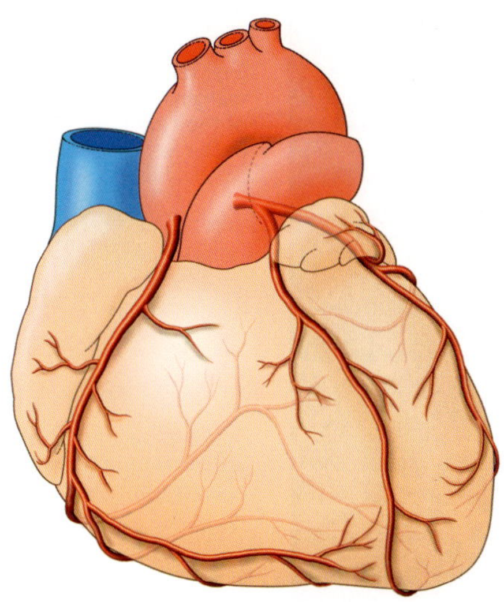

a

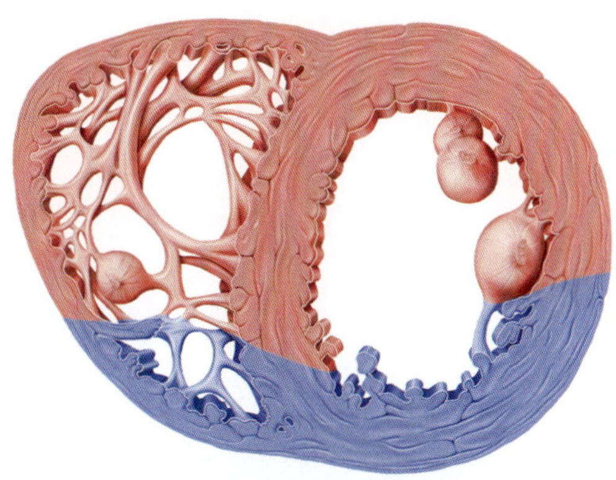

b Right dominance: the right coronary artery supplies the posterior wall of the right and left ventricles and the interventricular septum.

Principal variants in the **blood supply of the posterior wall of the heart and interventricular septum**: **a**, viewed from the front; **b**, transverse section of the ventricles showing the territory of supply of the right (in *red*) and left (in *blue*) coronary arteries.

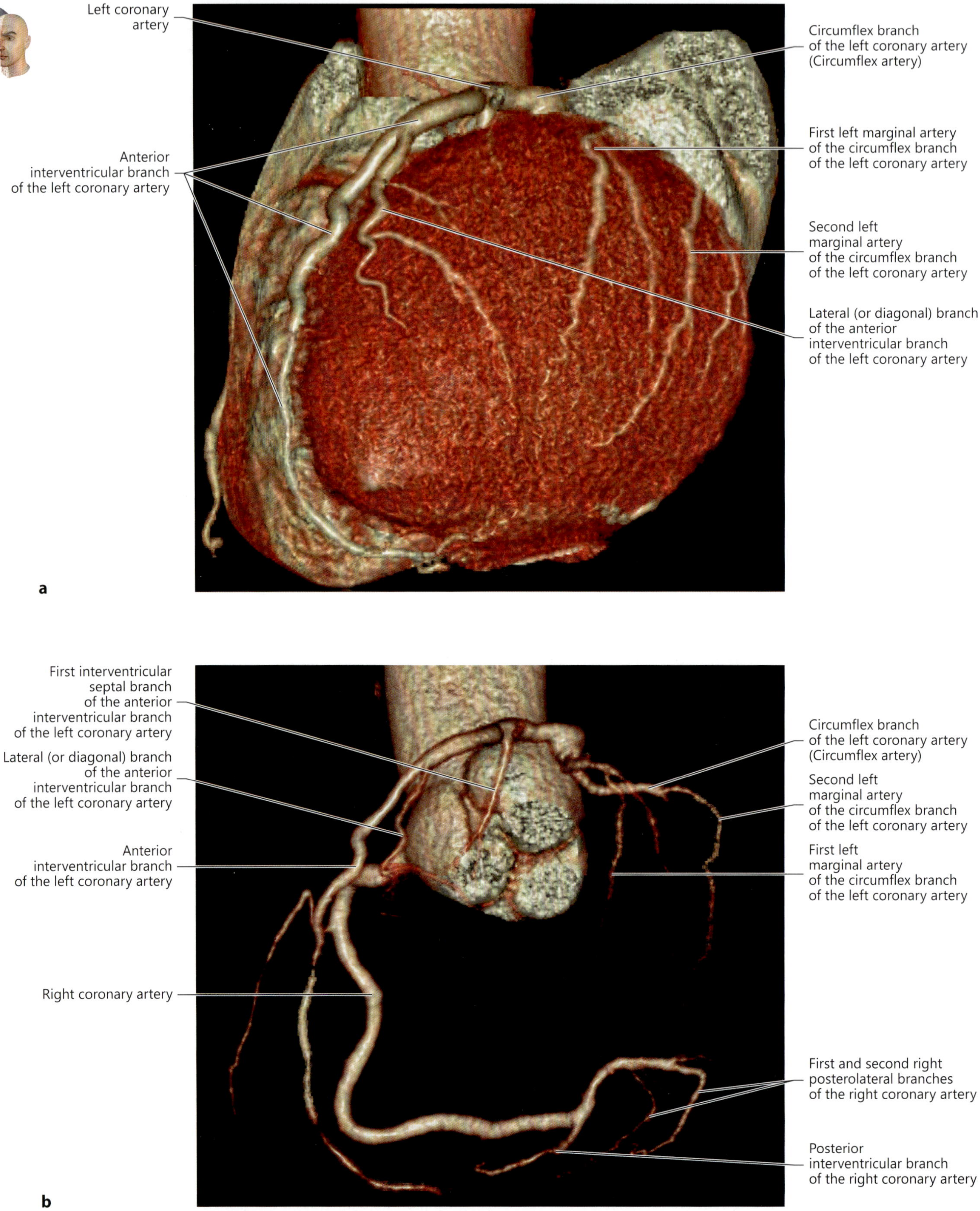

Three-dimensional images of a living human body, obtained by CT scan using a 3D volume rendering technique. **a**, The heart is viewed from the left (left or obtuse margin). The branches of the left coronary artery are highlighted. **b**, With the cardiac tissue extracted, also the right coronary artery and aortic sinuses are clearly displayed.

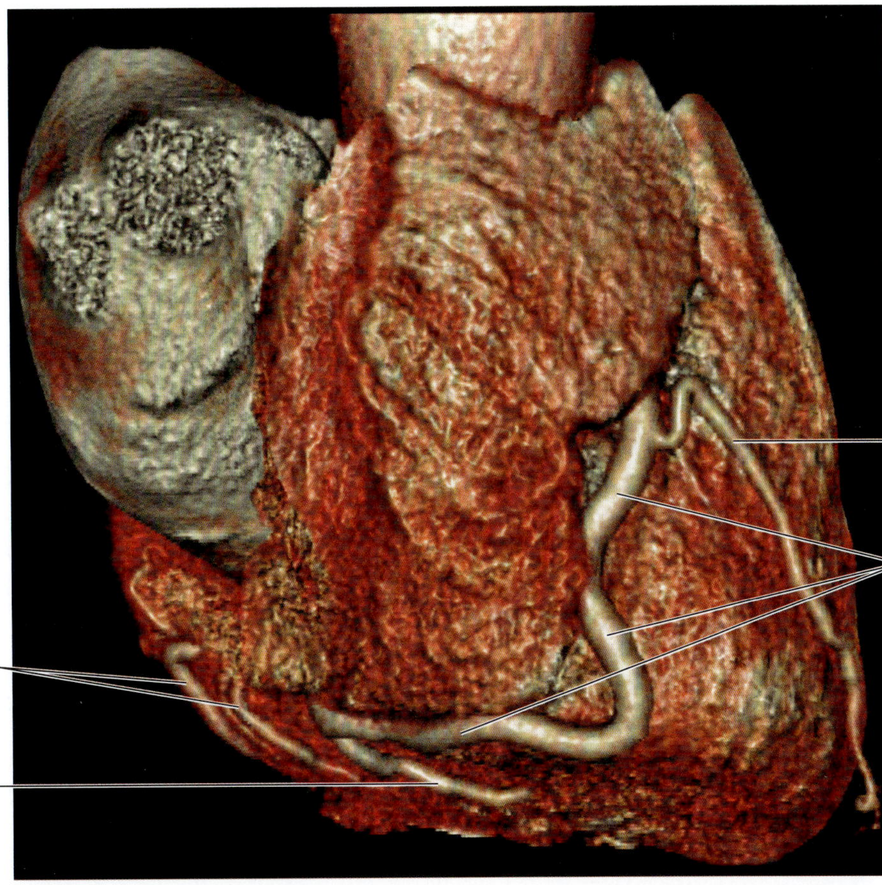

a

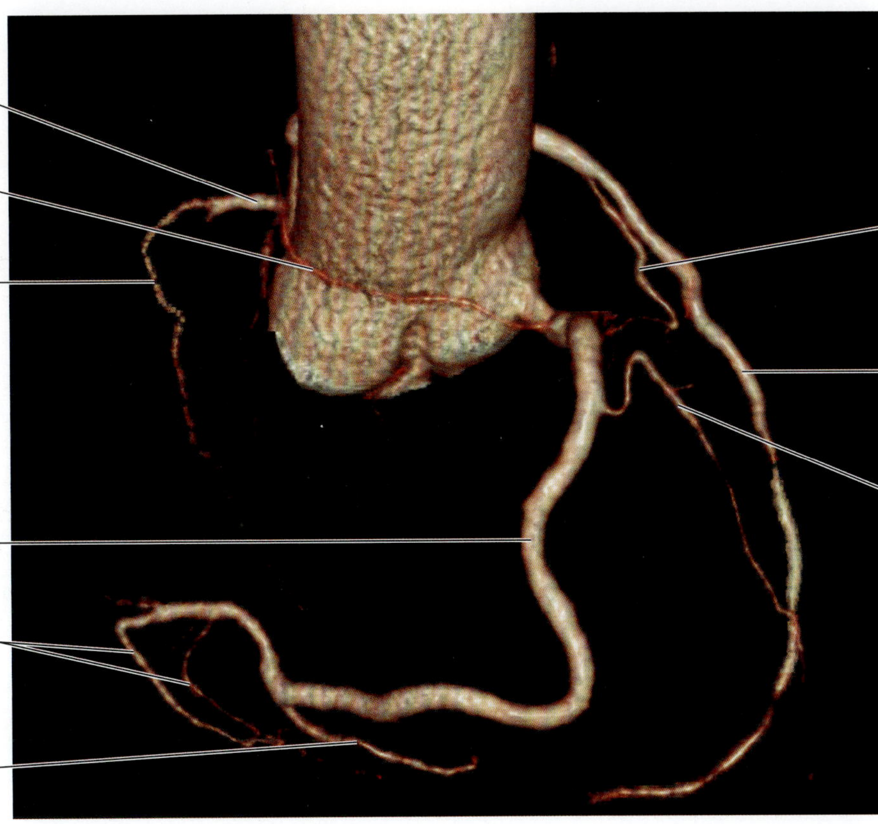

b

Three-dimensional images of a living human body, obtained by CT scan using a 3D volume rendering technique. **a**, The heart is viewed from the right (right or acute margin). The right coronary artery and some of its branches are displayed. **b**, With the cardiac tissue extracted, one can see the whole course of the right coronary artery and some branches of the left coronary artery.

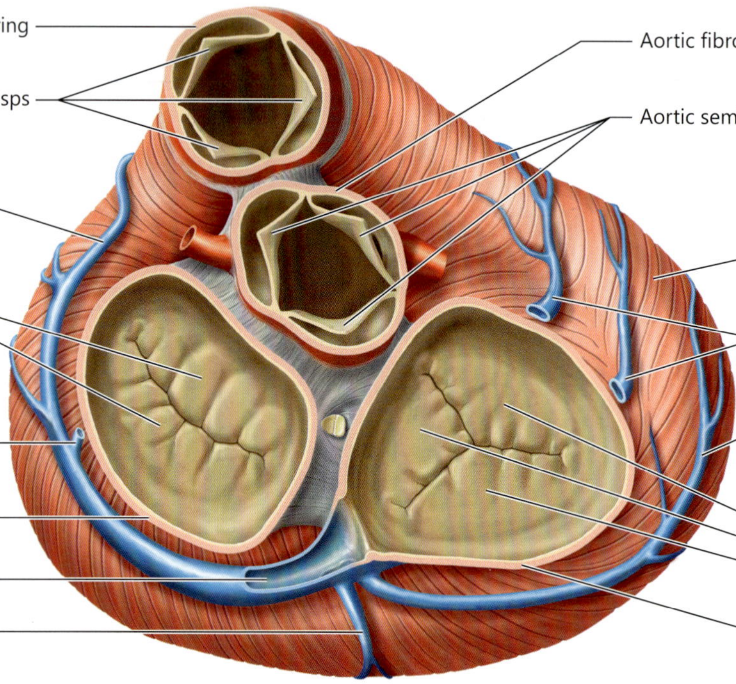

Course of the **cardiac veins** in the coronary sulcus visualized after removal of the atria.

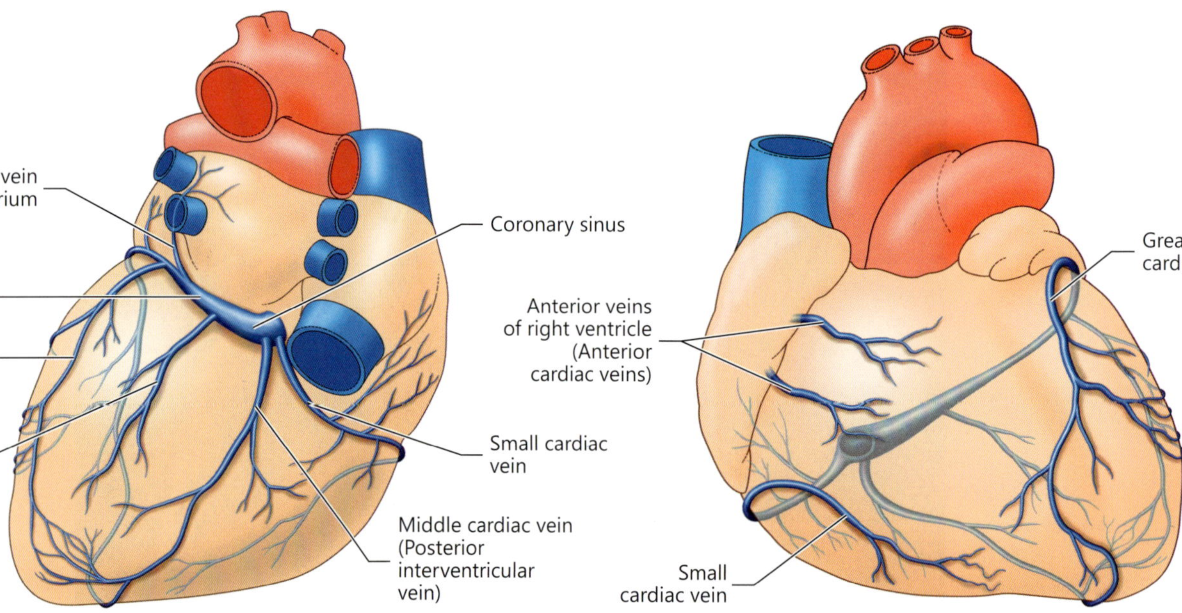

Territories of drainage of the principal **cardiac veins**. On the left, a posterior projection is shown; on the right, an anterior projection. With the myocardium drawn in transparency, one can see the distribution of the vessels over the whole surface of the heart.

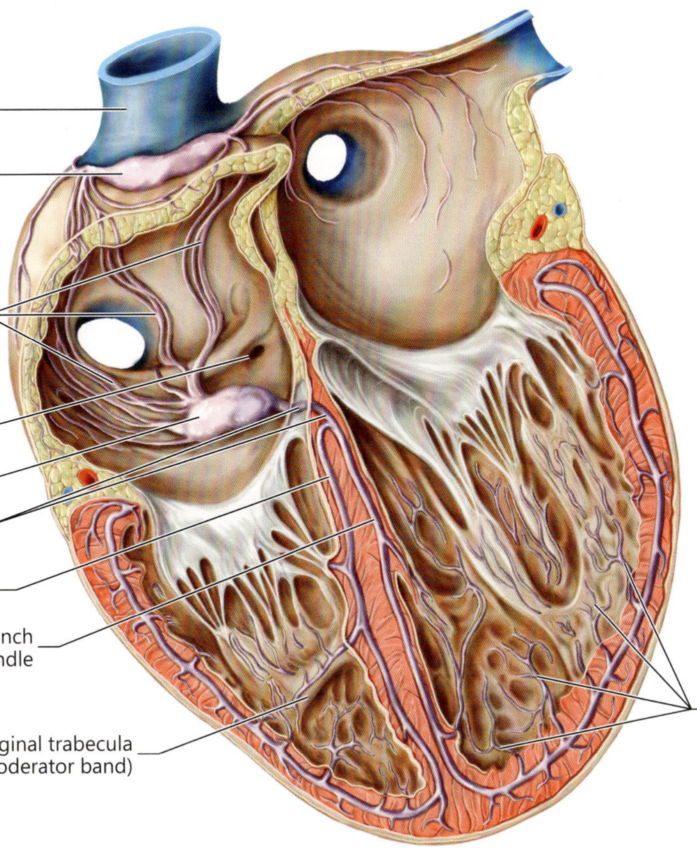

The **sinuatrial node** (SA node, pacemaker of the heart) is a structure formed of specific myocardium, with a semilunar shape, and approximately 10 mm in diameter. It has a more voluminous part situated between the opening of the superior vena cava and the crista terminalis and a thinner part extending downwards to the right. A series of myocardial bundles, which originate from the SA node and run on the anterior, posterior and lateral walls of the right atrium (internodal bundles), lead to the atrioventricular node (AV node). The AV node is situated in the right atrium, within Koch's triangle (see image below), in proximity to the right atrioventricular orifice. From the AV node departs the atrioventricular bundle (bundle of His) which, after crossing the fibrous skeleton of the heart, runs on the right side of the membranous part of the interventricular septum and separates into two branches (right and left). The right branch has a cylindrical form with a diameter of 1-2 mm. It runs on the right surface of the interventricular septum, first within the myocardium, and then in the subendocardial layer. It gives off a branch that enters the septomarginal trabecula (moderator band), which reaches the base of the anterior papillary muscle of the right ventricle. The left branch has the form of a flat tape. It first runs in the subendocardial layer to the left of the interventricular septum, and then divides into two or more branches that lead to the papillary muscles of the left ventricle.

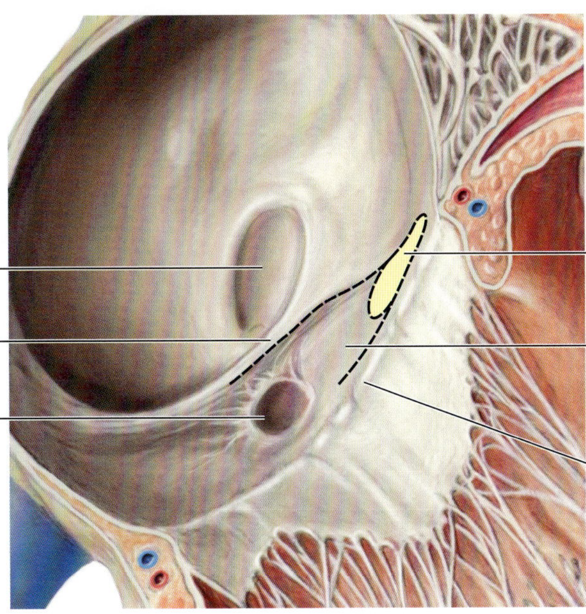

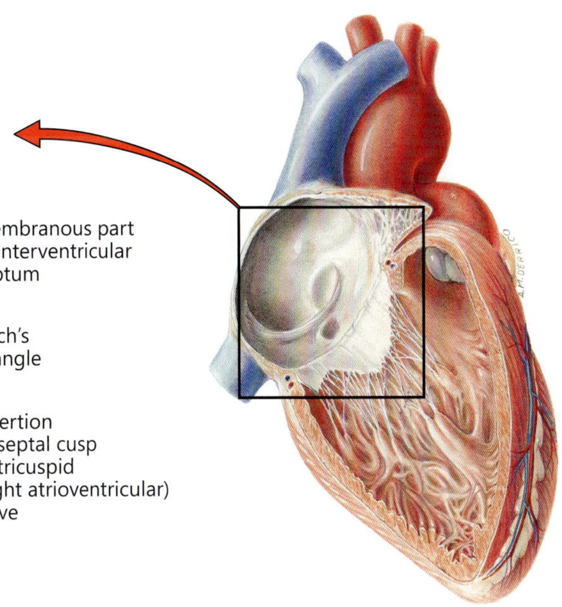

Koch's Triangle. Demarcates the area in which the atrioventricular node is situated.

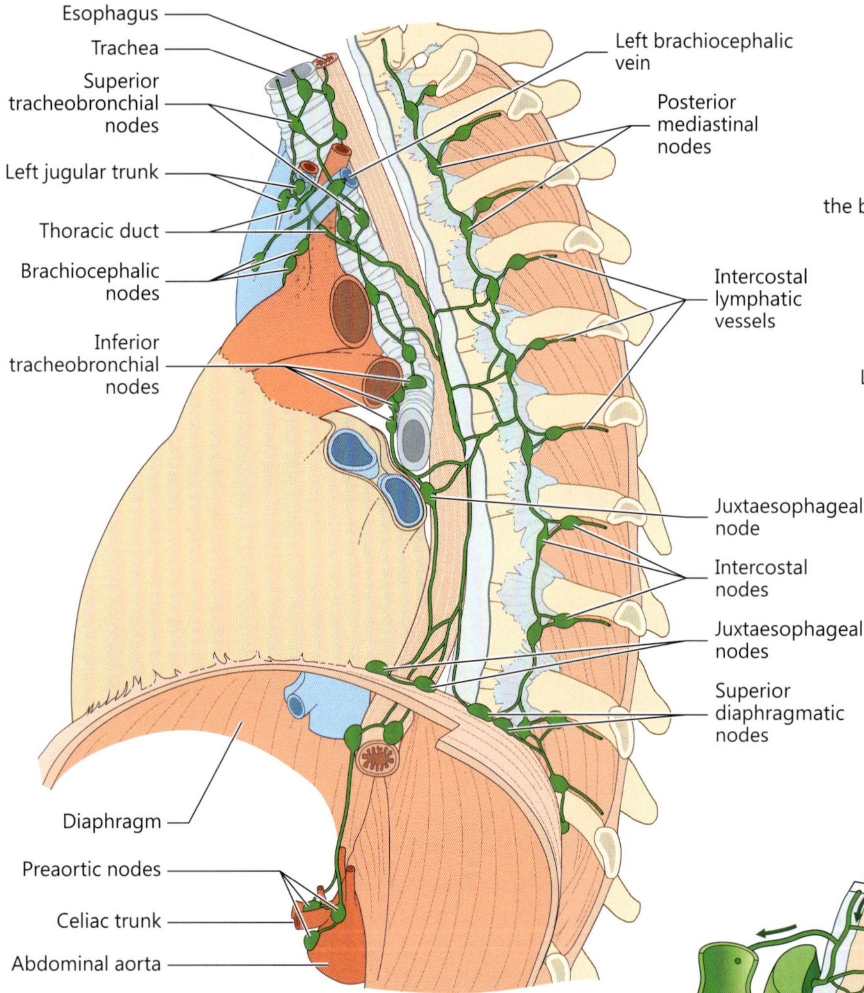

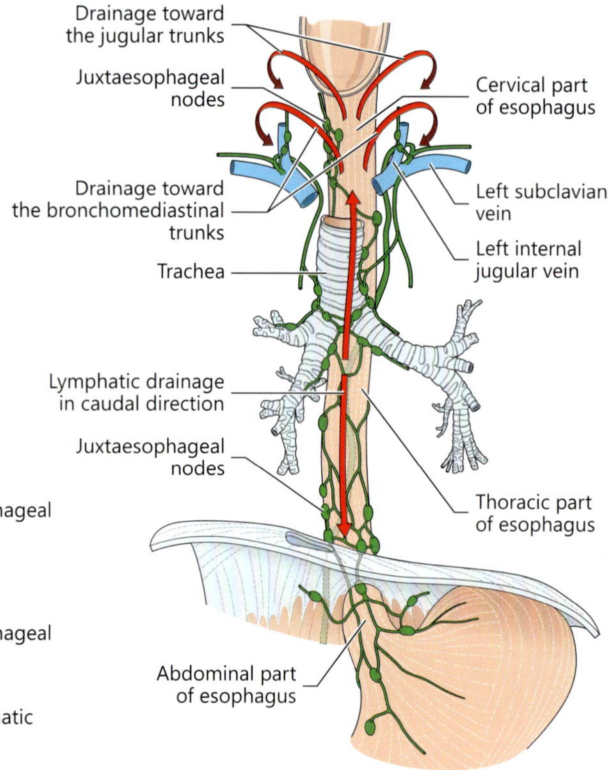

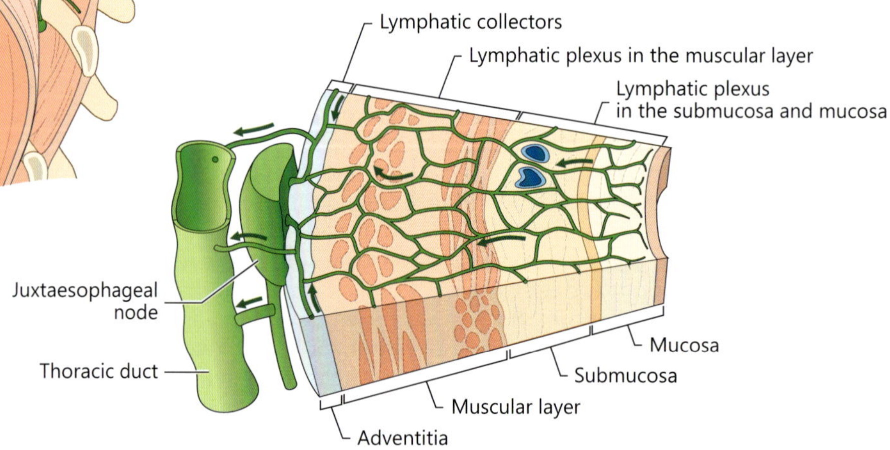

In the three images the **lymph nodes of the thorax** are represented in lateral and frontal projections and in a close-up detail of the transected esophageal wall. Arrows indicate the direction of **lymphatic flow**.

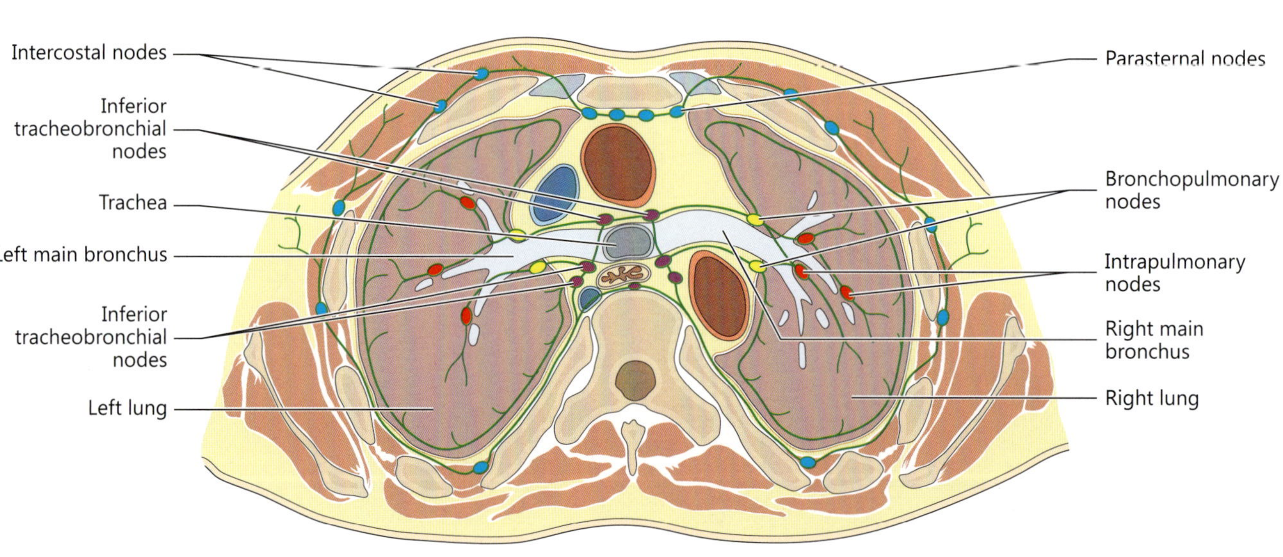

Principal **lymph nodes of the thorax** viewed in transverse section at the level of T IV.

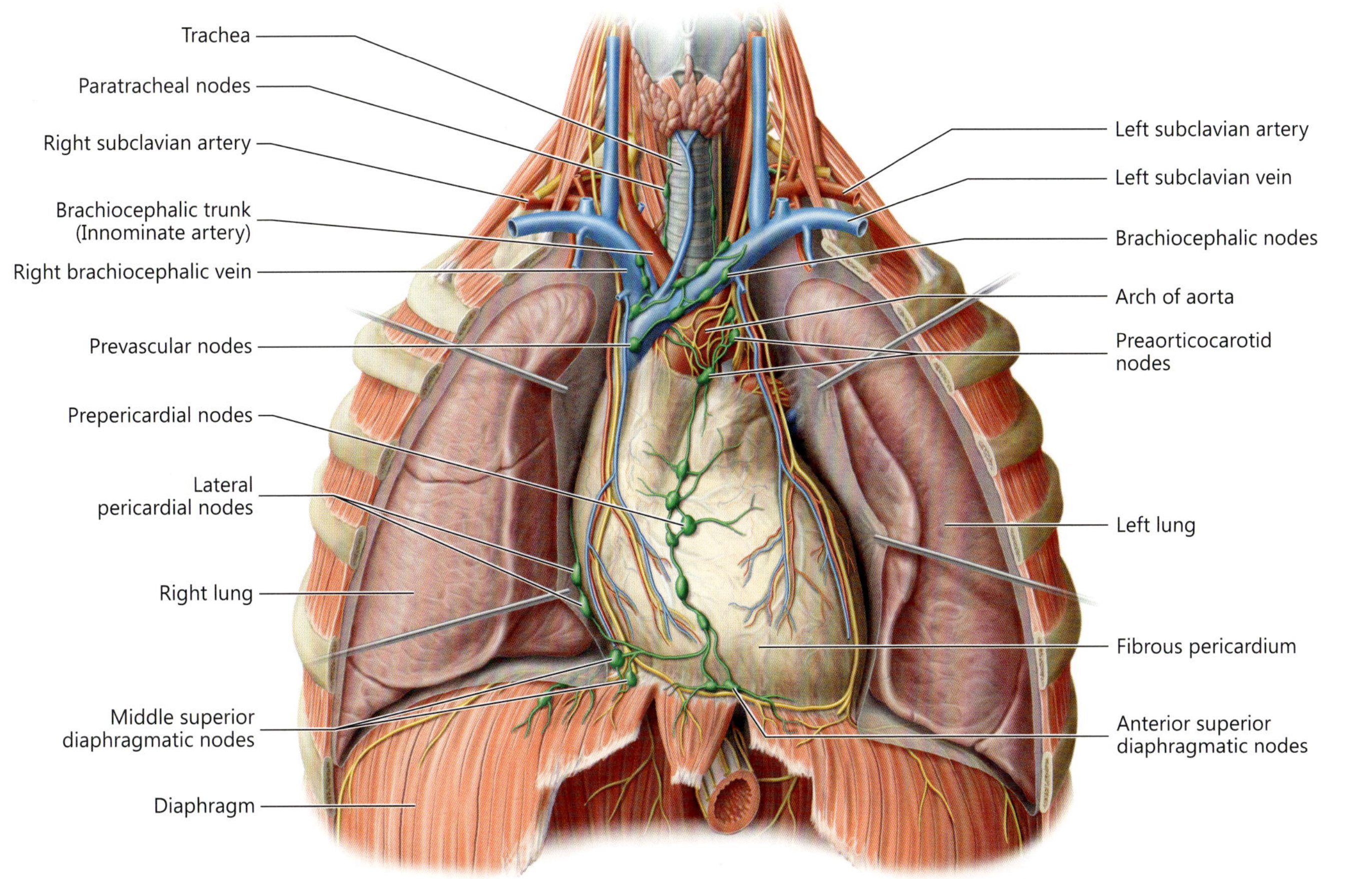

Middle and anterior mediastinal nodes.

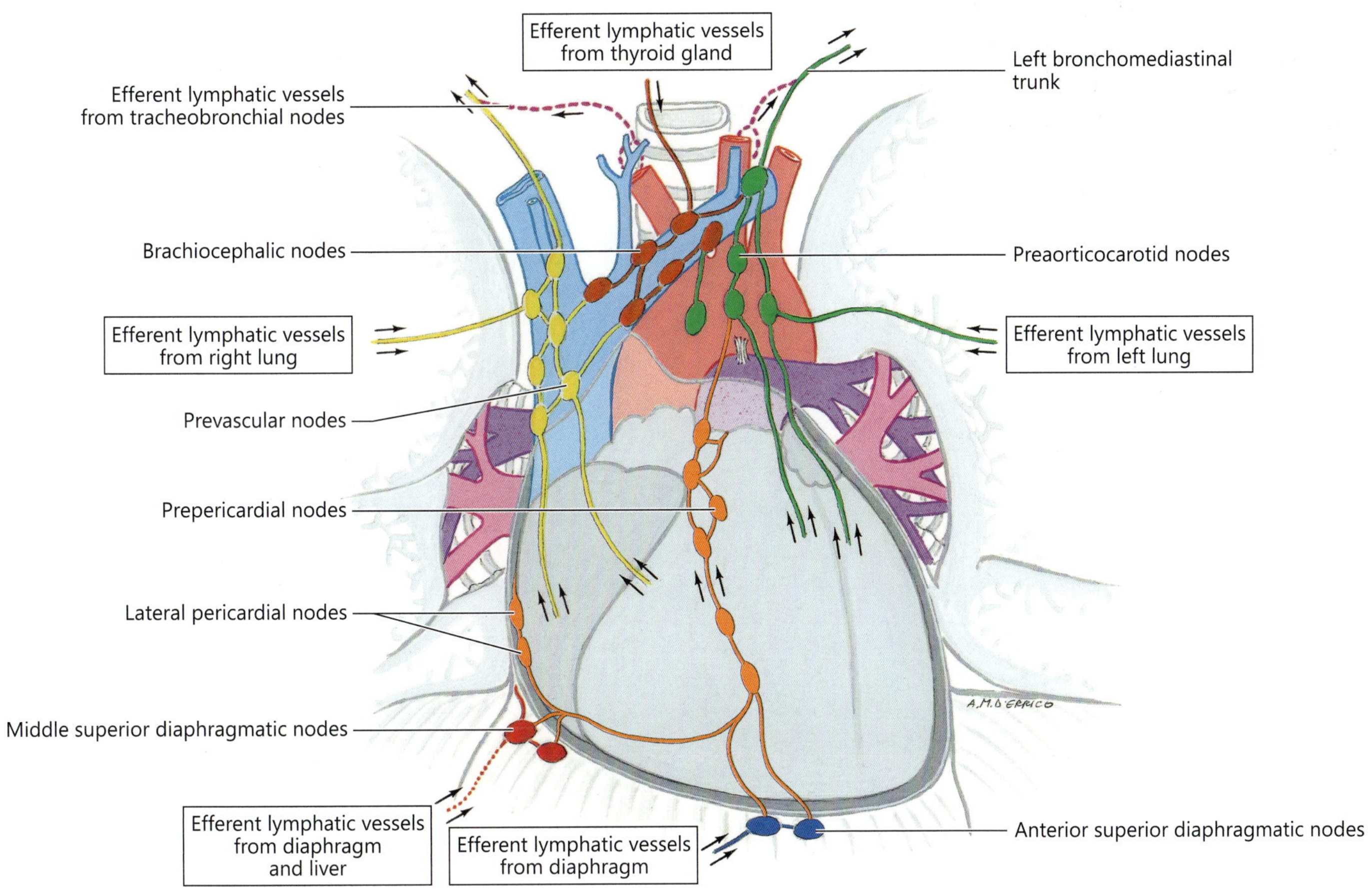

Superior and diaphragmatic mediastinal nodes. The principal pathways of drainage are indicated.

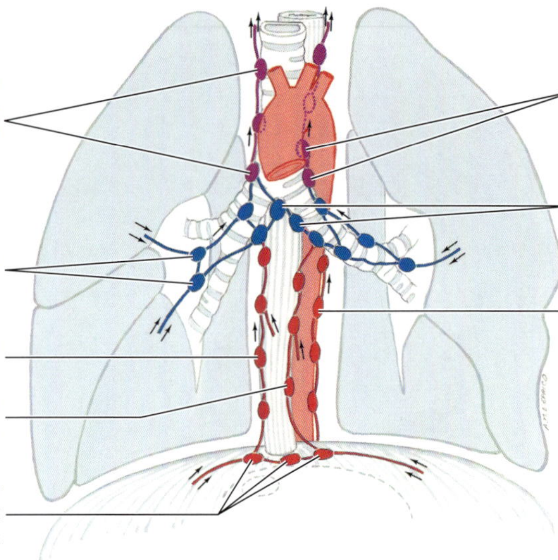

Schematic representation showing the **posterior mediastinal nodes** (in *red*), including the juxtaesophageal, interaorticoesophageal, juxta-aortic and superior diaphragmatic nodes, the **bronchopulmonary** and **inferior tracheobronchial nodes** (in *blue*), and the **superior tracheobronchial** and **paratracheal nodes** (in *purple*). The efferent collectors of the tracheobronchial nodes lead to the bronchomediastinal trunks. The arrows indicate the lymphatic drainage from the organs and the lymphatic flow towards the principal collecting trunks.

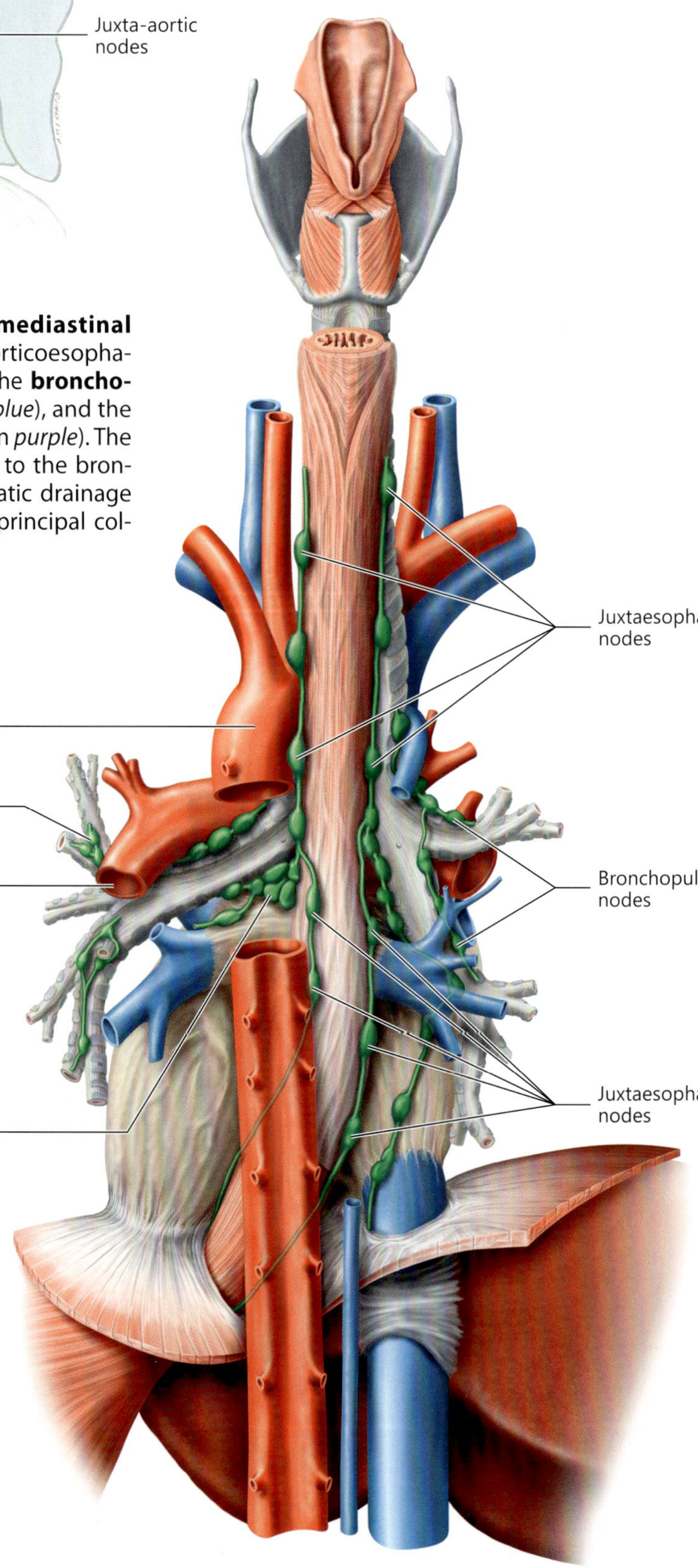

Distribution of the principal **lymph node chains of the posterior mediastinum**, viewed from behind.

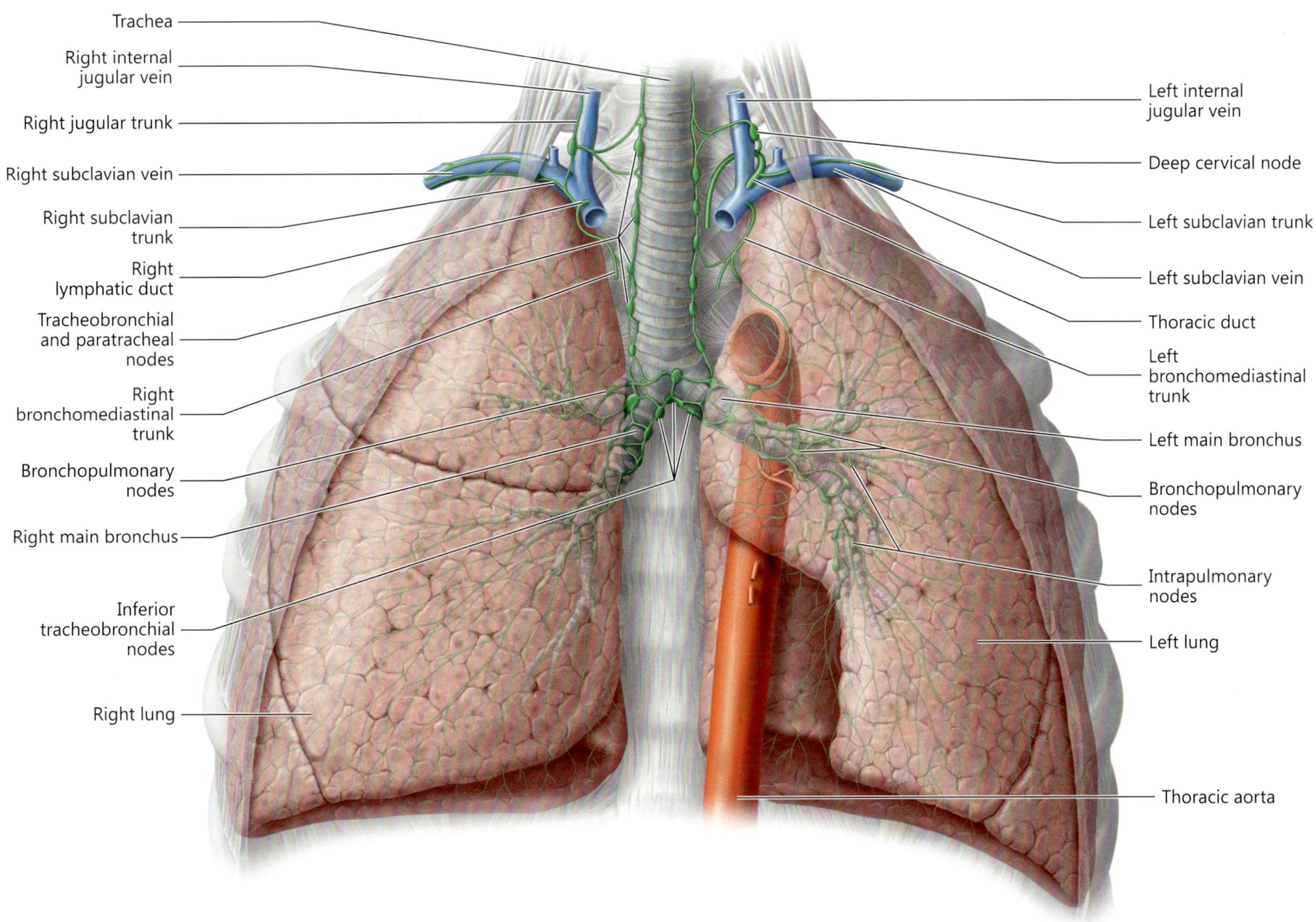

Lymphatic drainage of trachea, bronchi and lungs.

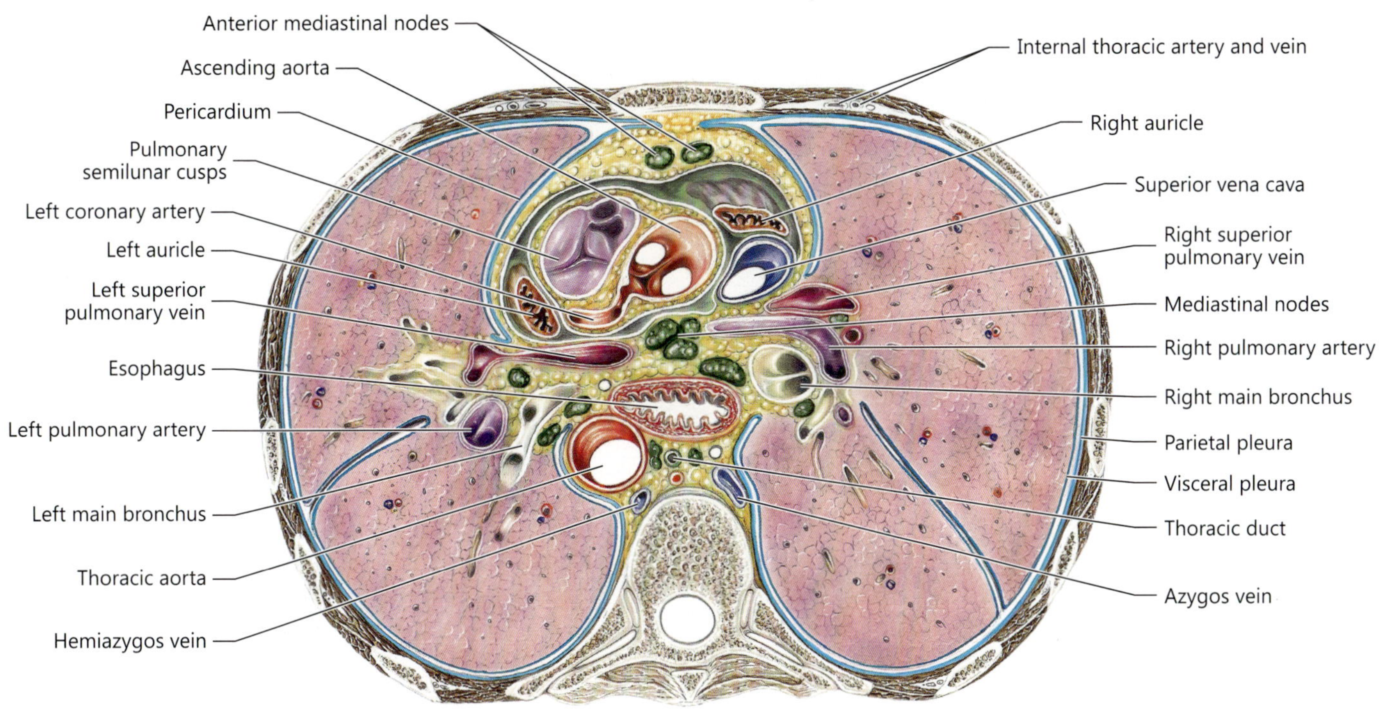

Transverse section passing through the fifth thoracic vertebra. Schematic representation of the **mediastinal nodes** in proximity to the tracheal bifurcation.

Schematic representation of the **innervation of the heart**. Parasympathetic and sympathetic fibers, both afferent and efferent, play a role in the innervation of the heart; they constitute the cardiac plexus. From the cardiac plexus originate fascicles of nerve fibers that travel to the heart, reaching the atrial and ventricular myocardium and the wall of the great vessels.

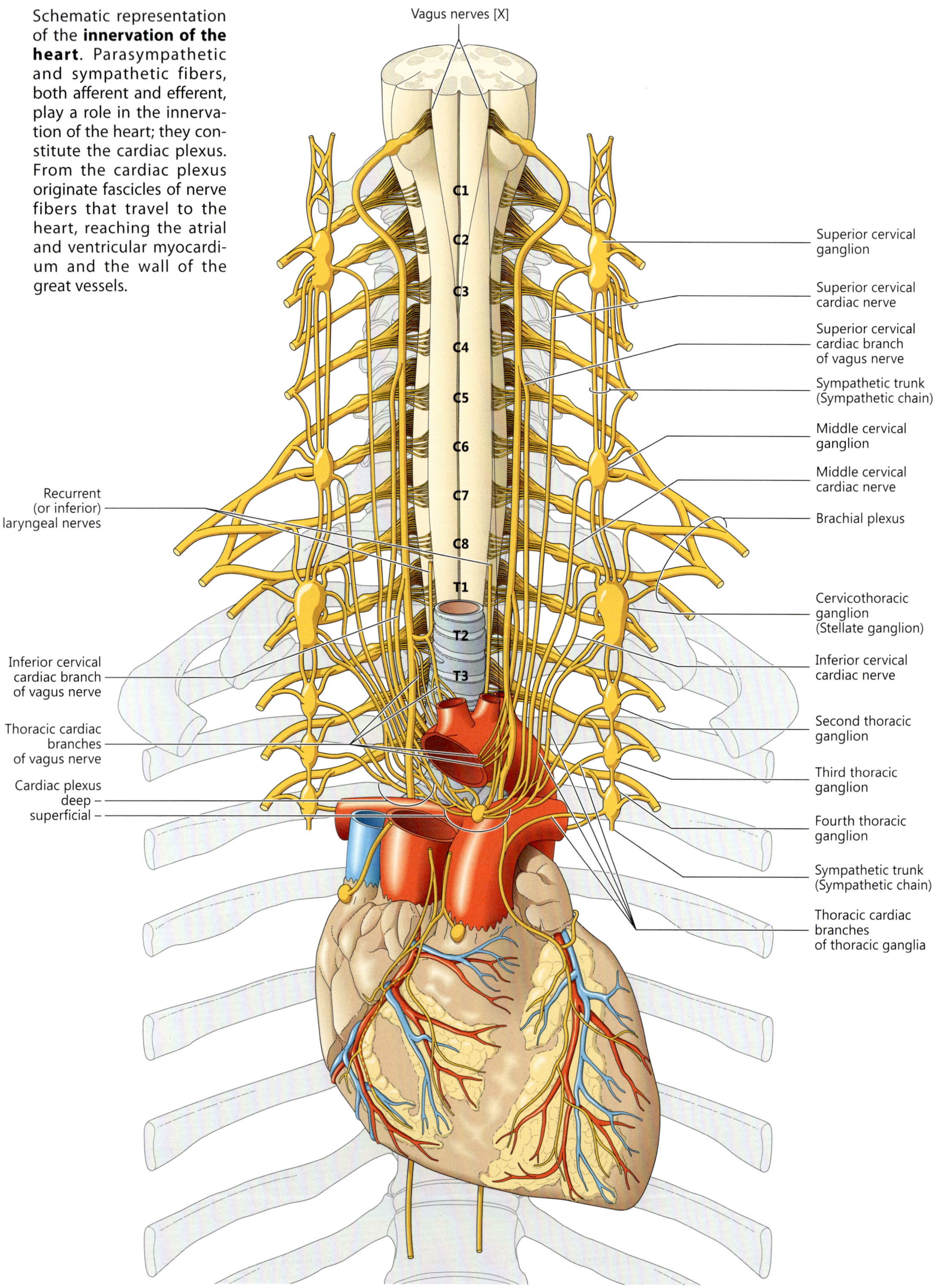

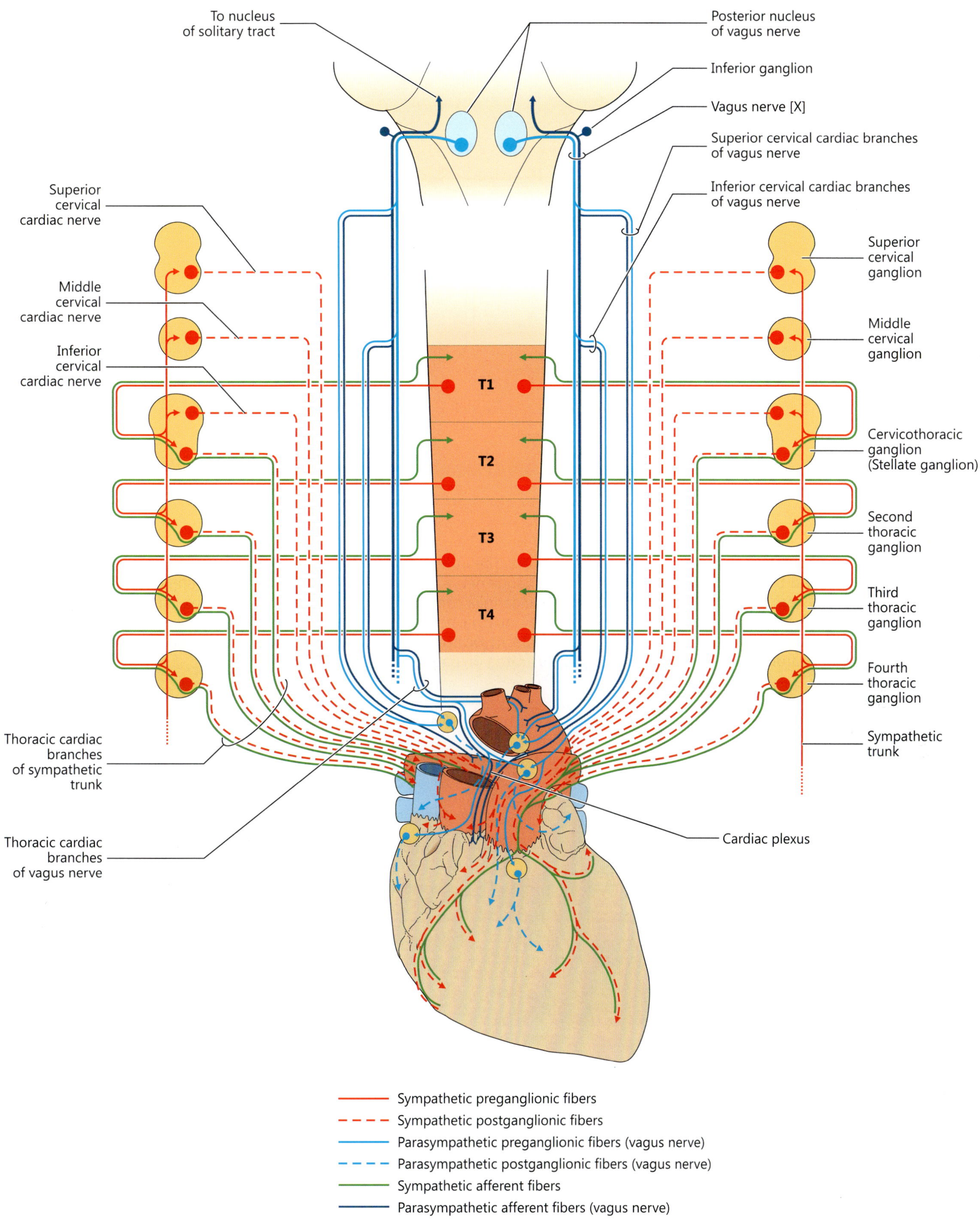

Schematic representation of the **innervation of the heart**. Detail of the composition of the nerve fibers that arrive at and depart from the cardiac plexus.

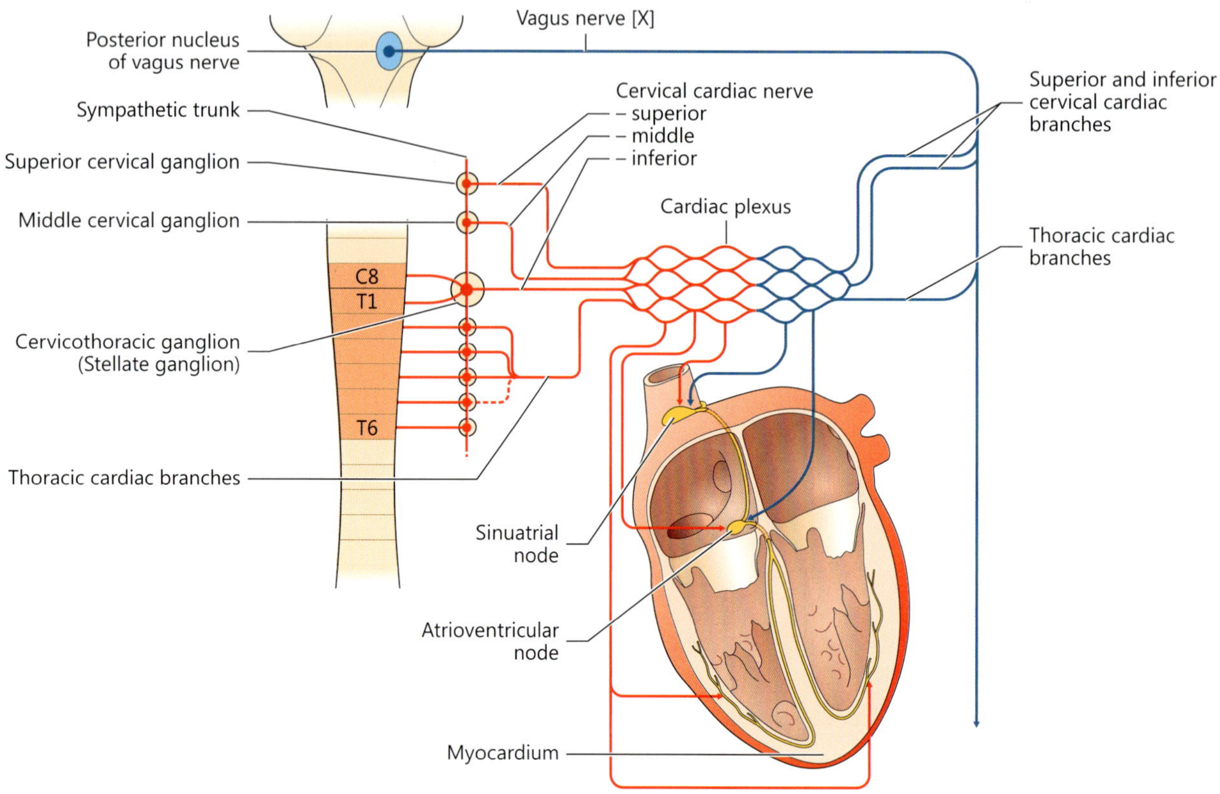

Schematic representation of the **innervation of the heart**. The innervation of the parasympathetic nervous system is carried out by cervical and thoracic collateral branches of the vagus nerve that travel to the cardiac plexus. Branches of the sympathetic nervous system coming from cervical and thoracic ganglia constitute the cardiac plexus. From the cardiac plexus depart branches of the parasympathetic nervous system for the sinuatrial node and atrioventricular node, and branches of the sympathetic system for the sinuatrial node, atrioventricular node, myocardium and coronary vessels. The cardiac conduction system, which generates cardiac impulses autonomously, is illustrated on page 357.

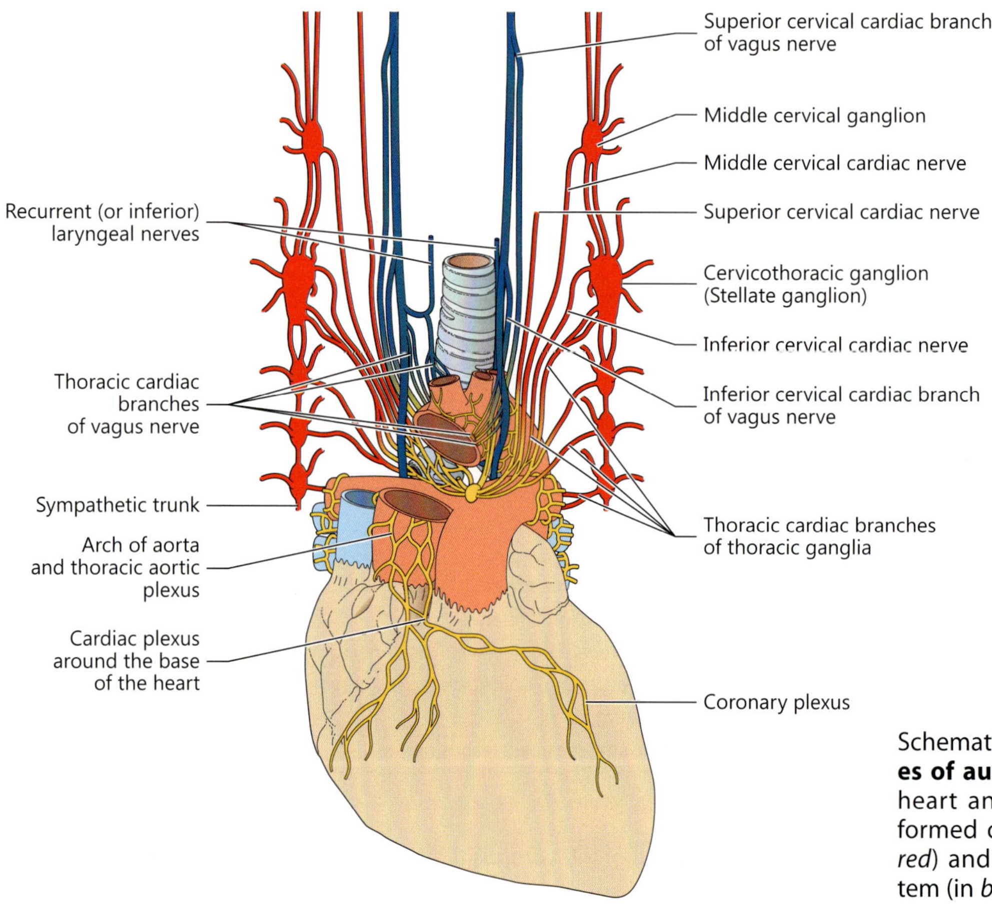

Schematic representation of the **plexuses of autonomic fibers** present on the heart and adjacent vessels, which are formed of fibers of the sympathetic (in *red*) and parasympathetic nervous system (in *blue*).

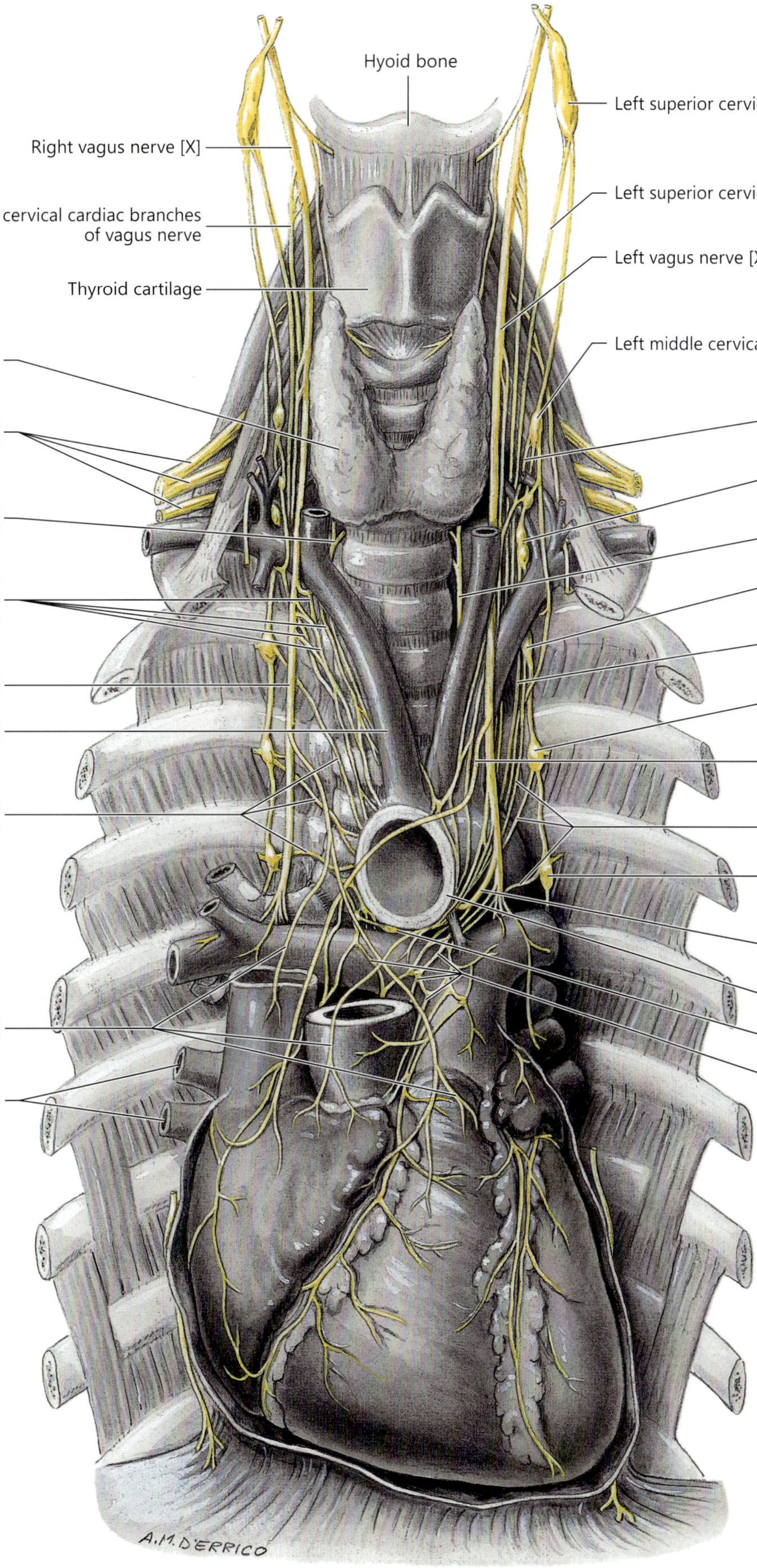

Schematic representation of the **innervation of the heart**. Through resection of the arch of the aorta, it is possible to see the exact location of the cardiac plexus, situated in correspondence to the base of the heart, between the arch of the aorta and the point of division of the pulmonary trunk. Removing the pericardium, one can see fascicles of nerve fibers accompanying the right and left coronary arteries, which travel to innervate the atrial and ventricular myocardium.

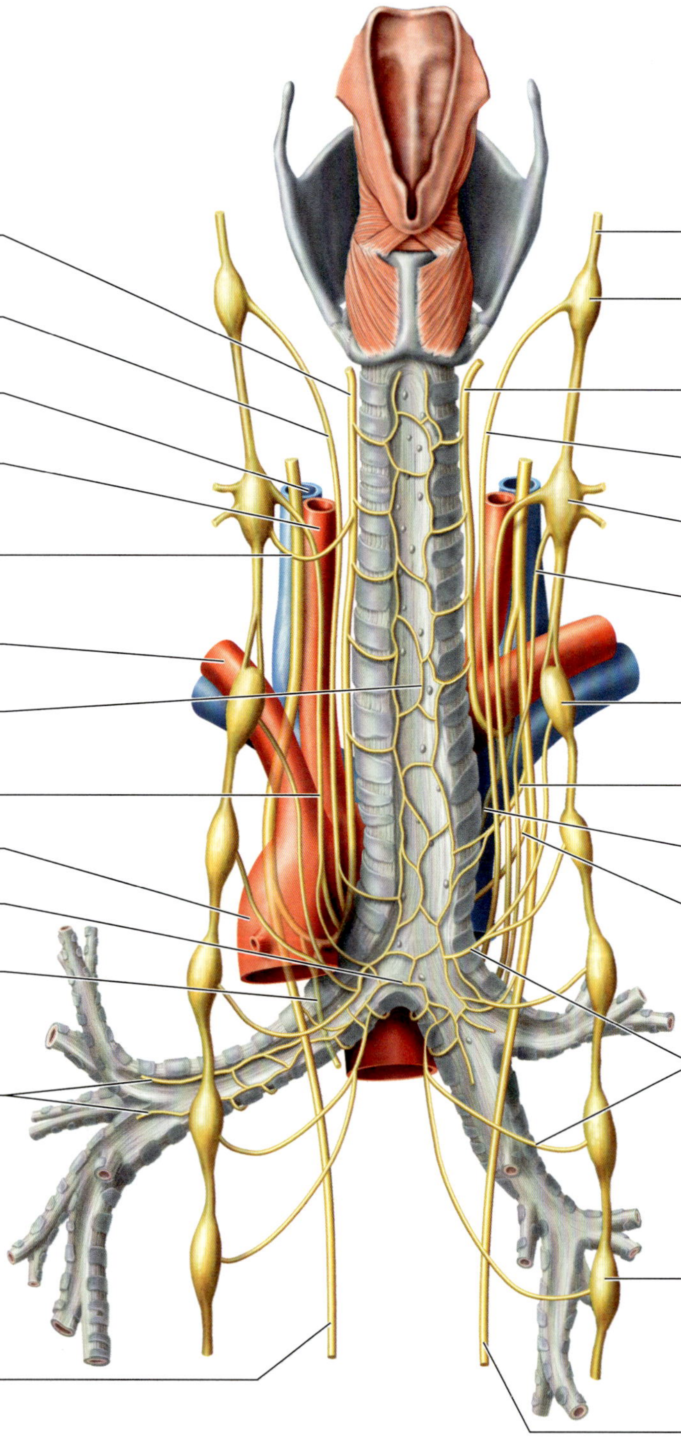

Representation of the **innervation of the heart**, posterior view. Note the course of the thoracic cardiac branches, coming from the vagus nerve, which join the cardiac plexus.

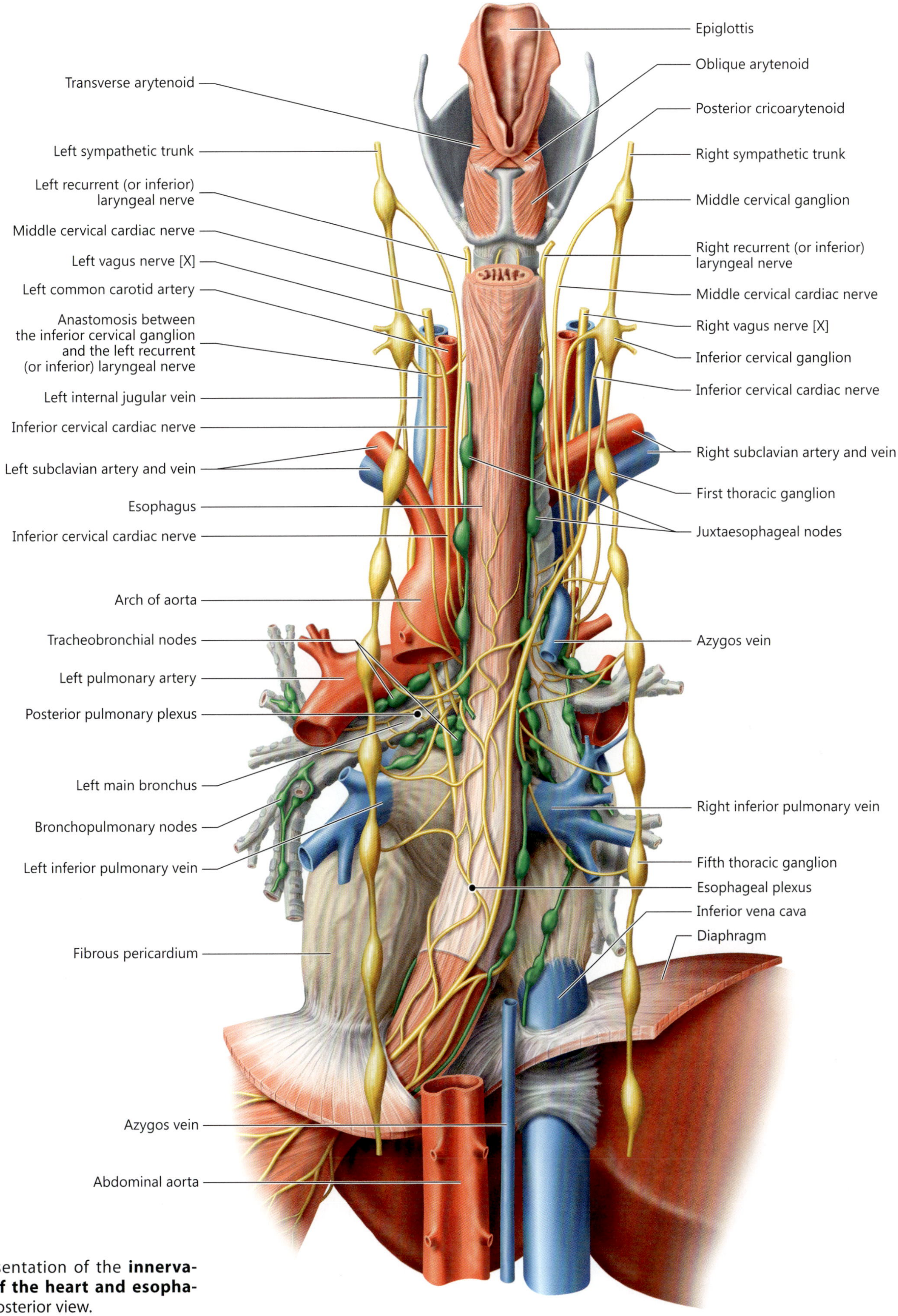

Representation of the **innervation of the heart and esophagus**, posterior view.

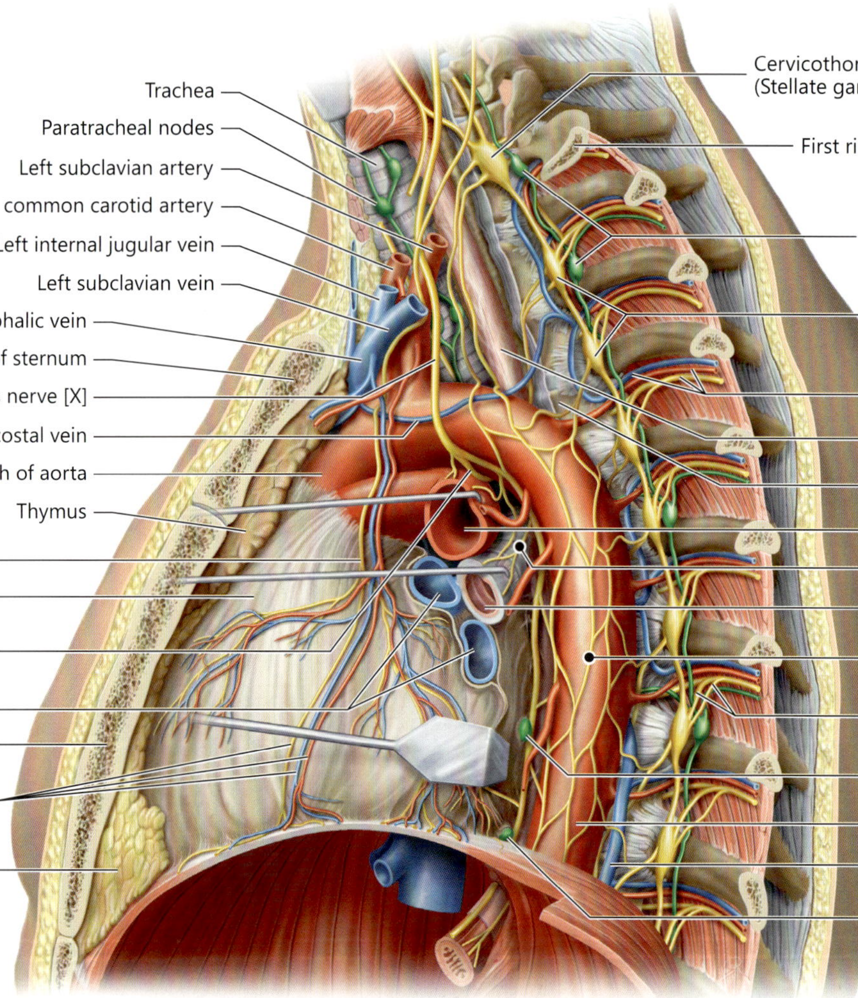

Schematic representation of the **innervation of the heart**, left lateral view. From the cervicothoracic (stellate) ganglion arise nerve fibers that descend towards the cardiac plexus. The pericardium is innervated by small branches coming from the right and left phrenic nerve.

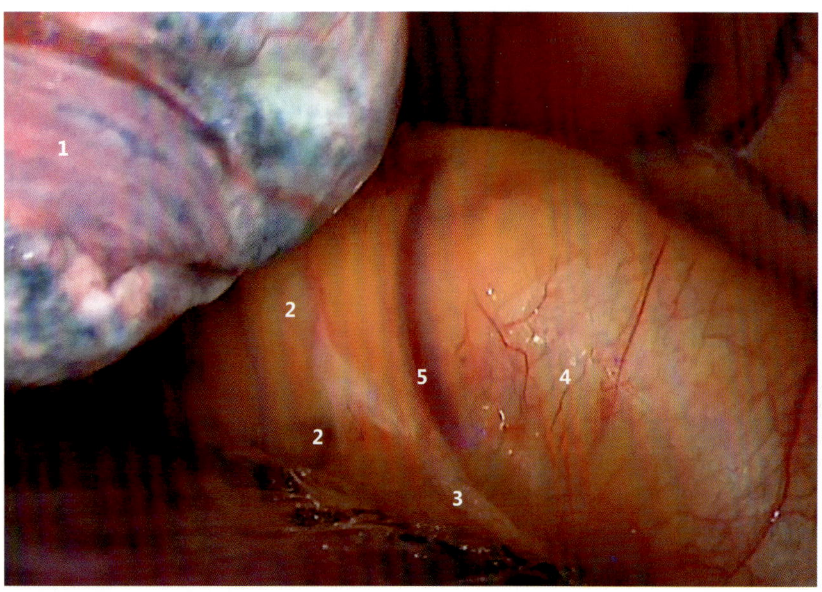

Image of the **arch of the aorta** obtained in the course of a thoracoscopy for diagnostic purposes. The endoscope is placed between the parietal and visceral layers of the pleura. View from above. One can observe the course of the vagus nerve on the lateral surface of the vessel.

1 Left lung
2 Vagus nerve [X]
3 Recurrent laryngeal nerve
4 Arch of aorta
5 Vasa vasorum

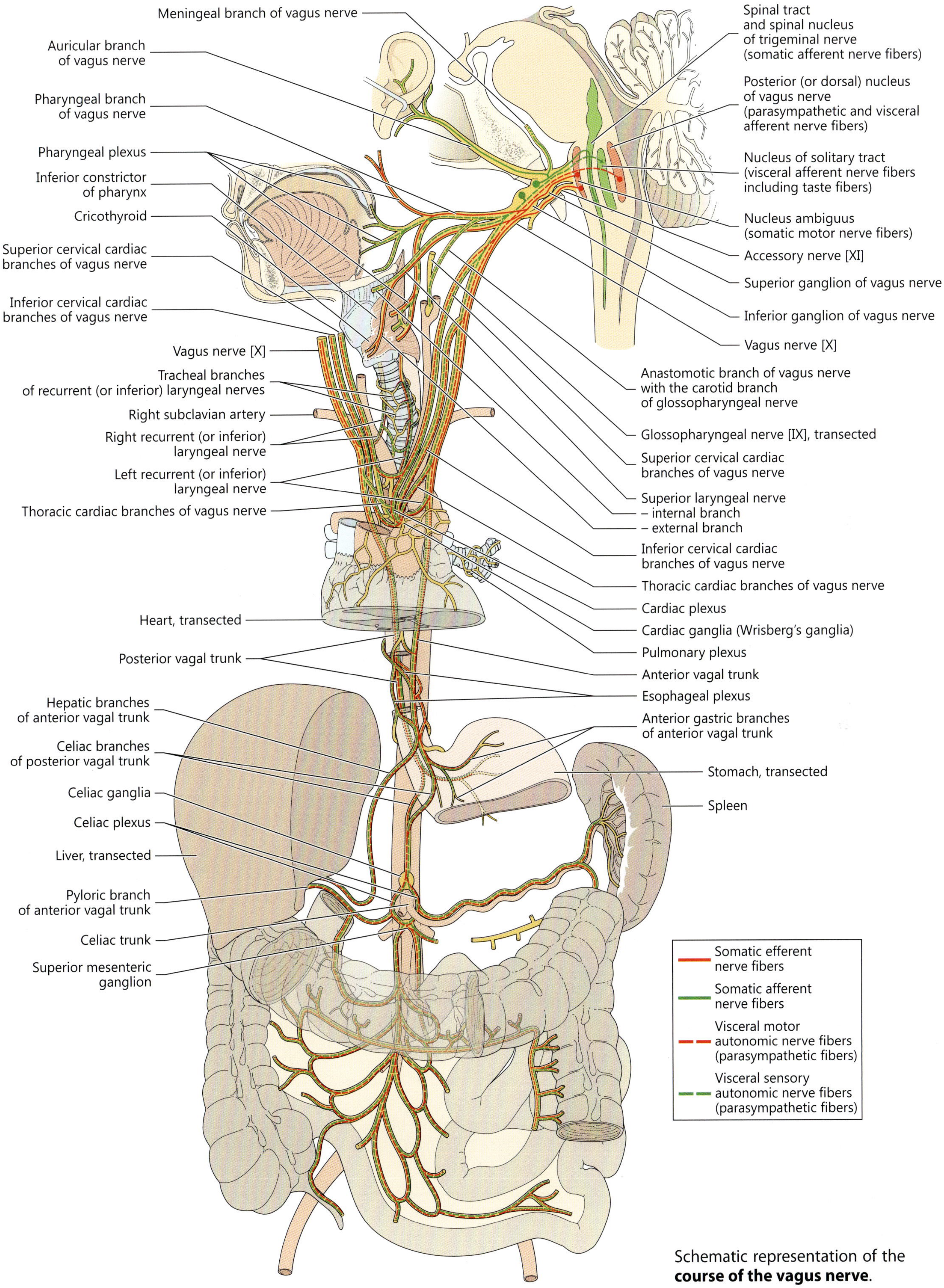

Schematic representation of the **course of the vagus nerve.**

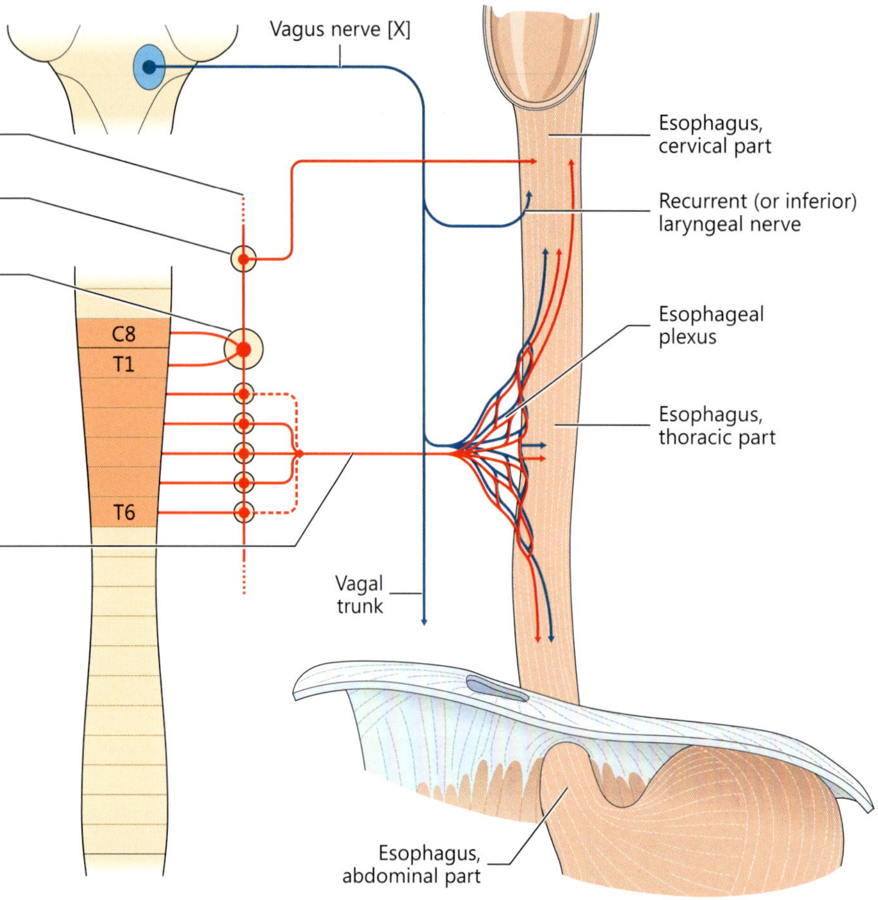

Schematic representation of the **innervation of the esophagus**. The parasympathetic nervous system innervation is carried out by esophageal branches of the laryngeal nerve coming from the vagus nerve. The fibers of the vagus nerve combine to form the esophageal plexus. From the thoracic ganglia of the sympathetic nervous system arise fibers that combine to form the esophageal plexus.

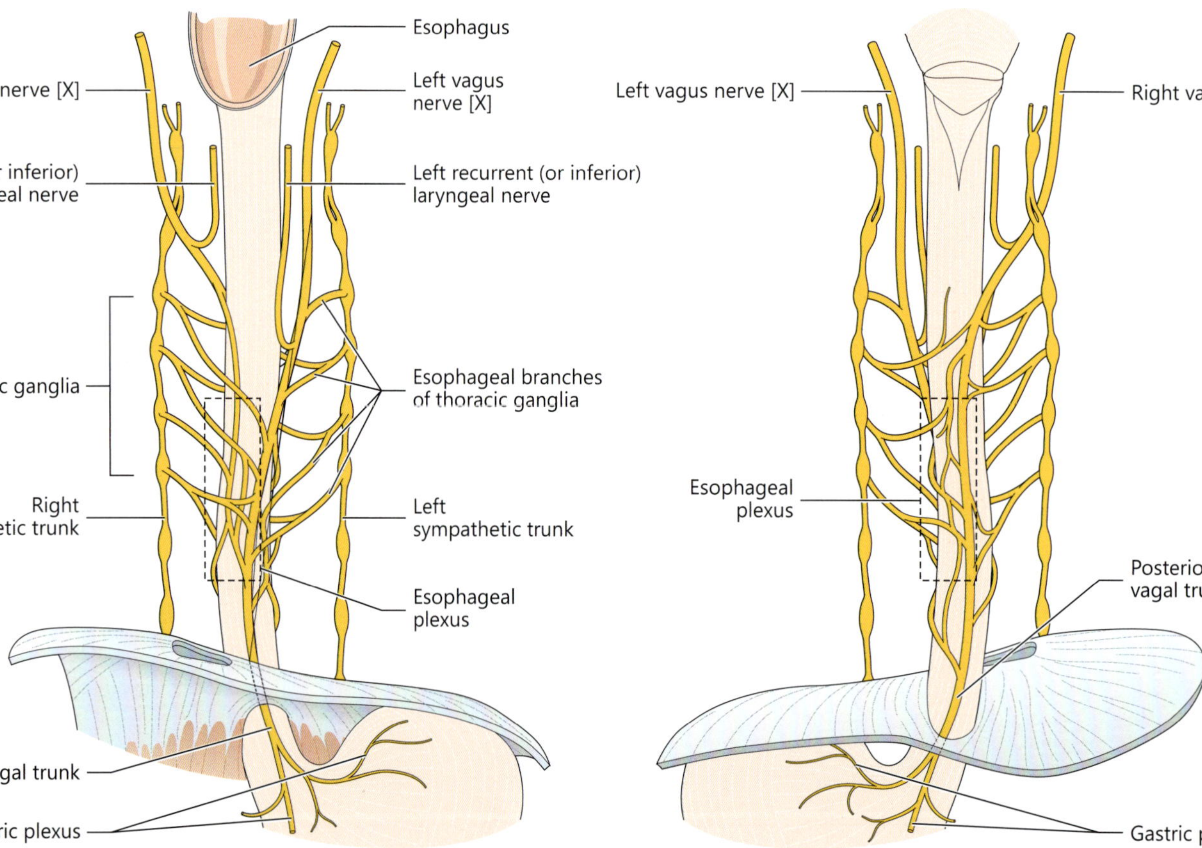

Schematic representation of the course of the (right and left) **vagus nerves** and their ramifications, which form the **plexuses of autonomic fibers on the esophagus**. Anterior and posterior views.

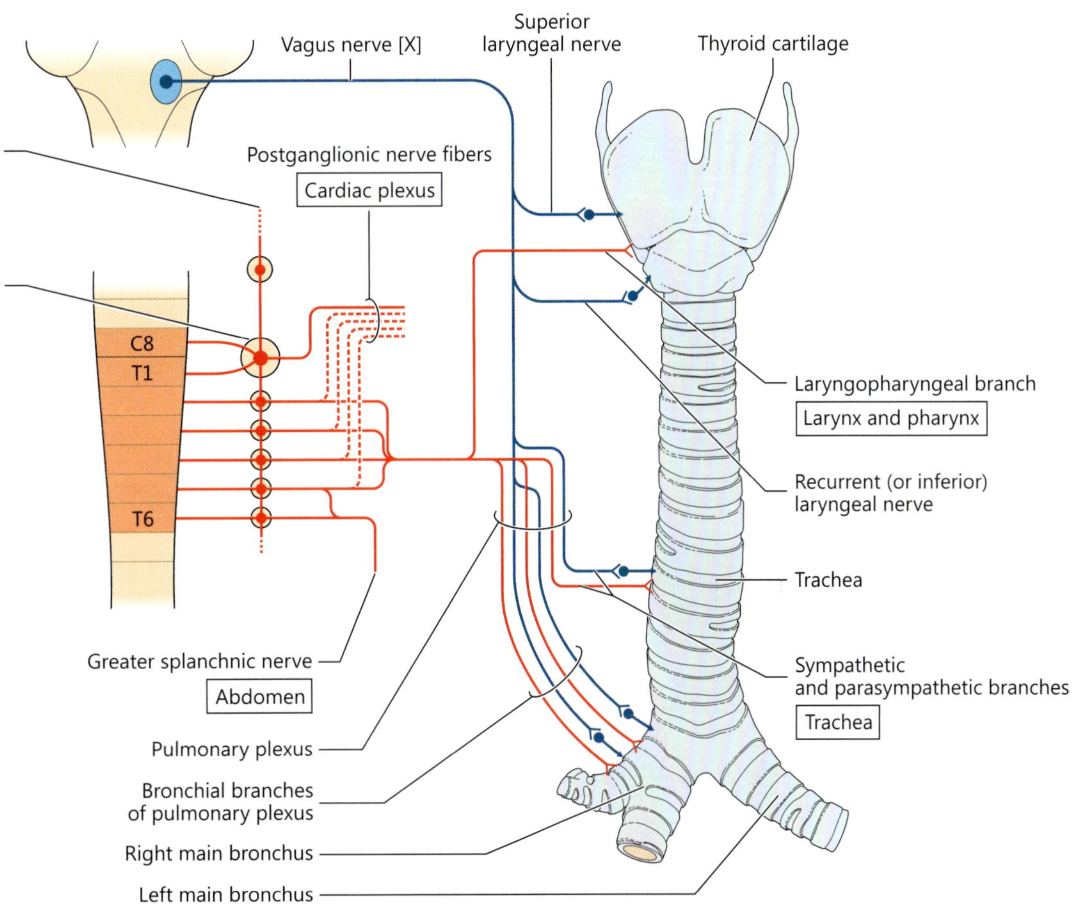

Schematic representation of the **innervation of the trachea and bronchial tree**. The parasympathetic nervous system innervation takes place through the laryngeal nerves, branches of the vagus nerve. The sympathetic nervous system innervation takes place through a few fibers towards the trachea and numerous postganglionic branches of the thoracic ganglia (thoracic pulmonary branches), which combine to form the pulmonary plexus.

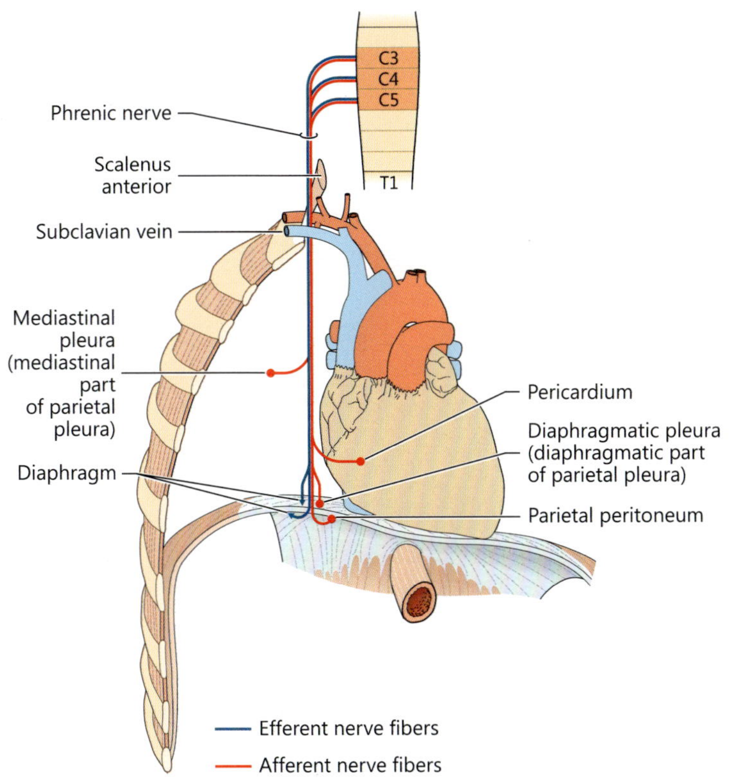

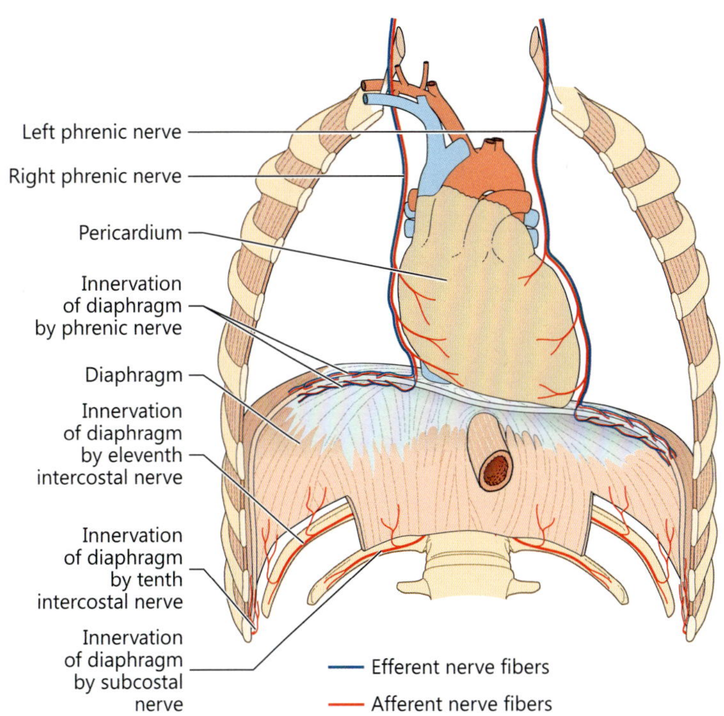

The **innervation of the diaphragm and pericardium** is carried out by the phrenic nerve (origin from C3-C5). The motor innervation of the diaphragm takes place also through the intercostal nerves X and XI and the subcostal nerve T12.

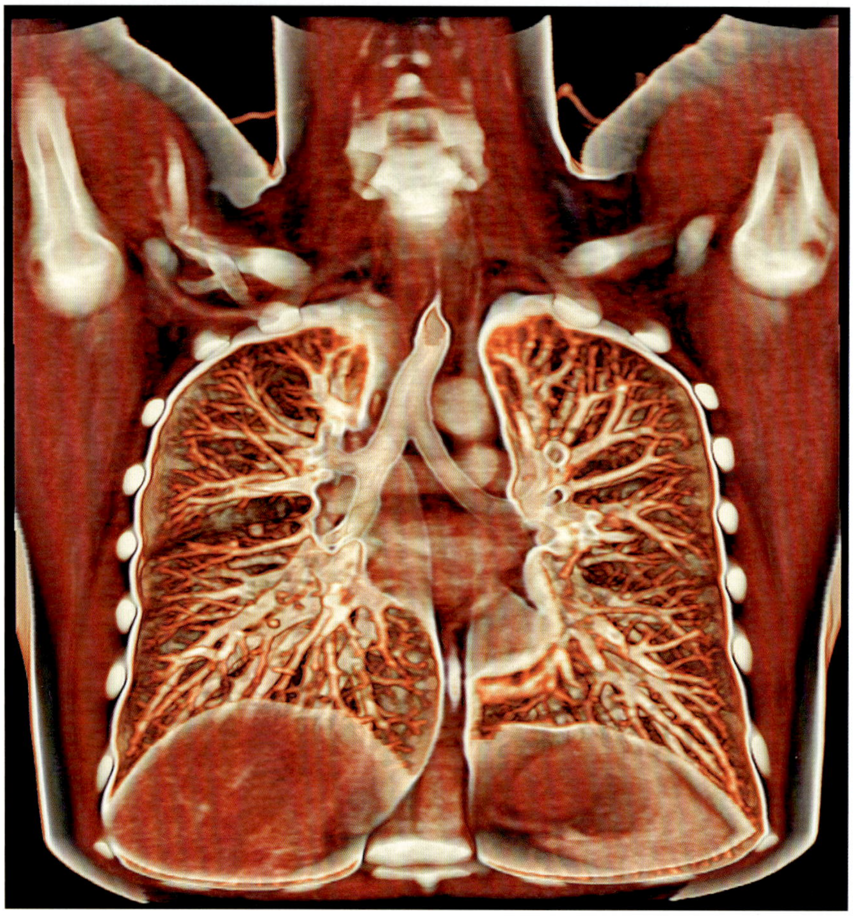

The lungs are contained within the **pleural compartments** inside the thoracic cavity (three-dimensional image of a living human body, obtained by CT scan using a 3D volume rendering technique).

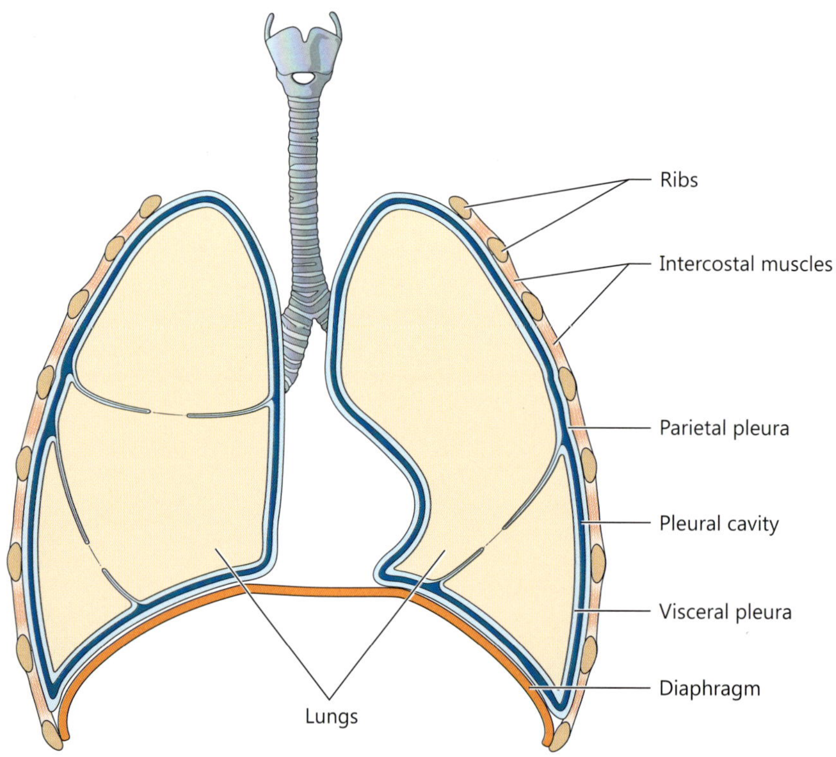

The **pleurae** consist of two layers: the parietal layer adheres closely to the endothoracic fascia, while the visceral layer adheres to the lung surface, extending into the pulmonary fissures. The two layers reflect one onto the other at the level of the hilum.

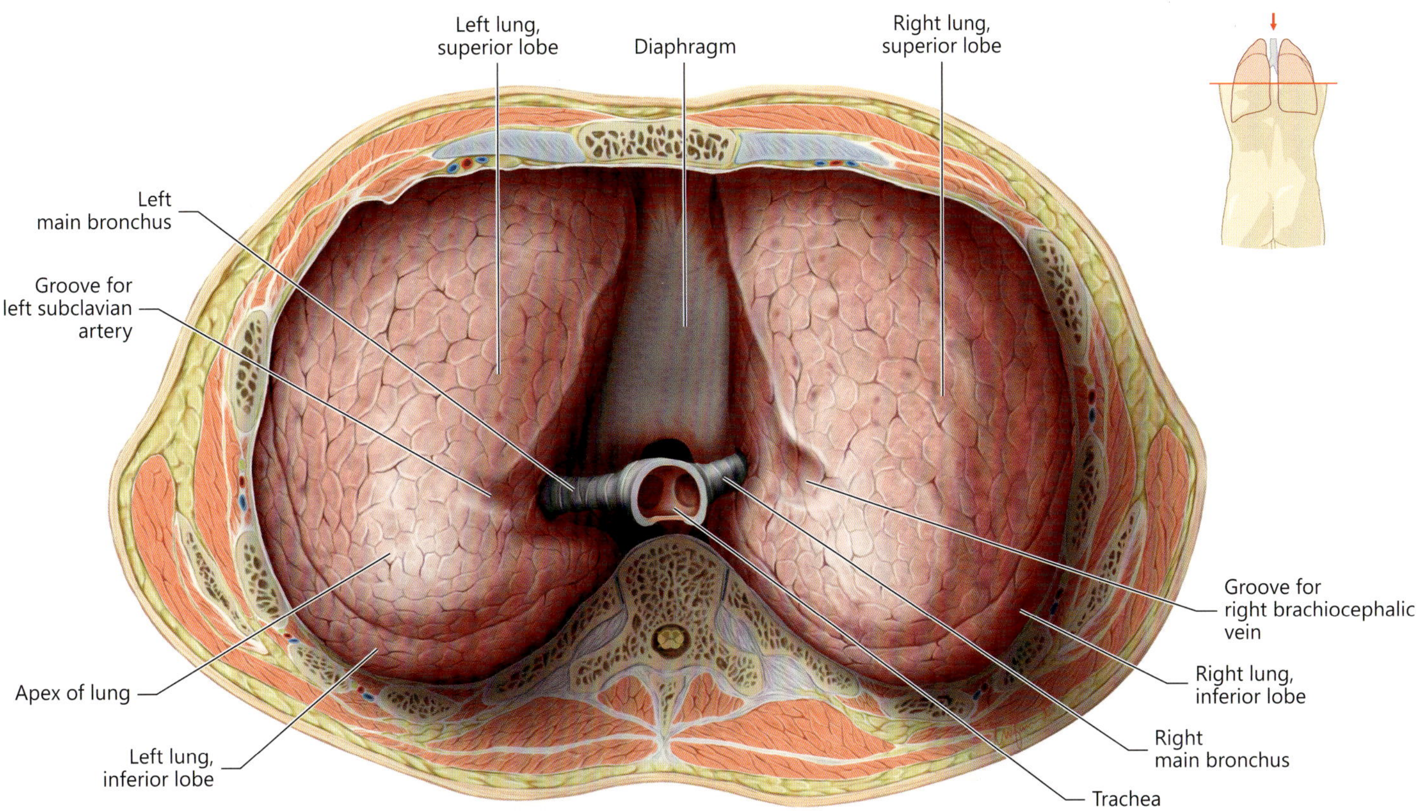

Lungs. View from above. The thoracic cage has been transected at the level of T V. The space of the mediastinum has been evacuated with the exception of the trachea.

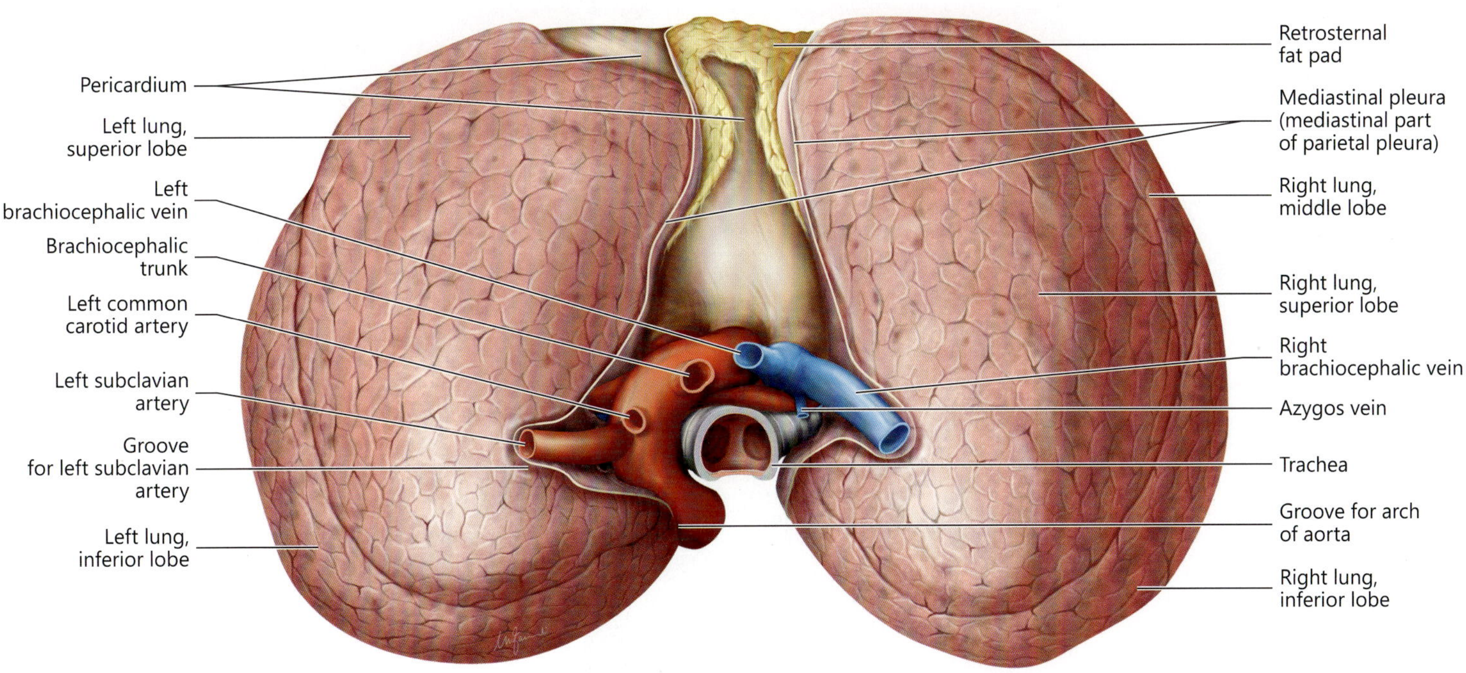

Lungs. View from above. The two mediastinal pleurae separate the pleural compartments from the mediastinum. On the medial surface of the lungs, the great vessels of the mediastinum and the heart leave deep impressions.

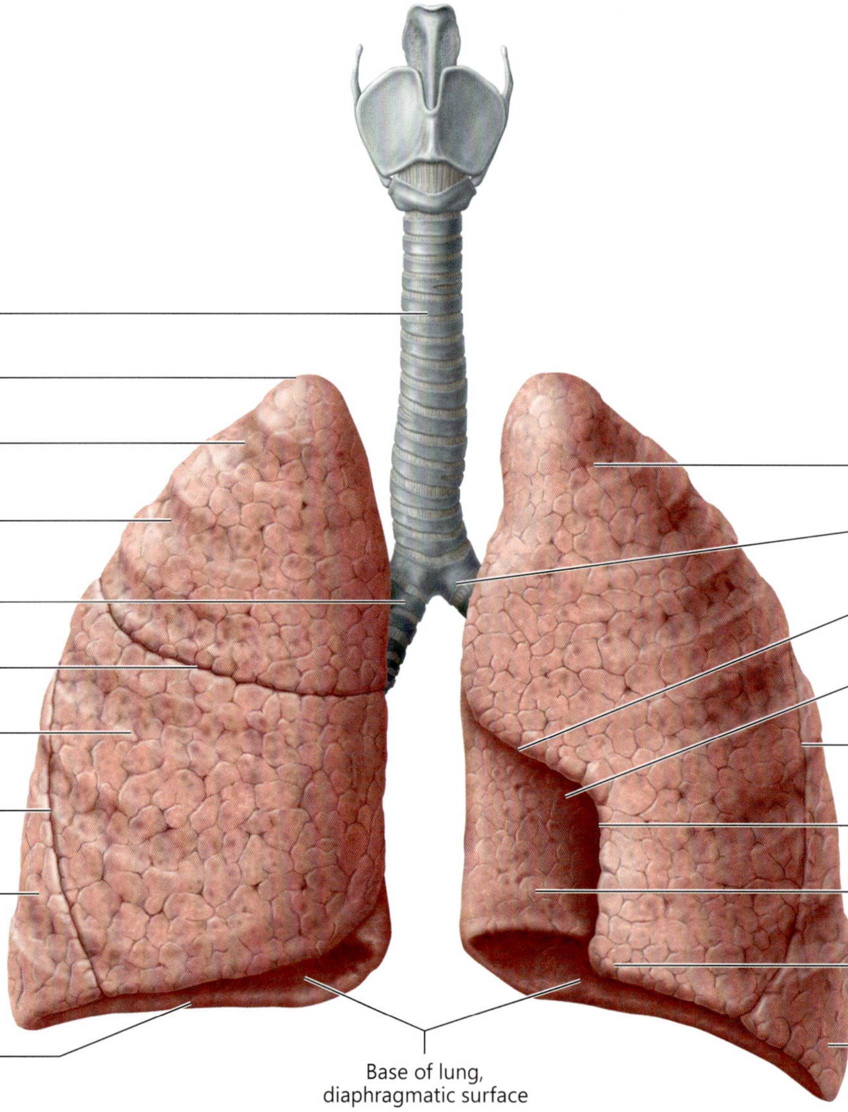

Lungs. Anterior view. One can see the pathway of the right pulmonary fissures and of the left pulmonary fissure. The left lung, smaller than the contralateral lung, presents only two lobes and contains the heart, which leaves the deep cardiac impression. The anterior border of the lung presents a notch (cardiac notch of the left lung), which renders it asymmetrical with respect to the contralateral one. The base of the lungs is concave towards the top and follows the line of the diaphragm. On the lateral surface of the lung, one can see the costal impressions created by the ribs.

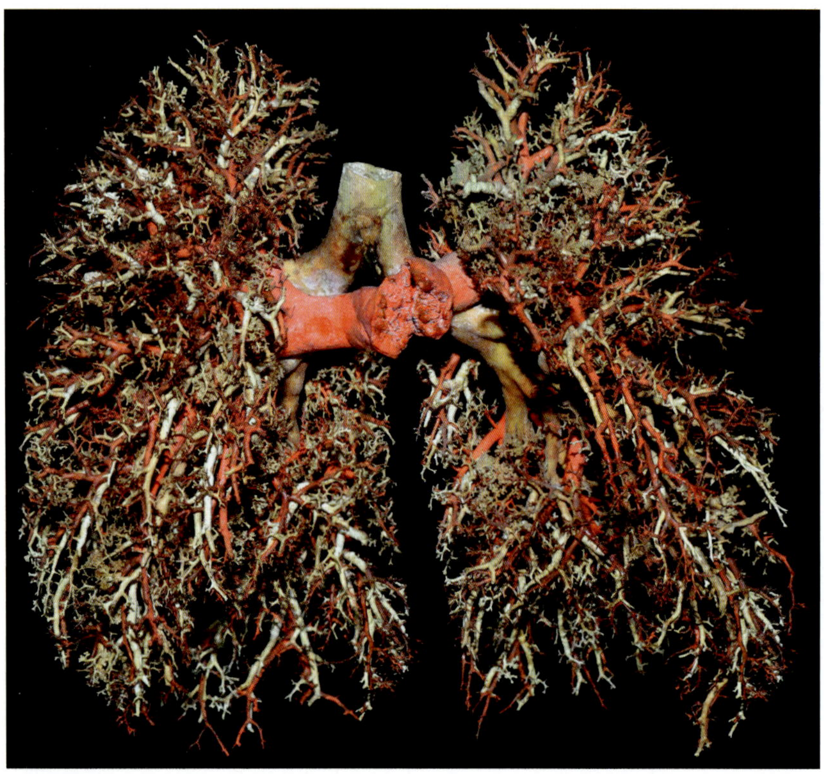

Tracheobronchial tree. Cast, anterior projection. In *yellow*, trachea and bronchial tree; in *red*, pulmonary trunk and its ramifications (courtesy of D. Sasse, Collezione anatomica, Basilea).

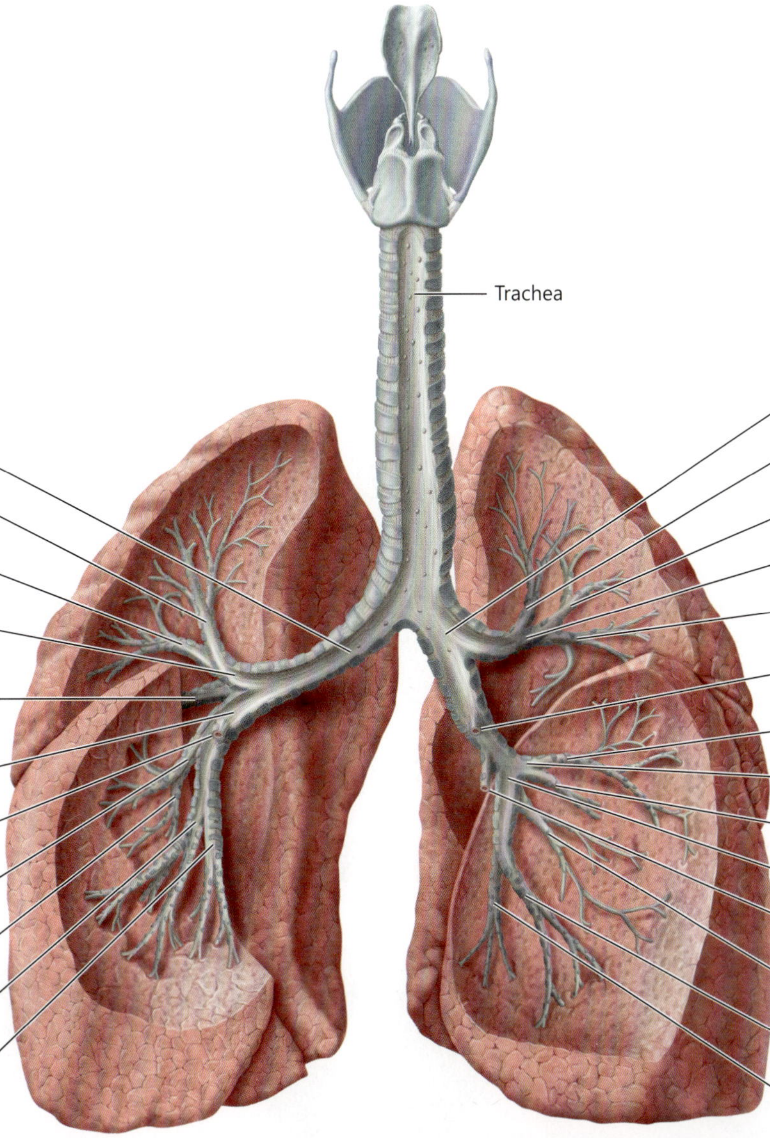

Tracheobronchial tree. Posterior view. Removal of part of the lung parenchyma makes it possible to see the ramifications of the bronchial tree.

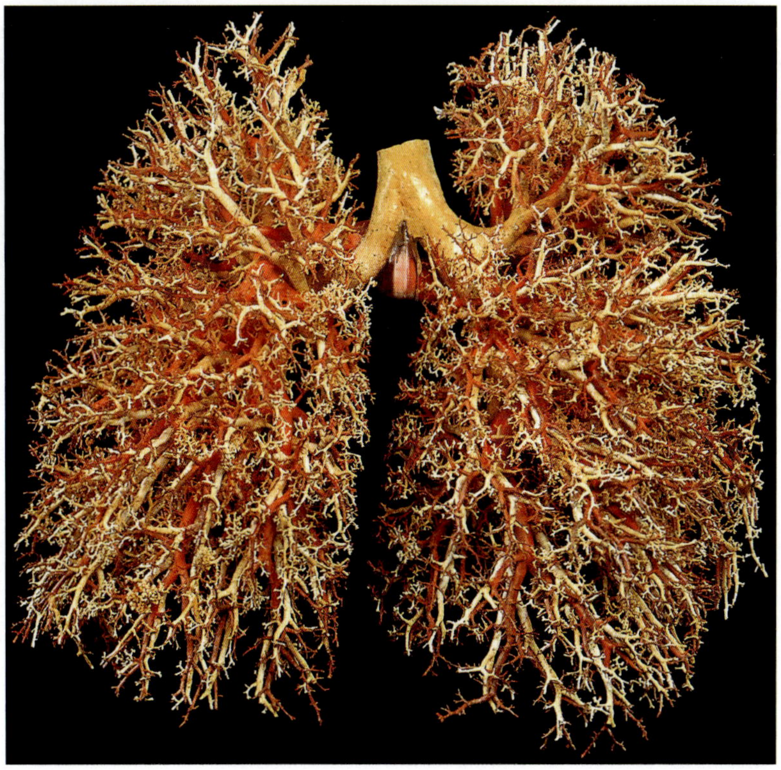

Tracheobronchial tree. Cast, posterior projection. In *yellow*, trachea and bronchial tree; in *red*, pulmonary trunk and its ramifications (courtesy of D. Sasse, Collezione anatomica, Basilea).

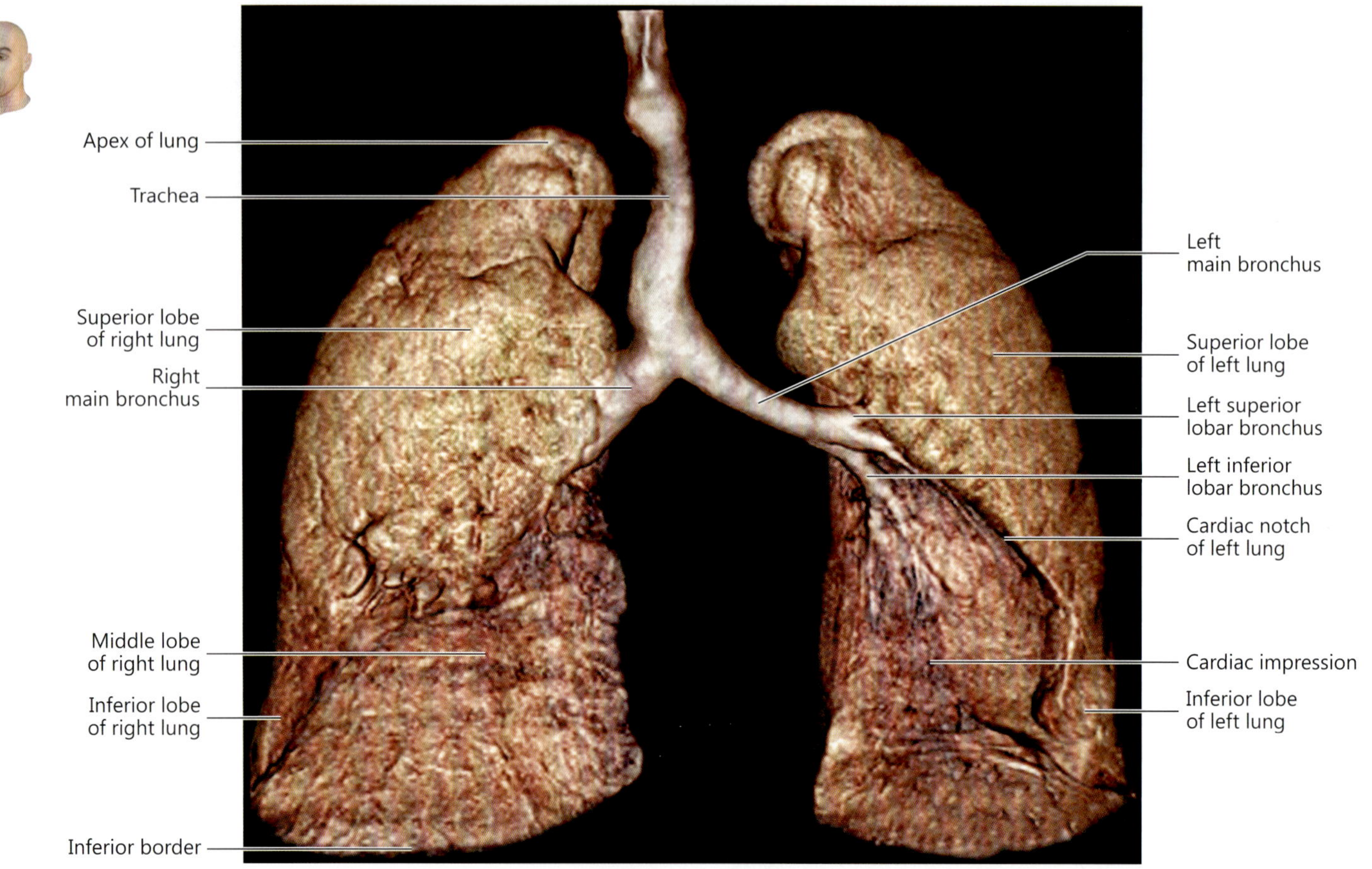

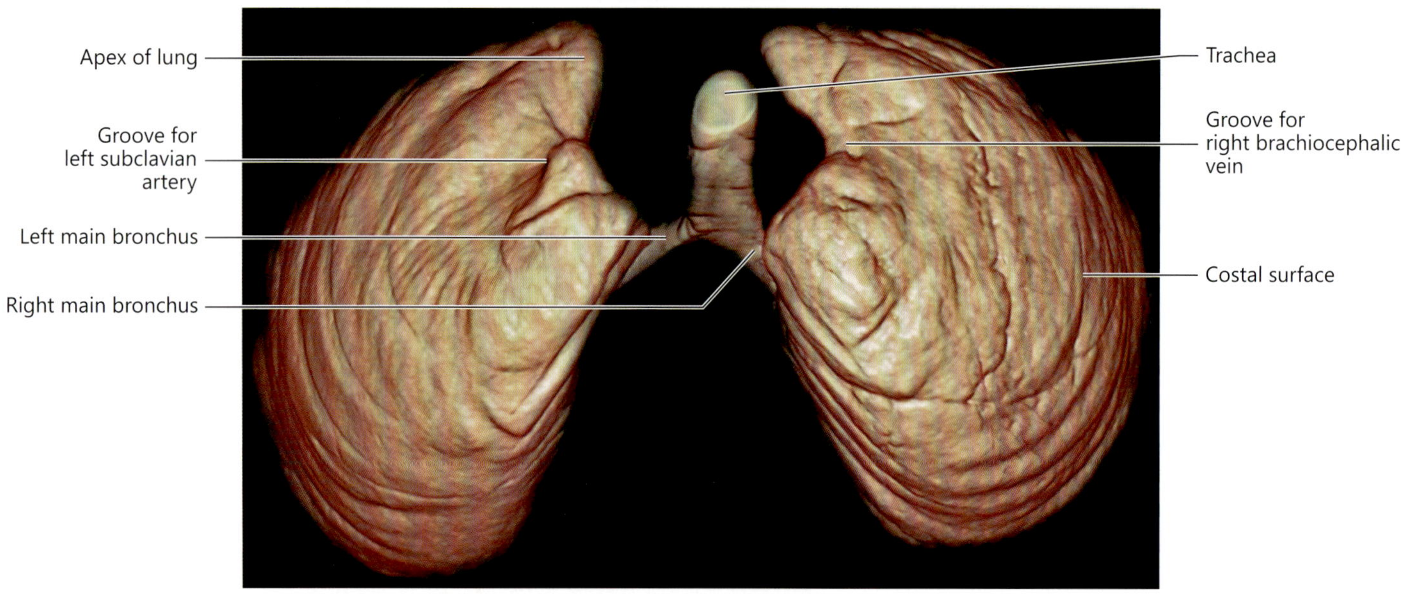

Three-dimensional images of a living human body, obtained by CT scan using a 3D volume rendering technique, showing the **lungs**. Above, anterior view; below, view from above.

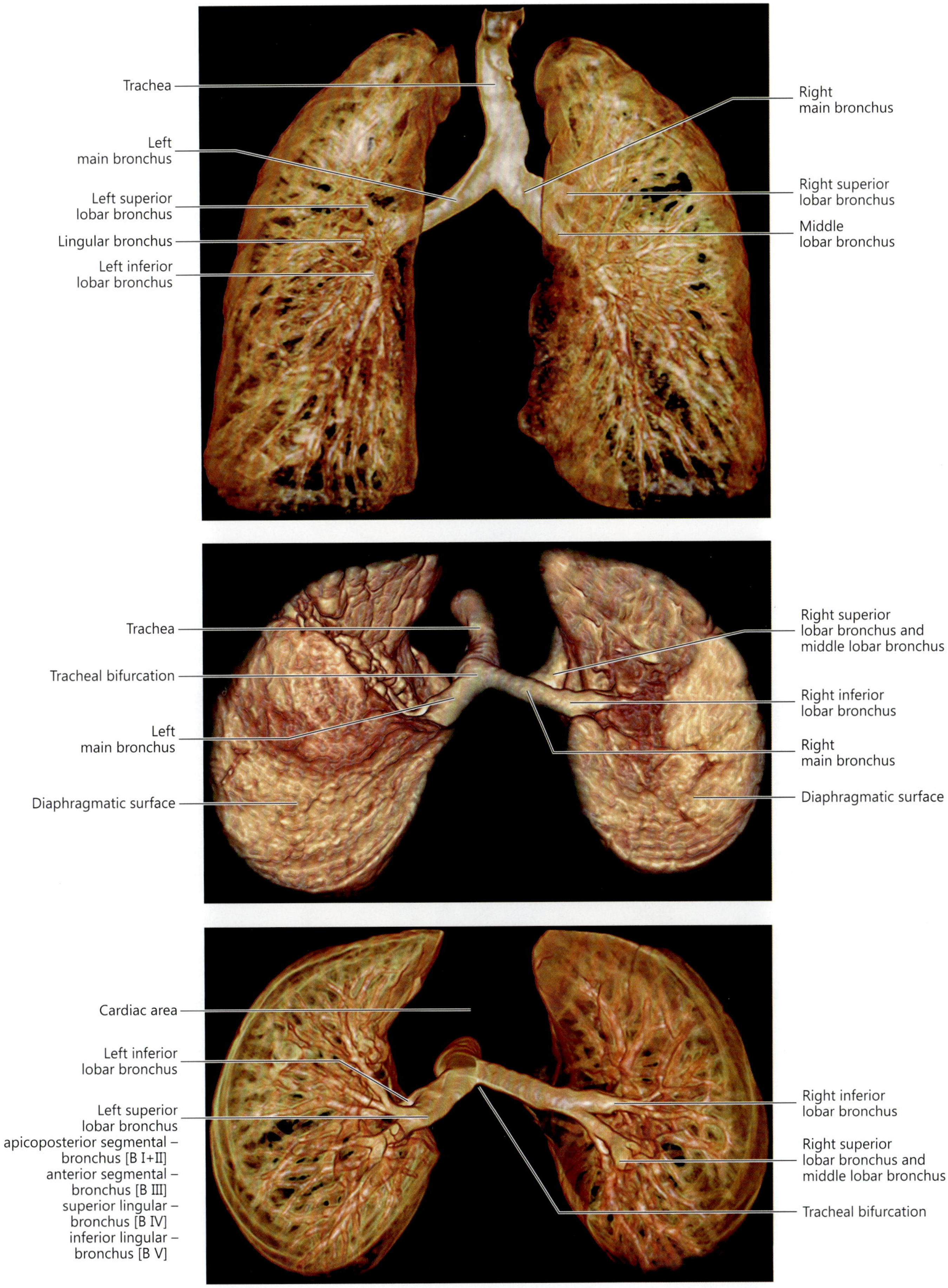

Three-dimensional images of a living human body, obtained by CT scan using a 3D volume rendering technique, showing the **lungs**. At the top, posterior view. The plane makes it possible to see the ramifications of the bronchial tree. In the center, view from the base of the lungs. At the bottom, same projection as the preceding but with removal of part of the lung parenchyma in order to display the bronchial ramifications.

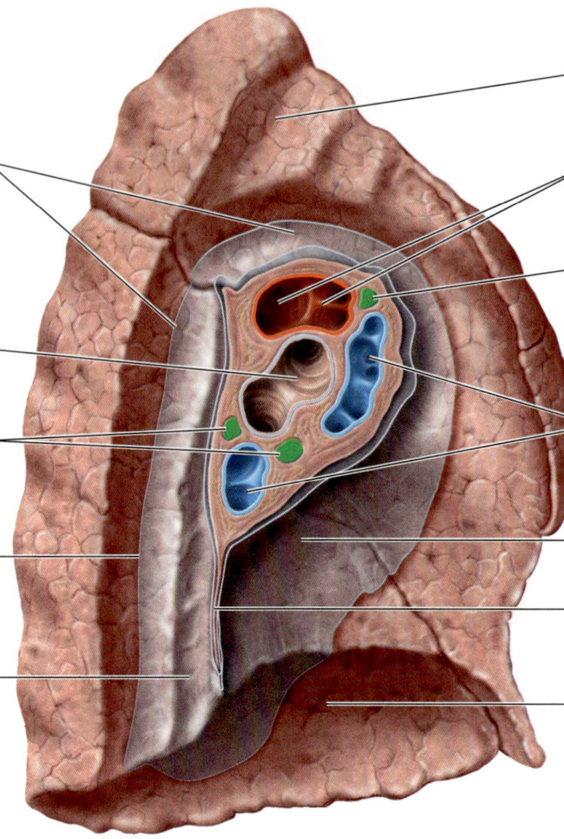

a

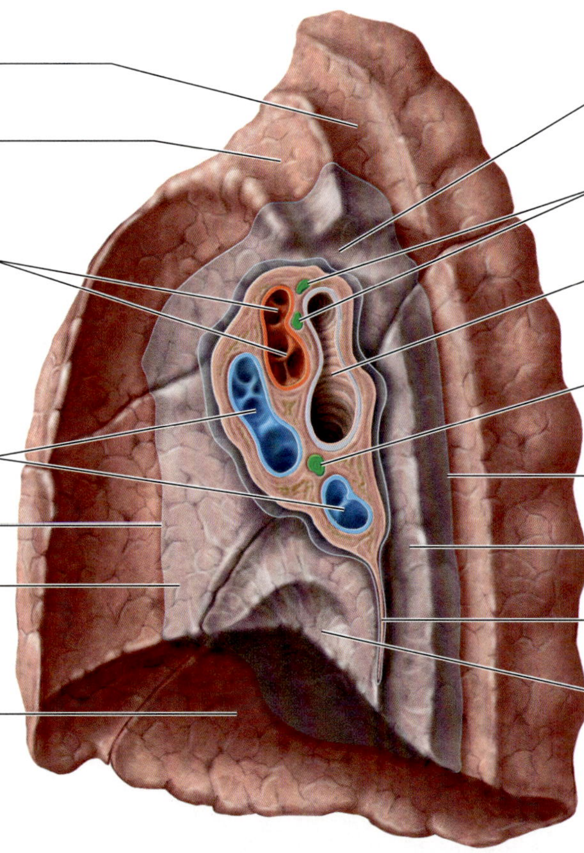

b

Lungs. a, Mediastinal surface of the left lung; **b**, mediastinal surface of the right lung. One can clearly see the deep impressions created by the structures of the mediastinum and by the thoracic vertebrae. One can also see the structures of the hilum and the position of the pulmonary arteries and veins relative to the bronchi. On the left, the pulmonary arteries are situated at a higher level than the bronchi, compared to the right hilum. The reflection of the parietal pleural layer onto the visceral one (not shown) at the level of the hilum contributes to the formation of the pulmonary (triangular) ligament.

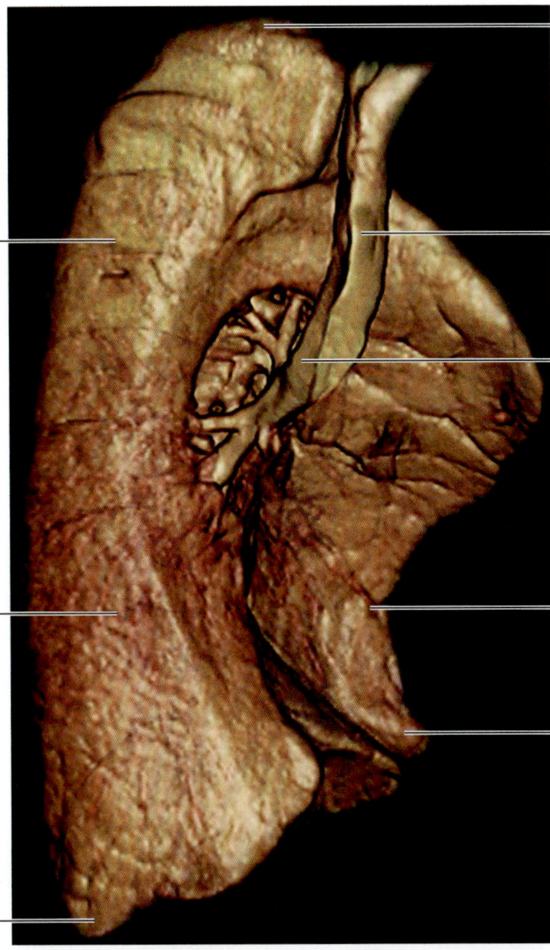

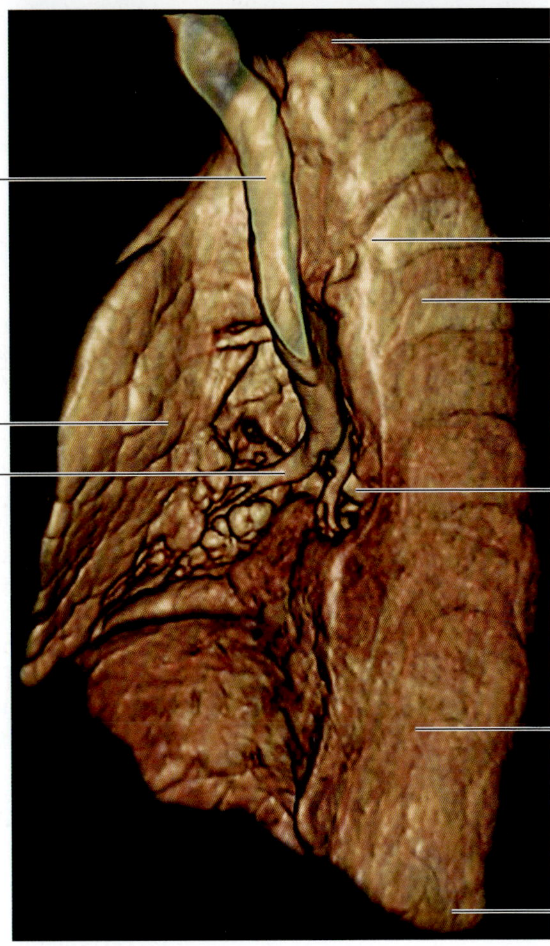

Three-dimensional images of a living human body, obtained by CT scan using a 3D volume rendering technique, showing the **lungs**. Above, medial view of the left lung. Below, medial view of the right lung.

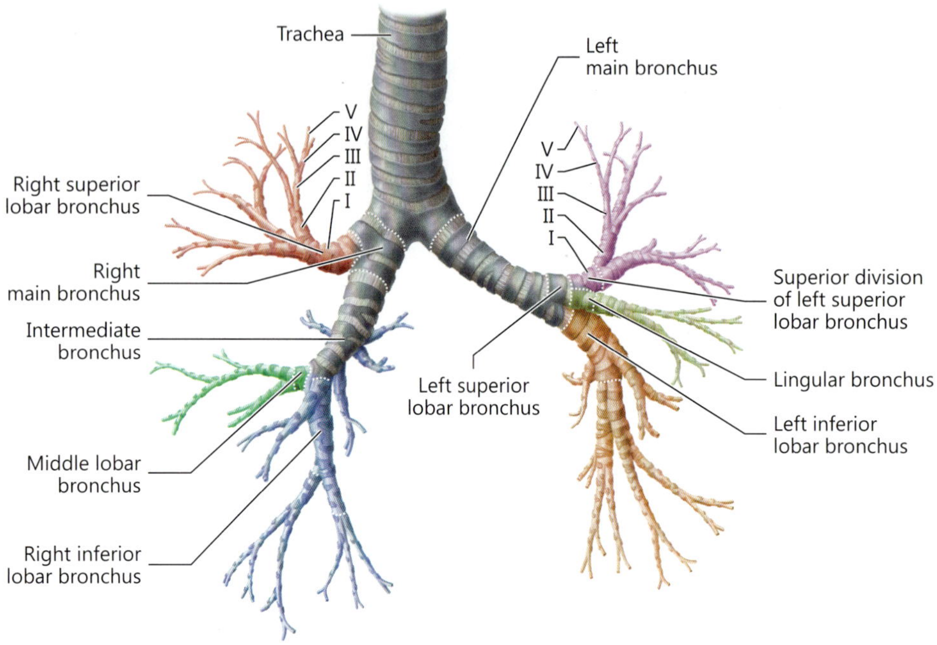

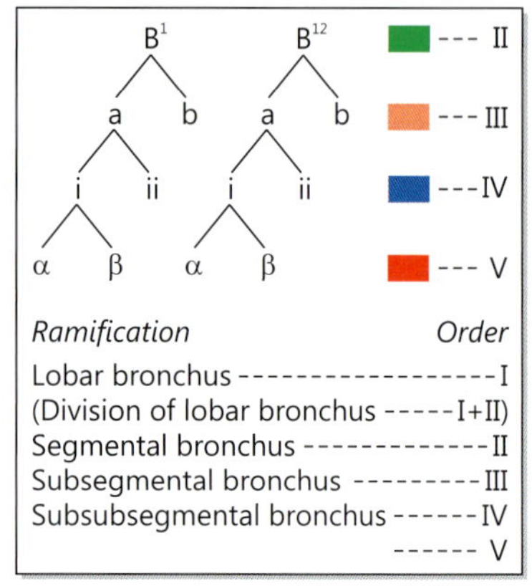

Ikeda's classification with indication of the order of ramifications (I, II, III, IV and V) and the color code utilized in the figure below on the left.

Right lung

Superior lobe
- 1 Apical segmental bronchus [B I]
- 2 Posterior segmental bronchus [B II]
- 3 Anterior segmental bronchus [B III]

Middle lobe
- 4b Lateral segmental bronchus [B IV]
- 5b Medial segmental bronchus [B V]

Inferior lobe
- 6 Superior segmental bronchus [B VI]
- 7 Medial basal segmental bronchus [B VII]
- 8 Anterior basal segmental bronchus [B VIII]
- 9 Lateral basal segmental bronchus [B IX]
- 10 Posterior basal segmental bronchus [B X]

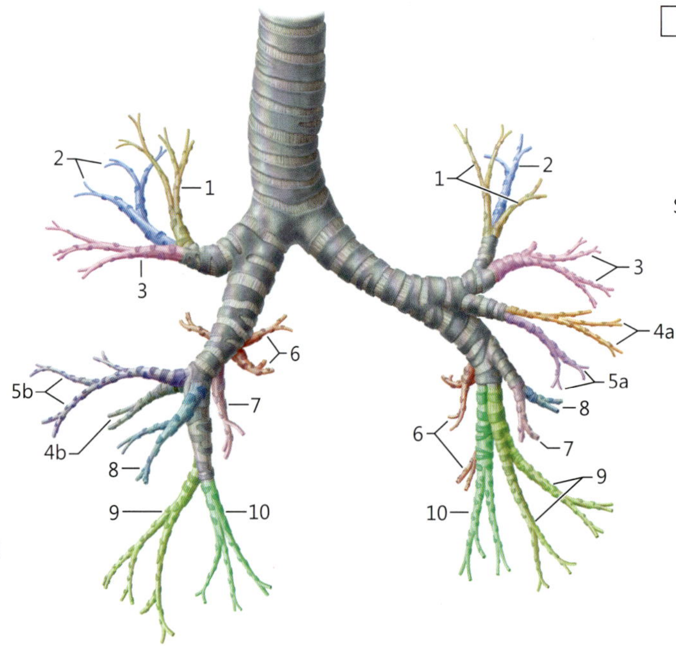

Left lung

Superior lobe
- 1 Apical segmental bronchus [B I] (Apicoposterior segmental bronchus [B I+II])
- 2 Posterior segmental bronchus [B II] (Apicoposterior segmental bronchus [B I+II])
- 3 Anterior segmental bronchus [B III]
- 4a Superior lingular bronchus [B IV]
- 5a Inferior lingular bronchus [B V]

Inferior lobe
- 6 Superior segmental bronchus [B VI]
- 7 Medial basal segmental bronchus [B VII]
- 8 Anterior basal segmental bronchus [B VIII]
- 9 Lateral basal segmental bronchus [B IX]
- 10 Posterior basal segmental bronchus [B X]

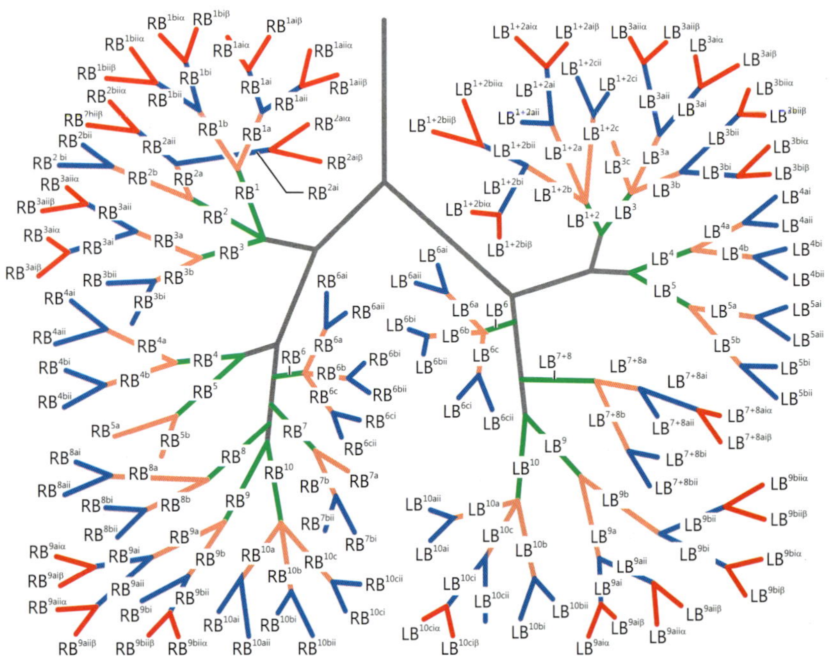

Nomenclature for describing the **lobar**, **segmental** and **subsegmental ramifications of the bronchi**. *Jackson-Huber* (figure at the top): the bronchi are named based on their spatial orientation (right/left, superior/inferior, anterior/posterior). *Boyden*: the classification reflects the subdivision of the bronchial tree (and of the accompanying arteries and veins) as it is observed during development. The segmental bronchi (order II) are indicated with the letter B followed by a number from 1 to 10 (1-3 superior lobe, 4-5 middle or lingular node, 6-10 inferior lobe). The introduction of flexible fiberoptic bronchoscopy by *Ikeda* has enabled a precise classification of the ramifications downstream of order II bronchi on the right (R) and left (L) side: the subsegmental ones (order III) are indicated by the letter a, b, c; the ramifications of order IV by i (anterior) and ii (posterior); and order V ramifications by α and β. The figure at the center shows the correspondence between the classifications of Jackson-Huber and Boyden regarding the segmental bronchi, while the figure on the side and the table above show the subsegmental classification of Ikeda.

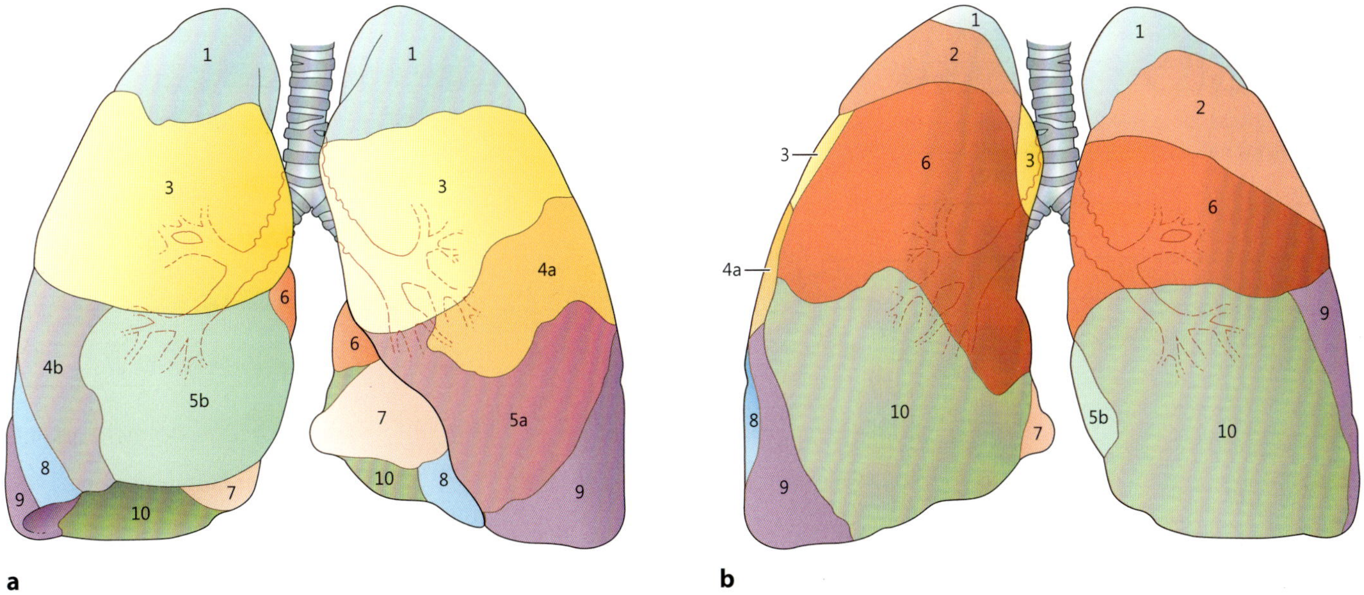

Pulmonary zones (colors correspond to those indicated in the preceding figure). **a**, Anterior projection; **b**, posterior projection.

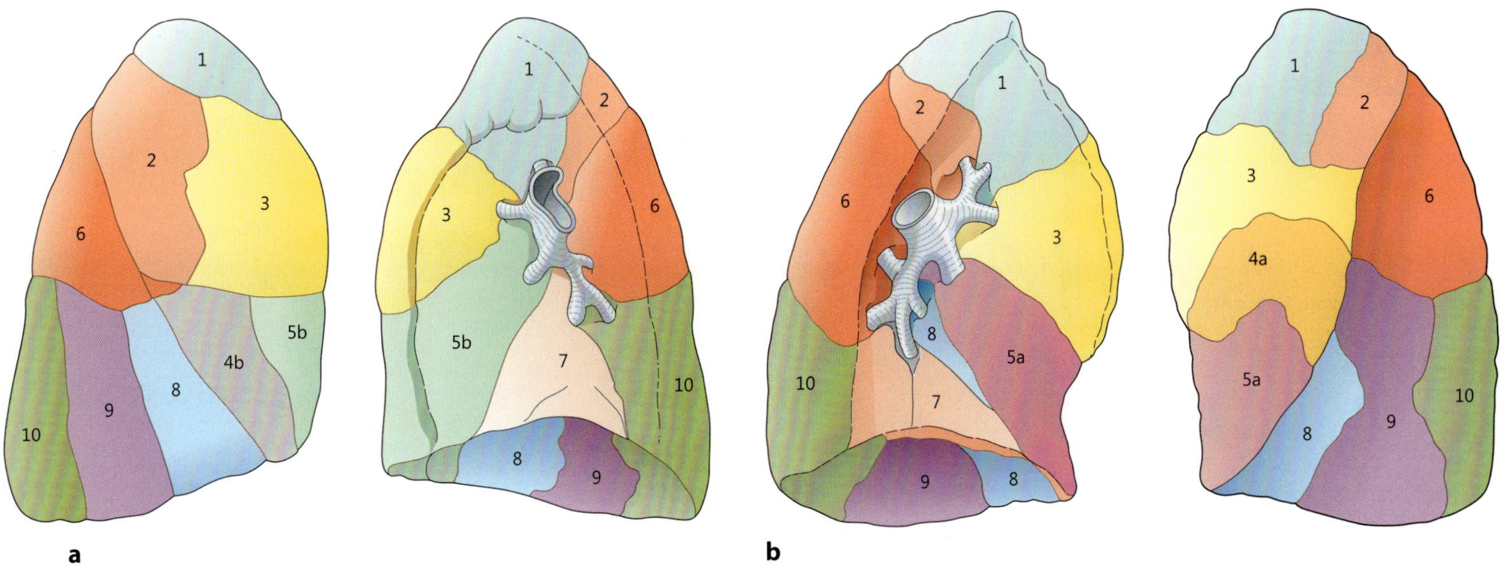

Pulmonary zones. **a**, Lateral and mediastinal surface of the right lung; **b**, mediastinal and lateral surface of the left lung.

PULMONARY LOBES	*RIGHT BRONCHIAL TREE*			*LEFT BRONCHIAL TREE*		
	JACKSON-HUBER	*BOYDEN*	*IKEDA*	*JACKSON-HUBER*	*BOYDEN*	*IKEDA*
Superior lobe	Apical	B^1	RB^{1a}, RB^{1b} + ramifications (i, α)	Superior division		
	Posterior	B^2	RB^{2a}, RB^{2b} + ramifications (i, α)	apicoposterior	B^1, B^2	LB^{1+2a} + ramifications (i, α)
	Anterior	B^3	RB^{3a}, RB^{3b} + ramifications (i, α)	apicoanterior	B^3	LB^{3a}, LB^{3b} + ramifications (i, α)
				Lingular division		
				superior	B^4	LB^{4a}, LB^{4b} + ramifications (i, α)
				inferior	B^5	LB^{4a}, LB^{4b} + ramifications (i, α)
Middle lobe	Lateral	B^4	RB^{4a}, RB^{4b} + ramifications (i, α)			
	Medial	B^5	RB^{5a}, RB^{5b} + ramifications (i, α)			
Inferior lobe	Superior	B^6	RB^{6a}, RB^{6b} + ramifications (i, α)	Superior	B^6	LB^{6a}, LB^{6b} + ramifications (i, α)
	Medial basal	B^7	RB^{7a}, RB^{7b} + ramifications (i, α)	Anteromedial	B^7, B^8	LB^{7+8a} + ramifications (i, α)
	Anterior basal	B^8	RB^{8a}, RB^{8b} + ramifications (i, α)	Lateral basal	B^9	LB^{9a}, LB^{9b} + ramifications (i, α)
	Lateral basal	B^9	RB^{9a}, RB^{9b} + ramifications (i, α)	Posterior basal	B^{10}	LB^{10a}, LB^{10b} + ramifications (i, α)
	Posterior basal	B^{10}	RB^{10a}, RB^{10b} + ramifications (i, α)			

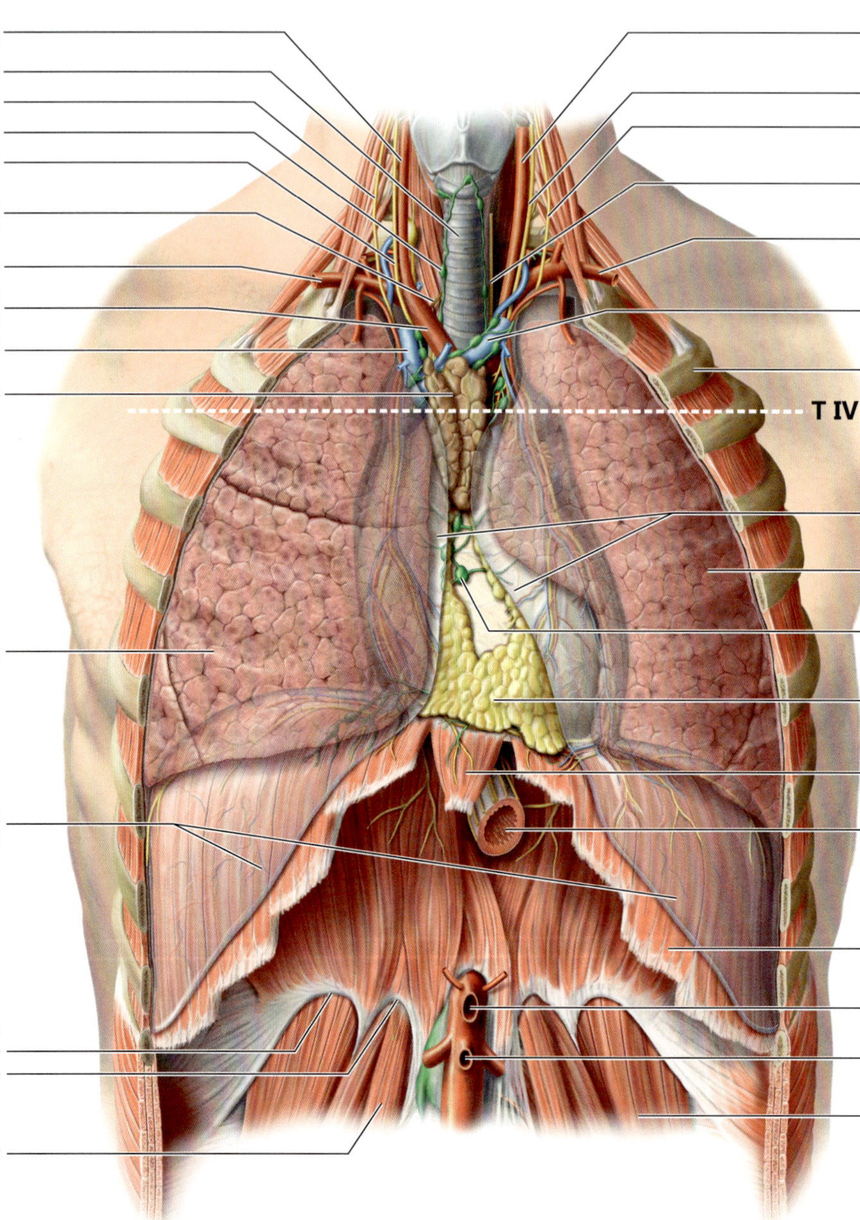

Anterior view of the **pleural lining of the lungs**, after resection of the anterior wall of the thoracic cage. In transparency, it is possible to see the course of the anterior and inferior borders of the lungs. The pleura exceeds the boundaries of the lung and extends downwards into the cavity formed between the diaphragm and the ribs (costodiaphragmatic recesses); forwards, it proceeds in front of the pericardium (costomediastinal recesses).

Pleurae

PLEURA	DESCRIPTION	VASCULARIZATION, LYMPHATIC DRAINAGE, INNERVATION
Visceral (pulmonary)	Membrane (serosa and subserosa) investing the surface of the lung penetrating into the depths of the interlobar fissures. At the level of the hilum of the lung it invests a short tract of the root of the lung, whereupon it continues in the mediastinal part of the parietal pleura	Bronchial arteries; pulmonary veins, bronchial veins. Bronchopulmonary nodes. Pulmonary plexus (sympathetic trunk)
Parietal		Intercostal arteries, internal thoracic artery, musculophrenic artery; superior vena cava. Intercostal, parasternal, superior diaphragmatic and celiac nodes. Intercostal, phrenic, vagus nerves and sympathetic trunk
– costal part (costal or costovertebral pleura)	Extending over the internal surface of the sternum, ribs, transversus thoracis, intercostal muscles, and lateral surface of the thoracic vertebrae, it continues medially in the mediastinal part, superiorly in the cervical pleura, and inferiorly in the diaphragmatic part	
– diaphragmatic part (diaphragmatic pleura)	Adhering to the diaphragm, it continues superiorly in the costal part and medially in the mediastinal part	
– mediastinal part (mediastinal pleura)	Extending between the sternum and vertebral column, it delimits the mediastinum, forming at the level of the root of the lung the pulmonary ligament	
– cervical pleura (dome of pleura)	Continuation upwards of the costal pleura to the point of covering the apex of lung	

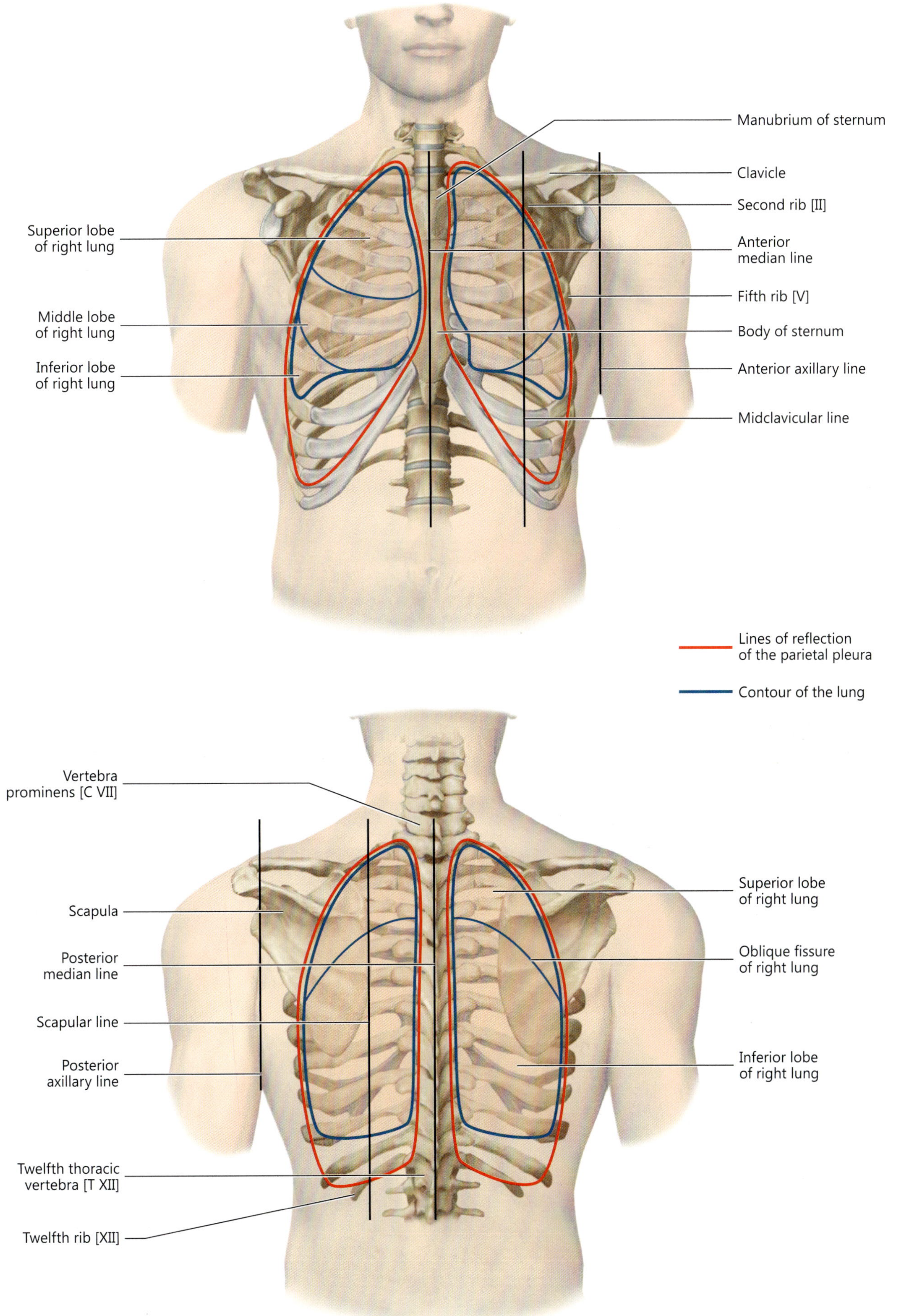

Pleural compartments. Projections onto the thoracic cage of the pulmonary (*blue*) and pleural (*red*) borders and fissures.

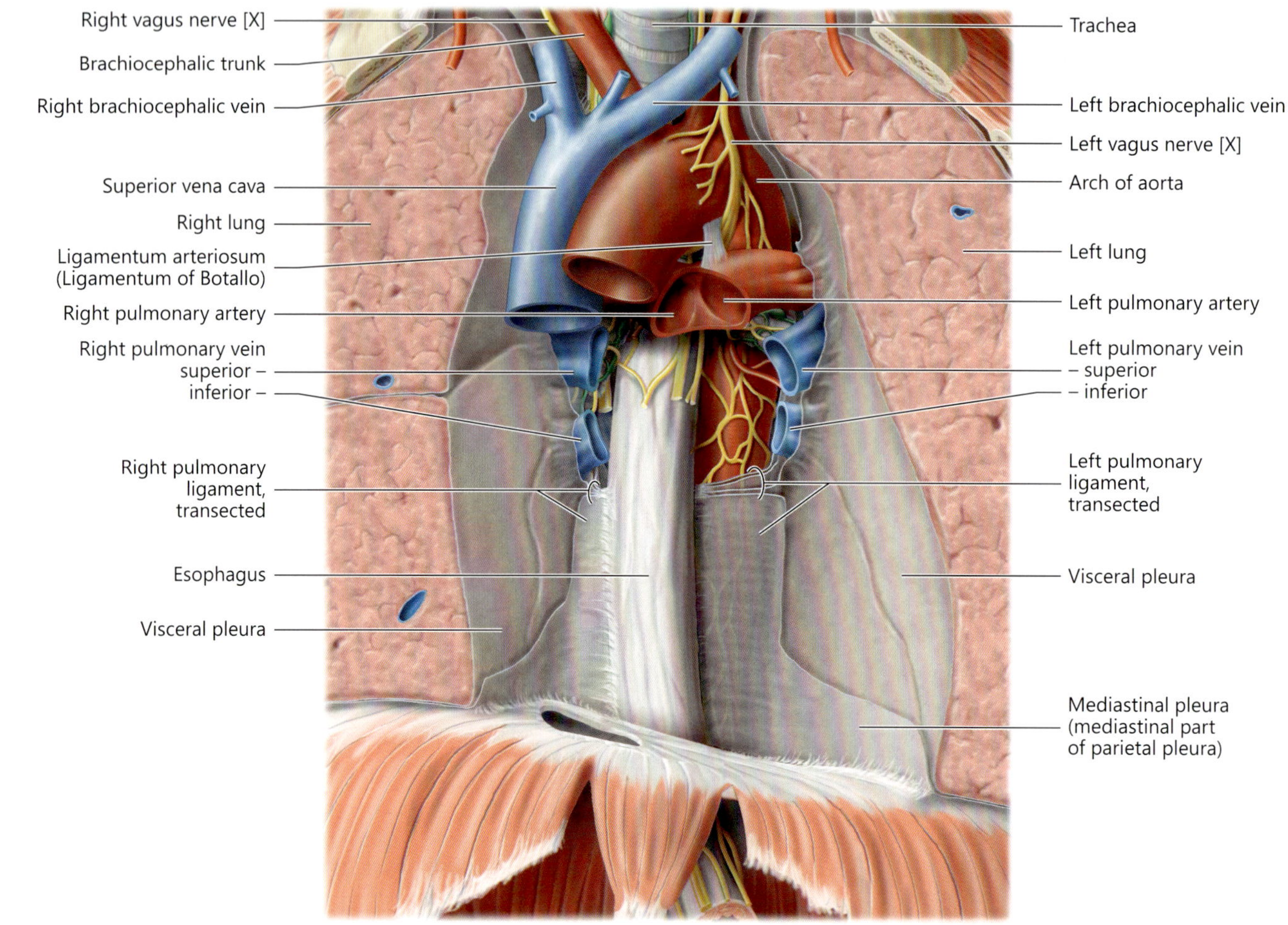

Frontal transection of the mediastinum. The great vessels of the pulmonary hilum and of the heart have been conserved. The **pulmonary ligament** is formed by the two reflections of mediastinal parietal pleura onto visceral pleura. The two reflections are located in front of and behind the hilum of the lung, respectively. Below the hilum, the two pleural reflections come together forming a ligament that extends medially to the lateral wall of the esophagus and below continues with the diaphragmatic pleura. By shifting the lung laterally, the pulmonary ligament is pulled, assuming a typical triangular shape.

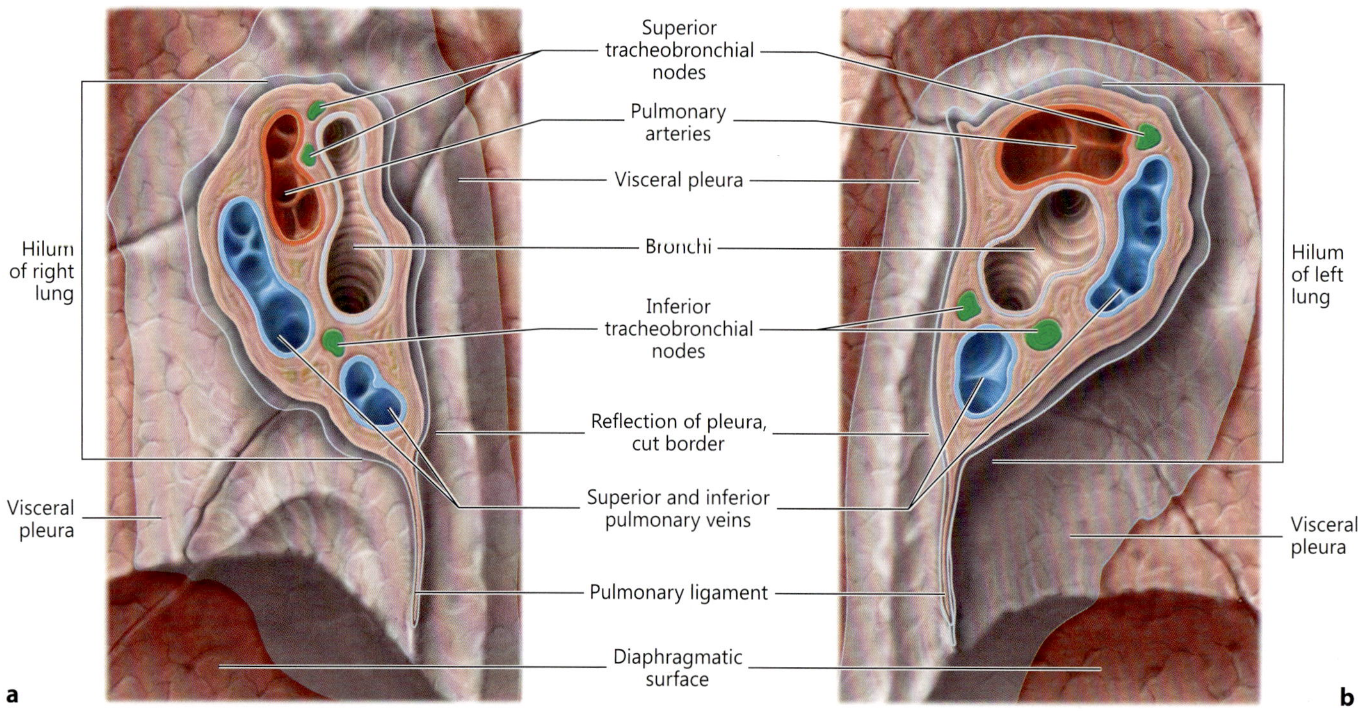

a, **Hilum of the right lung**; **b**, **hilum of the left lung**. In these images the **pulmonary ligament** (triangular ligament) appears in sagittal section.

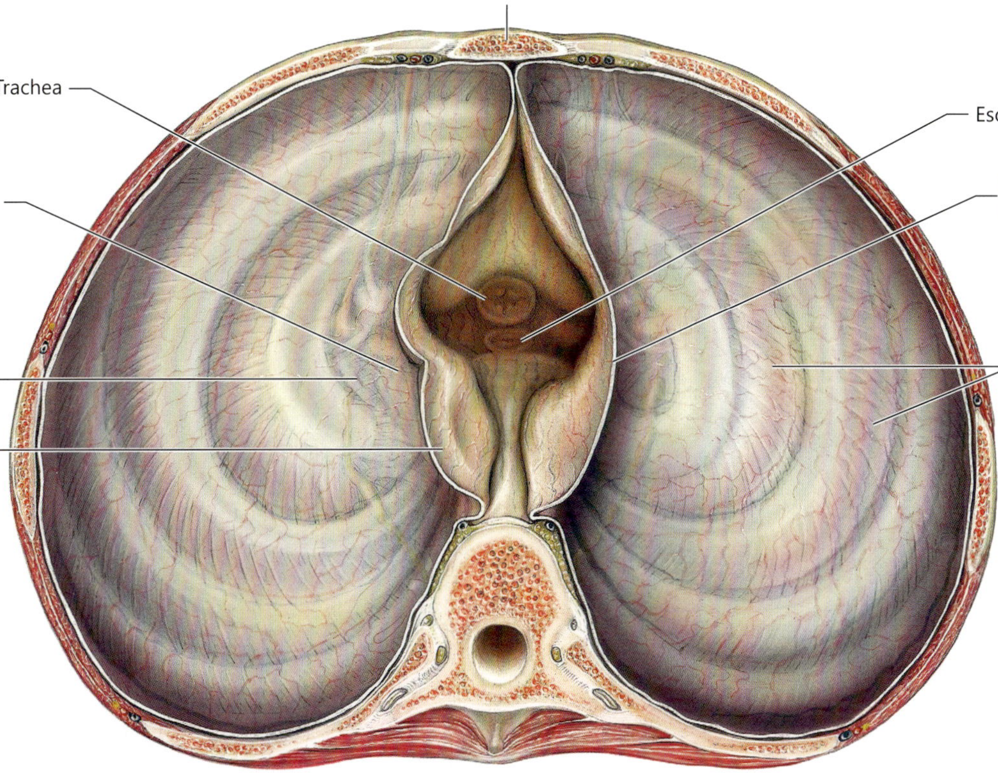

In this image one can see the **cervical pleurae** (domes of pleura) and the right and left **mediastinal pleurae**, viewed from below, after resection of the thorax, removal of the lungs and visceral pleural layers, and partial evacuation of the mediastinum.

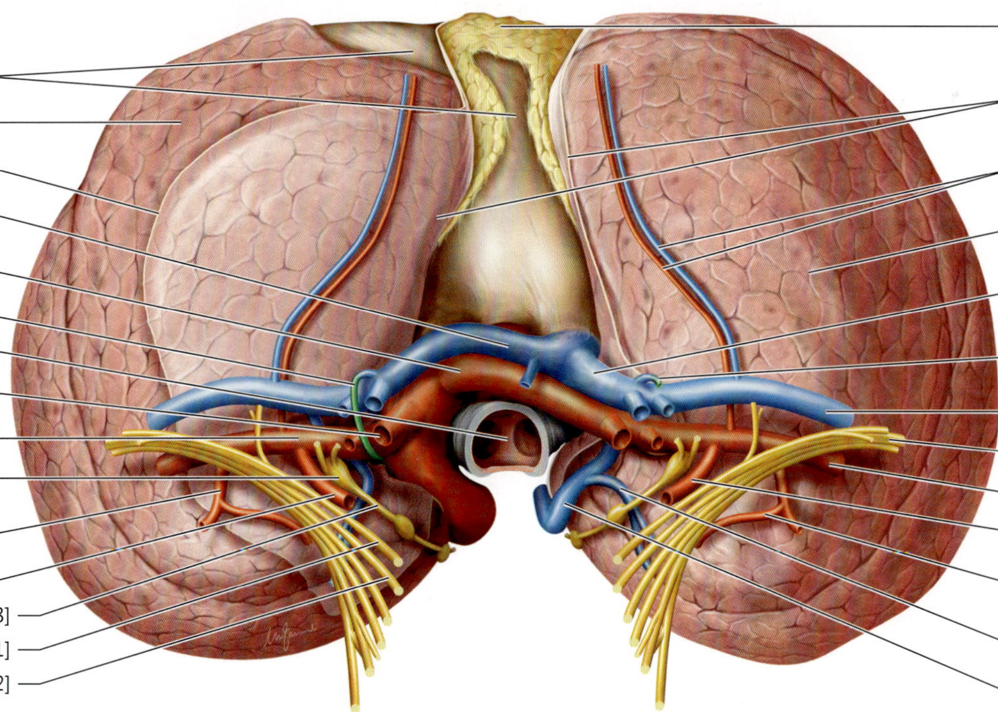

Relationship between the pulmonary apexes mediated by the **cervical pleurae**. In tumors of the apex of the lung (Pancoast tumor), an impairment of these structures is at the base of the typical symptomatologic features. In Bernard-Horner syndrome, impairment of the cervicothoracic (stellate) ganglion provokes palpebral ptosis, miosis, pseudoenophthalmos, and homolateral facial anhidrosis. In the Pancoast syndrome, these symptoms are associated with manifestations linked to the infiltration of the eighth cervical nerve and of the first and second thoracic nerve (pain in the shoulder and on the medial side of the upper limb). Impairment of the lymphatic ducts or of the subclavian veins can provoke lymphedema in the drainage sites or edema of the upper limb, respectively; impairment of the subclavian artery can manifest with cyanosis at the extremities of the upper limb.

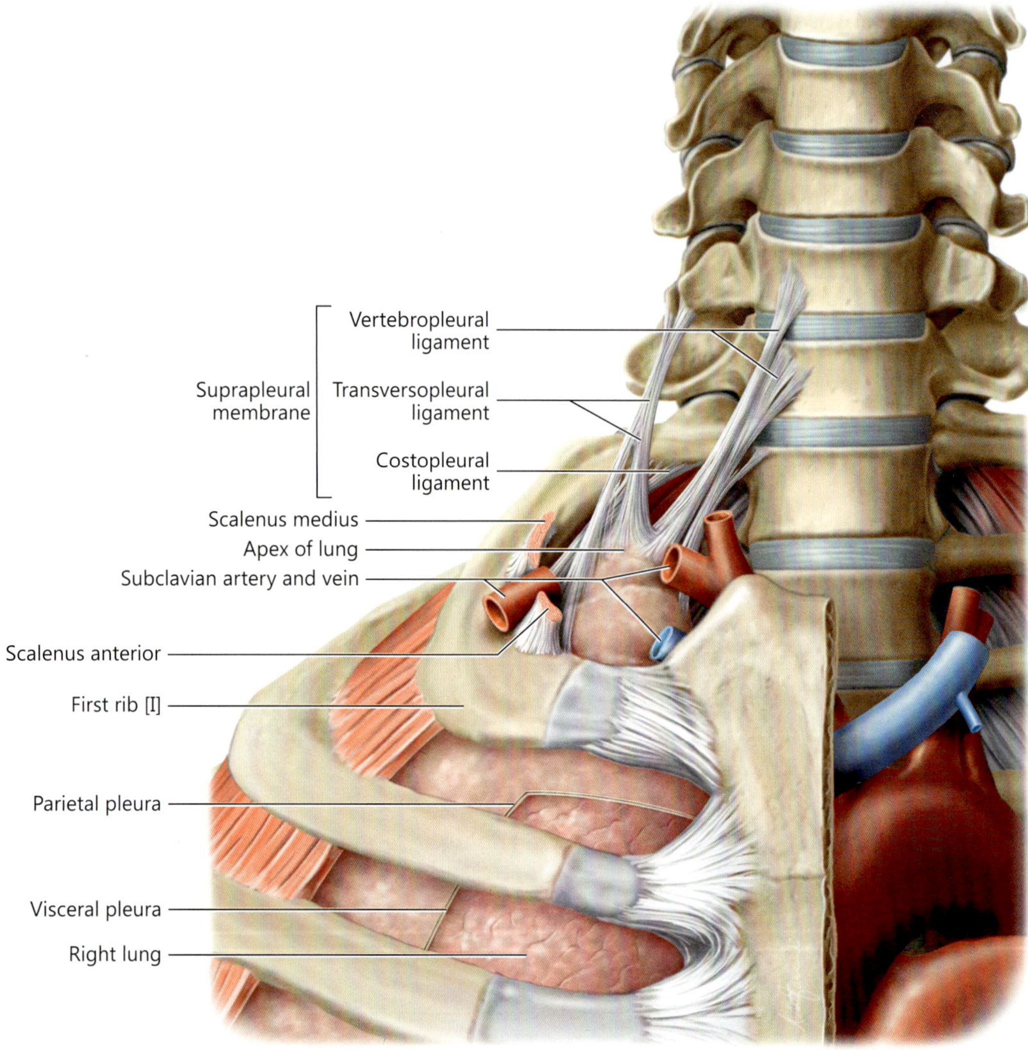

Schematic representation of the principal **means of attachment of the cervical pleura**.

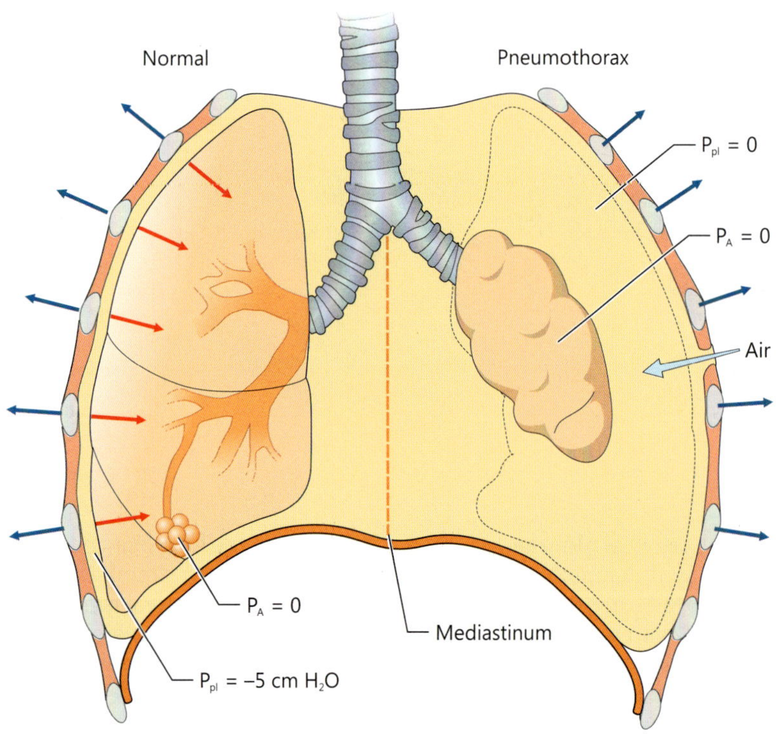

Rupture of the lung or of the thoracic wall, which places the pleural cavity in communication with atmospheric air, produces the condition known as **pneumothorax**, in which the transpulmonary pressure becomes zero and the lung's tendency to elastic recoil provokes its collapse. The barrier effect of the mediastinum impedes the collapse of the contralateral lung. In humans, the two pleural cavities (right and left) are not in communication with each other and, thus, in the case of pneumothorax, ventilation is nevertheless assured by the healthy lung.

The withdrawal of fragments of pulmonary tissue (**biopsy**) or the drainage of fluids or air from the pleural cavity is performed by the insertion of bioptic needles or needle-cannula through the intercostal spaces (**a1**). The procedure must take into account the position of the intercostal vascular and nervous structures. Needle biopsies involve inserting the needle on the superior border of the underlying rib. The procedure is often guided by a radiographic examination or CT scan.

Thoracentesis (**a2**) is a procedure used to drain fluids that have accumulated in the pleural recesses. The technique involves the insertion of a needle-cannula through an intercostal space. The patient is in a seated position and the upper limit of the pleural effusion is determined by percussion; local anesthesia is performed with a needle of reduced caliber and length in proximity to the zone of insertion of the thoracentesis needle. The insertion of the thoracentesis needle is performed 1 or 2 intercostal spaces below the upper limit of the effusion; the best site is between the posterior axillary line and a line placed 6-7 centimeters from the posterior median line. The thoracentesis needle is inserted at the level of the upper border of the inferior rib of the selected intercostal space. The needle, after being inserted a few centimeters aspirating repeatedly to verify if it has reached the effusion, is then positioned horizontally in the pleural cavity.

b, The positioning for **endopleural drainage**, indicated for the aspiration of fluids (gaseous in the case of pneumothorax, liquid in the case of effusions) from the pleural cavity, takes place through the introduction of a multi-fenestrated silicone catheter, with or without an introducer device, which penetrates through the skin and subcutaneous layer on the upper border of the underlying rib, in order to avoid lesions of the intercostal neurovascular bundle. When an introducer is used, as in the figure, it will penetrate through the intercostal muscles and proceed until it reaches the pleural cavity, whereupon it will implant the multi-fenestrated drainage.

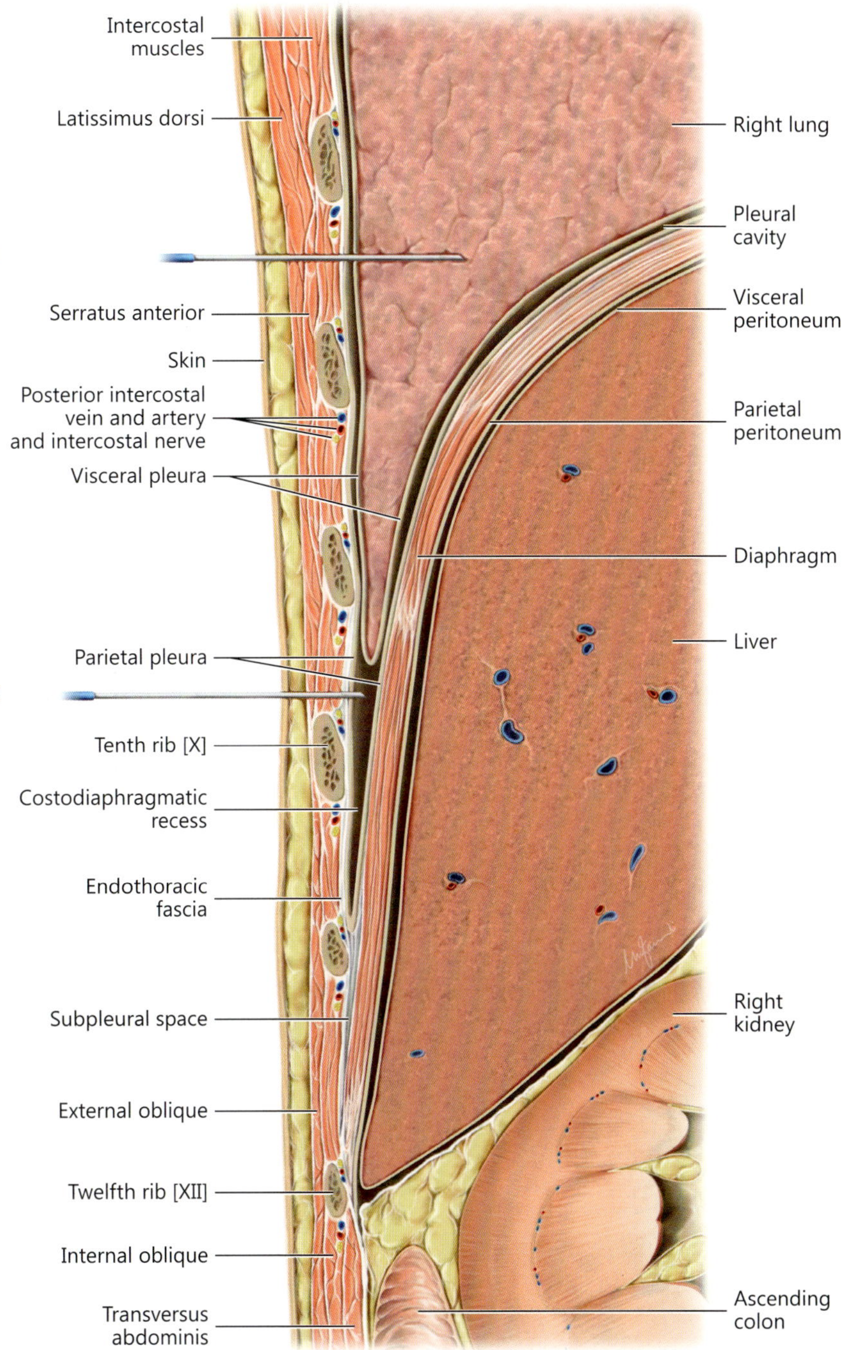

a

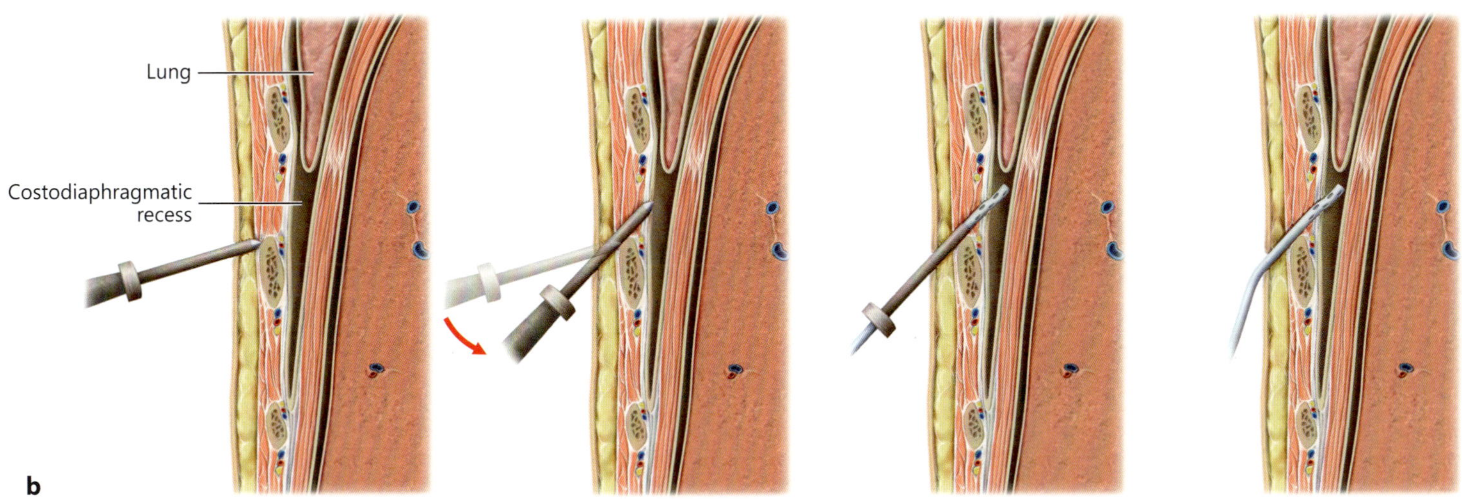

b

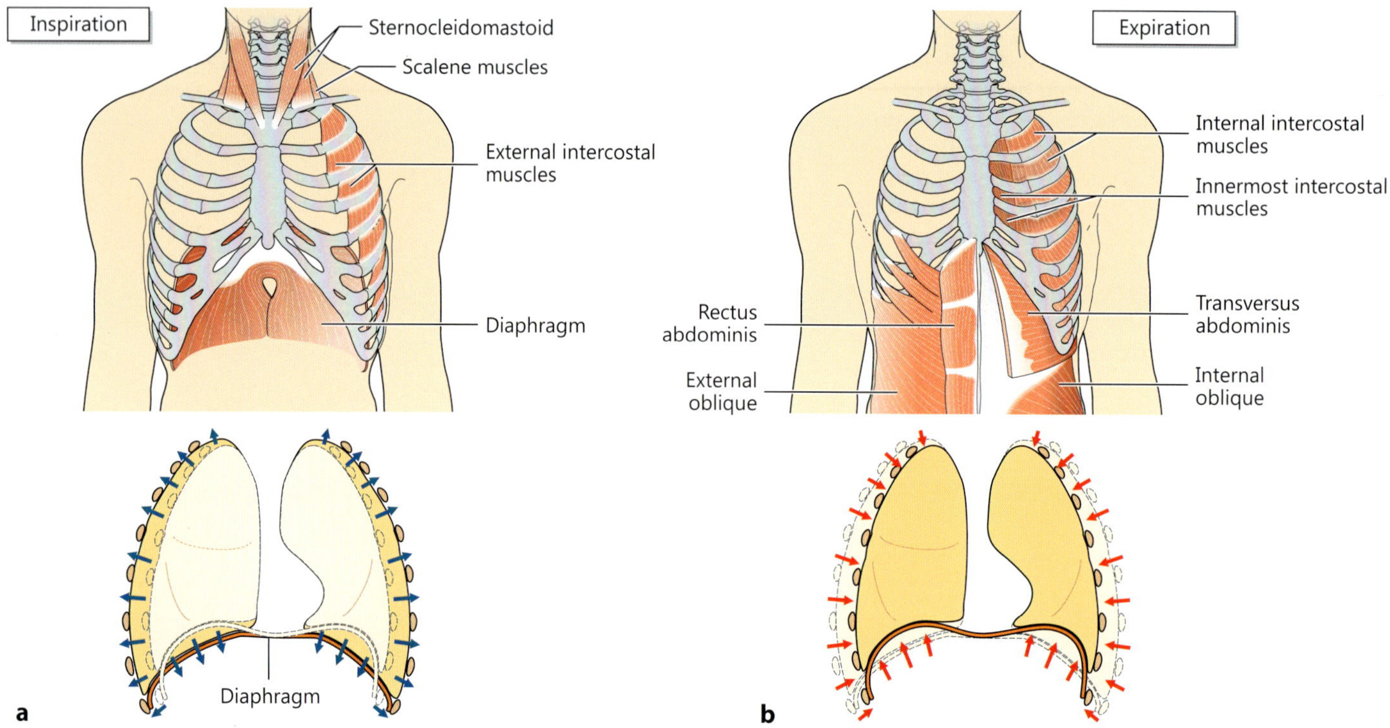

Flat muscle bundles run between two neighboring ribs, constituting the **intercostal musculature**. The external intercostal muscles of the posterior and lateral surface of the thoracic cage raise the ribs (**a**, inspiration); the internal intercostal muscles of the anterior surface lower the ribs (**b**, expiration).

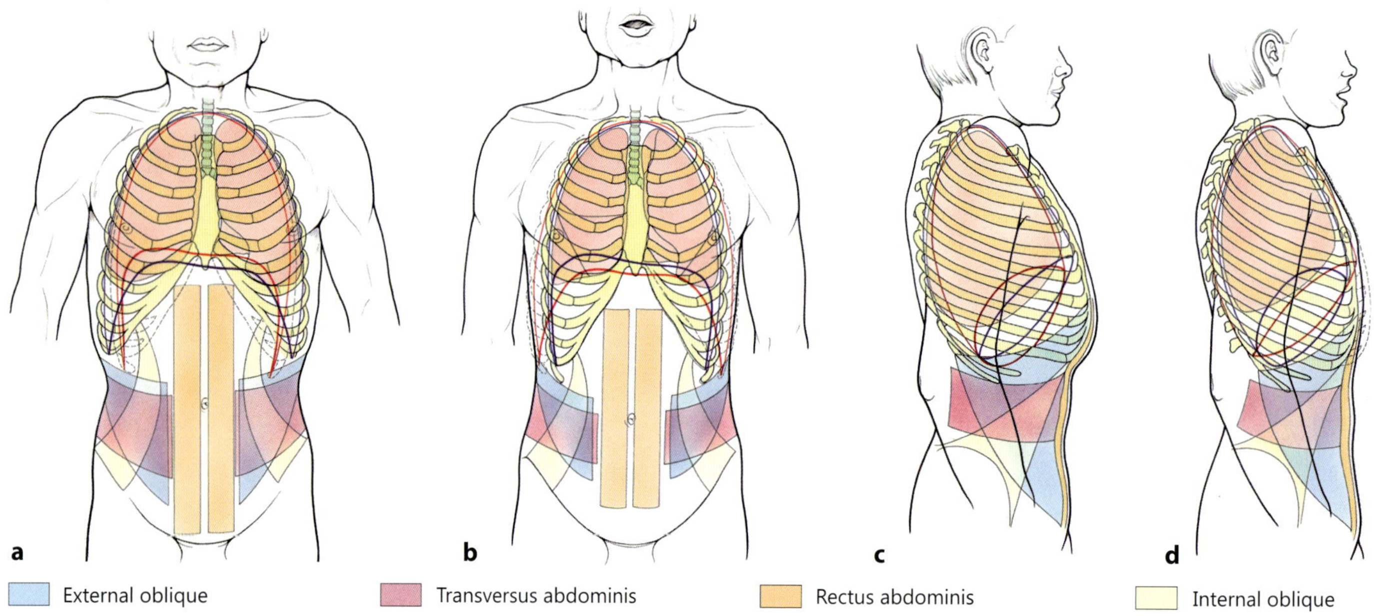

INSPIRATORY MUSCLES	*EXPIRATORY MUSCLES*
• Principal muscles: – diaphragm – external intercostal muscles – scalene muscles	• Principal muscles: – diaphragm – internal intercostal muscles – innermost intercostal muscles
• Secondary (accessory) muscles: – sternocleidomastoid – levatores costarum – serratus posterior superior – subclavius – pectoralis minor and pectoralis major – serratus anterior – latissimus dorsi – trapezius – levator scapulae – rhomboid major and rhomboid minor – muscles of back proper (erector spinae)	• Secondary muscles: – quadratus lumborum – transversus thoracis – subcostales – serratus posterior inferior – muscles of abdomen → A deficit of their muscle tone has major repercussions on respiratory function and, from this perspective, they can be considered as principal expiratory muscles. They act, however, as secondary expiratory muscles, pushing the contents of the abdominal cavity against the diaphragm, so reducing the thoracic cavity

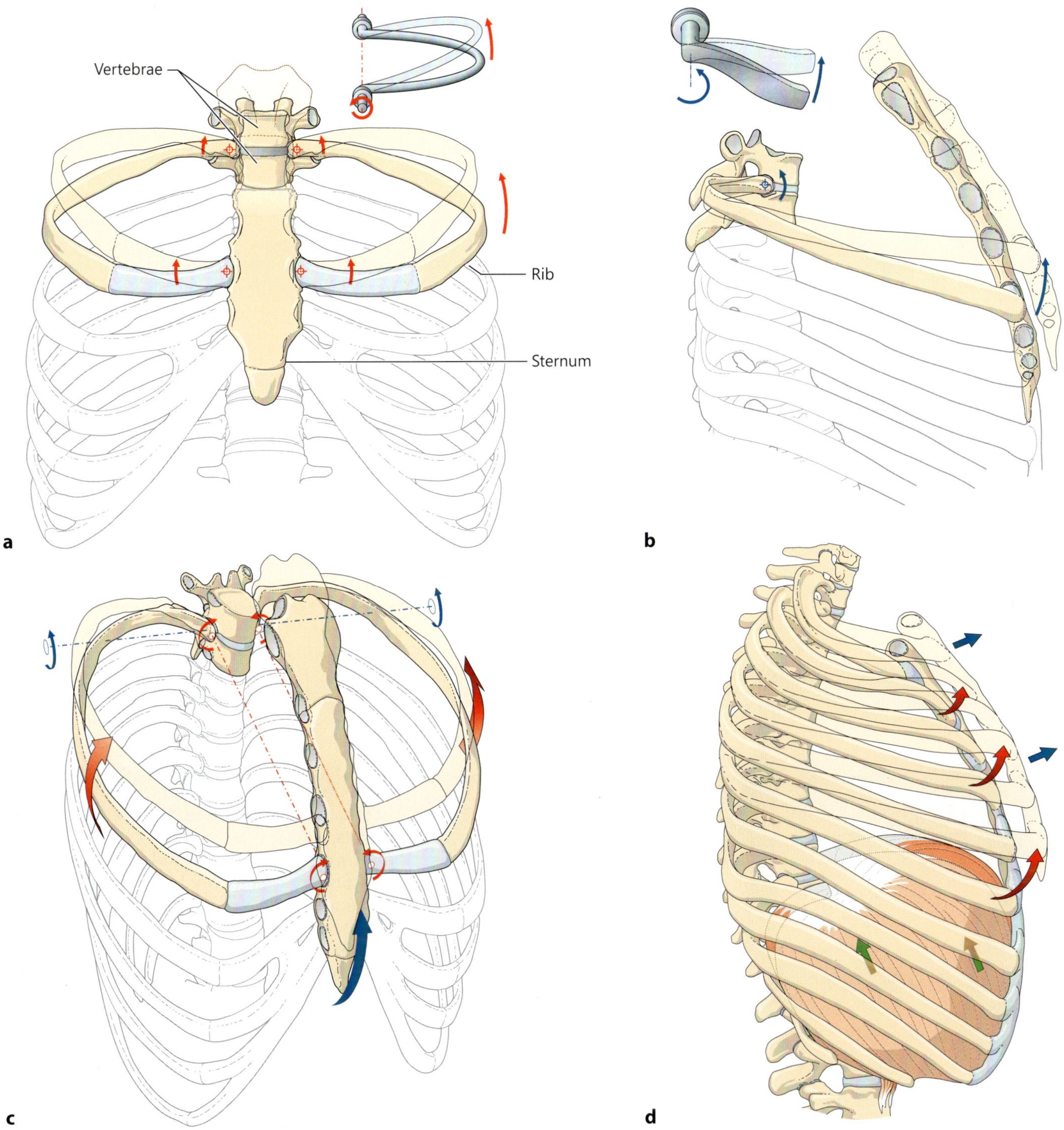

Respiration is based on a coordinated action of the diaphragm and the abdominal, thoracic and cervical muscles. The goal of the action of these muscles is to increase (inspiration) or reduce (expiration) the sagittal, vertical and transverse diameters of the thoracic cavity. In breathing at rest, their function is linked prevalently to the excursions of the diaphragm. In inspiration, the excursion downwards of the central tendon of the diaphragm is favored by the relaxation of the abdominal muscles. Once the maximum excursion consented by the residual abdominal pressure has been reached, a further contraction of the fibers of the diaphragm with respect to the blocked central tendon enables the ribs to be raised (**a**, **b**, **d** in the above figure). Elevation of the ribs enables the transverse (**a**, **c** in the above figure) and sagittal (**b**, **d** in the above figure) diameters of the thoracic cage to increase. The widening of the transverse diameter is the fruit of a movement analogous to lifting the handle of a bucket, which involves the costovertebral joints, from the 2nd to 12th, and the sternocostal joints, with the exclusion of the first. The widening of the sagittal diameter is, instead, linked to the raising of the sternum consequent upon the elevation of the ribs, with a movement that can be compared to that of a handle. The raising of the ribs is aided by the action of the external intercostal muscles (as illustrated in the figure above on the preceding page). The action is made more effective by the activity of the scalene muscles and sternocleidomastoid, which lift and hold the first rib. Expiration relies on the action of the internal intercostal muscles and the diaphragm. In the case of forced expiration, also the muscles of the abdomen (rectus abdominis, external oblique, internal oblique and transversus abdominis) enter into play. By contracting, they determine an increase of the intra-abdominal pressure, further raising the central tendon of the diaphragm, and they lower the ribs.

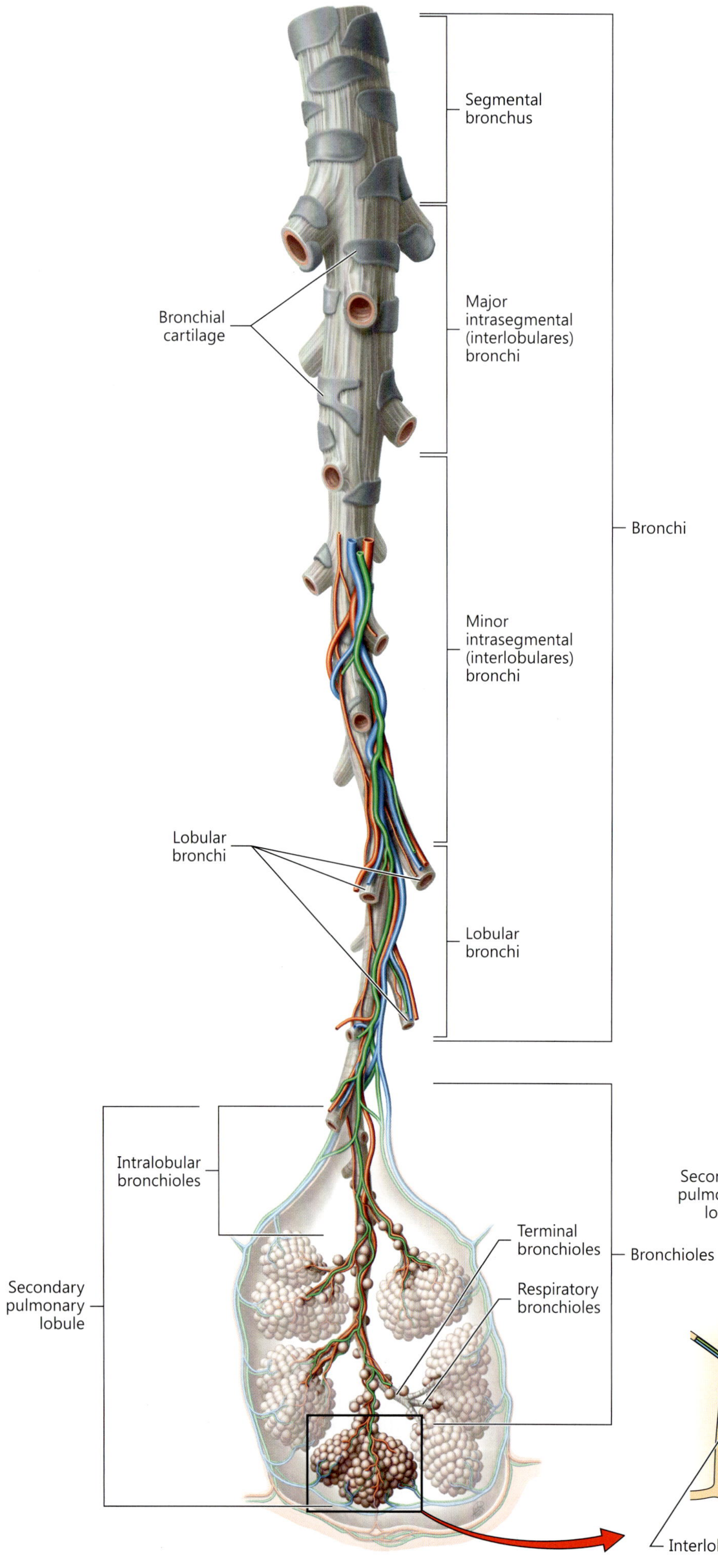

Schematic description of the final ramifications of the **bronchial tree**. The **pulmonary acinus** is formed of a group of alveoli which are intercommunicating through the alveolar pores. Furthermore, through the canals of Lambert a collateral ventilation is created, which interconnects all the pulmonary acini with the terminal bronchioles. Each acinus is aerated by a respiratory bronchiole, which, in turn, is one of the ramifications of a terminal bronchiole. The structure of the acini is completed by a dense satellite vascularization of the airways.

The **secondary pulmonary lobule** (today more simply called **pulmonary lobule**) is the smallest unit of the lung surrounded by connective tissue and has the following characteristics:

- it is distal to a small bronchiole
- 3-5 terminal bronchioles penetrate into it (for illustrative clarity, each drawing shows just one terminal bronchiole for each secondary pulmonary lobule)
- it includes a dozen pulmonary acini which are generated from these terminal bronchioles
- it has a polyhedral form with septa which are clearly visible in the peripheral (pleural) pulmonary lobules while they are thinner and partially discontinuous in the central pulmonary lobules (they become clearly visible also in the central lobules following fibrous diseases)
- it has a diameter of 1-2.5 cm (mean: 1.1-1.7 cm)
- in the interlobular septa run the smallest ramifications of the pulmonary veins and lymphatic vessels; other lymphatic vessels form in the peribronchovascular interstitium and then ascend the bronchial tree with the pulmonary arteries.

The **primary pulmonary lobule** is contained in the secondary pulmonary lobule and includes the alveolar ducts, the alveolar sacs and the alveoli distal to the last respiratory bronchiole (together with the vessels, nerves and associated connective tissue). It is estimated that each secondary pulmonary lobule is composed of 30-50 primary pulmonary lobules. The term "primary pulmonary lobule" is little used.

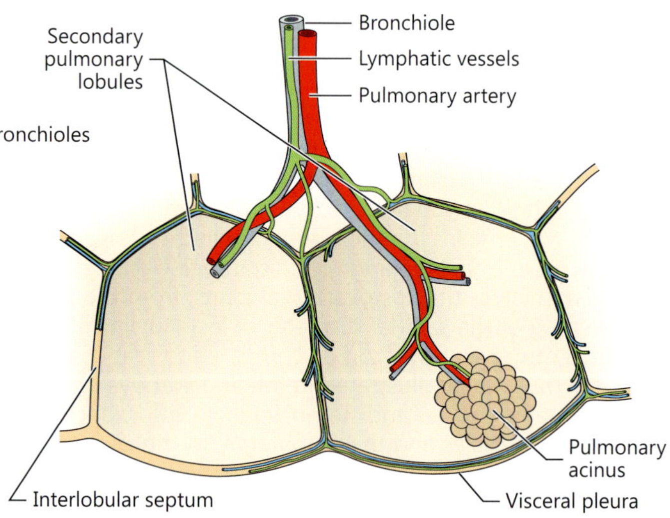

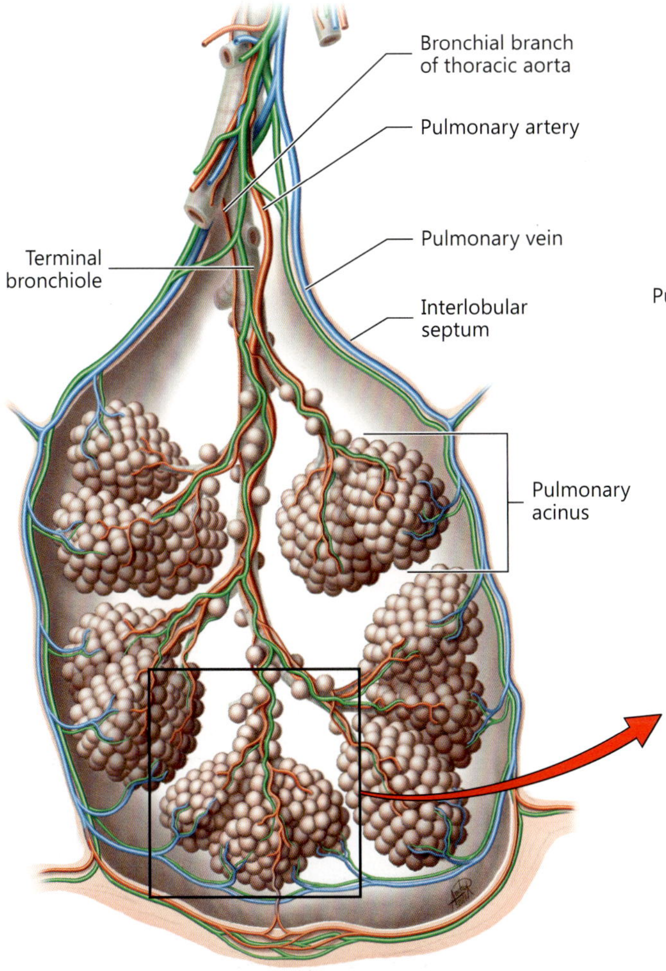

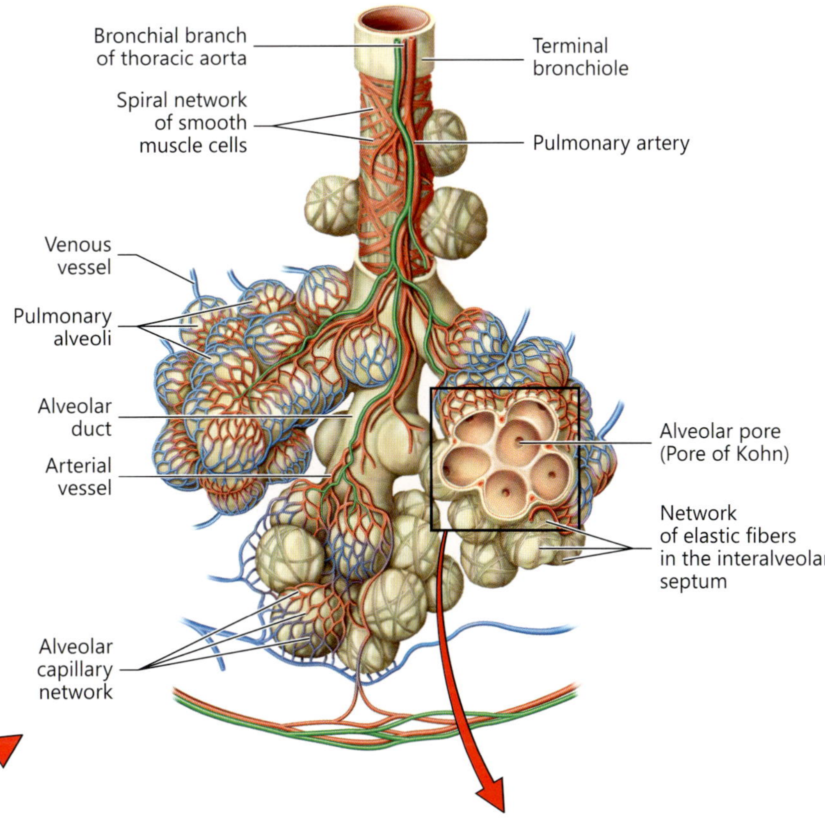

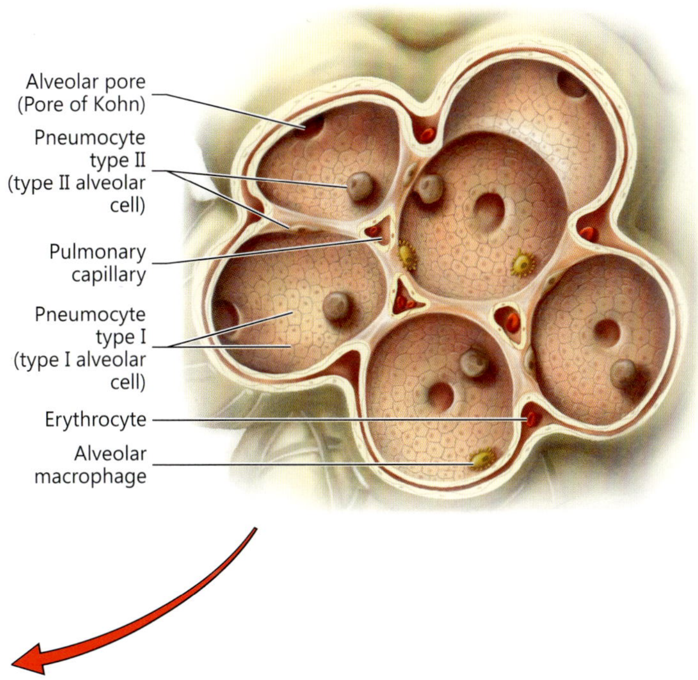

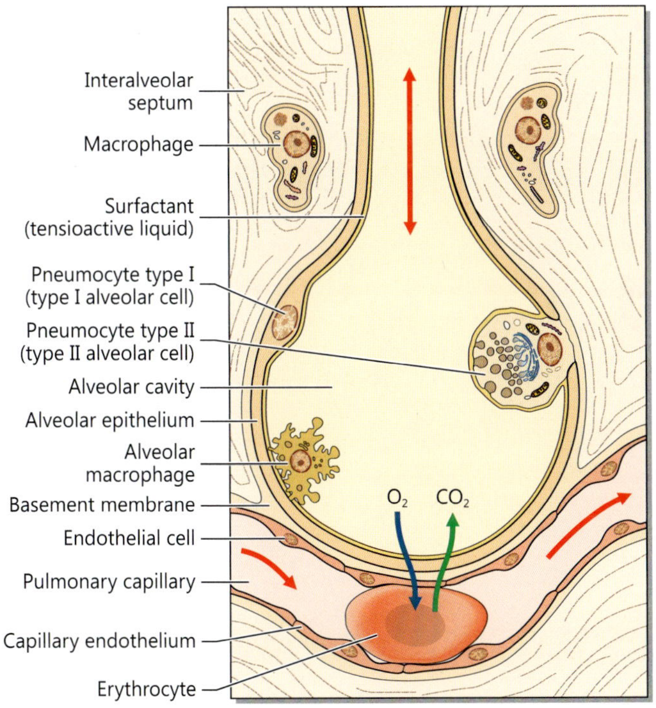

Schematic representation of a **pulmonary alveolus** and of the **blood-air barrier**.

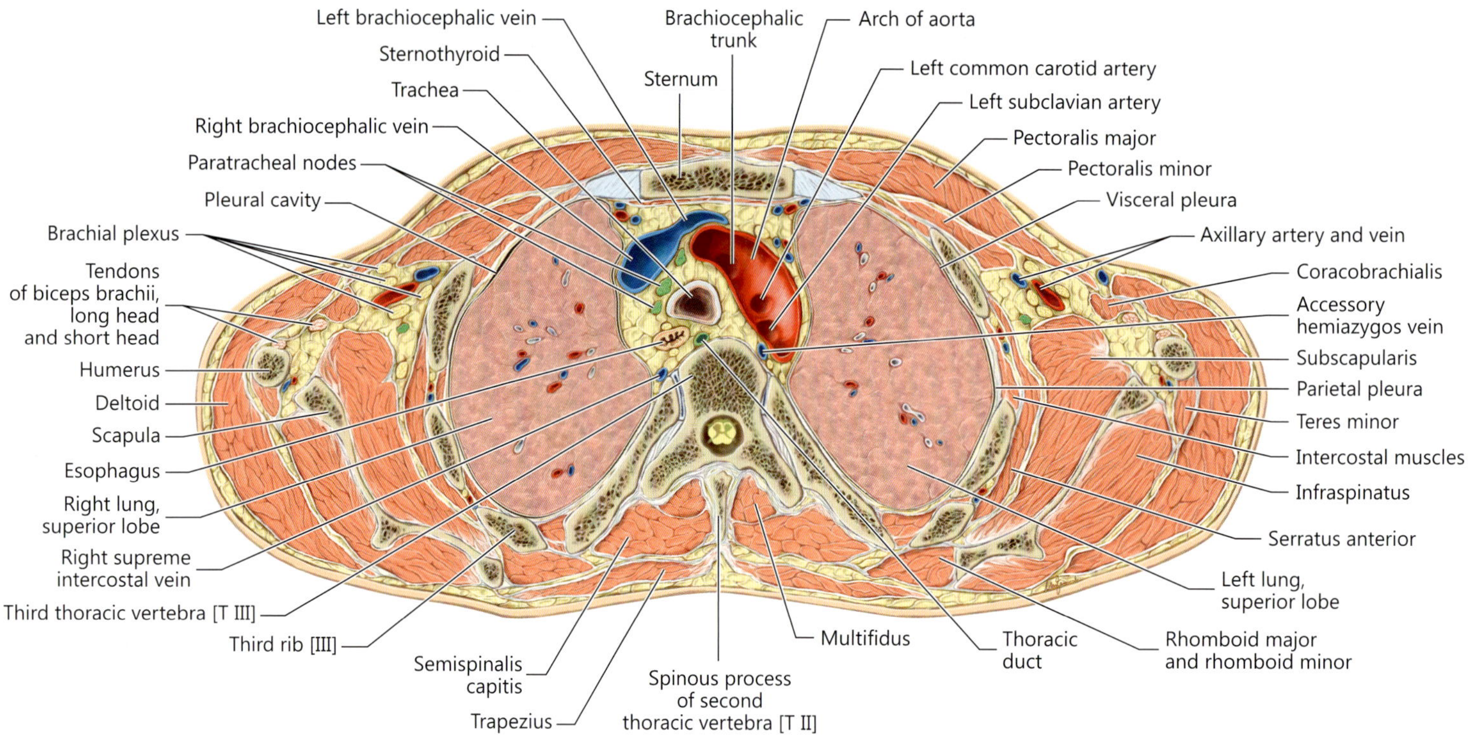

Thoracic cavity. Transverse section at the level of the arch of the aorta, viewed from below.

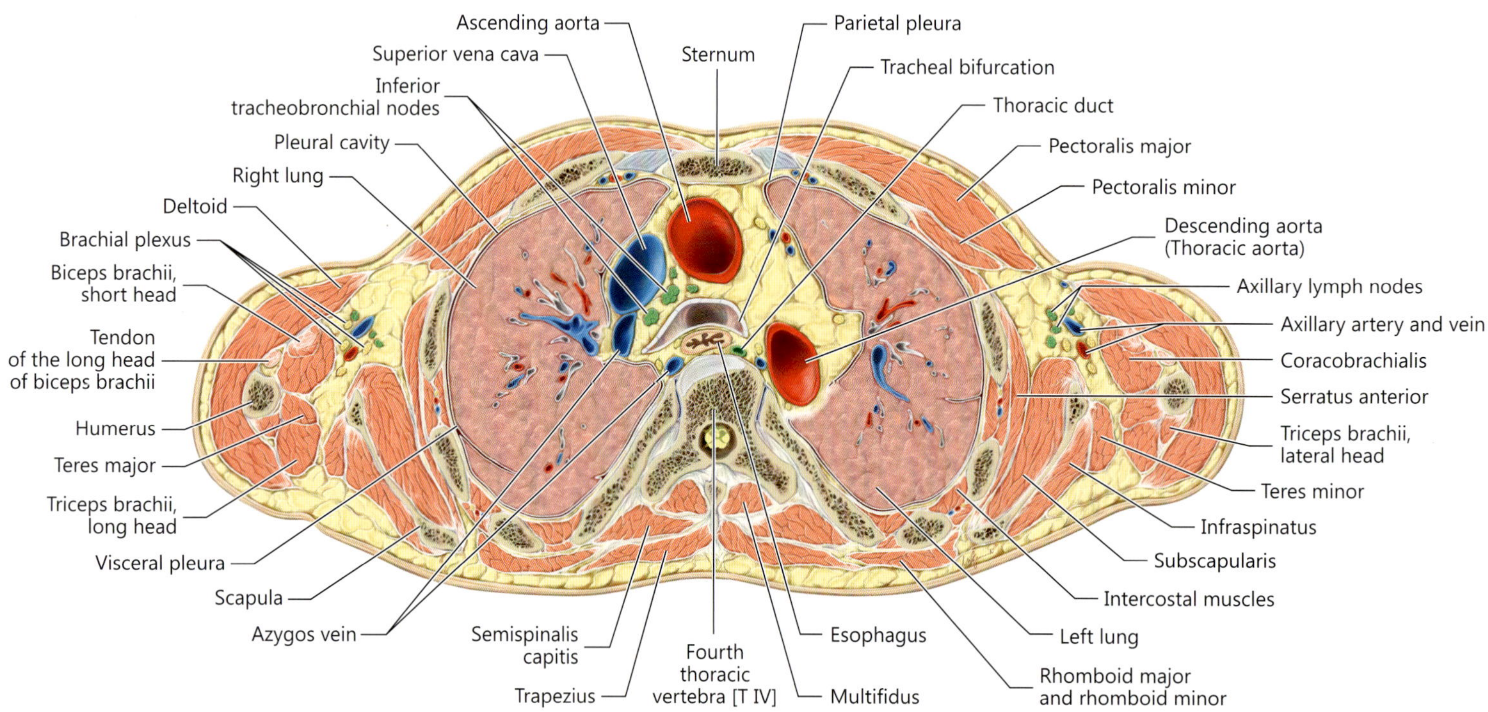

Thoracic cavity. Transverse section at the level of the fourth thoracic vertebra, viewed from below.

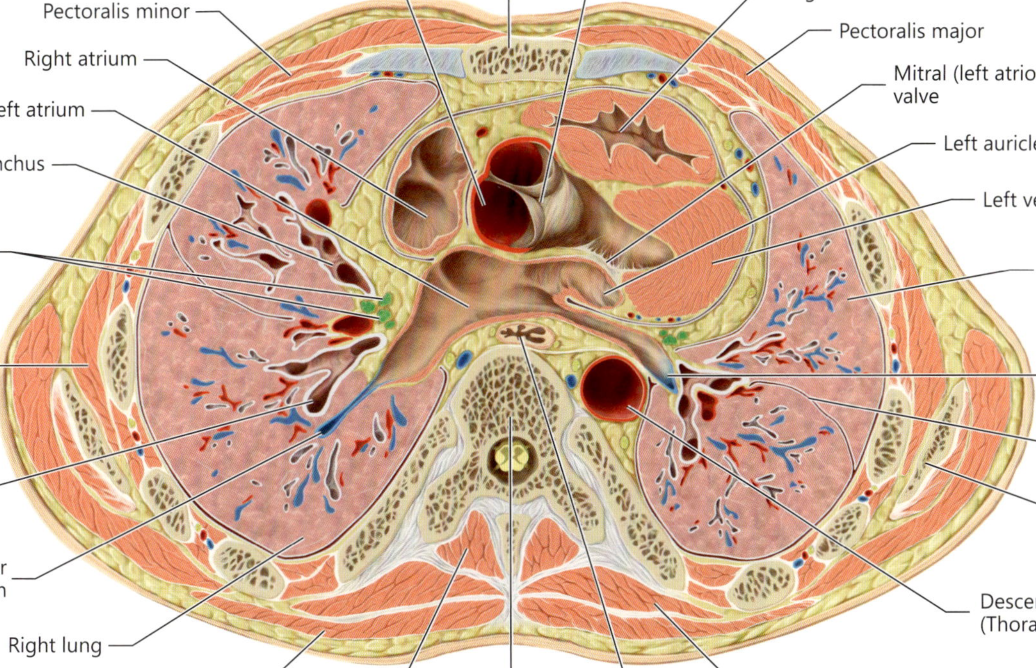

Thoracic cavity. Transverse section at the level of T VII, viewed from below.

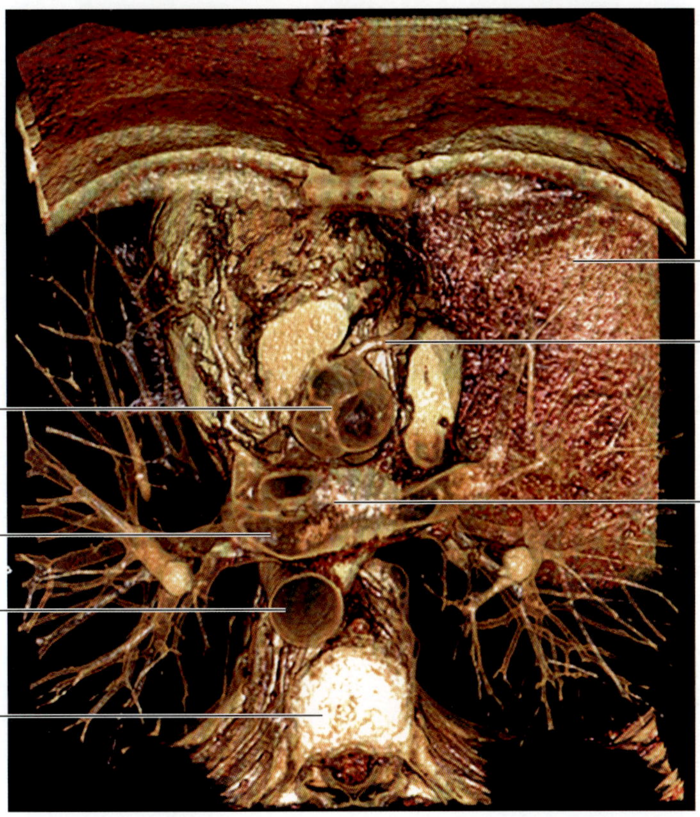

Three-dimensional image of a living human body, obtained by CT scan using a 3D volume rendering technique, showing the **organs of the thoracic cavity**, viewed from above, according to a plane passing through the seventh thoracic vertebra. The lungs and the diaphragm have been graphically removed in order to expose part of the diaphragmatic surface of the liver.

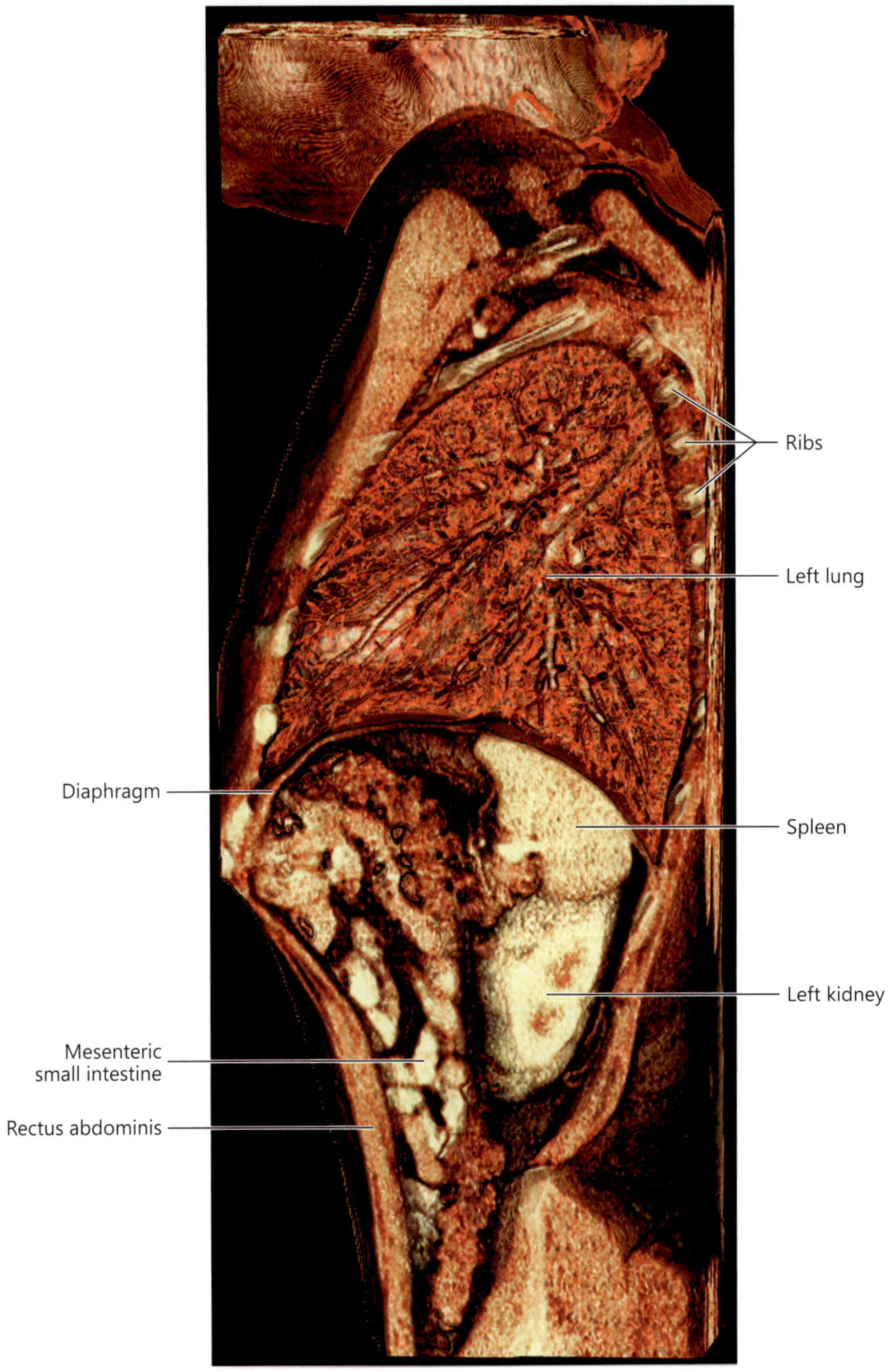

Three-dimensional image of a living human body, obtained using a 3D volume rendering technique. Left parasagittal section showing the position of the **organs of the abdominal and thoracic cavity**, in a plane passing through the spleen and the left kidney.

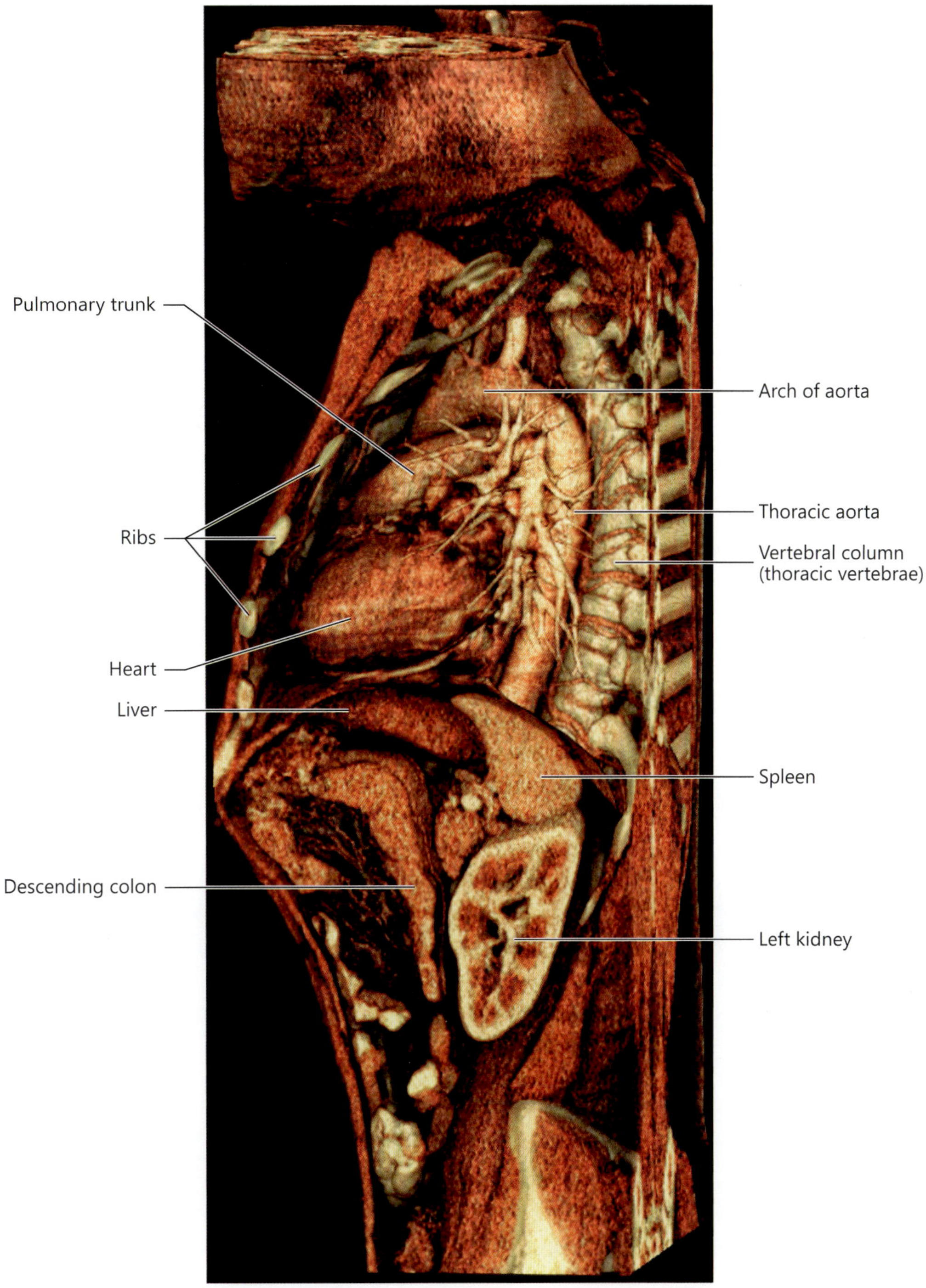

Three-dimensional image of a living human body, obtained using a 3D volume rendering technique. Left parasagittal section showing the position of the **organs of the abdominal and thoracic cavity**.

Index

This index provides that single entry words are organized under the relative structures (i.e. Artery(ies), Bone(s), Muscle(s), etc.). For example, the single entry word "Humerus" is under "Bone(s)" or the single entry word "Latissimus dorsi" is under "Muscle(s)". This concerns also structures like ducts, prominence, tracts, etc. Organs and regional structures (i.e. "Colon") have their main entries and subentries. Page numbers with "t" refer to tables.

A

Abdomen, 371
Acinus
– pulmonary, 390, 391
Airways, 125
Alveolus
– dental, 135
– pulmonary, 391
– –, surfactant, 391
Ampulla
– bony, anterior, 194
– –, lateral, 194
– –, posterior, 194
– membranous, anterior, 195
– –, lateral, 195
– –, posterior, 195
Anastomosis
– cilioretinal, 177
Angle
– iridocorneal, 176, 179
– –, spaces, 179
– sternal, 297
Ansa
– cervicalis, 75, 76, 94t, 133, 225, 227, 270, 272
– –, root(s), 272
– –, –, inferior, 76, 109, 110, 112, 133, 225
– –, –, superior, 76, 109, 112, 128, 133, 225
– –, –, superior and inferior, 110
– of hypoglossal nerve, *see* Ansa, cervicalis
– subclavia, 226, 277, 278
Anulus
– fibrous, 345
– –, pulmonary, 345, 346, 352, 356
– of Zinn, *see* Ring, tendinous, common
Aponeurosis(es)
– epicranial, 52, 100, 120, 121
– lingual, 148
– palatine, 123
Arachnoid mater, 52
– cranial, 114
– granulation, 52
Arcade(s)
– dental, mandibular (or lower), 135
– –, maxillary (or upper), 135
Arch(es)
– alveolar, manibular (or lower), 135
– –, maxillary (or upper), 135
– palatoglossal, 122, 125
– palatopharyngeal, 122, 230
– palpebral, inferior, 162
– –, superior, 162, 173, 174
– venous, jugular, 42-44, 46, 96, 97, 102, 103, 222, 223
– zygomatic, 140, 148
Area
– cardiac, 377
– Kiesselbach's, 152
Areola, 280, 281
Arteriole, intramural coronary, 351
Artery(ies)
– acromiothoracic, *see* Artery(ies), thoracoacromial
– of ala of nose, *see* Artery(ies), nasal, lateral
– alveolar, inferior, 24, 25, 35t, 99, 112, 137, 141, 142
– –, –, mental branch, 96-99, 112, 128
– –, –, mylohyoid branch, 35t
– –, superior, anterior, 34t, 137
– –, –, posterior, 24, 25, 38t, 112, 114, 137, 141, 142
– angular, 16, 23, 27, 34t, 96, 97, 107-111, 162
– aorta, 248, 252, 255t, 298, 306, 334-338, 342, 348-350
– – abdominal, 247, 249, 252, 255t, 301, 302, 308-311, 324, 325, 358
– – –, branches, 252
– – arch, 16, 19, 217-221, 224, 225, 231, 240, 246-249, 253, 254, 255t, 277, 282, 288-295, 298, 299, 302, 307, 309-311, 315, 317, 321, 323-326, 328-340, 344, 359, 360, 364, 365, 367, 368, 384, 392, 395
– – –, branches, 221
– – –, –, collateral, 327
– – –, groove, 373, 378
– – ascending, 16-18, 20, 246-248, 254, 255t, 293, 299, 307, 327-329, 338, 343, 344, 347, 351, 392
– – descending, 219, 240, 244, 247, 249, 250, 254, 255t, 282, 298, 300, 315-317, 324, 325, 328, 334, 392, 393
– – –, abdominal branches, 252
– – –, thoracic branches, 252
– –, branches, 16
– – thoracic, 16-18, 20, 40, 244, 246-250, 254, 255t, 261, 282, 288-290, 292, 293, 298, 300, 301, 307, 309-311, 315-317, 321, 325, 327, 333, 392, 393, 395
– – –, branch(es), 247, 255t, 288, 289
– – –, –, bronchial, 246, 321, 327, 391
– – –, –, esophageal, 246, 321
– – –, –, mediastinal, 246
– – –, –, pericardial, 246, 330
– of arm, deep, *see* Artery(ies), profunda brachii
– auricular, deep, 24, 35t
– –, posterior, 17, 18, 20, 21t, 23-25, 27, 38t, 39t, 107-109, 143, 183
– –, –, branch(es), 183
– –, –, – auricular, 118-120
– –, –, – occipital, 118-120
– axillary 22, 220, 221, 247, 249, 260, 282, 392
– basilar, 16-18, 20, 21t, 25, 32, 33, 35t, 39t, 115
– brachial, 249, 282
– of brain, 39
– buccal, 35t, 98, 99, 111, 112, 141
– callosal, median, 37t
– callosomarginal, 17, 33, 35t, 115
– –, branches, cingular, 33
– –, –, paracentral, 33
– –, –, frontal, anteromedial, 33
– –, –, –, intermediomedial, 33
– –, –, –, posteromedial, 33
– caroticotympanic, 17, 35t, 191
– carotid, common, 16-20, 22-31, 34, 40t, 51, 99, 105, 106, 109-112, 114-116, 132, 154, 218-221, 226, 228-232, 234-236, 246-249, 253, 256t, 282, 289-297, 299, 309-312, 315-317, 321, 323, 326, 332, 334-340, 373, 382, 385, 392
– –, –, bifurcation, 23-25
– –, –, course and relations, 226
– –, external, 16-30, 35t, 40t, 51, 104, 105, 109, 111, 112, 124, 128, 130, 132, 137, 139, 141, 143, 183, 217, 220, 221, 228-230, 232, 233, 235, 236, 246
– –, –, collateral branches, 23

– –, –, terminal branches, 23
– –, internal, 16-33, 36t, 39t, 40t, 51, 52, 54, 55, 105, 106, 109-112, 121, 128, 130, 132, 133, 138, 139, 143, 159, 160, 162, 169, 171, 191, 193, 194, 217, 220, 221, 233, 235, 236, 246, 247
– –, –, cavernous part, 171
– –, –, cerebral part, 162
– –, –, cerebral, cavernous, petrous and cervical parts, 29
– –, –, tracts, communicating (distal supraclinoid), ophthalmic (proximal supraclinoid), clinoid, cavernous and precavernous, 29
– celiac, *see* Trunk(s), celiac
– central, retinal, 35t, 161, 162, 171, 177, 178
– –, anterolateral, 34t
– –, anteromedial, 34t
– –, posterolateral, 38t
– –, posteromedial, 38t
– cerebellar, inferior, anterior, 16-18, 20, 21t, 32, 33, 34t
– –, –, posterior, 17, 18, 20, 21t, 32, 33, 38t
– –, superior, 16-18, 20, 21t, 25, 32, 33, 39t
– cerebral, 52
– –, anterior, 16-18, 20, 21t, 25, 29, 32, 33, 34t, 39t, 115
– –, –, terminal branches, 33
– –, middle, 16-18, 20, 21t, 29, 32, 33, 37t, 39t
– –, –, anterior temporal branch, 33, 114
– –, –, branch to angular gyrus, 17, 33
– –, –, middle temporal branch, 33, 114
– –, –, posterior temporal branch, 33, 114
– –, posterior, 16-18, 20, 21t, 25, 32, 33, 38t, 39t
– –, –, P3 segment, *see* Artery(ies), occipital, lateral
– –, –, P4 segment, *see* Artery(ies), occipital, medial
– –, –, terminal branches, 33
– cervical, ascending, 17-20, 22, 40t, 98, 103, 104, 110-112, 218, 219, 249
– –, –, spinal branches, 40t
– –, deep, 22, 40t, 119-121
– –, superficial, 17-20, 22, 41t, 110, 218-220, 249
– –, transverse, 16, 18, 19t, 20, 22, 41t
– choroidal, anterior, 17, 18, 20, 21t, 32, 34t, 39t
– ciliary, anterior, 34t, 161, 162, 174, 177, 178
– –, posterior, 177
– –, –, lateral long, 177
– –, –, long, 36t, 161, 162, 178
– –, –, short, 39t, 161, 162, 177, 178
– cilioretinal, *see* Anastomosis, cilioretinal
– circumferential, short, 38t
– circumflex, *see* Artery(ies), coronary, left, circumflex branch
– –, iliac, superficial, 260
– cochlear, common, 194, 196
– collicular, 35t
– commissural, median, 37t
– communicating, anterior, 17, 18, 20, 21t, 32, 34t, 39t
– –, posterior, 17, 18, 20, 21t, 25, 32, 38t, 39t
– conjunctival, anterior, 34t, 177, 178
– –, posterior, 38t
– coronary, 17, 18, 20, 246, 247, 256t, 294, 329, 336-338, 343-346, 350-355
– –, branches, 247, 294, 336, 337, 344, 350-355
– –, epicardial, 351
– –, left, circumflex branch, 256t, 350-355
– –, –, anterior interventricular branch (LAD, left anterior descendens artery), 329, 334, 336, 350-355
– –, right, posterior interventricular branch, 256t, 337, 350-352, 354, 355
– cricothyroid, 40t
– dental, anterior, *see* Artery(ies), alveolar, superior, anterior
– –, inferior, *see* Artery(ies), alveolar, inferior
– –, posterior, *see* Artery(ies), alveolar, superior, posterior
– epigastric, inferior, 260
– –, superior, 247, 249, 257t, 260
– episcleral, 35t, 177
– esophageal, 40t
– ethmoidal, anterior, 24, 25, 34t, 115, 116, 143, 152, 156, 162, 173, 174
– –, –, branches, anterior lateral nasal, 152
– –, –, –, anterior septal, 152, 156
– –, posterior, 24, 25, 38t, 115, 143, 152, 156, 162, 172
– facial, 16-18, 20-25, 27, 30, 35t, 96-98, 103-106, 109-112, 124, 129, 139, 140, 143, 217, 228-230, 233
– –, deep, *see* Artery(ies), maxillary
– –, tonsillar branch, 146, 147
– frontal, *see* Artery(ies), supratrochlear
– frontobasal, 17
– –, lateral, 33, 36t
– –, medial, 33, 36t, 115
– hyaloid, 35t
– hypophysial, inferior, 35t
– –, superior, 39t
– infrahyoid, 40t
– infraorbital, 25, 36t, 97, 98, 114, 141, 142, 160
– innominate, *see* Trunk(s), brachiocephalic
– insular, 36t
– intercostal, 301, 302, 305, 308-312, 333
– –, anterior, *see also* Artery(ies), thoracic, internal, branches, anterior intercostal
– –, –, first, 22
– –, –, second, 22
– –, posterior, 220, 246-251, 257t, 261, 282, 286, 287, 321
– –, –, branch(es), 250, 251, 261, 321
– –, –, –, lateral cutaneous, 282
– –, –, first, 17, 18, 20, 22
– –, –, first and second, 16, 255t
– –, –, second, 17, 18, 20, 22
– –, –, twelfth, *see* Artery(ies), subcostal
– –, supreme (superior), 16-18, 20, 22, 41t, 220, 246, 247, 249, 250, 257t, 286, 287, 301-304, 333, 385
– internal auditory, *see* Artery(ies), labyrinthine
– interventricular, anterior, *see* Artery(ies), coronary, left, anterior interventricular branch
– –, posterior, *see* Artery(ies), coronary, right, posterior interventricular branch
– intramural, 351
– labial, inferior (inferior labial branch of facial artery), 23, 27, 35t
– –, superior, 23, 27, 39t, 110, 111, 152, 156, 162
– labyrinthine, 17, 32, 36t, 116, 194, 196
– lacrimal, 25, 36t, 159-162, 171, 172
– –, recurrent meningeal branch, 162
– laryngeal, inferior, 40t
– –, superior, 41t 128, 230, 232
– lingual, 17, 18, 20-25, 27, 36t, 110-112, 114, 115, 126, 128, 130, 132, 143, 229, 230, 232, 233
– –, branches, 129, 146, 147
– –, deep, 24, 35t, 123, 129, 130
– –, dorsal, 35t
– lingular, 246, 322
– –, inferior, 246
– –, superior, 246
– middle lobar, 246, 322
– –, inferior, 246
– –, superior, 246
– lumbar, 249
– mammary, external, *see* Artery(ies), thoracic, lateral
– –, internal, *see* Artery(ies), thoracic, internal
– mammillary, 36t
– mandibular, *see* Artery(ies), alveolar, inferior
– masseteric, 24, 36t
– maxillary, 17, 18, 20, 21t, 23-25, 27, 30, 36t, 111, 112, 137, 141-143
– –, external, *see* Artery(ies), facial
– –, internal, *see* Artery(ies), maxillary
– –, portion, mandibular, 25

– –, –, pterygoid, 25
– –, –, pterygopalatine, 25
– –, pterygoid branches, 24, 141
– medullary, segmental, 250
– meningeal, middle, 24, 25, 37t, 141, 142, 162, 173, 174
– –, –, frontal branch, 23-25, 116
– –, –, parietal branch, 23-25, 116
– –, posterior, 25, 27, 38t
– mesencephalic, 17, 37t
– mesenteric, inferior, 249
– –, superior, 246, 247, 249, 288-297, 382
– muscular, 37t, 161, 162
– musculophrenic, 247, 249, 256t
– mylohyoid, 41t
– nasal, dorsal, 25, 35t, 98, 107-109, 114, 160-162, 171
– –, external, *see* Artery(ies), nasal, dorsal
– –, lateral, 36t
– –, – posterior, 24, 38t, 143, 152
– –, – –, inferior, 116
– –, – –, superior, 116
– nasopalatine, *see* Artery(ies), sphenopalatine
– nutrient, 250
– occipital, 17, 18, 20-25, 27, 37t, 41t, 107-112, 118, 120, 121, 130, 143, 228-230
– –, lateral, 36t
– –, medial, 36t
– –, –, calcarine branch, 17, 33
– –, –, parietal branch, 33
– –, –, parieto-occipital branch, 17
– –, meningeal branch, 25
– –, sternocleidomastoid branch, 112
– ophthalmic, 17, 18, 20, 21t, 25, 32, 37t, 152, 156, 161, 162, 171-174
– –, muscular branches, *see* Artery(ies), muscular
– –, recurrent meningeal branch, 173, 174
– orbitofrontal, lateral, *see* Artery(ies), frontobasal, lateral
– –, medial, *see* Artery(ies), frontobasal, medial
– ovarian, 249
– palatine, ascending, 35t, 40t
– –, descending, 35t, 40t
– –, greater, 24, 35t, 116, 152, 156
– –, lesser, 36t, 123, 146
– palpebral, lateral, 36t, 162, 173, 174
– –, medial, 36t, 161, 162
– parietal, anterior, 17, 33, 34t, 114
– –, posterior, 17, 33, 38t
– perforating, anterior, 34t
– pericallosal, 17, 33, 37t, 115
– –, paracentral branch, 17
– –, precuneal branch, 17, 33
– pericardiacophrenic, 247, 252, 256t, 295, 303-305, 310-312, 330, 333
– –, branches, 247
– pericardial, *see* Artery(ies), aorta, thoracic, branch(es), pericardial
– pharyngeal, ascending, 17-20, 23-25, 27, 30, 35t, 40t, 112, 228, 229
– phrenic, inferior, 246-249, 252
– –, superior, 246, 247, 252, 257t
– –, –, branches, 252
– polar frontal, 17, 33, 37t
– – temporal, 37t
– pontine, 17, 32, 37t
– prefrontal, 17, 33, 38t, 114
– preoptic, 38t
– profunda brachii, 249, 282
– of pterygoid canal, 17, 37t
– pterygomeningeal, 38t
– pulmonary, 218, 219, 246, 256t, 292-294, 300-312, 316, 317, 322-330, 332, 333, 335-338, 340, 360, 378, 384, 390, 391
– –, basal part, 300
– quadrigeminal, *see* Artery(ies), collicular
– radicular, anterior, 250
– –, posterior, 250
– ranine, *see* Artery(ies), lingual, deep
– renal, 249
– scapular, dorsal, 40t, 249
– –, transverse, *see* Artery(ies), suprascapular
– segmental, anterior, 246, 322
– –, apical, 246, 322
– –, basal, anterior, 246, 322
– –, –, lateral, 246, 300, 322
– –, –, medial, 246, 322
– –, –, posterior, 246, 300, 322
– –, lateral, 246, 322
– –, medial, 246, 322
– –, posterior, 246, 322
– –, superior, 246, 322
– sphenopalatine, 24, 39t, 115, 141-143, 152, 156
– –, posterior septal branches, 24, 143, 152, 156
– sphenospinal, *see* Artery(ies), meningeal, middle
– spinal, 40t, 41t
– –, anterior, 16-18, 20, 21t, 32, 34t, 40t, 115, 250, 255t, 257t
– –, dorsal, *see* Artery(ies), spinal, posterior
– –, posterior, 17, 18, 20, 21t, 32, 33, 38t, 41t, 250, 256t, 257t
– –, segmental branches, 250
– –, ventral, *see* Artery(ies), spinal, anterior
– sternocleidomastoid, 41t
– striate, medial, distal, 35t
– –, –, proximal, 38t
– subcostal, 249, 256t, 257t
– of sulcus, central, 17, 33, 37t, 114
– –, postcentral, 33, 37t
– –, precentral, 17, 33, 37t, 114
– suprachiasmatic, 39t
– suprahyoid, 41t
– supraoptic, 39t
– supraorbital, 25, 39t, 96-99, 160-162, 172, 173
– suprascapular, 17-19, 20, 22, 41t, 98, 104, 109-112, 218-220, 249, 282
– supratrochlear, 25, 39t, 114, 161, 162, 172, 173, 174
– subclavian, 16-20, 22, 41t, 51, 99, 105, 106, 112-116, 218-221, 225-232, 246-249, 253, 256t, 282, 289-300, 302-305, 309-311, 315-317, 321, 323-326, 332-340, 359, 373, 376, 382, 385, 386, 392
– –, course and relations, 226
– –, groove, 373
– sublingual, 24, 39t, 124, 129, 130
– submental, 23, 25, 39t, 41t, 96-99, 128
– subscapular, 246, 247, 249, 282
– stylomastoid, 39t, 190, 191
– temporal, anterior, 34t
– –, deep, anterior, 17, 24, 34t, 111, 112, 141
– –, –, posterior, 17, 24, 38t, 111, 112, 141
– –, middle, 17, 37t
– –, –, groove, 188
– –, superficial, 16-18, 20, 21t, 23-25, 27, 39t, 52, 96, 97, 104, 110-112, 118, 119, 141, 183
– –, –, branches, 183
– –, –, –, anterior auricular, 187
– –, –, –, frontal, 23, 107-109, 118, 183, 187
– –, –, –, parietal, 23, 107-109, 118, 183, 187
– testicular, 249
– thalamogeniculate, 39t
– thalamoperforating, 39t
– thalamotuberal, 39t
– thoracic, internal, 16-20, 22, 41t, 220, 221, 226, 246-250, 252, 255t, 257t, 260, 282, 297, 303, 304, 333, 385
– –, –, branches, 247, 249, 260, 282
– –, –, –, anterior intercostal, 247, 249 250, 255t, 297
– –, lateral, 246, 247, 249, 256t, 260, 282
– –, –, branches, 280, 282, 284
– – long, *see* Artery(ies), thoracic, lateral
– –, superior, 246, 247, 249, 257t, 282
– –, twelfth, *see* Artery(ies), subcostal
– thoracoacromial, 22, 246, 247, 249, 257t, 282
– –, branch(es), 249, 282
– thoracodorsal, 246, 247, 257t
– thyroid ima, 41t, 257t
– thyroid, inferior, 16-19, 20, 22, 40t, 98, 99, 104, 105, 113, 217, 219, 220, 228, 231, 234, 246, 247

– –, –, branches, 319
– –, superior, 16-20, 22-25, 27, 41t, 104, 105, 109-112, 217, 219, 220, 221, 226, 228, 229, 231, 246
– of tongue, deep, *see* Artery(ies), lingual, deep
– tonsillar, 41t
– transverse, cervical, 16-20, 22, 41t, 97-99, 103, 104, 106, 109-112, 120, 220, 221, 246, 247, 249
– –, facial, 23, 39t, 97, 139, 183
– of tuber cinereum, 37t
– tympanic, anterior, 24, 34t, 190
– –, inferior, 36t, 191
– –, posterior, 38t, 190
– –, superior, 39t
– uncal, 39t
– vertebral, 16-20, 22-25, 27-33, 35, 39t, 41t, 51, 54, 112, 114-116, 119-121, 220, 221, 227, 233, 234, 246, 247, 249, 257t, 282, 385
– –, lateral medullary branches, 33
– vestibular, 194
– –, anterior, 196
– vestibulocochlear, 194, 196
– vidian, *see* Artery(ies), of pterygoid canal
– zygomatico-orbital, 23, 39t, 107-109, 183
Auricle, 5, 181, 182, 189, 192, 197
–, arteries, 183
–, cartilage, 182
–, innervation, 186
–, lymphatic drainage, 185
–, lymphatic networks, 185
–, veins, 184
Axis
– optic, 177
– visual, 177

B

Blood-air barrier, 391
Bone(s)
– alveolar, 136
– atlas [C I], 121, 200
– –, lateral mass, 31
– –, posterior arch, 31
– axis [C II], 233
– –, dens, 31, 192
– choana, 125, 145
– clavicle, 31, 49, 101, 117, 221, 240, 383
– ethmoid, 150, 151
– frontal, 144, 158
– –, nasal part, 150
– –, orbital surface, 55, 150
– –, squamous part, 149, 150
– –, zygomatic process, 150
– humerus, 392
– hyoid, 26, 27, 30, 67, 76, 100, 104-106, 125, 127, 128, 200, 203, 205, 208-210, 220, 221, 222, 224-226, 235, 314, 315
– –, body, 124, 201, 202-206, 210
– –, horn, greater, 127, 201, 202-209
– –, –, lesser, 127, 202-207
– nasal, 125, 144, 149
– occipital, 144
– palatine, 149
– rib(s), 286-296, 301-305, 308-312, 335, 372, 383, 392, 394
– –, false [VIII-X], 297
– –, true [I-VII], 297
– scapula, 253, 254, 383, 392, 393
– sphenoid, 159, 160, 170
– –, body, 125, 149
– –, greater wing, orbital surface, 150
– –, lesser wing, 55, 150
– –, sella turcica, 54, 149, 170
– –, –, dorsum sellae, 194
– sternum, 218, 219, 250, 253, 254, 324, 325, 334, 385, 392, 393
– –, body, 297, 301-305, 307-312, 333, 368, 383
– –, manubrium, 297, 301-305, 307-312, 333, 335, 368, 383
– –, xiphoid process, 238, 297, 301, 302, 304, 305, 307-312, 333
– temporal, 188, 195
– –, mastoid process, 188
– –, petrous part, 188
– –, squamous part, 188
– –, styloid process, 30, 124, 188
– –, tympanic part, 188
– –, zygomatic process, 188, 150
– vomer, 31, 99, 148-150, 155
– zygomatic, 150
– –, orbital surface, 150
Border
– alveolar, 136
– inferior of neck, 2, 238
Brain
–, arteries, 39
–, –, of the base, 32
–, cerebral veins, 63
Branch(es)
– cardiac, cervical, inferior, 364
– –, –, superior, 364
– –, thoracic, 364
Breast, 280-282
–, adipose tissue, 280, 281
–, areolar tubercles, 280
–, arteries, 282
–, blood supply, 282
–, conformation and structure, 280, 281
–, drainage, lymphatic, 284
–, –, physiologic, 285
–, –, venous, 283
–, inframammary sulcus, 238, 280
–, lactiferous sinuses, 281
–, lymph nodes, 284, 285
–, nerves, 285
–, ring of smooth muscle, 281
–, suspensory ligament, 281
–, veins, 283
Bronchiole(s), 390
– intralobular, 390
– respiratory, 390
– terminal, 390, 391
Bronchus(hi), 199, 390
– epiarterial, *see* Bronchus(hi), lobar, superior
– intermediate, 333, 380
– intrapulmonary, 380
– intrasegmental, major, 390
– –, minor, 390
– lingular, 199, 319, 320, 377, 380
– –, inferior [B V], 318, 375, 377, 380
– –, superior [B IV], 318, 332, 375, 377, 380
– lobar, 199
– –, inferior, 318-320, 332, 375-377, 379, 380, 393
– –, middle, 298, 318-320, 375, 377, 379, 380, 393
– –, superior, 218, 298, 301-305, 318-320, 333, 375-377, 379, 380
– lobular, 390
– main, 199, 218, 219, 290, 298, 301-305, 308-312, 315, 316, 318-322, 324, 325, 332, 333, 358, 361, 371, 373, 374-378, 380
– –, left, 358, 367, 368
–, ramification, lobar, 380
–, –, segmental, 380
–, –, subsegmental, 380
– segmental, 199, 390
– –, anterior [B III], 318, 375, 377, 379, 380
– –, apical [B I], 318, 375, 380
– –, apicoposterior [B I + II], 298, 318, 375, 377, 379, 380
– –, basal, anterior [B VIII], 375, 380
– –, –, lateral [B IX], 318, 375, 380
– –, –, medial [B VII], 318, 375, 380
– –, –, posterior [B X], 318, 375, 380
– –, lateral [B IV], 318, 375
– –, medial [B V], 318, 375, 380
– –, posterior [B II], 318, 375, 380
– –, superior [B VI], 318, 375, 380
Bud, taste, 131
Bulb
– aortic, 344
– of jugular vein, inferior, 99, 105
– olfactory, 115, 116, 143, 155, 156
Bundle
– atrioventricular, 345, 346, 352, 357
– of His, *see* Bundle, atrioventricular
– of neck, neurovascular, 106
Bursa, pharyngeal, 146

C

Canal(s)
– alveolar, 83t
– carotid, 83t, 195
– condylar, 83t
– diploic, 83t
– external collector, 178
– facial, 83t
– for auditory tube, 83t
– for tensor tympani, 83t
– hyaloid, 177
– hypoglossal, 83t
– incisive, 83t, 149
– infraorbital, 83t, 99
– mandibular, 83t
– musculotubal, 83t
– nasolacrimal, 83t
– optic, 83t
– palatine, greater, 83t
– –, lesser, 83t
– palatovaginal, 83t
– pharyngeal, *see* Canal(s), palatovaginal
– pterygoid, 83t
– pterygopalatine, *see* Canal(s), palatine, greater
– root (pulp canal), 136
– semicircular, 193, 197
– –, anterior, 188, 193-195, 197
– –, common bony limb, 194
– –, lateral, 193-195, 197
– –, membranous, 192
– –, posterior, 193-195, 197
– vidian, *see* Canal(s), pterygoid
– vomerobasilar, *see* Canal(s), vomerorostral
– vomerorostral, 83t
– vomerovaginal, 83t
Canaliculus(li)
– caroticotympanic, 83t
– for chorda tympani, 83t
– cochlear, 83t
– lacrimal, inferior, 158
– –, superior, 158
– mastoid, 83t
– tympanic, 83t
– vestibular, 83t
Capillary, pulmonary, 391
Carotid body, 132, 138
Cartilage
– alar, major, 149
– –, minor, 149
– arytenoid, 199, 203, 205-210, 212, 214-216, 313, 319
– –, apex, 212
– –, articular surface (for the cricoid cartilage), 212, 215
– –, colliculus, 212
– –, fovea, oblong, 212
– –, –, triangular, 212
– –, process, muscular, 212
– –, –, vocal, 212
– –, surface, anterolateral, 212
– –, –, medial, 212
– –, –, posterior, 212
– bronchial, 390
– corniculate, 199, 203, 205-210, 212, 319
– costal, 297
– cricoid, 145, 199, 202-210, 213, 215, 216, 226, 230, 232, 313-315, 318, 319
– –, arch, 125, 203, 207, 215
– –, area of insertion for the lateral cricoarytenoid, 211
– –, fossa of the lamina, 211
– –, lamina, 203, 207, 215
– –, –, crest, 206, 211
– –, surface, arytenoid articular, 214
– –, –, thyroid articular, 211
– cuneiform, 203, 210, 212
– epiglottic, 125, 145, 202, 203, 205, 206, 208-210, 216, 313, 319
– laryngeal, 204
– septal nasal, 149
– thyroid, 27, 30, 105, 125, 127, 128, 145, 199, 202-210, 213, 215, 216, 218, 219, 221, 226, 230, 232, 235, 301, 302, 308-314, 318, 319, 324, 325, 365, 371
– –, border, inferior, 213
– –, –, superior, 213
– –, horn, inferior, 202-207, 212
– –, –, superior, 201-209
– – of larynx, 26, 220, 225
– –, oblique line, 211
– –, thyroid tubercle, inferior, 211
– –, – –, superior, 211
– tracheal, 203, 205, 206-210, 318, 319
– triticeal, 209, 210
Caruncle
– lacrimal, 5, 158
– sublingual, 123, 128
Cavity(ies)
– abdominal, 240, 244, 388
– –, organs, 394, 395
– alveolar, 136, 391
– of concha, 182
– infraglottic, 208, 210
– Meckel's, 12t
– nasal, 143, 145, 150-157
– –, conformation and structure, 157
– –, mucosa, 151
– –, subdivision, 157
– –, true, 157
– oral, 122, 129
– –, conformation and structure, 123-125
– orbital, 150, 161, 164, 165, 167, 169, 171-174
– pleural, 244, 251, 372, 387, 392
– rhombencephalon, 12t, 13t
– thoracic, 239, 240, 251, 330, 372, 388, 392, 393
– –, organs, 393-395
– –, topographic anatomy, 240
– tympanic, 195
Cecum, vestibular, 195
Cell(s)
– alveolar, type I, *see* Pneumocyte type I
– –, type II, *see* Pneumocyte type II
– ethmoidal, 99, 150, 151
– –, anterior, 151
– –, middle, 151
– –, posterior, 151
– hair, inner, 198
– –, outer, 198
– mastoid, 228-230
– tubal air, 188
Cerebellum, 53, 87, 115
–, tentorium cerebelli, 55, 82
Chain(s)
– lymph node, cervical, 65
– –, –, transverse, *see* Chain(s), horizontal, inferior
– –, deep, 68
– –, horizontal, inferior, 67, 68
– –, –, superior, 67, 68
– –, superficial, 67, 68
– –, supraclavicular, *see* Chain(s), horizontal, inferior
– – vertical, 67, 68
– sympathetic, 274, 277; *see also* Trunk(s), sympathetic
Chamber
– anterior, 177-179
– posterior, 177, 178
Choroid, 177-180
Circle
– cerebral arterial, 20, 32, 39t
– of Zinn-Haller, 177
Circulation
– coronary, 247
– pulmonary, large, 323, 325
– –, –, vessels, 253, 255, 321
– –, small, vessels, 253, 255
Cisterna chyli (chyle cistern), 265, 266, 287, 288
Cochlea, 181, 192-195, 197, 198
–, aqueduct, 193, 194, 197
–, base, 194, 198
–, cupula, 194
Collectors, lymphatic, 358
–, –, lateral, 166
–, –, medial, 166
Colon, ascending, 387
–, descending, 395
Column
– vertebral, 334, 395
– – dorsal, 250
Compartment(s), 11
– carotid, *see* Compartment(s), vascular
– cerebellar, *see* Cavity(ies), rhombencephalon
– cerebral, 12t
– fascial, 11
– hypophyseal, 12t

– masseteric, 12t
– parotid, 12t, 139, 140, 144
– pleural, 243, 244, 372, 383
– –, blood supply, 243
– –, boundaries, 243
– –, content, 243
– –, innervation, 243
– –, lymphatic drainage, 243
– –, vascular formations, 244
– prefascial, 12t
– retrofascial, 13t
– sternocleidomastoid, 7t, 14t
– sublingual, 13t
– submandibular, 14t, 140
– supraclavicular, 3, 7t, 14t
– temporal, 13t
– tonsillar, 13t
– vascular, 3, 7t, 11, 14t
Concha, nasal, 157
– nasal (turbinate), inferior, 99, 148, 150-153, 155, 156, 230
– –, –, ethmoidal process, 150
– –, lymphatic network, 154
– –, middle, 99, 148, 150-153, 155, 156, 230
– –, superior, 150, 152, 153, 155, 156
Confluence of sinuses (torcula Herophili), 52, 57t
Conjunctiva, 159, 176, 178
– bulbar, 168, 179
– –, lymphatic capillaries, 166
– palpebral, 168, 173, 174, 176
Conus, arteriosus (infundibulum), 334, 336, 339
– elasticus, 206-208, 210, 214
Cord, spinal, 115, 233, 250, 261, 275
– –, arterial circulation, 250
–, sympathetic, *see* Trunk(s), sympathetic
Cornea, 166, 176-179
–, limbus, *see* Junction, corneoscleral
–, substantia propria, 178, 179
Corona ciliaris, 180
Cranium
–, bony structures,144
–, calvaria, 52
Crest
– frontal, 150
– iliac, 245
– nasal, 149
– supraventricular, 338, 339, 341, 345
– tegmental of temporal bone, 188
Crista
– terminalis, 339
– galli, 149-151
Cupula
– diaphragmatic, 240
– pleural, 226, 245, 382, 385, 386
– –, means of attachment, 386
Cusps
– aortic semilunar, 299, 338, 339, 343-346, 356
– –, nodule, 338, 339, 343
– pulmonary semilunar, 338, 339, 345, 346, 356, 361
Cymba conchae, 182

D

Dentine, 136
Dentition, 136
Desmodentium (periodontal fiber), 136
Diaphragm, 240, 244, 246-248, 252, 258, 266, 289-296, 304-307, 310-316, 324, 325, 330, 335, 358, 359, 367, 371-373, 382, 387-389, 394
–, blood supply, 252
–, central tendon, 289, 304, 333
–, cupula, 245
–, inferior limit, 245
–, innervation, 371
–, part, costal, 289-292
–, –, lumbar, 289-292, 297
–, –, sternal, 293-296, 382
Diencephalon, 115
Disc, optic, 177
Diverticulum
– epibronchial, 314
– epiphrenic, 314
– Zenker's, 314
Dome of pleura, *see* Cupula, pleural
Duct(s)
– alveolar, 391
– cochlear, 192, 195
– endolymphatic, 195, 197
– intralobular, 280
– lactiferous, 280, 281
– lymphatic, 217, 218, 224, 265, 266, 269, 361, 385
– membranous semicircular, *see* Canal(s), semicircular, membranous
– nasolacrimal, 158
– –, opening, 158
– parotid, 98, 124, 139
– saccular, 195
– sublingual, 128
– – minor, 128
– – –, orifices, 123
– submandibular, 114, 115, 123, 124, 129
– thoracic, 66, 99, 105, 106, 217, 219, 224, 226, 252, 265, 266, 269, 274, 287, 288, 358, 361, 392
– utricular, 195
Ductus reuniens, 195
Duodenum, 245
Dura mater, 52, 121, 170
– – cranial, 114

E

Ear, 5, 181-198
–, antihelix, 5, 182
–, antitragus, 5, 182
–, auditory ossicles, 181, 191-193, 197
–, –, muscles, 192
–, auricle, 5, 181, 182, 189, 192, 197
–, auricular tubercle, 5, 182
–, bone structure, 188-191
–, concha of auricle, 5
– external, 181, 192
– –, cartilaginous parts, 181
– –, general structure, 5
– –, innervation, 187
– –, lymphatic drainage, 187
– –, vascularization, 187
–, external acoustic meatus, 5, 181, 182, 188, 189, 192, 193, 195, 197
–, groove of helix, 5, 182
–, helix, 5, 182
–, –, crus, 5, 182
–, –, groove, 5, 182
–, –, tail, 182
– internal, 181, 189, 192, 193, 195, 198
–, intertragic incisure, 5
–, lobule of auricle, 5
–, lymphatic drainage, 185
– middle, 181, 189, 192, 193
–, nerves, 186
–, stapes, 88, 189-191
–, –, base, 191
–, –, head, 190, 191
–, –, limb, anterior, 191
–, –, –, posterior, 191
–, tragus, 5
–, triangular fossa, 5, 182
–, veins, 184
–, vestibule, 192, 193
Eminence, pyramidal, 190, 191
Emmetropia, 180
Endocardium, 351
Endopleural drainage, 387
Endothelium
– of anterior chamber, 176, 178
– capillary, 391
Epicardium, *see* Pericardium, serous
Epiglottis, 125, 199, 204, 205, 207, 210, 230, 232, 367
–, margin, 214
Epithelium
– alveolar, 391
– bathyprismatic transitional, 157
– conjunctival, 179
– corneal, 176, 178, 179
– investing, 157
– keratinized stratified pavimentous, 157
– pseudostratified ciliated, 157
– – with olfactory cells, 157
Esophagus, 106, 125, 145, 200, 216, 217, 220, 222, 224, 225, 228, 229, 234, 244, 248, 252, 254, 274, 289-293, 301, 302, 304, 305, 308-314, 316, 317, 319, 325, 326, 333, 334, 358, 367, 368, 384, 385, 392, 393

–, adventitia, 216, 313, 314, 358
–, aggregated lymphoid nodules (MALT), 314
–, groove, 378, 379
–, innervation, 367, 370
–, lumen, 314
–, mucosa, 216, 313, 319, 358
–, muscular layer (coat), 216, 230, 232, 313, 314, 319, 358
–, – –, circular layer, 313, 314, 319
–, – –, longitudinal layer, 313, 314, 319
–, part, abdominal, 2. 291-297, 310, 311, 315, 324, 325, 333, 358, 370, 382
–, –, cervical, 324, 325, 358, 370
–, –, thoracic, 315, 324, 358
–, position, 313
–, serosa, 313
–, structure, 216, 314
–, submucosa, 216, 313, 314, 358
–, topographic relations, 315, 316, 317
–, venous plexus, 314
–, wall, 314
Expiration, 388
Extension
– of pretracheal layer of cervical fascia, 97, 103
Eye, 5, 158-165, 169, 180
–, arteries, 161, 162
–, emmetropic, 180
–, eyeball, 176-180
–, –, conjunctiva, 159, 176, 178
–, –, inferior tarsus and superior tarsus, 159, 160
–, –, fascial sheath, 179
–, eyebrow, 5, 158, 176
–, eyelid(s), inferior, 5, 158
–, –, lateral lymphatic pathways, 166
–, –, medial lymphatic pathways, 166
–, –, superficial lymphatic network, 166
–, –, superior, 5, 158, 176
–, general structure, 5
–, innervation, 171-174
–, lacrimal caruncle, 5, 158
–, lacus lacrimalis, 5, 158
–, lymphatic drainage, 166
–, muscles, 159, 160
–, myopic, 180
–, nerves, 167, 168
–, –, cranial, 170
–, plica semilunaris, 5, 158
–, position and structure, 158
–, structure of the anterior (iridociliary) part of the vascular layer, 179
–, superciliary arch, *see* Eye, eyebrow
–, vascularization, 171-174
–, veins, 163-165
Eyeball, 176-178, 180, 192
–, blood circulation, 177
–, blood vessels, 178
–, equator, 177
–, external axis, 177
–, protective apparatus, 158
Eyelash, 176

F

Falx
– cerebri, 52, 54, 55, 82, 115
– septi, 340
Fascia(e), 10
– alar, 10, 234
– cervical, 10
– – investing layer (superficial layer), 10, 96, 97, 102, 103, 234
– – pretracheal layer, 10, 97, 98, 103, 104, 234
– – prevertebral layer, 10, 234
– endothoracic, 251, 387
– nuchal, 10, 111, 113, 234
– parotid, 139, 140, 185, 187
– pectoral, 281
– pharyngeal, 147, 230, 232
– pharyngobasilar, 125
– superficial, 281
– –, layer, deep, 281
– –, –, superficial, 281
Fastigium, 115
Fat
–, body, pre-epiglottic, 125, 207, 208
–, pad, retrosternal, 244, 252, 296, 304, 311, 331, 333, 368, 373, 382, 385
– pericardial, 330
– retrobulbar, 172
Fiber(s)
– alveologingival, 136
– apical, 136
– alveolar crest, 136
– dentogingival, 136
– sympathetic, visceral, motor, 79
– –, –, sensory, 79
– –, postganglionic, 78, 276
– interdental, 136
– parasympathetic, postganglionic, 78, 276
– preganglionic, 78, 276
– oblique, 136
– horizontal, 136
– zonular, 178, 180
Fissure
– orbital, inferior, 83t, 99, 150
– –, superior, 83t, 99, 167, 150
– palpebral, 158
– petrosquamous, 188
– petrotympanic, 83t, 188
– pulmonary, 244
– tympanomastoid, 83t, 188
Flank, *see* Region(s), abdominal, lateral
Fold(s)
– aryepiglottic, 203, 210, 216, 230, 313
– fimbriated, 123, 128
– glossoepiglottic, lateral, 125
– –, median, 125, 232
– semilunar, 158
– sublingual, 123
– transverse palatine, 122
– vestibular, 208, 210, 214
– vocal, 125, 145, 208, 210, 214
Foramen(ina)
– apical, 136
– cecum, 84t
– cribriform, 84t
– etmoidal, anterior, 84t
– –, posterior, 84t
– frontal, 84t
– jugular, 28, 84t, 105, 193
– incisive, anterior, 84t
– –, posterior, 84t
– infraorbital, 84t
– lacerum, anterior, 84t
– –, posterior, *see* Foramen(ina), jugular
– magnum, 84t
– mandibular, 84t
– mastoid, 84t, 188
– mental, 84t
– occipital, great, *see* Foramen(ina), magnum
– optic, 84t, 99
– ovale, 84t, 193
– palatine, greater, 84t, 123
– –, lesser, 84t, 123
– parietal, 84t
– petrosum, 84t
– rotundum, 84t
– sphenoidal emissary, 84t
– sphenopalatine, 84t
– spinosum, 84t, 193
– stylomastoid, 84t, 87
– supraorbital, 84t
– for superior laryngeal artery and superior laryngeal nerve, 201, 202, 204-206, 208
– thyroid, 127t
– vertebral, 31
– zygomatico-orbital, 84t
– zygomaticofacial, 84t
– zygomaticotemporal, 84t
Fornix, 115
–, body, 33
– superior conjunctival, 176
Fossa
– cranial, anterior, 55, 172
– –, middle, 55, 172
– –, posterior (cerebellar), 55
– infraclavicular, 238, 239
– infratemporal, 140, 141, 142
– jugular, *see* Fossa, suprasternal
– mandibular, 188
– ovalis, 339, 357
– –, limbus, 339
– piriform, 208, 210, 230
– pterygopalatine, 143, 151
– retromandibular, 6

- supraclavicular, greater, 6, 7t
- –, lesser, 6, 7t
- suprasternal, 6, 7t
- triangular, 182, 215
Fovea centralis, 177
Frenulum
- of lower lip, 123
- of tongue, 123
- of upper lip, 123

G

Ganglion(a)
- aorticorenal, 78, 276
- cardiac, 365, 369
- celiac, 78, 276, 369
- cervical, inferior, 78, 94t, 132, 138, 217, 227, 276, 277, 366, 367
- –, middle, 78, 79, 94t, 169, 227-230, 274, 276, 277, 362-364, 366, 367, 370
- –, – left, 365
- –, – of sympathetic trunk, 106
- –, superior, 78, 79, 94t, 132, 138, 139, 169, 217, 225, 227-229, 274, 276, 277, 362-364
- –, – left, 365
- –, – of sympathetic trunk, 106
- cervicothoracic, 79, 169, 218, 219, 226, 274, 287, 288, 301-305, 308-312, 362-365, 368, 370, 371, 385
- ciliary, 78, 79, 85, 86, 167-171, 174, 276
- –, branch to ciliary ganglion, 167-169
- –, communicating branch with ciliary ganglion, 167-169
- –, sympathetic root, 167-169
- cochlear, 196, 198
- Corti's, *see* Ganglion(a), cochlear
- Gasser's, *see* Ganglion(a), trigeminal
- geniculate, 87, 88, 191
- impar, 78, 276
- inferior, 363
- – of vagus nerve, 113
- lumbar, 78
- mesenteric, inferior, 78, 276
- –, superior, 78, 276, 369
- otic, 78, 79, 132, 276
- –, parasympathetic root, *see* Nerve(s), petrosal, lesser
- pelvic, parasympathetic root, *see* Nerve(s), splanchnic, pelvic
- preaortic, 79
- pterygopalatine. 78, 79, 85, 88, 116, 137, 138, 143, 155, 156, 276
- sacral, 78
- Scarpa's, *see* Ganglion(a),vestibular
- spinal (or dorsal root ganglion), 275
- spiral, *see* Ganglion(a), cochlear
- stellate, *see* Ganglion(a), cervicothoracic
- sublingual, 79, 132
- submandibular, 78, 79, 85, 88, 113, 129, 130, 132
- sympathetic thoracic, 277
- of sympathetic trunk, 302, 368
- thoracic, 276, 362, 363, 365-367, 371
- –, branches, 362
- –, –, esophageal, 370
- –, –, thoracic cardiac, 364, 365
- –, –, thoracic pulmonary, 366
- –, –, visceral, 275
- – of sympathetic trunk, 274
- trigeminal, 79, 82, 85, 86, 132, 137, 138, 143, 167-169, 171, 173, 174
- vestibular, 194, 196
- Wrisberg's, *see* Ganglion(a), cardiac
Gingiva, 136
Gland(s)
- accessory, 281
- areolar, 280
- ciliary, 176
- esophageal, 314
- labial, 122
- –, inferior, 122
- – superior, 122
- lacrimal, 88, 98, 138, 160-162, 168, 171-174
- –, accessory, 176
- –, –, excretory duct, 176
- –, excretory ducts, 158
- –, orbital part, 158
- –, palpebral part, 158
- lingual, 129, 131
- –, anterior, 123, 126, 128, 129
- mammary, 280, 282, 283
- –, axillary process, 280
- –, duct(s), extralobular terminal, 281
- –, –, intralobular terminal, 281
- –, –, lobular, 281
- –, ductule, 281
- –, fibroglandular ridge, 281
- –, lobules, 280, 281
- –, terminal duct lobular unit (TDLU), 281
- nasal, 157
- palatine, 123
- parathyroid, 228, 229
- –, configuration and relations, 231
- –, inferior, 231
- –, superior, 231
- parotid, 67, 79, 98, 102-106, 108, 117, 124, 129, 132, 140, 148, 160, 185, 187, 233
- – accessory, 124
- pineal (pineal body), 33, 115
- pituitary, 32, 55, 115, 170
- sebaceous, 176, 281
- sublingual, 99, 114-116, 123, 124, 128, 129, 132, 148, 233
- submandibular, 88, 99, 103, 114-116, 124, 128, 129, 132, 140, 148
- tarsal, 176
- –, excretory duct, 176
- thyroid, 31, 67, 104, 105, 128, 213, 220-222, 224, 225, 228, 229, 231, 234, 274, 330, 365
- –, configuration and relations, 231
- –, lobe, 226
- von Ebner's, *see* Gland(s), lingual
Glottis, 210
–, rima glottidis, 210, 214

H

Hamulus, pterygoid, 149
Head, 96-101, 107-116, 118-120, 140
–, arteries, 16, 17, 20, 34t-39t
–, –, territories of supply, 21t, 34t-39t
–, compartment(s), boundaries and contents, 12t, 13t
–, – cerebellar, *see* Head, compartment(s), rhombencephalon cavity
–, – cerebral, 12t
–, – hypophyseal, 12t
–, – masseteric, 12t
–, – Meckel's cavity, 12t
–, – parotid, 12t
–, – prefascial, 12t
–, – retrofascial, 13t
–, – rhombencephalon cavity, 13t
–, – sublingual, 13t
–, – temporal, 13t
–, – tonsillar, 13t
–, cutaneous territories of innervation, 80, 81
–, lymph nodes, 65, 68-71, 72t
–, lymphatic groups, 67, 74
–, nerves, 89t-93t
–, region(s), 3
–, – buccal, 3, 4
–, – cheek, *see* Head, region(s), buccal
–, – chin, *see* Head, region(s), mental
–, – facial, 3, 4
–, – frontal, 3, 4
–, – infraorbital, 3, 4
–, – infratemporal, 3, 4
–, – mental, 3, 4
–, – mouth, *see* Head, region(s), oral
–, – nasal, 3, 4
–, – occipital, 3, 4
–, – oral, 3, 4
–, – orbital, 3, 4
–, – parietal, 3, 4
–, – parotid, 4
–, – parotid-masseteric, 4
–, –, subdivision and boundaries, 4
–, – temporal, 3, 4
–, – zygomatic, 3, 4
–, space(s)
–, – anterior subparotid, 12t

–, – lateral pharyngeal, *see* Head, space(s), parapharyngeal
–, – lateropharyngeal, *see* Head, space(s), parapharyngeal
–, – leptomeningeal, 12t
–, – masticator, 12t
–, – maxillopharyngeal, *see* Head, space(s), parapharyngeal
–, – parapharyngeal, 12t
–, – paratonsillar, *see* Head, space(s), anterior subparotid
–, – peripharyngeal, *see* Head, space(s), parapharyngeal
–, – pharyngomaxillary, *see* Head, space(s), parapharyngeal
–, – prestyloid, *see* Head, space(s), parapharyngeal
–, – retropharyngeal, 13t
–, – retrostyloid, *see* Head, space(s), parapharyngeal
–, – retrovisceral, *see* Head, space(s), retropharyngeal
–, – subdural, 13t
–, superficial boundaries, 2
–, supraorbital margin, 2
–, vascularization, 16
–, veins, 16, 42-45, 48, 59t-63t
–, venous sinuses, 45
Heart, 244, 247, 248, 294, 307, 317, 323, 328-334, 336, 337, 340-343, 345-351, 354, 355, 369, 395
–, apex, 334, 336, 338-340, 351
–, atrium, 240, 254, 259, 298, 299, 306, 317, 328, 332, 334-342, 344, 350, 351, 393
–, –, anterior surface, 338
–, –, cavities, 339-342
–, –, vestibule (roof), 332, 337, 338
–, auricle, 326, 327, 329, 336, 338-340, 342, 344, 347, 350, 351, 361, 393
–, band, Torrent-Guasp, *see* Heart, band, ventricular myocardial
–, –, ventricular myocardial, 348, 349
–, base, 332, 338
–, cardiac muscles, 347-350
–, –, atrial, 347
–, –, ventricular, 347
–, cardiac veins, 356
–, cavities, blood flow, 345
–, chordae tendineae, 339, 340, 343
–, conduction system, 352, 357
–, –, arterial vascularization, 352
–, coronary arteries, 352, 353
–, external conformation, 336, 337
–, fibrous skeleton, 345, 346
–, innervation, 362-368
–, internal configuration, 338, 340-344
–, interventricular septum, 353
–, –, blood supply, 353
–, margin, acute, *see* Heart, margin, right
–, –, right, 336, 337, 343, 353
–, –, obtuse, *see* Heart, margin, left
–, –, left, 336-338, 343, 353
–, myocardial fibers, 350
–, plexuses of autonomic fibers, 364
–, sulcus, interventricular, anterior, 262t, 336, 338, 339, 343, 347
–, –, –, posterior, 263t, 337, 340, 343, 347
–, –, terminalis cordis, 338, 347
–, surface, diaphragmatic (inferior), 332, 337, 353
–, –, anterior (sternocostal), 336, 353
–, topographic relations, 328-333
–, trabecula(e) carneae, 338, 339, 343, 353
–, – septomarginal, 338
–, tract(s) internodal, 357
–, valves, 345, 346
–, –, diastole, 345
–, –, sites of auscultation, 346
–, –, systole, 345
–, vessels, arteries, 351, 352
–, –, –, anatomic variants, 352
–, –, cardiac, 350, 351
–, –, of left (obtuse) margin, 351-355
–, –, veins, 351
–, ventricle, 240, 248, 254, 298, 299, 306, 328, 332, 334-337, 339-342, 344, 350, 351, 393
–, –, base, 346
–, –, cavity, 338-343, 353
–, –, conus arteriosus, 338
–, –, wall, 340, 353
–, –, –, anterior, 343
–, –, – posterior, 343
–, vortex, 347
–, wall(s), posterior, 353
–, –, –, blood supply, 353
–, – ventricular, 343
Helicotrema, 198
Hiatus
– aortic, 289, 303, 304
– esophageal, 289, 313
– for greater petrosal nerve, 84t
– for lesser petrosal nerve, 84t
– semilunaris (or semilunar groove), 150
Hypermetropia, 180
Hypochondrium, 239

I

Incus, 189-191
–, body, 191
–, lenticular process, 191
–, long limb, 190, 191
–, short limb, 190, 191
Inspiration, 388
Intestine, mesenteric small, 394
Iris, 159, 178, 180
–, anterior surface, 179
–, major circulus arteriosus, 162, 174, 177, 178
–, minor circulus arteriosus, 177, 178
–, pigmented epithelium, 176, 179
–, pupillary margin, 179
–, stroma, 179
Isthmus
– of cartilaginous auricle, 182
– of fauces, 122, 145-147
– –, mucosa, 147

J

Joint(s)
– cricoarytenoid, 206-209
– cricothyroid, 204-206
– –, capsule, 206, 207
– sternocostal, 297, 307, 340
Junction
– esophagogastric, 313
– corneoscleral, 166, 176-180
– –, marginal vascular loops, 178

K

Kidney, 244, 245, 394, 395
– left, 245, 394, 395
– right, 244, 245, 387

L

Labyrinth
– bony, 193, 194
– –, cavity, 193
– –, vestibule, 192, 193
– –, –, aqueduct, 188, 193, 194
– –, –, crest, impression, 194
– cochlear, 181, 195, 196
– ethmoidal, 151
– membranous, 195, 196
– vestibular, 181, 195, 196
–, vein(s), 43
Lacus lacrimalis, 158
Lamella, median fibroelastic, 100
Lamina
– basal, 198
– capillary, 177
– of cricoid cartilage, 125
– limiting, anterior, 178
– –, posterior, 178, 179
– papyracea, *see* Bone(s), ethmoid, plate, orbital
– propria, 157
– – of labial mucosa, 122
– spiral, osseous, 198
– –, secondary, impression, 194
– tragal, 182
– vascular, 177

Laryngeal inlet, 125, 145, 210, 230, 232
Laryngopharynx, 145, 232
–, muscular layer, 230, 232
Larynx, 203, 205-212, 214, 215, 221, 223, 371
–, cartilage(s), 211, 212
–, – thyroid, 26, 222, 224
–, external configuration, 202
–, functional aspects, 214, 215
–, muscles, 201-210
–, structures, 201-210
Layer
– of pleura, parietal, 251
– –, visceral, 251
Lens, 176-180
–, axis, 179
–, capsule, 179
–, concentric lamellae, 179
–, conformation, 179
–, cortex, 179
–, epithelium, 179
–, equator, 179
–, nucleus, 179
–, pole, anterior, 179
–, –, posterior, 179
–, radii, 179
–, substance, 179
–, surface, anterior, 179
–, –, posterior, 179
Ligament(s)
– anular, 199, 203, 205, 206, 318, 319
– arcuate, lateral, 289-297, 382
– –, medial, 289-297, 382
– arteriosum, 293, 336, 338, 384
– aryepiglottic, 208
– of Botallo, *see* Ligament(s), arteriosum
– costopleural, 386
– cricoarytenoid, 207
– cricothyroid, 201
– – median, 202-204, 208, 214
– cricotracheal, 202-206
– hyoepiglottic, 125, 208, 209
– of incus, superior, 190
– of malleus, superior, 190
– nuchae, 110-114, 119-121, 233, 234
– palpebral, lateral, 100, 160
– –, medial, 100, 158, 160
– pulmonary, 292, 305, 312, 378, 384
– posterior of incus, 190
– spiral, 198
– stylohyoid, 114-116, 146, 147
– thyroepiglottic, 125, 206, 207, 209
– thyrohyoid, lateral, 201-210
– –, median, 125, 201-204, 208, 209
– transversopleural, 386
– triangular, *see* Ligament(s), pulmonary
– vertebropleural, 386
– vestibular, 208-210
– vocal, 203, 206-210, 214, 215
Limen nasi, 152, 153, 155, 156
Line(s)
– anterior, axillary, 238, 383
– horizontal, between the acromioclavicular joints passing over C VII, 2
– –, passing over the clavicle, 2
– median, anterior, 383
– –, posterior, 383
– midclavicular, 238, 244, 383
– nuchal, superior, 2
– oblique, 204
– – of thyroid cartilage, 211
– paravertebral, 244
– passing over the medial border of scapula, 238
– passing over the third rib, 238
– pericraniocervical, 2
– posterior, axillary, 383
– scapular 244, 383
– sternal, 238, 244
– thoracoabdominal, 238
Liver, 244, 306, 307, 317, 395
–, lobe(s), 245
Lobe, frontal, 99, 115
Lobule, pulmonary, 390
Lung(s), 244, 245, 251, 253, 254, 288-296, 299, 301, 302, 330, 335, 344, 358, 359, 372, 374-380, 382, 384, 386, 387, 392, 394
–, apex, 240, 244, 245, 332, 373, 374, 376, 379, 386
–, base, 244, 374, 379
–, biopsy, 387
–, border, anterior, 244, 374
–, –, inferior, 245, 301, 302, 374, 376
–, cardiac notch, 374, 376, 379
–, circulation, 322, 323, 325
–, conformation, 373
–, contour, 383
–, fissure(s), 374
–, –, horizontal, 245, 344
–, –, oblique, 245, 301, 302, 332, 383, 393
–, hilum, 240, 254, 384
–, impression cardiac, 301, 302, 308, 309, 374, 376, 378, 379
–, –, costal, 374, 378
–, –, vertebral, 378
–, lingula, 301, 302, 374, 379
–, lobe(s), 381
–, –, inferior, 244, 245, 328, 332, 373, 374, 376, 379, 380, 383
–, –, middle, 244, 245, 328, 373, 374, 376, 380, 383
–, –, superior, 244, 245, 328, 332, 373, 374, 376, 379, 380, 383, 385, 392
–, pleural lining, 382
–, pulmonary segments, 381
–, pulmonary zones, 381
–, respiratory dynamics, 388, 389
–, root of lung, 248, 306, 307
–, surface, costal, 376
–, –, diaphragmatic, 308, 309, 377, 378, 384
–, –, lateral, 381
–, –, mediastinal, 374, 378, 381
Lymph node(s)
– accessory, 66, 68, 70, 73t, 74t, 109, 110
– of accessory nerve, *see* Lymph node(s), accessory
– anterior jugular, *see* Lymph node(s), cervical, anterior, superficial
– aortopulmonary window, *see* Lymph node(s), subaortic
– of arch of azygos vein, 266-268
– ascending aorta, *see* Lymph node(s), para-aortic
– auricular, anterior, *see* Lymph node(s), preauricular
– axillary, 67, 266, 392
– – anterior, *see* Lymph node(s), pectoral
– – apical, 284, 285
– – central, 265, 284, 285
– – lateral, *see* Lymph node(s), humeral
– – posterior, *see* Lymph node(s), subscapular
– brachiocephalic, 217-219, 224, 266-268, 295, 358, 359
– bronchopulmonary, 266, 358, 360, 361
– – left, 268t
– – right, 268t
– buccinator, 67, 68, 70, 72t, 109, 110
– carinal, *see* Lymph node(s), tracheobronchial, inferior
– celiac, 265
– cervical, anterior, 67, 73t
– –, –, deep, 66, 71, 73t, 74t, 111-113
– –, –, superficial, 67-69, 73t, 96, 102, 108
– –, deep, 361
– –, lateral, 67, 73t, 265
– –, –, deep, 67, 70, 73t, 104, 105, 109, 110, 118, 154, 185, 187, 217-219, 224, 228, 265
– –, –, –, inferior, 67, 73t, 74t, 99
– –, –, –, middle, 73t, 74t
– –, –, –, superior, 67, 73t, 74t, 99
– –, –, superficial, 66-69, 73t, 96, 102, 103, 107, 108
– –, nuchal, 118
– deltopectoral, 265, 284
– diaphragmatic, superior, 266, 268t, 295, 358, 360
– –, –, anterior, 359
– –, –, middle, 359
– epigastric, 265
– facial, 66-68, 70, 72t
– hilar, *see* Lymph node(s), bronchopulmonary
– –, left, *see* Lymph node(s), bronchopulmonary, left
– –, right, *see* Lymph node(s), tracheobronchial, superior, right

– humeral, 265, 285
– iliac, common, 266
– infra-auricular, *see* Lymph node(s), parotid, deep
– infraclavicular; *see* Lymph node(s), deltopectoral
– infrahyoid, 66, 67, 71, 73t, 111-113, 217-219, 224
– interaorticoesophageal, *see* Lymph node(s), juxtaesophageal
– intercostal, 265, 268t, 301-304, 308-312, 333, 358
– –, anterior, 266
– –, posterior, 266, 287
– interlobar, 268t
– interpectoral, 284
– intraglandular, 67, 68, 70, 72t, 108, 109
– intrapulmonary, 266, 268t, 358, 361
– jugular, anterior, *see* Lymph node(s), cervical, anterior, superficial
– –, external, *see* Lymph node(s), cervical, lateral, superficial
– –, internal, *see* Lymph node(s), cervical, lateral, deep
– jugulo-omohyoid, 67, 70, 73t, 74t, 109
– jugulodigastric 67, 70, 73t, 74t, 109, 154, 185, 187, 217, 224
– juxta-aortic, 266-268, 290-292, 360
– juxtaesophageal, 74t, 106, 217-219, 265-268, 290-293, 358, 360
– of ligamentum arteriosum, 266-268
– lingual, 67, 71, 72t, 113, 130
– lobar, 268t
– lumboaortic, 265, 266
– malar, 67-70, 72t, 107-110
– mandibular 67, 68, 70, 72t, 109
– mastoid, 65-70, 72t, 107-110, 118, 185, 187, 224
– mediastinal, 268t, 331, 359-361, 382
– – anterior, 266, 268t, 295, 296, 331, 361, 382
– – –, diaphragmatic, 268t
– – inferior, 268t
– – – and middle, 295, 296, 331, 382
– – posterior, 218, 219, 266, 268t, 358, 360
– – –, diaphragmatic, 268t
– – superior, 267t, 268t, 359
– nasolabial, 67-70, 72t, 107-110
– occipital, 65-70, 72t, 107-109, 118
– para-aortic, 265-268
– paraesophageal, *see* Lymph node(s), juxtaesophageal
– paramammary, 265, 268t, 284
– parasternal, 265, 266, 268t, 284, 285, 358
– paratracheal, 66, 67, 71, 73t, 74t, 99, 105, 106, 113, 217, 224, 265, 266, 268t, 291-297, 301-305, 308-312, 359-361, 382, 392
– –, inferior, 267t, 268t
– –, superior, 218, 267t, 268t
– parotid, 66
– –, deep, 67, 68, 70, 72t, 97, 102, 103, 108, 166, 185, 187, 217, 224
– –, superficial, 67-70, 72t, 96, 107, 185, 187, 217, 224
– pectoral, 265, 284, 285
– pericardial, lateral, 266, 268t, 359
– of phrenic nerve, *see* Lymph node(s), para-aortic
– postaortic, 266
– posterior, *see* Lymph node(s), subscapular
– of posterior triangle, *see* Lymph node(s), accessory
– preaortic, 266, 358
– preaorticocarotid, 217, 224, 266, 267t, 268t, 359
– preauricular, 65, 67, 68, 70, 72t, 108, 166
– prelaryngeal, 66, 67, 71, 73t, 74t, 111-113, 217-219, 224
– prepericardial, 266, 269t, 359
– pretracheal, 66, 67, 71, 73t, 74t, 99, 105, 111-113, 217-219, 224
– prevascular, 266, 267t, 269t, 359
– prevertebral, 266, 267t, 269t
– pulmonary ligament, 266, 267t, 269t
– retroarticular, *see* Lymph node(s), mastoid
– retropharyngeal, 66-68, 71, 73t, 154, 228
– retrotracheal, 266, 267t, 269t
– segmental, 268t
– subaortic, 266, 267t, 269t
– subcarinal, 267t, 269t
– submandibular, 65-68, 70, 72t, 74t, 103, 104, 109, 110, 128, 154, 166, 217-219, 265
– submental, 65-68, 70, 72t, 74t, 103, 109-111, 217, 218, 219, 265
– subparotid, 70, 72t
– subscapular, 265, 284, 285
– subsegmental, 268t
– supraclavicular, 65-68, 70, 73t, 74t, 109, 217, 224, 265, 285
– thoracic, parietal, 268t
– –, visceral 268t
– thyroid, 66, 71, 73t, 74t, 111-113, 217, 224
– tracheobronchial, 266, 269t, 361
– –, inferior, 217, 224, 269t, 291, 358, 360, 361, 378, 384, 392
– –, superior, 219, 291, 358, 360, 378, 384
– –, –, left, 269t
– –, –, right, 269t
– transverse cervical artery, *see* Lymph node(s), supraclavicular
– of transverse cervical chain, *see* Lymph node(s), supraclavicular
– of transverse chain, *see* Lymph node(s), brachiocephalic
Lymphatic groups, 66, 266

M

Macrophage, alveolar, 391
Macula
– cribrosa media, 188
– – superior, 188
– of retina, 177
MALT (mucosae associated lymphoid tissue), 314
Malleus, 181, 189, 191
–, handle, 190, 191
–, head, 190, 191
–, neck, 191
–, process, anterior, 190, 191
–, –, lateral, 191
–, –, long, *see* Malleus, process, anterior
–, –, short, *see* Malleus, process, lateral
–, –, spatulate, 191
Mammography, 281
Mandible, 27, 30, 125, 128, 134, 144, 233, 235, 236
–, alveolar arches, 135
–, body, 2, 8
–, ramus, 31, 148, 233
Margin, costal, 238
Matter
– gray, 275
– white, 52
Maxilla, 27, 30, 125, 134, 149
–, palatine process, 148, 149
Meatus
– acoustic, external, 84, 181, 182, 188, 189, 192, 193, 195, 197
– –, –, bony part, 181
– –, –, cartilaginous, 181
– –, internal, 84, 193, 198
– –, –, fundus, transverse crest, 198
– nasal, inferior, 148, 150
– –, middle, 148, 150
– –, superior, 150
Mediastinum, 240-242, 244, 248, 306, 307, 319, 328-330, 332, 334
–, arteries, 246, 247
–, contents, 242
–, formations, vascular, 244
–, –, visceral, 244
–, great vessels, 321-327
–, lymph node chains, 358, 360
–, lymph nodes, 359-362
–, subdivision, 241, 242
–, topographic anatomy, 241, 242, 244
–, topographic relations, 321-325
–, vessels, 246-248
Membrane(s)
– atlanto-occipital, 121
– –, anterior, 125

– basement, 391
– hyoglossal, 127
– quadrangular, 208, 210
– suprapleural, 386
– tectorial, 198
– thyrohyoid, 114-116, 201, 202, 204-208, 210, 226, 230, 232, 314
– tympanic, 181, 189, 190, 192, 193, 197
– vestibular (or vestibular surface), 198
Midbrain, tegmentum, 115
Modiolus, 198
–, spiral canal, 198
Mouth, 122-137, 142, 144
–, angle of mouth, 5
–, buccal fat pad, 12, 140
–, lip, lower, 5, 123
–, –, upper, 5, 123, 125, 152, 153, 155, 156
–, lips, general structure, 5
–, floor, 128
–, –, muscles, 148
–, oral fissure, 5
–, oral vestibule, 123, 139
–, philtrum, 5
–, sulcus, mentolabial, 5
–, –, nasolabial, 5
Mucosa
– nasal, 157
– –, vascular network, 156
– olfactory, 157
– oral (mucous membrane of mouth), 124
– peritonsillar, 147
– respiratory region, 153, 156, 157
– sublingual, 125
Muscle(s)
– of abdomen, 388
– antitragicus, 182
– arytenoid, oblique, 202, 203, 205-207, 210, 216, 230, 232, 313, 367
– –, –, aryepiglottic part 205
– –, transverse, 201, 203-208, 210, 216, 230, 232, 313, 367
– of auricle, oblique, 182
– –, transverse, 182
– auricularis, anterior, 182, 184-186
– –, posterior, 182-187
– –, superior, 182-187
– of back proper (erector spinae), 388
– biceps brachii, 392
– buccinator, 98-100, 124, 139, 140, 148
– caninus, *see* Muscle(s), levator anguli oris
– ciliary, 176, 178, 179
– constrictor (of pharynx), inferior, 114, 200, 228, 229, 234, 301, 302, 308-312, 314, 324, 325
– –, –, cricopharyngeal part, 216, 313, 314
– –, –, thyropharyngeal part, 210, 314
– –, middle, 114, 124, 200, 216, 228, 229, 232, 233, 313, 314
– –, –, ceratopharyngeal part, 314
– –, –, chondropharyngeal part, 314
– –, superior, 123, 146, 147, 200, 216, 228-230, 233, 313
– coracobrachialis, 392
– corrugator supercilii, 98, 100, 160
– cricoarytenoid, lateral, 203, 206, 207, 209, 210
– –, posterior, 201, 203-207, 216, 230, 232, 313, 367
– cricopharyngeus, *see* Muscle(s), constrictor (of pharynx), inferior, cricopharyngeal part
– cricothyroid, 105, 114, 200-202, 204, 207, 209, 210
– cutaneous, *see* Muscle(s), facial
– deltoid, 392
– depressor anguli oris, 100, 101, 117, 233
– – labii inferioris, 100, 233
– – septi nasi, 100
– digastric, 101, 103, 104-106, 117, 124, 127, 128, 130, 139, 139, 148, 154, 228, 229, 230, 233
– dilator pupillae, 176, 178, 179
– epicranius, 117, *see also* Muscle(s), occipitofrontalis
– expiratory, 388
– –, principal, 388
– –, secondary, 388
– eye, 175
– of eyeball, extraocular, 159, 160, 175
– –, inferior oblique, 158-161, 170, 175
– –, inferior rectus, 159-161, 170, 175
– –, lateral rectus, 159-161, 168, 170, 172, 175, 177
– –, medial rectus, 160, 161, 168, 170, 175, 177
– –, superior rectus, 159, 160, 161, 168, 170, 172, 173, 175
– facial, 100, 101, 117
– genioglossus, 124-128, 133, 148, 201, 202, 233
– geniohyoid, 76, 105, 106, 124, 125, 127, 128, 133, 272
– glossopharyngeal, 123
– helicis, major, 182
– –, minor, 182
– hyoglossus, 124, 126-128, 130, 133, 148, 201, 202, 233
– infrahyoid, 201
– infraspinatus, 392
– inspiratory, 388
– –, principal, 388
– –, secondary, 388
– intercostal, 301-305, 308-312, 333, 372, 385, 392
– –, external, 250, 251, 286-289, 297, 388
– –, innermost, 251, 388
– –, internal, 250, 286, 287, 388
– interspinales cervicis, 121
– intertransversarii, cervical, medial posterior, 121
– latissimus dorsi, 388
– levator anguli oris, 98, 100
– – costarum, 388
– – labii superioris, 100
– – – alaeque nasi, 100
– – palpebrae superioris, 159-161, 172, 173, 175, 176
– – scapulae, 119, 120, 120, 121, 144, 221, 234, 388
– – veli palatini, 138, 146, 193, 230
– longissimus, cervicis, 234
– –, capitis, 120, 121, 233
– longus, colli, 106, 113, 200, 226, 233, 234, 286-288
– –, capitis, 200, 233
– masseter, 101, 110, 117, 124, 140, 144, 148, 233, 98
– masticatory, 117
– mentalis, 100, 233
– mimic, *see* Muscle(s), facial
– multifidus, 392, 393
– –, cervicis, 120, 121, 234
– mylohyoid, 103-106, 125, 127, 128, 144, 145, 148, 233
– nasalis, 100, 101, 117, 144
– oblique, external, 388
– –, internal, 388
– –, superior, 159-161, 168, 170, 175
– –, –, trochlea, 159-161, 163, 167
– obliquus capitis, inferior, 119, 120, 233
– –, superior, 119
– occipitofrontalis, 98, 100, 101, 110, 111, 121
– omohyoid, 97, 98, 103-105, 133, 201, 221, 234, 272
– orbicularis, oculi, 100, 101, 110, 111, 117, 144, 158, 159, 166, 176
– –, oris, 99-101, 117, 122
– –, –, labial part, 144
– palatoglossus, 114, 123, 128, 146, 232
– palatopharyngeus, 114, 123, 216, 230, 232, 233, 313
– papillary, 341, 342
– –, anterior, 338-340, 343, 348, 353
– –, –, apex, 343
– –, –, base, 343
– –, posterior, 338-340, 343, 348, 353
– –, septal, 338
– pectinati, 347
– pectoralis major, 281, 388, 392, 393
– – –, investing layer, 280
– – minor, 281, 392, 393
– pharyngoepiglotticus, 230, 232
– phrenoesophageal, 313
– platysma, 96, 100, 102, 103, 107, 233, 234
– prevertebral, 200
– procerus, 100
– psoas major, 286-297, 382

– pterygoid, lateral, 141, 230
– –, medial, 230, 233
– quadratus labii inferioris, *see* Muscle(s), depressor labii inferioris
– – – superioris, *see* Muscle(s), levator labii superioris
– – lumborum, 286-297, 382, 388
– rectus abdominis, 388, 394
– – capitis anterior, 200
– – – lateralis, 200
– – – posterior major, 119, 120
– – – – minor, 120
– rhomboid major, 388, 392
– – minor, 388, 392
– risorius, 100, 101, 117
– salpingopharyngeus, 146, 216, 230, 313
– scalenus, 286-288, 297, 388
– –, anterior, 98, 99, 104-106, 200, 221, 226, 234, 286-288, 297, 386
– –, medius, 98, 99, 104-106, 200, 221, 226, 234, 286-288, 297, 386
– –, posterior, 98, 99, 104, 105, 106, 200, 221, 226, 234, 286, 287, 288, 297
– semispinalis, cervicis, 120, 121, 234
– –, thoracis, 393
– –, capitis, 118, 119, 120, 121, 233, 234, 274, 392
– serratus anterior, 387, 388, 392, 393
– – posterior inferior, 388
– – – superior, 388
– sphincter, pupillae, 176, 178-179
– splenius, 67
– –, cervicis, 234
– –, capitis, 119-121, 233, 234
– stapedius, 190-193
– sternocleidomastoid, 31, 96-99, 101-105, 117-119, 121, 124, 139, 144, 154, 233, 234, 388
– sternohyoid, 76, 104, 105, 133, 201, 234, 272
– sternothyroid, 98, 99, 104, 105, 133, 201, 234, 272, 392, 76
– styloglossus, 105, 106, 123, 124, 128, 130, 132, 133, 139, 146, 233
– stylohyoid, 103-106, 124, 127, 128, 130, 139, 233
– styloid, 139
– stylopharyngeus, 124, 130, 132, 139, 147, 154, 216, 229, 230, 233, 313, 314
– subclavius, 388
– subcostales, 286, 287, 388
– subscapularis, 392
– temporalis, 101, 110, 117, 144
– tensor, tympani, 189, 191, 192, 193
– –, veli palatini, 230
– teres major, 392
– – minor, 392
– thyroarytenoid, 203, 207, 209, 210, 216, 313
– –, medial bundle, *see* Muscle(s), vocalis
– –, thyroepiglottic part, 209
– thyrohyoid, 76, 104, 105, 133, 201, 272
– thyropharyngeus, *see* Muscle(s), constrictor (of pharynx), inferior, thyropharyngeal part
– of tongue, extrinsic, 124
– –, intrinsic, 131, 133
– –, longitudinal, inferior, 126, 148
– –, –, superior, 126, 148
– –, transverse, 126, 148
– –, vertical, 126, 148
– trachealis, 205, 319
– tracheoesophageal, 319
– tragicus, 182
– transversus, thoracis, 388
– –, abdominis, 286-288, 388
– trapezius, 76, 97, 101, 103, 117-120, 144, 154, 221, 233, 234, 388, 392, 393
– triangularis labiorum, *see* Muscle(s), depressor anguli oris
– triceps brachii, 392
– uvulae, 138, 216, 230, 313
– vocalis, 206, 207, 209, 210
– zygomaticus major, 100, 101, 117
– – minor, 100
Myocardium, 351, 364
– atrial, 347
– –, horizontal interauricular bundle, 347
– –, transverse bundles, *see* Myocardium, atrial, horizontal interauricular bundle
– –, vertical bundles, 347
– ventricular, 343, 346, 347
– –, anterior common bundles, 346, 352, 356
– –, posterior common bundles, 346, 352
Myopia, 180

N

Nasopharynx, 145
Neck, 96-101, 104-116, 118-120, 144, 199, 216-221, 225, 228-233
–, arteries, 16, 17, 40t, 41t, 220, 221
–, –, territories of supply, 19
–, carotid sheath, 10
–, compartment(s), 11
–, –, boundaries and contents, 14t, 15t
–, –, carotid, 3, 7, 11t, 14t; *see also* Neck, compartment(s), vascular
–, –, fascial, 11
–, –, sternocleidomastoid, 7t, 14t
–, –, supraclavicular, 3, 7t, 14t
–, –, submandibular, 14t
–, –, vascular, 3, 7t, 11, 14t
–, –, visceral, 3, 7t, 11, 14t, 15t
–, cutaneous territories of innervation, 81
–, fascia(e), 10
–, – alar, 10
–, – cervical, 10
–, – –, investing layer, 10
–, – –, pretracheal layer, 10
–, – –, prevertebral layer, 10
–, –, nuchal, 10
–, fossa, jugular, *see* Neck, fossa, suprasternal
–, –, suprasternal, 6, 7
–, fossa, retromandibular, 6
–, –, supraclavicular, greater, 6, 7t, 9
–, –, –, lesser, 6, 7t
–, lymph node chains, 68
–, lymph nodes, 65, 69-71
–, –, deep, 224
–, lymphatic groups, 67, 74
–, nerves, 218, 219, 225
–, region(s), 3, 6, 239
–, –, carotid, *see* Neck, region(s), sternocleidomastoid
–, –, cervical, anterior, 3, 6, 8
–, –, –, lateral, 3, 6, 7t, 8, 9
–, –, –, posterior, 3, 6, 7t, 11
–, –, infrahyoid, 3, 6, 7t
–, –, nuchal, *see* Neck, region(s), cervical, posterior
–, –, subdivision and boundaries, 6, 7t
–, –, supraclavicular, *see* Neck, region(s), cervical, lateral
–, –, suprahyoid, 3, 6
–, –, sternocleidomastoid, 3, 6t, 7t
–, sections, 233
–, space, carotid, *see* Neck, compartment(s), vascular
–, –, "danger", 14t
–, –, lateral vascular, *see* Neck, compartment(s), vascular
–, –, pre-epiglottic, 14t
–, –, prevertebral, 14t
–, –, previsceral, *see* Neck, space, visceral
–, –, retroesophageal, 14t
–, –, retrovisceral, *see* Neck, space, retroesophageal
–, –, suprasternal, 14t
–, –, visceral, *see* Neck, compartment(s), visceral
–, superficial boundaries, 2
–, superficial layer, *see* Neck, fascia(e), cervical, investing layer
–, topographic relations, 217-219, 226
–, triangle, anterior, *see* Neck, region(s), cervical, anterior
–, –, carotid, 6-9
–, –, digastric, *see* Neck, triangle, submandibular
–, –, muscular, 6-9
–, –, occipital, 6-9
–, –, omoclavicular, 6-9
–, –, omotracheal, *see* Neck, triangle, muscular

–, –, posterior, *see* Neck, region(s), cervical, lateral
–, –, subclavian, *see* Neck, triangle, omoclavicular
–, –, submandibular, 6, 8, 9t
–, –, submental, 6, 8
–, –, subdivision, boundaries, 8, 9
–, –, supraclavicular, *see* Neck, triangle, omoclavicular
–, vascularization, 16
–, vessels, 218, 219, 235, 236
–, vein(s), 16, 42, 43, 46, 47, 48, 63, 103, 222, 223
Nerve(s)
– abducens [VI], 32, 82, 89t, 159-161, 167, 168, 170, 170, 171, 174, 228, 230
– accessory [XI] (spinal accesory nerve), 32, 75, 76, 82, 94t, 103-106, 109-112, 116, 119, 120, 217, 228-230, 233, 270, 272, 369
– –, external branch, 118
– alveolar, 136
– –, inferior, 85, 86, 90t, 99, 128, 137, 141, 142, 233
– –, –, inferior dental plexus, inferior dental branches, 85
– –, superior, 85, 86, 92t, 137, 143
– –, –, branches, 137
– ampullary, anterior, 89t
– –, lateral, 90t, 194
– –, posterior, 92t, 194
– –, superior, 194
– anal, inferior, 271
– anococcygeal, 271
– auricular, anterior, 89t
– –, posterior, 87, 88, 92t, 109
– –, great, 75, 76, 80, 81, 90t, 102, 107, 108, 110, 111, 118, 119, 119, 120, 186, 187, 225, 227, 270, 272
– –, –, branches, 186
– auriculotemporal, 79, 80, 85, 86, 89t, 96, 97, 107-109, 132, 141, 142, 186, 187
– axillary, 75, 77, 270, 273
– of Block, *see* Nerve(s), maxillary, branches, ganglionic, to pterygopalatine ganglion
– buccal, 80, 85, 89t, 98, 99, 112, 141, 142
– cardiac, cervical, 364
– –, –, inferior, 278t, 362-367
– –, –, middle (great cardiac nerve), 278t, 279t, 362-367
– –, –, superior, 218, 219, 279t, 362, 363-365
– caroticotympanic, 89t
– carotid, external, 89t
– –, internal, 90t
– cervical [C1-C8], 76, 77, 94t, 115, 133, 233, 234, 272, 273, 285, 385
– –, cutaneous, *see* Nerve(s), cervical, transverse
– –, rami, 80, 81, 106, 110-113, 118, 120, 121, 133, 225, 227, 285
– –, transverse, 75, 76, 80, 81, 95t, 96, 102, 107-112, 225, 227, 270, 272
– ciliary, long, 91t, 167, 178
– –, short, 85, 92t, 167-169
– clunial, inferior, 271
– cochlear [VIII], 89t, 193, 194, 196-198
– cranial, 32, 82, 89t
– cutaneous, 80
– –, lateral, of thigh, 271
– –, –, femoral, *see* Nerve(s), cutaneous, lateral, of thigh
– –, medial, of arm, 75, 77, 270, 273, 285
– –, –, of forearm, 75, 77, 270, 273, 285
– –, perforating [S2, S3], 271
– –, posterior, femoral, *see* Nerve(s), cutaneous, posterior, of thigh
– –, –, of thigh [S1, S2, S3], 271
– encephalic, *see* Nerve(s), cranial
– ethmoidal, anterior, 85, 89t, 116, 155, 156, 167, 168
– –, –, branches, 80, 107-109, 115, 116, 143, 155
– –, posterior, 92t, 167, 168
– –, –, branches, 116
– to external acoustic meatus, 92t
– facial [VII], 32, 78, 81, 82, 87, 88, 89t, 98, 110, 116, 139, 142, 181, 186, 187, 190, 191, 193, 194, 228-230, 276
– –, branches, 87, 88, 107, 108, 109, 114, 115, 124
– –, cervicofacial trunk, 87
– –, parotid plexus, 109
– –, temporofacial trunk, 87
– femoral, 271
– fibular, common, 271
– frontal, 85, 86, 89t, 99, 167, 168, 172, 173, 174
– to geniohyoid, 75, 76, 95t, 270, 272
– genitofemoral, 271
– glossopalatine, *see* Nerve(s), intermediate [VII]
– glossopharyngeal [IX], 32, 76, 78, 81, 82, 89t, 94t, 106, 112, 113, 116, 123, 130, 146, 147, 217, 228-230, 232, 233, 272, 276, 369
– –, branches, 132, 232, 369
– –, inferior ganglion, 132
– –, superior ganglion, 132
– gluteal, inferior [L5, S1, S2], 271
– –, superior [L4, L5, S1], 271
– hypoglossal [XII], 32, 75, 76, 82, 90t, 110-113, 116, 128-130, 133, 217, 225, 227-230, 233, 270, 272
– –, venous plexus of canal, 82
– iliohypogastric, 271
– ilioinguinal, 271
– iliopubic, *see* Nerve(s), iliohypogastric
– infraorbital, 80, 85, 86, 90t, 97, 98, 99, 137, 138, 160, 167, 168, 171
– –, branches, 110, 111
– infratrochlear, 80, 85, 86, 90t, 96, 97, 167, 168, 171, 172, 173, 174
– intercostal [T1-T12], 75, 77, 250, 251, 270, 271, 271, 273, 275, 277, 278t, 285, 287, 297, 301, 302, 305, 308, 309, 310, 311, 312, 333, 368, 371
– –, branches, 77, 271, 273, 275, 278t, 285
– –, pathway, 250, 251
– –, twelfth, *see* Nerve(s), subcostal
– intercostobrachial [T2], 271, 278t
– intermediate [VII], 88, 90t, 228, 229, 230
– internal respiratory nerve of Bell, *see* Nerve(s), phrenic
– jugular, 94t
– lacrimal, 80, 90t, 138, 167-169, 171-173
– –, communicating branch with zygomatic nerve, 167, 168, 172-174
– laryngeal, 371
– –, inferior, *see* Nerve(s), laryngeal, recurrent
– –, recurrent, 94t, 99, 105, 106, 217-219, 225, 226, 228, 229, 231, 234, 274, 277, 279t, 289-297, 302, 310, 311, 319, 333, 362, 364-371, 382
– –, –, branches, 319, 369, 366
– –, superior, 94t, 217-219, 225, 228-232, 277, 371
– –, –, branches, 369
– to lateral pterygoid, 85, 93t, 141, 142
– to levator ani and ischiococcygeus, 271
– lingual, 79, 85, 88, 91t, 113-115, 123, 126, 128-130, 132, 137, 139, 141, 142, 233
– to longus capitis, 76, 272
– to longus capitis and longus colli, 75, 76, 270, 272
– to longus colli, 272
– mandibular [V3], 81, 82, 85, 86, 91t, 113, 114, 128, 137, 142, 143, 167-169, 171, 186, 187
– –, meningeal branch, 82, 91t, 116, 173
masseteric, 85, 91t, 141, 142
– maxillary [V2], 81, 82, 85, 86, 91t, 137, 143, 155, 156, 167-171, 173, 174
– –, branches, 82, 91t, 115, 143, 155
– –, –, ganglionic, to pterygopalatine ganglion, 91t, 143, 155
– to medial pterygoid, 85, 93t
– median, 75, 77, 270, 273
– mental, 80, 85, 91t, 97-99, 128
– –, branches, 96-98
– musculocutaneous, 75, 77, 270, 273, 285
– to mylohyoid, 95t, 128
– nasal, inferior lateral posterior, 116
– nasociliary, 85, 91t, 137, 159, 160, 161, 167, 168, 169, 171, 174
– nasopalatine, 82, 91t, 115, 143, 155, 156
– obturator, 271

- to obturator internus [L5-S2], 271
- occipital, greater, 75, 80, 81, 90t, 107, 108, 118, 119, 120, 121, 270, 274
- -, -, branches, 118
- -, lesser, 75, 76, 80, 81, 90t, 107, 108, 118-120, 225, 227, 270, 272, 274
- -, third, 75, 80, 81, 92t, 118-121, 270, 274
- oculomotor [III], 32, 55, 78, 82, 91t, 115, 159, 160, 167-171, 174, 276
- -, branches, 160, 161, 167, 168, 169, 173, 174
- olfactory [I], 32, 82, 92t, 99, 115, 116, 143, 155, 156, 168, 172-174
- -, olfactory bulb, 32
- -, olfactory tract, 32
- to omohyoid, 75, 76, 95t, 270, 272
- ophthalmic [V1], 81, 82, 85, 86, 92t, 137, 167-171
- optic [II], 32, 55, 82, 92t, 99, 115, 155, 156, 159-162, 165, 167, 168, 170-175, 177, 178
- palatine, greater, 82, 90t, 116, 143, 155
- -, -, branches, 155
- -, lesser, 82, 91t, 123, 143, 155, 156
- pectoral, lateral, 75, 77, 270, 273, 278t, 279t, 285
- -, medial, 75, 77, 270, 273, 278t, 279t, 285
- to pectoralis major, *see* Nerve(s), pectoral, lateral
- to pectoralis minor, *see* Nerve(s), pectoral, medial
- petrosal, deep, 82, 89t, 138, 143
- -, greater, 82, 88, 90t, 138, 143, 191
- -, -, superficial, *see* Nerve(s), petrosal, greater
- -, lesser, 82, 91t, 132, 173, 191
- pharyngeal, 82, 143
- phrenic, 75-77, 97-99, 103-106, 109-112, 225, 226, 227, 252, 270, 272, 273, 278t, 279t, 285, 295-297, 303-305, 310, 312, 330, 333, 368, 371, 382
- -, accessory, 278t
- -, branches, 330
- -, inferior rootlets, 330
- -, superior rootlets, 330
- pneumogastric, *see* Nerve(s), vagus
- of pterygoid canal, 90, 138, 143, 155
- pterygopalatine, *see* Nerve(s), maxillary, branches, ganglionic, to pterygopalatine ganglion
- pudendal [S2, S3, S4], 78, 271, 276
- to quadratus femoris [L4, L5, S1], 271
- radial, 75, 77, 270, 273, 285
- rectal, inferior, *see* Nerve(s), anal, inferior
- to rectus capitis anterior, 76, 270, 272
- to rectus capitis lateralis, 76, 270, 272
- to rectus capitis lateralis, longus capitis and rectus capitis anterior, 75
- saccular, 92t, 194
- to scalene muscles and levator scapulae, 76, 75, 270, 272
- scapular, dorsal, 75, 77, 270, 273, 278t, 279t
- -, posterior, *see* Nerve(s), scapular, dorsal
- of Scarpa, *see* Nerve(s), nasopalatine
- sciatic [L4, L5, S1, S2, S3], 271
- sphenopalatine, *see* Nerve(s), maxillary, branches, ganglionic, to pterygopalatine ganglion
- spinal, 75, 79, 261, 270, 271, 274, 275, 278t, 279t
- -, ramus(i), anterior, 75, 270, 271
- -, -, communicans, white, 275, 301-305, 308-312, 333, 368
- -, -, -, gray, 275, 301-305, 308-312, 333, 368
- -, -, posterior, 75, 270, 271, 274, 274
- -, root(s), 79, 275
- -, thoracic, 169
- - -, rami, 275
- spinosus, *see* Nerve(s), mandibular, meningeal branch
- splanchnic, 287, 288
- -, greater, 78, 252, 274, 276, 277, 278t, 301, 302, 303, 304, 305, 308, 309, 333, 371
- -, least, 78, 252, 276, 287, 288
- -, lesser, 78, 252, 276-278
- -, lowest, *see* Nerve(s), splanchnic, least
- -, lumbar, 2. 78, 276
- -, pelvic, 78, 276
- -, sacral, 78, 276
- to stapedius, 88, 93t
- statoacoustic, *see* Nerve(s), vestibulocochlear [VIII]
- to sternohyoid, 75, 76, 95t, 270, 272
- to sternothyroid, 75, 76, 95t, 270, 272
- stylohyoid branch, 88
- subclavian, 75, 77, 270, 273, 279t
- subcostal, 271, 277-279, 371
- sublingual, 92t
- suboccipital (posterior ramus of the first cervical nerve), 75, 94t, 120, 121, 270
- subscapular, lower, 75, 77, 270, 273
- -, upper, 75, 77, 270, 273
- supraclavicular, 75-77, 96, 102, 109-111, 225, 227, 270, 272, 273, 285
- -, anterior, *see* Nerve(s), supraclavicular, medial
- -, intermediate, 107, 108, 278t
- -, lateral, 107, 108, 278t
- -, middle, *see* Nerve(s), supraclavicular, intermediate
- -, medial, 107, 108, 278t
- -, common trunk, 112
- supraorbital, 80, 81, 86, 92t, 98, 99, 160, 167, 168, 172
- -, branches, 96, 97, 107-109
- suprascapular, 75, 77, 109, 111, 112, 270, 273
- supratrochlear, 80, 81, 92t, 96-98, 107-109, 160, 167, 172
- -, branches, 167
- temporal, deep, 85, 89t, 141, 142
- to tensor tympani, 93t
- to tensor veli palatini, 93t
- terminal, 93t
- thoracic [T1-T12], 76, 77, 272, 275, 279t, 285, 385
- -, long (nerve to serratus anterior), 75, 77, 225, 227, 270, 273, 278t, 285
- -, rami, 111-113, 278t, 285
- thoracodorsal (long subscapular nerve), 75, 77, 227, 270, 273, 279t, 285, 340, 341, 347, 350, 351
- to thyrohyoid, 75, 76, 95t, 270, 272
- tibial (internal popliteal nerve), 271
- to trapezius, 225, 227
- trigeminal [V], 32, 55, 81, 85, 86, 93t, 138, 169, 228, 229, 230, 369
- -, first branch, *see* Nerve(s), ophthalmic [V1]
- -, nucleus, mesencephalic, 86
- -, -, motor, 86
- -, -, sensory, principal, 86
- -, -, spinal, 86, 369
- -, second branch, *see* Nerve(s), maxillary [V2]
- -, spinal tract, 369
- -, third branch, *see* Nerve(s), mandibular [V3]
- trochlear [IV], 32, 55, 82, 93t, 167, 168, 170-173
- tympanic (Jacobson's nerve), 93t, 132
- -, branches, 88
- ulnar, 75, 77, 270, 273, 285
- utricular, 93t, 194
- utriculoampullary, 93t
- vagus [X], 32, 76, 78, 81, 82, 93t, 95, 98, 99, 104-106, 111-113, 116, 217-219, 225, 226, 228-234, 252, 270, 272, 274, 276-279, 289-297, 303-305, 310-312, 330, 333, 362-371, 382, 384
- -, branches, 75, 76, 110, 111, 112, 113, 116, 226, 228, 278, 301-305, 329, 362-366, 369
- -, course, 369
- -, inferior ganglion, 112, 228, 229, 230, 369
- -, posterior nucleus, 364
- -, superior ganglion, 369
- vertebral, 93t, 95t
- vestibular [VIII], 93t, 193, 194, 196, 197
- -, canaliculus for the superior part, 188

– vestibulocochlear [VIII], 32, 82, 93, 116, 181, 193, 197, 228-230
– vidian, *see* Nerve(s), of pterygoid canal
– vomeronasal, 93t
– Wrisberg's, *see* Nerve(s), intermediate [VII]
– zygomatic, 85, 86, 93t, 98, 99, 138, 167, 168
– –, branches, 80, 160, 167, 168
Network
–, capillary, alveolar, 391
–, lymphatic, radial, 166
Neurocranium, 54
Nipple, 280, 281
Node
– atrioventricular, 352, 357, 364
– sinuatrial, 352, 357, 364
Nodules, lymphoid, pharyngeal, 147
Nose, 5
–, ala, 5
–, –, fibroadipose tissue, 149
–, apex, 5
–, artery(ies), 152
–, –, dorsal, 25
–, conformation and structure, 149
–, dorsum, 5
–, external, 149
–, –, general structure, 5
–, innervation, 156
–, lymphatic drainage, 154, 156
–, naris, 5
–, nerves, 155
–, root, 5
–, vascularization, 156
–, veins, 153
–, vestibule, 152, 156
–, –, lymphatic network, 154
Notch
– of cardiac apex, 336, 338
– frontal, *see* Foramen(ina), frontal
– interarytenoid, 206, 230, 232
– jugular, 238, 297
– –, superior border, 213
– mastoid (digastric fossa), 188
– Santorini's, 182
– superior thyroid, 201-204, 207, 212
– supraorbital, *see* Foramen(ina), supraorbital
Nucleus(i)
– of abducens nerve, 170
– accessory of oculomotor nerve, 169, 170
– ambiguus, 132, 369
– cochlear, 197
– Edinger-Westphal, *see* Nucleus(i), accessory of oculomotor nerve
– of facial nerve, motor, 88, 138
– of hypoglossal nerve, 133
– lacrimal, 88
– motor of trigeminal nerve, 169
– of oculomotor nerve, 170
– principal sensory of trigeminal nerve, 169
– salivatory, inferior, 132
– –, superior, 88, 132, 138
– of solitary tract, 88, 132
– of trochlear nerve, 170
– vestibular, 197

O

Odontoblasts, 136
Ora serrata, 176, 177, 179, 180
Orbiculus ciliaris, 180
Orbit, 151
–, nerves, 167
–, medial wall, 162, 165, 168, 170
–, vault, 172
Organ(s)
– of Corti, *see* Organ(s), spiral
– of lacrimal apparatus, 158
– spiral, 198
– supramesocolic, 245
– retroperitoneal, 245
– vestibulocochlear, 181, 197
Orifice
– atrioventricular, 339, 340, 348
– submandibular, 123
Oropharynx, 145, 233

P

Palate, 122
–, hard, 123, 148, 151-153, 155, 156
–, mucosa, 148
–, soft, 122, 123, 125, 145, 152, 153, 155, 156
Papilla(e), 131
– filiform, 125, 131
– foliate, 125, 131
– fungiform, 125, 131
– incisive, 122
– lacrimal, inferior, 158
– –, superior, 158
– vallate, 125, 131, 232
Paranasal sinuses, 150, 151
Pericardium, 252, 293-295, 329, 330, 332, 335, 344, 361, 371, 373, 385
–, apex, 335
–, base, 335
– fibrous, 303-305, 310-312, 333, 359, 367, 368
–, innervation, 371
–, posterior wall, 335
– serous, 335, 343, 351
– –, layer, parietal, 335
– –, – visceral, 335, 343
Pericranium, 52
Periorbita, 172
Periosteum, 157
Peritoneum
– parietal, 371, 387
– visceral, 313, 387
Pharynx, 67, 122, 200, 230, 316, 371
–, mucosa, 230
–, muscles, 200
Pia mater, 32, 52
Plate
– of ethmoid, cribriform 55, 149, 151
– –, orbital, 150, 151, 155
– –, perpendicular, 149-151
– of pterygoid process, lateral, 149
– –, medial, 149
Pleura(e), 251, 305, 372, 382, 385, 386
– cervical, *see* Cupula, pleural
– costal, *see* Pleura(e), parietal, costal part
– diaphragmatic, *see* Pleura(e), parietal, diaphragmatic part
–, innervation, 382
–, line of reflection, 245
–, lymphatic drainage, 382
– mediastinal, 305, 335, 373, 382, 384, 385
– parietal, 244, 251, 252, 330, 361, 372, 382, 386, 387, 392
– –, boundaries, 244
– –, costal part, 305, 312, 382
– –, diaphragmatic part, 288, 301, 302, 312, 382
– –, lines of reflection, 383
– –, mediastinal part, *see* Pleura(e), mediastinal
– pulmonary, *see* Pleura(e), visceral
–, reflection, 384
–, topography, 382-384
–, vascularization, 382
– visceral, 251, 361, 372, 378, 382, 384, 386, 387, 390, 392
Plexus(es)
– aortic, thoracic, 217, 225, 293, 310, 311, 312, 333, 364, 368
of Auerbach, *see* Plexus(es), myenteric
– basilar, 42-47, 50, 52, 54, 55, 57t, 165, 173, 174
– brachial, 75, 77, 95, 225, 270, 273, 330, 362, 365, 385, 392
– –, cord(s), 77, 273, 285
– –, – anterior ramus, 77
– –, – lateral, 77
– –, – medial, 77
– –, – posterior, 77
– –, – roots, 76, 77, 227, 272, 273, 285
– –, – trunks, 77, 97, 98, 99, 103, 104, 105, 106, 226, 227, 273, 285
– cardiac, 293, 344, 362-365, 369, 371
– celiac, 369
– cervical, 75, 76, 81, 95, 225, 227, 270, 272
– –, branches, 109

– –, roots, 76, 227, 272
– coccygeal, 271
– coronary, 364
– esophageal, 225, 289-291, 293, 303, 304, 333, 367, 368, 370
– hypogastric, inferior (pelvic plexus), 78, 276
– –, superior (presacral nerve), 78, 276
– internal carotid, 143, 191
– lumbar, 271
– of Meissner, *see* Plexus(es), submucous
– myenteric, 314
– parotid, 87
– – of facial nerve, 88, 97, 109
– – –, branch(es), buccal, 96, 97
– – –, –, cervical, 96, 97
– – –, –, mandibular, 96, 97
– – –, –, temporal, 96, 97
– – –, –, zygomatic, 96, 97
– pharyngeal, 230, 232, 369
– pterygoid, 48-50, 111, 137
– pulmonary, 291, 293, 368, 366, 367, 369, 371
– renal, 78, 276
– sacral, 271
– submucous, 314
– venous, 232
– –, internal carotid, 46
– –, suboccipital, 121
– –, superficial, 153, 156
– –, vertebral, external (of Batson), anterior, 261
– –, –, –, posterior, 121
– –, –, internal (of Batson), anterior, 261
– –, –, –, posterior, 121, 261
Pneumocyte type I, 391
– – II, 391
Pneumothorax, 386
Pons, 115
Pore
– alveolar (pore of Kohn), 391
– taste, 131
Predentine, 136
Process(es)
– anterior clinoid, 170
– ciliary, 176, 178-180
– –, vascular plexuses, 177
– frontal of maxilla, 158
– muscular, 207
– retroarticular, *see* Tubercle(s), zygomatic, posterior
– vocal, 207
– xiphoid, 238, 297, 301, 302, 304, 305, 307-312, 333
Prominence
– of facial canal, 88
– laryngeal, 201-204
– of lateral semicircular canal, 88
Punctum, lacrimal, 158
Pupil, 159, 177, 180

R

Raphe
– palatine, 122, 123
– pharyngeal, 200, 228, 229, 314
– pterygomandibular, 123, 139, 146
Recess(es)
– azygoesophageal, 305
– costodiaphragmatic (parietal pleura, diaphragmatic part), 245, 252, 296, 305, 312, 382, 387
– costomediastinal, 252, 296, 331, 382
– elliptical, 194
– epitympanic, 189, 192
– –, cupular part, 189
– interaortoesophageal, 312
– saccular, *see* Recess(es), spherical
– spherical, 194
– utricular, *see* Recess(es), elliptical
Region(s)
– abdominal, lateral, 239
– buccal, 3, 4
– carotid, *see* Region(s), sternocleidomastoid
– cervical, anterior, 3, 6, 8, 102
– –, lateral, 3, 6-9
– –, posterior, 3, 6, 7, 11
– cheek, *see* Region(s), buccal
– chin, *see* Region(s), mental
– costal, 238
– crural, posterior, 3, 6, 7, 11
– deltoide, 239
– dorsal, *see* Region(s), vertebral
– epigastric (epigastric fossa), 239
– facial, 3, 4
– frontal, 3, 4
– of head, 3
– hypochondrium, 239
– infraclavicular, 238
– infrahyoid, 3, 6, 7
– inframammary, 239
– infraorbital, 3, 4
– infrascapular, 238, 239
– infratemporal, 3, 4
– lumbar, 239
– mammary, 239
– mental, 3, 4
– mouth, *see* Region(s), oral
– nasal, 3, 4
– of neck, 6, 7
– nucal, *see* Region(s), cervical, posterior
– occipital, 3, 4
– oral, 3, 4
– orbital, 3, 4
– parietal, 3, 4
– parotid (parotid-masseteric), 3, 4
– pectoral, 238, 239
– –, lateral, 238, 239
– presternal, 238, 239
– scapular, 238, 239
– suprahyoid, 3, 6, 7
– supraclavicular, *see* Region(s), cervical, lateral
– suprascapular, 239
– sternocleidomastoid, 3, 6, 7
– temporal, 3, 4
– of thorax, 238, 239
– umbilical, 239
– vertebral, 238, 239
– zygomatic, 3, 4
Respiration, 389
Retina, 177, 180
–, nonvisual, 177
–, part, ciliary, 178
–, –, iridial, 178
–, –, optic, 177, 180
Rima glottidis, 210, 214, 215
Ring
– cartilaginous, *see* Cartilage, tracheal
– fibrous, aortic, 345, 346, 352, 356
– –, left, 345, 346, 352, 356
– –, right, 345, 346, 352, 356
– pericorneal lymphatic, 166
– pharyngeal lymphoid, 147
– tendinous, common, 159-163, 167, 168, 170, 172-174
– –, –, of extraocular muscles, 99
– Waldeyer's, *see* Ring, pharyngeal lymphoid

S

Sac
– conjunctival, 176
– endolymphatic, 193, 195, 197
– lacrimal, 98, 151, 158
– –, venous plexus, 163
– pericardial, 333, 335
Saccule, 195
Scala
– media, 198
– tympani, 198
– vestibuli, 198
Sclera, 176-178, 180
–, corneoscleral part, 178
–, substantia propria, 179
–, trabecular tissue, 179
–, uveal part, 178
–, venous sinus, 176-179
Septum(a)
– interalveolar, 391
– interatrial, 339-341
– interglandular, 140
– interlobular, 390, 391
– interventricular, membranous part, 339, 341, 343, 345, 353, 357
– lingual, 126, 127, 148, 233
– nasal, 115, 148-150, 153, 230
– –, cartilage, 125, 149, 155
– –, mucosa, 125, 152, 155

– orbital, 98, 160, 176
Sheath, carotid, 10, 103, 104, 234
Sinus(es)
– aortic, 343, 393
– carotid, 19, 22-25, 132, 138, 221
– cavernous, 42-48, 50, 52-55, 57t, 164, 165, 170, 171, 173, 174
– coronary, 259, 264, 332, 335, 337, 340, 341, 345-347, 350, 351, 356
– –, affluent branches, 259
– –, anterior, *see* Sinus(es), intercavernous, anterior
– –, opening, 339, 357
– –, posterior, *see* Sinus(es), intercavernous, posterior
– –, valve, 339
– frontal, 99, 114-116, 149-151, 159, 160
– –, opening, 150
– –, septum, 99, 150
– Haller's, *see* Sinus(es), pericardial, oblique
– intercavernous, anterior, 42-45, 47, 52, 54, 55, 57t, 165, 173, 174
– –, posterior, 43-47, 52, 54, 55, 57t, 165, 173, 174
– lactiferous, 280, 281
– marginal, 43-47, 57t
– maxillary, 99, 114, 137, 148, 150, 151, 158-160
– –, medial (nasal) wall, 151
– –, mucosa, 151
– –, opening in the semilunar groove, 150
– occipital, 42-47, 52, 54, 57t, 116
– pericardial, oblique, 335
– –, transverse, 335
– petrosal, inferior, 42-47, 50, 52, 54, 55, 57t, 116, 164, 165, 173, 174
– –, superior, 42-48, 50, 52, 54, 55, 58t, 116, 164, 165, 173, 174, 194
– petrosquamous, 43-47, 57t
– sagittal
– –, inferior, 43-48, 50, 52-56, 57t, 115
– –, superior, 30, 42-48, 50, 52-56, 58t, 99, 114-116
– – –, confluence, 44, 46
– sigmoid, 28-30, 42-48, 50-55, 58t, 116, 194, 228-230
– sphenoidal, 115, 116, 125, 149, 151, 170
– –, septum, 170
– sphenoparietal, 42-47, 50, 52-55, 58t, 116, 165, 172-174
– straight, 30, 42, 43, 45-48, 50-56, 58, 116
– –, confluence, 44, 46
– transverse, 16, 28, 29, 42-48, 50-56, 58t, 114-116
– of Valsalva, *see* Sinus(es), aortic
– venosus, 30, 42-47
– –, dural, 42, 44, 45, 47, 48, 50-54
– –, of head, 45
– –, scleral, 176-179
Skin, 52, 334
Space(s)
– "danger", 14t
– epidural, 52, 261
– extradural, *see* Space(s), epidural
– lateropharyngeal, *see* Space(s), parapharyngeal
– leptomeningeal, 12t
– masticator, 13t
– maxillopharyngeal, *see* Space(s), parapharyngeal
– parapharyngeal, 13t
– –, nerves, 228, 229
– –, vessels, 228, 229
– paratonsillar, *see* Space(s), subparotid, anterior
– peripharyngeal, *see* Space(s), parapharyngeal
– pharyngeal, lateral, *see* Space(s), parapharyngeal
– pharyngomaxillary, *see* Space(s), parapharyngeal
– pre-epiglottic, 14t
– prestyloid, *see* Space(s), parapharyngeal
– prevertebral, 14t
– previsceral, *see* Space(s), visceral
– retroesophageal (retrovisceral space), 14t
– retromammary, 281
– retropharyngeal (retrovisceral space), 13t, 233
– retrostyloid, *see* Space(s), parapharyngeal
– subarachnoid, 52
– subdural, 13t, 52
– subparotid, anterior, 12t
– suprasternal, 14t
– vascular, lateral, *see* Compartment(s), vascular
– visceral, 3, 7t, 10, 11, 15t
Spine nasal, anterior, 149
Spleen, 245, 369, 394, 395
Stomach, 244, 245, 313, 369
Stria vascularis, 198
Sulcus(i)
– coronary 336, 337
– inframammary, 238, 280
– interatrial, 337, 338
– interventricular, anterior, 336, 338, 339, 343, 347
– –, posterior, 337, 340, 343, 347
– tympanic, 195
Suture(s)
– frontonasal (nasion), 2
– frontozygomatic, 2
Syphon, carotid, 29
System
– auditory, 181
– nervous, autonomic, 78, 79
– –, –, parasympathetic part, 78, 79, 276-279, 370, 371;
– –, –, sympathetic part, 78, 276-279, 370, 371
– –, peripheral, 85

T

Tarsus
– inferior, 159, 160
– superior, 159, 160, 176
Tegmen tympani, 181, 190
Tendon(s)
– of biceps brachii, 392
– of infundibulum, 345, 346, 352
– of levator palpebrae superioris, 176
– of stapedius, 88
– of superior oblique, 159-161, 163, 167
– of tensor tympani, 189-191
– Todaro's, 357
Thoracentesis, 387
Thoracic cage, 240, 244, 245, 346, 383
– –, surface projection of the heart, 328
Thorax, 238, 248, 316, 392-394
–, arteries, 255t-257t
–, contents, 286-312
–, ganglia, 275
–, ganglionic chains, 274
–, intercostal musculature, 388
–, lymph nodes, 267-269, 358
–, lymphatic drainage, 265-267, 269
–, lymphatic ducts, 265, 266
–, lymphatic flow, 358
–, lymphatic groups, 265, 266, 268, 269
–, nerves, 270-279
–, parietal blood supply, 249
–, parietal cava-caval anastomoses, 260
–, regions, 238, 239
–, topographic anatomy, 238, 239
–, veins, 258, 259, 262t-264t
–, vessels, 16, 250-264
Thymus, 244, 296, 304, 305, 311, 331, 333, 368, 382
–, cervical cornua, 330
, lobes, 330
Thyroid gland, 31, 67, 104, 105, 128, 213, 220-222, 224, 225, 228, 229, 231, 234, 274, 330, 365
– articular surface, 206
Tissue
– adipose, subpericardial, 343
– connective, 319
– subcutaneous, 96
Tongue, 99, 122, 145
–, apex, 125, 128, 232
–, conformation and structure, 126, 127
–, body, 125, 148
–, dorsum, 122, 123, 125, 230, 232
–, foramen cecum, 125
–, inferior surface, 127
–, innervation, 129, 130, 132, 133
–, margin, 125

–, mucosa, 131
–, muscles, 148
–, nerves, 130
–, papillae, 131
–, root, 125, 127, 208, 230, 232
–, topographic relations, 128
–, midline groove, 125
–, terminal sulcus, 125, 232
–, surface, 131
–, –, dorsal, 125
–, vascularization, 129, 130
–, vessels, 130
Tonsil
– lingual, 125, 145-147, 230, 232
– palatine, 122, 123, 125, 139, 145, 147, 230, 232, 233
– –, neurovascular peduncles, 147
– pharyngeal, 125, 145-147
– tubal, 147
Tooth (teeth)
– canines, 134, 135
–, conformation and structure, 134, 135, 136
– deciduous, 134
–, dental pulp, 136
–, – –, vessels, 136
–, enamel, 136
–, incisors, 134, 135
–, – central, 134, 135
–, – lateral, 134, 135
–, innervation, 137
–, molars, 134-136
–, –, first, 134, 135
–, –, second, 134, 135
–, –, third, 99, 134, 135, 148
– permanent, 134, 136
–, premolars, 134-136
–, –, first, 134, 135
–, –, second, 134, 135
–, surface, distal, 135
–, –, lingual, 135
–, –, mesial, 135
–, –, vestibular, 135
–, vascularization, 137
Trachea, 31, 125, 145, 199-210, 220-222, 224, 225, 234, 244, 253, 254, 290-298, 301-305, 308-312, 314-321, 323-326, 328, 358, 359, 361, 368, 371, 373-380, 382, 384, 385, 392
–, bronchial branches, 320
–, bronchial subdivisions, 318
–, cervical part, 320
–, conformation, 318, 319
–, innervation, 371
–, membranous wall, 205, 206, 208, 209, 319, 332
–, position and structure, 199
–, thoracic part, 320
–, tracheal bifurcation, 199, 290, 318, 320, 332, 377, 392
Tracheotomy, 213
Tract(s)
– digestive, 125
– olfactory, 155
– solitary, nucleus, 363, 369
Tree
– bronchial, 329, 344, 390
– –, innervation, 371
– –, structure, 391
– –, subdivisions, 381
– tracheobronchial, 374, 375
– venous, jugular, external, 46
– –, –, internal, 46
Triangle
– anterior of neck, 3, 6, 8
– carotid, 6-9
– clavipectoral, 238, 239
– deltopectoral, *see* Triangle, clavipectoral
– digastric, *see* Triangle, submandibular
– Killian, 216, 313, 314
– Koch's, 357
– Laimer, 216, 313, 314
– muscular, 6-9
– occipital, 6-9
– omoclavicular, 6-9
– omotracheal, *see* Triangle, muscular
– posterior of neck, 6-9
– subclavian, *see* Triangle, omoclavicular
– submandibular, 6, 8, 9
– submental, 6, 8
– supraclavicular, *see* Triangle, omoclavicular
Trigone, fibrous, 345, 346, 352
Trunk(s),
– brachiocephalic, 16-20, 40t, 220, 221, 228-230, 232, 244, 246-249, 253, 255t, 257t, 282, 289-296, 299, 302, 306, 307, 315, 321, 323, 326, 329, 331, 332, 334-339, 337, 359, 365, 373, 382, 384, 385, 392
– bronchomediastinal, 217, 224, 265, 266, 269, 358-361
– celiac, 246-249, 252, 265, 288-297, 301, 302, 304, 308-311, 358, 369, 382
– cervicofacial, 87, 102, 103, 141, 142
– costocervical, 16-20, 22, 40t, 220, 221, 246, 247, 249, 255t, 385
– intestinal, 265, 266
– jugular, 66, 67, 98, 99, 104-106, 217, 224, 265, 266, 358, 361
– lumbar, 265, 266
– lumbosacral, 271
– lymphatic, aboral, 116, 154
– –, rostral, 116, 154
– pulmonary, 218, 219, 240, 246, 248, 257, 292, 299, 322-327, 329, 334-336, 338, 340, 342, 344, 347-351, 395
– subclavian, 66, 217, 224, 265, 266, 269, 284, 361
– sympathetic, 77, 78, 106, 113, 217, 227-230, 234, 252, 273-275, 276, 277, 362-364, 366, 367, 370, 371
– –, branches, esophageal, 278t
– –, –, thoracic cardiac 329, 363
– –, –, thoracic pulmonary, 279t
– –, cervical segment, 227
– –, ganglion(a), 225, 288, 301, 303-305, 308-311, 333
– –, –, middle cervical, 226
– –, –, thoracic, 287
– –, thoracic segment, 279t
– thyrocervical, 16-20, 22, 40, 41t, 98, 99, 104-106, 110-112, 218-221, 231, 246, 247, 249, 282
– vagal, anterior, 289-293, 369, 370
– –, posterior, 369, 370
Tube
– auditory, *see* Tube, pharyngotympanic
– Eustachian, *see* Tube, pharyngotympanic
– pharyngotympanic, 88, 145, 146, 181, 189-191, 193, 197
– –, cartilage, 230
– –, cartilaginous part, 193
– –, pharyngeal opening, 145
Tubercle(s)
– areolar, 280
– articular, 188
– auricular, 5, 182
– corniculate, 208, 210, 214, 216, 230, 232, 313
– cuneiform, 208, 210, 214, 216, 230, 232, 313
– Darwin's, *see* Tubercle(s), auricular
– epiglottic, 210
– Montgomery's, *see* Tubercle(s), areolar
– thyroid, inferior 204, 211
–, –, superior, 204, 211
– zygomatic, posterior, 188
Tympanum
–, chorda tympani, 79, 82, 88, 132, 190, 191
–, tympanic cavity, 88, 189, 190
–, –, arterial blood supply, 191
–, –, medial wall, 193
–, tympanic membrane, 181, 189, 190, 192, 193, 197

U

Utricle, 195
Uvula, 122, 123, 125, 145, 230

V

Valve(s)
– aortic, 254, 299, 344-346, 352, 393
– –, auscultation site, 346
– –, cusps, 343

– –, radiation of the murmur, 346
– atrioventricular, right, *see* Valve(s), tricuspid
– –, left, *see* Valve(s), mitral
– of coronary sinus, 339
– of inferior vena cava, 339
– mitral, 340, 341, 343-346, 352, 356, 393
– –, auscultation site, 346
– –, radiation of the murmur, 346
– nasal, 157
– pulmonary, 338, 345, 346, 352
– –, auscultation site, 346
– –, conus arteriosus, 338
– –, radiation of the murmur, 346
– tricuspid, 338, 339, 345, 346, 352, 356, 357
– –, auscultation site, 346
– –, radiation of the murmur, 346
Vasa vasorum, 368
Vein(s)
– acromiothoracic, *see* Vein(s), thoracoacromial
– alveolar, inferior, 49, 60t, 99, 137
– –, posterior superior, 137
– anastomotic, inferior, 56, 60t, 114
– –, small, *see* Vein(s), anastomotic, inferior
– –, superior, 56, 62t
– angular, 42, 43, 44, 45, 46, 48-50, 59t, 96, 97, 113, 114, 163, 164, 171
– anterior of right ventricle, 259, 262t, 264, 322, 350, 351, 356
– – of septum pellucidum, 115
– apical, 259, 322
– apicoposterior, 259, 322
– aqueous, 178
– atrial, 259
– auricular, anterior, 59t, 184
– –, posterior, 42-46, 48, 49, 62t, 101, 107-109, 117-120, 124, 139, 184
– axillary, 222, 260 283, 392
– azygos, 42, 218, 222, 223, 250, 252, 254, 258, 259, 261, 262t, 283, 286-288, 301-306, 316, 317, 321, 324, 327, 332-334, 373, 378,385, 392
– –, arch, 301-306, 333
– –, nuchal, 118, 119
– basal, 56, 59t
– –, anterior, 259, 322
– –, common, 259, 322
– –, inferior, 259, 322
– –, superior, 259, 322
– basilic, 260
– basivertebral, 261, 262t
– brachial, 283
– brachiocephalic (brachiocephalic venous trunk), 16, 42-44, 46, 63, 111, 113-116, 217, 219, 222-224, 226, 244, 253, 259, 262t, 283, 294-296, 299, 302-305, 309-311, 321, 323, 329-331, 333, 336-340, 344, 358, 359, 373, 382, 384, 385, 392
– –, groove, 378
– of brainstem, 61t, 63t
– bronchial, 259, 262t, 321
– cardiac, anterior, *see* Vein(s), anterior of right ventricle
– –, great, 259, 262t, 264t, 335-338, 350, 351, 356
– –, innominate, *see* Vein(s), brachiocephalic
– –, middle, 259, 263t, 264t, 335, 337, 350, 351, 356
– –, small, 259, 263t, 264t, 335, 350, 351, 356
– cephalic, 260, 283
– cerebellar, 59t, 63t
– –, inferior of cerebellar hemisphere, 60t
– –, precentral, 62t
– –, superior of cerebellar hemisphere, 63t
– cerebral, anterior, 56, 59t, 115
– –, deep, 59t
– –, deep middle, 59t
– –, great, 33, 54-56, 59t, 60t, 115
– –, inferior, 60t
– –, internal, 56, 60t, 115
– –, superficial, 62t
– –, superficial middle, 50, 54, 56, 62t, 114
– –, superior, 52, 53, 56, 62t, 114, 115
– cervical, ascending, 63t
– –, deep, 43, 44, 46-48, 50, 63t, 113, 114, 119-222, 223
– –, superficial, 107, 108
– –, transverse, 42-44, 46, 47, 49, 64t, 222, 259
– choroid, inferior, 60t
– –, superior, 62t
– ciliary, 59t
– –, anterior, 59t, 177, 178
– cochlear, 59t
– of cochlear aqueduct, 46, 61t, 194
– common modiolar, 59t, 196
– communicating, 103
– conjunctival, 59t
– – anterior, 177
– coronary, small, *see* Vein(s), anterior of right ventricle
– cricothyroid, 49
– dental, inferior, *see* Vein(s), alveolar, inferior
– diploic, 46, 52, 116
– – frontal, 54, 60t
– – occipital, 61t
– – temporal, anterior, 54, 59t
– – –, posterior, 54, 62t
– dorsal, 258, 261
– emissary, 52
– – condylar, 59t, 121
– – of foramen lacerum, 59t
– – of foramen of Vesalius, 59t
– – of foramen ovale, 164, 165
– – mastoid, 48, 61t, 121
– – occipital, 48, 50, 61t, 121
– – parietal, 48, 50, 61t
– epigastric, inferior, 260
– –, deep, *see* Vein(s), epigastric, inferior
– –, superficial, 260
– –, superior, 259, 260, 264t
– episcleral, 59t, 177
– esophageal, 259, 262t
– ethmoidal, 60t, 153, 165, 172-174
– facial, 42-46, 48-50, 60t, 63, 96-98, 101, 103-106, 110, 111, 113, 114, 117, 124, 129, 130, 140, 144, 164, 171, 217, 222, 233
– – common, 42-44, 46-50, 59t, 63, 105, 106, 109-111, 124, 128, 222
– – deep, 49, 60t, 111, 113, 114
– –, posterior, *see* Vein(s), retromandibular
– – transverse, 49, 63t
– of foramen cecum, 153, 156
– of Galen, *see* Vein(s), cerebral, great
– of head, 42-45
– hemiazygos, 223, 252, 258, 259, 262t, 264t, 283, 286, 287, 308-312, 316, 317, 321, 325, 333
– – accessory, 42, 225, 250, 251, 258, 259, 261, 262t, 264t, 286, 287, 308, 319, 321, 392
– hepatic, 310, 311, 333
– iliac, circumflex, superficial, 260
– –, common, 258
– iliolumbar, 258
– infraorbital, 163-165
– innominate of Vieussens, *see* Vein(s), anterior of right ventricle
– insular, 56
– intercollicular, 61t
– intercostal, anterior, 250, 259, 262t, 283, 297
– –, posterior, 250, 251, 258, 259, 261, 263t, 286, 287, 301, 302, 305, 308-312, 321, 261, 333
– –, superior, 250, 259, 263t, 309-312, 333
– – supreme, 258, 259, 264t, 283, 286, 287, 301-304, 321, 326, 333, 385, 392
– interpeduncular, 61t
– interventricular, anterior, 259, 336, 338
– – posterior, *see* Vein(s), cardiac, middle
– intervertebral, 261, 262t
– jugular, anterior, 42-44, 46-48, 64, 102, 108, 144, 222, 223, 234
– –, external, 16, 42-44, 46-50, 60t, 64t, 97-99, 102-106, 108-111, 113-117, 124, 139, 140, 144, 184, 222, 223, 234, 259, 283
– –, –, posterior, 64t, 107, 108, 117, 144, 223
– –, inferior bulb, 106, 223, 265

– –, internal, 16, 19, 27, 30, 31, 42-44, 46-51, 60t, 63t, 64t, 70, 104-106, 109-111, 113-116, 121, 124, 128, 130, 139, 140, 154, 191, 194, 218, 219, 222, 223, 226, 228-234, 236, 259, 283, 309-312, 315-317, 332, 333, 358
– –, superior bulb, 48, 50, 53, 190
– Labbé's, *see* Vein(s), anastomotic, inferior
– labial, inferior, 48-50, 60t
– –, superior, 48-50, 62t, 114, 153, 156
– labyrinthine, 43-46, 61t, 116, 194, 196
– lacrimale, 61t, 163-165, 174
– laryngeal, inferior, 43, 46, 47, 64t
– –, superior, 43, 44, 46, 47, 49, 64t, 128, 230, 232
– lateral mesencephalic, 61t
– of lateral recess of fourth ventricle, 61t
– lingual, 42-46, 49, 61t, 114, 115, 123, 126, 128, 129
– –, deep, 59t, 129
– –, dorsal, 59t
– lingular, 259, 322
– lumbar, 258
– – ascending, 258
– marginal, 259, 335, 337, 350, 351, 356
– Marshall's, *see* Vein(s), oblique of left atrium
– maxillary, 43-46, 48-50, 61t, 111, 137, 184, 187
– mediastinal, 223, 259, 263t, 264
– of medulla oblongata, 61t
– medullary, anterolateral, 61t
– –, anteromedian, 61t
– –, dorsal, 61t
– –, posteromedian, 61t
– – transverse, 61t
– meningeal, 46, 61t
– – middle, 50, 54, 61t
– middle lobe, 259, 322
– muscular (muscular branches of ophthalmic veins), 163, 164
– musculophrenic, 259, 263t
– nasal, anterior lateral, 153
– –, external, 60t, 164
– –, inferior lateral posterior, 116, 153
– –, superior lateral posterior, 116, 153
– nasofrontal, 61t, 163-165, 171-174
– of neck, 42, 43, 46, 47, 103
– nutrient, 261
– oblique of left atrium, 259, 263t, 350, 351, 356
– occipital, 48, 49, 61t, 64, 107-109, 118
– ophthalmic, inferior, 43-46, 60t, 163-165, 171
– –, superior, 43-46, 48, 50, 55, 62t, 98, 113, 160, 163-165, 171, 174
– of orbit, 163
– palatine, external, 60t
– –, greater, 153
– palpebral, inferior, 60t
– –, superior, 63t
– paraumbilical, 260
– parotid, 61t
– of penis, superficial, 260
– pericardiacophrenic, 252, 259, 263t, 295, 303-305, 310-312, 330, 333
– pericardial, 223, 259, 263t, 330
– petrosal, 59, 61t
– pharyngeal, 42-44, 46, 47, 64t, 109, 110
– phrenic, inferior, 259
– –, superior, 259, 264t
– pontine, anterolateral, 62t
– –, anteromedian, 62t
– –, lateral, 62t
– –, transverse, 62t
– pontomesencephalic, 61t
– posterior of left ventricle, 259, 263t, 322, 335, 350, 351, 356
– of pterygoid canal, 61t
– pterygoid plexus, 62t
– pulmonary, 218, 219, 248, 254, 259, 263t, 292, 293, 298-305, 308-312, 316, 317, 322, 324, 325, 328, 332-335, 337, 338, 350, 351, 378, 384, 391, 393
– ranine, *see* Vein(s), lingual, deep
– retinal, central, 59t, 177, 178
– retromandibular, 42-46, 48-50, 62t, 64t, 101, 103-105, 110, 111, 117, 128, 140, 144, 184, 187, 222
– –, posterior division, 117, 184
– of Rosenthal, *see* Vein(s), basal
– saphenous, great, 260
– –, long, *see* Vein(s), saphenous, great
– sphenopalatine, 153
– spinal, 261, 262t
– –, anterior, 115, 262t
– –, posterior, 115, 262t
– of spinal cord, 261
– sternocleidomastoid, 43, 44, 46, 47, 64t
– stylomastoid, 62t
– subclavian, 42-44, 46, 64t, 219, 222, 223, 226, 228-232, 259, 264t, 283, 309-312, 315-317, 324, 325, 332, 333, 358, 385, 386
– subcostal, 259, 264t
– sublingual, 62t, 124
– submental, 48-50, 62t, 96-99, 110, 111, 113, 128, 130, 144
– subscapular, 283
– superficial Sylvian, *see* Vein(s), cerebral, superficial middle
– superior, 259, 322
– supraorbital, 49, 63t, 96-99, 107-109, 160, 163-165, 173, 174
– suprascapular, 43, 44, 46, 47, 49, 64t, 108, 283
– supratrochlear, 49, 63t, 107-109, 164
– temporal, deep, 59t, 111
– –, middle, 61t
– –, superficial, 42-46, 48-50, 52, 62t, 96, 97, 107-111, 117-119, 144
– –, –, frontal and parietal branches, 48, 118, 184, 187
– thalamostriate, inferior, 60t
– –, superior, 63t, 115
– Thebesian, *see* Vein(s), cardiac, smallest
– thoracic, internal, 41t, 42-44, 46, 222, 223, 226, 250, 252, 259, 260, 262t, 283, 297, 385
– –, –, perforating branches, 260, 283
– –, lateral, 42, 259, 260, 263t, 283
– thoracoacromial, 264t, 283
– –, branches, 283
– thoracoepigastric, 260
– thymic, 223, 259, 264t
– thyroid, inferior, 40t, 42-44, 46, 47, 49, 64t, 98, 99, 104-106, 217-219, 222, 223, 226, 228, 259, 321
– –, middle, 42-44, 46, 47, 49, 50, 64t, 105, 106, 217, 222
– –, superior, 41t, 42-44, 46-50, 64t, 103-106, 217-219, 222, 223, 226, 228, 229
– of tongue, deep, *see* Vein(s), lingual, deep
– transverse of scapula, *see* Vein(s), suprascapular
– of Trolard, *see* Vein(s), anastomotic, superior
– tympanic, 63t
– vena cava, inferior, 240, 244, 252, 258, 259, 262t, 305, 306, 310, 311, 315, 316, 324, 325, 332, 333, 334, 335, 335, 337, 338, 339, 347, 350, 351, 378
– –, –, opening, 289-291, 313, 315
– –, –, valve, 339
– –, superior, 42-44, 46, 217, 218, 222-224, 231, 254, 258, 259, 264t, 283, 294, 295, 298, 299, 303-306, 315, 317, 321, 323, 324, 326, 328, 329, 330, 332, 334-340, 344, 347, 350, 351, 357, 378, 384, 392
– ventricular, 259
– of vermis, inferior, 59t, 60t
– –, superior, 59t, 63t
– vertebral, 42-44, 46-48, 50, 64t, 114-116, 222, 233, 234, 259
– vestibular, 63t
– of vestibular aqueduct, 61t, 194, 196
– vidian, *see* Vein(s), of pterygoid canal
– vorticose, 63t, 164, 165, 171, 173, 174, 177, 178
Ventricle, fourth, choroid plexus, 115
–, laryngeal, 208, 210
–, lateral, choroid plexus, 115
–, third, tela choroidea, 33
Vertebra(e)
– cervical, 145, 234
– –, spinous process, 121
– prominens [C VII], 234, 383
– –, spinous process, 245
– thoracic, 319, 334, 392, 393, 395
– –, body, 31, 307, 309-311, 333, 368

– –, spinous process, 31
– –, transverse process, 31
Vessel(s)
– alveolar, 136
– – and alveolar nerves, 136
– blood, of retina, 177
– coronary, 339
– dental pulp, 136
– gingival, 136
– intercostal, 250, 251
– lymphatic, 358, 390
– pericardiacophrenic, 302
– periodontal, 136
– pulmonary, 253, 255, 300
Vestibule, 157
– aortic, 339
– laryngeal, 208, 210
– nasal, 125, 152, 153-157
– oral, 123, 139
Viscerocranium (facial skeleton), 137

W

Willis, circle of, *see* Circle, cerebral arterial
Window
– duodenal, *see* Window, oval
– oval, 193
– –, impression, 194
– round, 193
– –, impression, 194

Z

Zinn, anulus of, *see* Ring, tendinous, common
Zonule, ciliary 176, 179, 180